Informatik aktuell

Herausgeber: W. Brauer
im Auftrag der Gesellschaft für Informatik (GI)

T0122625

Alexander Horsch   Thomas M. Deserno
Heinz Handels   Hans-Peter Meinzer
Thomas Tolxdorff (Hrsg.)

Bildverarbeitung
für die Medizin 2007

Algorithmen – Systeme – Anwendungen

Proceedings des Workshops
vom 25.–27. März 2007 in München

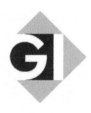

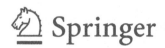 Springer

Herausgeber

Alexander Horsch
Technische Universität München, Klinikum rechts der Isar
Institut für Medizinische Statistik und Epidemiologie
Ismaninger Strasse 22, 81675 München

Thomas M. Deserno
Rheinisch-Westfälische Technische Hochschule Aachen
Institut für Medizinische Informatik
Pauwelsstrasse 30, 52057 Aachen

Heinz Handels
Universitätsklinikum Hamburg-Eppendorf
Institut für Medizinische Informatik
Martinistrasse 52, 20246 Hamburg

Hans-Peter Meinzer
Deutsches Krebsforschungszentrum
Abt. für Medizinische und Biologische Informatik / H0100
Im Neuenheimer Feld 280, 69120 Heidelberg

Thomas Tolxdorff
Charité – Universitätsmedizin Berlin
Institut für Medizinische Informatik
Campus Benjamin Franklin
Hindenburgdamm 30, 12200 Berlin

Bibliographische Information der Deutschen Bibliothek
Die Deutsche Bibliothek verzeichnet diese Publikation in der Deutschen Nationalbibliografie;
detaillierte bibliografische Daten sind im Internet über http://dnb.ddb.de abrufbar.

CR Subject Classification (1998):
A.0, H.3, I.4, I.5, J.3, H.3.1, I.2.10, I.3.3, I.3.5, I.3.7, I.3.8, I.6.3

ISSN 1431-472-X
ISBN-10 3-540-71090-6 Springer Berlin Heidelberg New York
ISBN-13 978-3-540-71090-5 Springer Berlin Heidelberg New York

Springer Berlin Heidelberg New York
Springer ist ein Unternehmen von Springer Science+Business Media

springer.de

© Springer-Verlag Berlin Heidelberg 2007
Printed in Germany

Satz: Reproduktionsfertige Vorlage vom Autor/Herausgeber
Gedruckt auf säurefreiem Papier   SPIN: 12025374   33/3180-543210

Veranstalter

IMSE	Institut für Medizinische Statistik und Epidemiologie
	Klinikum rechts der Isar der Technischen Universität München
BVMI	Berufsverband Medizinischer Informatiker e.V.
DAGM	Deutsche Arbeitsgemeinschaft für Mustererkennung
DGBMT	Fachgruppe Medizinische Informatik
	der Deutschen Gesellschaft für Biomedizinische Technik im VDE
GI	Fachgruppe Imaging und Visualisierungstechniken
	der Gesellschaft für Informatik
GMDS	Arbeitsgruppe Medizinische Bildverarbeitung der Gesellschaft
	für Medizinische Informatik, Biometrie und Epidemiologie
IEEE	Joint Chapter Engineering in Medicine and Biology, German Section

Tagungsleitung und -vorsitz

Prof. II Dr. Alexander Horsch

Institut für Medizinische Statistik und Epidemiologie
(Direktor: Prof. Klaus A. Kuhn)
Klinikum rechts der Isar der Technischen Universität München

Lokale Organisation

Dr. Andrea Bernklau
Dipl.-Phys. Andreas Enterrottacher
Dipl.-Inf. Gregor Lamla
Dipl.-Inf. Jörg Schlundt
Dipl.-Inf. Sebastian Wurst

Institut für Medizinische Statistik und Epidemiologie
Klinikum rechts der Isar der Technischen Universität München

Dipl.-Inf. Udo Poth
Frau Victoria Manzan

Rechenzentrum des Klinikum rechts der Isar

Prof. Dr. Dr. Karl-Hans Englmeier

GSF Forschungszentrum Neuherberg

Verteilte BVM-Organisation

Priv.-Doz. Dr. Thomas M. Deserno, Dipl.-Inform. Benedikt Fischer
Rheinisch-Westfälische Technische Hochschule Aachen (Tagungsband)

Prof. Dr. Heinz Handels, Dipl.-Ing. Martin Riemer
Universitätsklinikum Hamburg-Eppendorf (Begutachtung)

Prof. Dr. Hans-Peter Meinzer, Dipl.-Ing. Matthias Baumhauer
Deutsches Krebsforschungszentrum Heidelberg (Anmeldung)

Prof. Dr. Thomas Tolxdorff, Dagmar Stiller
Charité – Universitätsmedizin Berlin (Internetpräsenz)

Programmkomitee

Prof. Dr. Til Aach, RWTH Aachen
Prof. Dr. Dr. Johannes Bernarding, Universität Magdeburg
Dr. Wolfram Bunk, Max-Planck-Institut Garching
Prof. Dr. Thorsten M. Buzug, Universität zu Lübeck
Priv.-Doz. Dr. Thomas M. Deserno, RWTH Aachen
Prof. Dr. Hartmut Dickhaus, Universität Heidelberg
Dr. Jan Ehrhardt, Universitätsklinkum Hamburg-Eppendorf
Prof. Dr. Dr. Karl-Hans Englmeier, GSF Forschungszentrum Neuherberg
Prof. Dr. Bernd Fischer, Universität zu Lübeck
Prof. Dr. Heinz Handels, Universitätsklinkum Hamburg-Eppendorf
Priv.-Doz. Dr. Peter Hastreiter, Universität Erlangen-Nürnberg
Prof. Dr. Joachim Hornegger, Universität Erlangen-Nürnberg
Prof. II Dr. Alexander Horsch, TU München & Universität Tromsø, Norwegen
Prof. Dr. Peter Kneschaurek, Technische Universität München
Prof. Dr. Frithjof Kruggel, University of California, Irvine, USA
Prof. Dr. Dr. Hans-Gerd Lipinski, Fachhochschule Dortmund
Dr. Günter Lauritsch, Siemens AG, Medical Solutions, Forchheim
Prof. Dr. Tim Lüth, Technische Universität München
Prof. Dr. Hans-Peter Meinzer, Deutsches Krebsforschungszentrum Heidelberg
Prof. Dr. Heinrich Müller, Universität Dortmund
Prof. Dr. Nassir Navab, Technische Universität München
Dr. Stephan Nekolla, Technische Universität München
Prof. em. Dr. Heinrich Niemann, Universität Erlangen-Nürnberg
Prof. Dr. Dietrich Paulus, Universität Koblenz-Landau
Prof. Dr. Heinz-Otto Peitgen, Universität Bremen
Prof. Dr. Dr. Siegfried J. Pöppl, Universität zu Lübeck
Prof. Dr. Bernhard Preim, Universität Magdeburg
Dr. habil. Karl Rohr, Universität Heidelberg & DKFZ Heidelberg
Prof. Dr. Georgios Sakas, Fraunhofer Institut Darmstadt
Prof. Dr. Rainer Schubert, UMIT Innsbruck
Prof. Dr. Thomas Tolxdorff, Charité – Universitätsmedizin Berlin
Dr. Thomas Wittenberg, Fraunhofer Institut Erlangen
Dr. Ivo Wolf, Deutsches Krebsforschungszentrum Heidelberg

Preisträger des BVM-Workshops 2006 in Hamburg

Die BVM-Preise zeichnen besonders hervorragende Arbeiten aus. In 2006 wurden folgende Preisträger ausgewählt:

BVM-Preis 2006 für die beste wissenschaftliche Arbeit

1. Preis: *Jens von Berg, Cristian Lorenz*
A Statistical Geometric Model of the Heart

2. Preis: *René Werner, Jan Ehrhardt, Thorsten Frenzel, Dennis Säring, Daniel Low, Heinz Handels*
Rekonstruktion von 4D-CT-Daten aus räumlich-zeitlichen CT Segmentfolgen zur Analyse atmungsbedingter Organbewegungen

3. Preis: *Christian Kier, Karsten Meyer-Wiethe, Günter Seidel, Til Aach*
Ultraschall-Perfusionsbildgebung für die Schlaganfalldiagnostik auf Basis eines Modells für die Destruktionskinetik von Kontrastmittel

BVM-Preis 2006 für den besten Vortrag

1. Preis: *Astrid Franz, Ingwer C. Carlsen, Steffen Renisch*
An Adaptive Irregular Grid Approach using SIFT Features for Elastic Medical Image Registration

2. Preis: *May Oehler, Thorsten M. Buzug*
Maximum-Likelihood-Ansatz zur Metallartefaktreduktion bei der Computertomographie

3. Preis: *Patrick Jäger, Stefan Vogel, Achim Knepper, Thomas Kraus, Til Aach*
3D-Erkennung, Analyse und Visualisierung pleuraler Verdickungen in CT-Daten

BVM-Preis 2006 für die beste Posterpräsentation

1. Preis: *Tobias Heimann, Ivo Wolf, Hans-Peter Meinzer*
Automatische Erstellung von gleichmäßig verteilten Landmarken für statistische Formmodelle

2. Preis: *Jingfeng Han, Benjamin Berkels, Martin Rumpf, Joachim Hornegger, Marc Droske, Michael Fried, Jasmin Scorzin, Carlo Schaller*
A Variational Framework for Joint Image Registration, Denoising, and Edge Detection

3. Preis: a: *Dieter Hahn, Gabriele Wolz, Yiyong Sun, Frank Sauer, Joachim Hornegger, Torsten Kuwert, Chenyang Xu*
Utilizing Salient Region Features for 3D Multi-Modality Medical Image Registration
b: *Jan Ehrhardt, Dennis Säring, Heinz Handels*
Interpolation of Temporal Image Sequences by Optical-Flow-Based Registration

Vorwort

In diesem Jahr findet der Workshop Bildverarbeitung für die Medizin zum zweiten Mal in München statt. Er ist in dieser Form die zehnte Veranstaltung. Die Bedeutung des Themas Bildverarbeitung für die Medizin hat über die Jahre deutlich zugenommen. Die Bildverarbeitung ist eine Schlüsseltechnologie in verschiedenen medizinischen Bereichen wie etwa der Biomedizin, der Diagnoseunterstützung, der Therapieplanung und der bildgeführten Chirurgie.

Der BVM-Workshop konnte sich durch erfolgreiche Veranstaltungen in Aachen, Heidelberg, München, Lübeck, Leipzig, Erlangen, Berlin und Hamburg als ein zentrales interdisziplinäres Forum für die Präsentation und Diskussion von Methoden, Systemen und Anwendungen im Bereich der Medizinischen Bildverarbeitung etablieren. Ziel des Workshops ist die Darstellung aktueller Forschungsergebnisse und die Vertiefung der Gespräche zwischen Wissenschaftlern, Industrie und Anwendern. Der Workshop richtet sich ausdrücklich auch an Nachwuchswissenschaftler, die über ihre Diplom-, Promotions- und Habilitationsprojekte berichten wollen.

Der Workshop wird vom Institut für Medizinische Statistik und Epidemiologie der Technischen Universität München am Klinikum rechts der Isar ausgerichtet. Die Organisation ist wie gewohnt auf Fachkollegen aus Aachen, Berlin, Hamburg, Heidelberg und München verteilt, so dass die Organisatoren der vergangenen Jahre ihre Erfahrungen mit einfließen lassen können. Diese Aufgabenteilung bildet nicht nur eine starke Entlastung des lokalen Tagungsausrichters, sondern führt auch insgesamt zu einer Effizienzsteigerung.

Die etablierte webbasierte Einreichung und Begutachtung der Tagungsbeiträge hat sich auch diesmal wieder bewährt. Anhand anonymisierter Bewertungen durch jeweils drei Gutachter wurden aus 129 eingereichten Beiträgen 92 zur Präsentation ausgewählt: 46 Vorträge, 42 Poster und 4 Softwaredemonstrationen. Die Qualität der eingereichten Arbeiten war insgesamt sehr hoch. Die besten Arbeiten werden auch im Jahr 2007 mit BVM-Preisen ausgezeichnet.

Am Tag vor dem wissenschaftlichen Programm werden drei Tutorien angeboten: Prof. Dr. Karl-Hans Englmeier von der GSF in Neuherberg bei München wird ein Tutorium zum Thema *Virtuelle Realität in der Medizin* halten. Multidimensionale Visualisierungstechniken und virtuelle Realität sind heute bereits integraler Bestandteil in verschiedenen biomedizinischen Anwendungen. In diesem Tutorium werden Konzepte, Methoden und Technologien für die Visualisierung und virtuelle Realität vorgestellt und klassifiziert. Methoden zur effizienten, patientenspezifischen Visualisierung von Anatomie und Funktion werden beschrieben. Beispiele aus virtueller Endoskopie, morpho-funktionaler Visualisierung und biomechanische Analyse werden gezeigt.

Prof. Dr. Bernd Fischer und Priv.-Doz. Dr. Jan Modersitzki vom Insitut für Mathematik der Universität zu Lübeck werden ein Tutorium zum Thema *Medizinische Bildregistrierung* halten. Dieses hochaktuelle Thema der Bildverarbeitung hat in den letzten Jahren eine stürmische Entwicklung genommen. Ziel dieses Tutorials ist es, allgemeine Konzepte vorzustellen, die eine inhaltliche Einordnung von modernen medizinischen Bildregistrierungsverfahren erlauben. Insbesondere sollen die gängigen Verfahren übersichtlich dargestellt werden.

Im dritten Tutorium wird Dr. Philippe Lahorte vom Europäischen Patentamt in München zum Thema *Intellectual Property in Medical Imaging Research* referieren. Ziel dieses Tutoriums ist es, eine Einführung in das Gebiet des geistigen Eigentums allgemein und des Patentwesens im Besonderen zu geben und deren Bedeutung für die Forschung in der Medizinischen Bildverarbeitung aufzuzeigen. Es wird ein Überblick über verschiedene Formen geistigen Eigentums mit dem Schwerpunkt Patente gegeben. Die gesetzliche Bedeutung eines Patents wird ebenso diskutiert wie verschiedene Verfahren, ein Patent zu erlangen.

Besondere Höhepunkte des Workshops werden die beiden geladenen Vorträge sein. Den ersten Vortrag wird Prof. Dr.rer.nat. Dr.h.c. Gregor Morfill, Direktor des Max-Planck-Instituts für extraterrestrische Physik in Garching bei München zum Thema *Vom Kosmos zur Medizin – Bilder und ihre Auswertung* halten und dabei auf den Methodentransfer von Bilddatenanalysen in der extraterrestrischen Physik auf Fragestellungen in der Medizin anhand eindrucksvoller Beispiel eingehen. Den zweiten Vortrag wird Priv.-Doz. Dr.med. Nasreddin Abolmaali, Leiter der Gruppe „Biologische und Molekulare Bildgebung" des Kompetenzzentrums OncoRay (www.oncoray.de), zum Thema *Vom Molekül zum Patienten – Neue Bilder, neue Erkenntnis* halten. Dabei wird er den Bogen vom Zellsystem zum Patienten spannen und am Schwerpunkt Onkologie die Potentiale und Herausforderungen dieses faszinierenden neuen Gebietes der Bildverarbeitung darstellen.

Alle für den Workshop zur Präsentation ausgewählten 92 Beiträge wurden in diesem Tagungsband abgedruckt. Die Internetseiten des Workshops bieten ausführliche Informationen über das Programm und organisatorische Details rund um den Workshop. Sie sind abrufbar unter der Adresse:

http://bvm-workshop.org

Wie schon in den letzten Jahren, wurde der Tagungsband auch diesmal als LATEX-Projekt erstellt und in dieser Form an den Verlag übergeben. Von den 92 Beiträgen wurden lediglich 78 von den Autoren im LATEX-Format eingereicht (das sind 85% – 4 Beiträge weniger als im Vorjahr). Die 14 im Winword-Format abgefassten Arbeiten wurden konvertiert und nachbearbeitet. Die Vergabe von Schlagworten nahmen die Autoren selbst vor. Die Literaturverzeichnisse sämtlicher Beiträge wurden wieder mit BIBTEX generiert. Der gesamte Erstellungsprozess erfolgte ausschließlich über das Internet.

Die Herausgeber dieser Proceedings möchten allen herzlich danken, die zum Gelingen des BVM-Workshops 2007 beigetragen haben: Den Autoren für die rechtzeitige und formgerechte Einreichung ihrer qualitativ hochwertigen Arbeiten, dem Programmkomitee für die gründliche Begutachtung und den Referenten der Tutorien. Frau Dagmar Stiller vom Institut für Medizinische Informatik, Biometrie und Epidemiologie der Charité, Universitätsmedizin Berlin, danken wir für die engagierte Mithilfe bei der Erstellung und Pflege der Internetpräsentation.

Herrn Matthias Baumhauer vom DKFZ Heidelberg danken wir für die Pflege des BVM-Emailverteilers und der webgestützten Workshopanmeldung. Für die webbasierte Durchführung des Reviewingprozesses gebührt Herrn Dipl.-Ing. Martin Riemer vom Institut für Medizinische Informatik der Universität Hamburg unser Dank. Den Herren Dipl.-Inform. Bededikt Fischer und Markus Wolff vom Institut für Medizinische Informatik der RWTH Aachen danken wir für die tatkräftige Mitarbeit bei der Erstellung der Workshop-Proceedings. Dem Springer-Verlag, der nun schon den zehnten Tagungsband zu den BVM-Workshops herausbringt, wollen wir für die gute Kooperation ebenfalls unseren Dank aussprechen. Für die tatkräftige Mitwirkung bei der lokalen Organisation des Workshop gebührt Frau Victoria Manzan, Herrn Udo Poth, Prof. Karl-Hans Englmeier sowie den Kolleginnen und Kollegen des Instituts für Medizinische Statistik und Epidemiologie der TU München besonderer Dank.

Für die finanzielle Unterstützung bedanken wir uns ganz herzlich bei unserem Hauptsponsor Siemens, den weiteren Sponsoren Definiens, Sectra, ManaThea, TomTec und Creaso, sowie bei den Fachgesellschaften.

Wir wünschen allen Teilnehmerinnen und Teilnehmern des Workshops BVM 2007 lehrreiche Tutorials, viele interessante Vorträge, Gespräche an den Postern und der Industrieausstellung sowie interessante neue Kontakte zu Kolleginnen und Kollegen aus dem Bereich der Medizinischen Bildverarbeitung.

Januar 2007

Alexander Horsch (München)
Thomas M. Deserno, geb. Lehmann (Aachen)
Heinz Handels (Hamburg)
Hans-Peter Meinzer (Heidelberg)
Thomas Tolxdorff (Berlin)

Inhaltsverzeichnis

Die fortlaufende Nummer am linken Seitenrand entspricht den Beitragsnummern, wie sie im endgültigen Programm des Workshops zu finden sind. Dabei steht V für Vortrag, P für Poster und S für Softwaredemonstration.

3. Bildgebung I

4. Computer Assisted Diagnosis (CAD)

5. Registrierung I

6. Segmentierung I

7. Registrierung II

8. Therapieplanung I

9. Visualisierung I

10. Bildgebung II

11. Biomedizin II

12. Bildanalyse I

13. CAD und Endoskopie

14. Therapieplanung II

15. Visualisierung II

16. Therapie II

17. Segmentierung II

18. Bildanalyse II

19. Registrierung III

20. Bildgebung III

Ermittlung von räumlichen Proteinexpressionsmustern mittels Bildverarbeitung

Protein-Profiling stratifizierter Epithelien mittels Bildverarbeitung fluoreszent gefärbter Gewebeschnitte

Thora Pommerencke[1], Pascal Tomakidi[2], Hartmut Dickhaus[1], Niels Grabe[1]

[1]Institut für medizinische Biometrie und Informatik, Universität Heidelberg
[2]Poliklinik für Kieferorthopädie der Universität Heidelberg
Email: thora.pommerencke@med.uni-heidelberg.de

Zusammenfassung. Wir präsentieren hier erste Ergebnisse einer neuartigen und vollautomatischen Methode zur Ermittlung von räumlichen Proteinexpressionsmustern in stratifizierten Epithelien. Das Verfahren basiert auf der Bildanalyse von immunhistologisch gefärbten Gewebeschnitten. Exemplarisch wird die Anwendbarkeit dieses Verfahrens anhand der Expression von fünf Strukturproteinen demonstriert.

1 Einleitung

Äußere sowie innere Körperoberflächen werden von statifiziertem, epithelialem Gewebe bedeckt. Dieses unterliegt einem komplex regulierten Gleichgewicht (Homöostase) aus Proliferation, Differenzierung und Apoptose bei einer über die Zeit konstanten Morphologie, wobei in der Literatur vier Schichten unterschieden werden: Stratum Basale, S. Spinosum, S. Granulosum und S. Corneum [1, 2]. Störungen der Homöostase führen zu starken pathologischen Veränderungen wie der Schuppenflechte und epithelialen Tumoren [3]. Grundlage für die Diagnose und Therapie dieser pathologischen Veränderungen ist ein tiefes Verständnis dieses komplexen biologischen Systems. In diesem Zusammenhang haben die systembiologische Analyse sowie Modellierung zunehmend an Bedeutung gewonnen [4, 5, 6, 7]. Da die epitheliale Homöostase wesentlich durch die gezielte Proteinexpression vieler Proteine gleichzeitig gesteuert wird, besteht zur dynamischen Modellierung des Epithels der Bedarf an multiparametrischen (d.h. mehrere Proteine werden simultan betrachtet) und quantitativen Daten zur Proteinexpression in Abhängigkeit von der Zelldifferenzierung.

2 Stand der Forschung und Fortschritt durch den Beitrag

Gängige Verfahren zur quantitativen Messung der Proteinexpressionsmuster in der Zelle/Gewebe (Protein-Profiling) auf Basis von Protein-Arrays und 2D-Gel-Elektrophorese basieren auf der Homogenisierung von Gewebe, wodurch jedoch

Abb. 1. Bild der Markerfärbung (Desmoplakin) mit detektierter Epithelkontur ohne Stratum Corneum

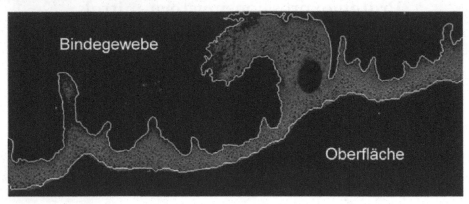

die Korrelation zwischen räumlicher Lage und Proteinexpression verloren geht [8, 9]. Neuere Verfahren wie z.B. das MALDI-Imaging bieten zwar eine Ortsauflösung, welche zur Zeit jedoch für die hier vorgestellte Anwendung noch zu gering ist [10]. Räumliche Beschreibungen der Proteinexpression entstammen in der Literatur daher hauptsächlich noch immer der mikroskopischen Analyse einzelner Gewebeschnitte durch einen Spezialisten. Die daraus resultierenden linguistischen und bildhaften Angaben lassen sich jedoch nur schwer in Parameter für Gewebesimulationen übersetzen [11]. Darüber hinaus sind die Daten unterschiedlicher Veröffentlichungen wegen mangelnder Standardisierung kaum vergleichbar. Aufgrund dieser unbefriedigenden Datenlage wurde ein neues Protein-Profiling-Verfahren entwickelt, welches die epitheliale Proteinexpression multiparametrisch und ortsauflösend durch automatische Bildanalyse gefärbter Gewebeschnitte quantifizieren kann.

3   Methoden

Experimentell wurden Schnitte cryokonservierter Gewebeproben von gesunden Patienten über eine fluoreszente Dreifachfärbung angefärbt. Dabei wird das interessierende Protein sowie das Kollagen-I als Bestandteil der extrazellulären Matrix im Bindegewebe über indirekte Immunfluoreszenz und die Zellkerne direkt chemisch mit DAPI (Diamidino-phenylindol) gefärbt. Da auf einem einzelnen Gewebeschnitt nur eine begrenzte Anzahl von Proteinen markiert werden können, wird die Analyse auf Serienschnitten durchgeführt, wodurch dieselbe Gewebeherkunft für jedes der Proteinexpressionsmuster gewährleistet ist.

Die Implementierung der Bildanalyse der digitalisierten Schnitte wurde mithilfe von Matlab 7.1 einschließlich der Image Processing Toolbox realisiert. In einem ersten Schritt wird das Epithel vollautomatisch segmentiert, wobei die Gewebekonturen über ein Phasenkontrastbild ermittelt werden. Die Abgrenzung des Epithels vom Bindegewebe erfolgt im wesentlichen über eine gezielte Canny-

Kantendetektion im Bild der Zellkernfärbung sowie der Auswahl von epithelialen Gewebebereichen anhand der Bindegewebsfärbung nahe den Kanten. Von der ermittelten Epithelmaske werden Bereiche starker Bindegewebsfärbung durch logisches NOT ausgeschlossen. Das segmentierte Epithel wird anschließend künstlich um etwa eine halbe Zellbreite in Richtung Bindegewebe dilatiert, um auch den zellfreien Raum zwischen Epithel und Bindegewebe, die Basalmembran, mit in die Analysen einschließen zu können. Das Stratum Corneum lässt sich über die Abwesenheit von Zellkernen ermitteln und gegebenenfalls ausschließen.

Die funktionale Abhängigkeit der Proteinexpression von der Differenzierung wird von uns über zwei verschiedene Maße beschrieben. Zum einen über die normierte Distanz d zum Bindegewebe (mit d = 0% direkt am Bindegewebe und d = 100 % an der Oberfläche), da sich differenzierende Zellen in Richtung Oberfläche bewegen. Zum anderen über die mittlere Intensität der Zellkernfärbung, welche die mittlere Zellkerndichte widerspiegelt. Diese nimmt durch die Vergrößerung der Zellen sowie die Auflösung des Zellkernes im Zuge der terminalen Differenzierung ab. Für das zellkernbasierte Maß wurde ein Glättungsverfahren entwickelt, bei dem das Bild der Zellkernfärbung mit einer annähernd rechteckigen Filtermatrix parallel zur Basalschicht gefaltet wird, dessen Breite und Höhe mit steigender Distanz zum Bindegewebe zunehmen (siehe Gleichung 1).

$$G(p) = \frac{\sum_{i=1}^{|N(p)|} E(N(p)_i)}{|N(p)|}$$

$$N(p) = \left\{ x \in M | M(x) \neq 0 \wedge d(x,p) \leq \frac{l_p}{2} \wedge |d(x,b(x)) - d(p,b(p))| \leq \frac{l_p}{4} \right\} \quad (1)$$

$$l_p = f \cdot d(p,b(p)) + l_{min}$$

E: Bild der Zellkernfärbung   G: geglättetes Bild
M: Epithelmaske   p: aktuell betrachtetes Pixel
f: Wachstumsfaktor l_{min}: Mindestkantenlänge der Filtermatrix
I(x): Wert von Pixel x in Bild I l_p: aktuelle Kantenlänge der Filtermatrix
N(p): Menge der Nachbarschaftspixel von p
d: Distanzfunktion, d(x,p) liefert euklidische Distanz zwischen Pixel x und p
b: b(p) liefert nächstes Bindegewebspixel zu p

Auf Basis dieser Differenzierungsmaße kann zu jeder „Differenzierungsstufe" die jeweilige mittlere Färbungsintensität des Markers ermittelt werden. Die Auftragung der normierten Markerintensität gegen das Differenzierungsmaß ergibt für jeden Marker ein charakteristisches Expressionsprofil.

4   Ergebnisse

Mit dem entwickelten Verfahren wurde hier beispielhaft die kombinatorische Expression von den fünf Strukturproteinen Desmoplakin (Dp), Filaggrin (Fil),

Abb. 2. Generierte Multi-Marker-Profile der humanen Epidermis ohne Stratum Corneum über den distanzbasierten Ansatz (links) und über den zellkernbasierten Ansatz (rechts)

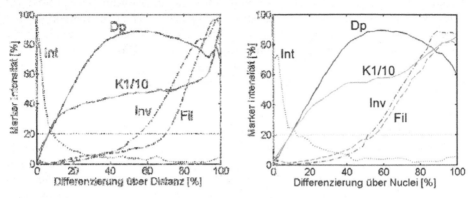

Integrin-$\alpha_6\beta_4$(Int), Involucrin (Inv) und Keratin 1/10 (K1/10) untersucht, die charakteristisch für die üblicherweise beschriebenen „Differenzierungsstufen" sind. Für die Analyse wurde eine epidermale Gewebeprobe (humane Haut) gewählt. In dem dargestellten Multi-Marker-Profil handelt es sich je Marker um ein gemitteltes Expressionsprofil aus mehreren Bilddatensätzen derselben Gewebeprobe.

5   Diskussion

Das realisierte Profiling-Verfahren ist in der Lage, erstmals automatisiert eine grobe quantitative und räumliche Beschreibung der Proteinexpression im Epithel zu liefern. Die ermittelten epidermalen Expressionsprofile stimmen mit den in der Literatur qualitativ beschriebenen überein. Für die Generierung der Profile sind die zugrunde liegenden „Differenzierungsstufen" beliebig groß oder klein wählbar. Dadurch kann eine sehr hohe räumliche Auflösung der Profile erzielt werden, welche eine kontinuierlichen Messung ohne a priori interpretative Unterteilung in die herkömmlichen vier Schichten.

Die beiden hier gewählten Differenzierungsmaße stellen eine erste Realisierung dar. Besonders in Bezug auf die Schärfe der Profile sind jedoch Verbesserungen denkbar. Inwieweit die Beschreibung des Differenzierungsgrades über die mittlere Anzahl an Zellkernen pro Fläche einen Vorteil gegenüber der Korrelation von Differenzierung und Distanz zum Bindegewebe bringt, muss durch die Analyse weiterer Datensätze überprüft werden. In den bisherigen Ergebnissen zeigt der zellkernbasierte Ansatz eine geringere statistische Sicherheit und ein schlechteres Auflösungsvermögen, doch ist bei komplexeren räumlichen Epithelstrukturen mit einer gestörten Differenzierungsschichtung ein robusteres Verhalten gegenüber dem distanzbasierten Ansatz zu erwarten.

Die vorgestellte Methodik zur Generierung von Expressionsprofilen bildet eine erste Grundlage für mathematische Beschreibungen der räumlichen Proteinexpression in stratifizierten Epithelien. Zum einen könnten die gemessenen funktionalen Abhängigkeiten in ein systembiologisches Modell der epithelialen Homöostase integriert werden. Zum anderen würden die ermittelten Beschreibungen der Expression einen statistischen Vergleich von Gewebeproben unterschiedlicher Gewebelokalisationen bzw. von pathologischem und Normalgewebe ermöglichen.

6 Danksagung

Die Bildakquise wurde am Nikon Imaging Center in Heidelberg durchgeführt.

Literaturverzeichnis

1. Candi E, Schmidt R, Melino G. The cornified envelope: A model of cell death in the skin. Nature 2005;6(4):328–338.
2. Fuchs E, Byrne C. The epidermis: Rising to the surface. Curr Opin Cell Biol 1994;4(5):725–736.
3. Carlos L, Junqueira U, Carneiro J. Histologie. Springer, Berlin; 2005.
4. Morel D, Marcelpoil R, Brugal G. A proliferation control network model: The simulation of two-dimensional epithelial homeostasis. Acta Biotheoretica 2001;49(4):219–234.
5. Rashbass J, Stekel D, Williams E. The use of a computer model to simulate epithelial pathologies. J Pathology 1996;179(3):333–9.
6. Walker D, Southgate J, et al GHill. Agent-based computational modelling of epithelial cell monolayers. IEEE/ACM Trans Nanobioscience 2004;3(3):153–163.
7. Grabe N, Neuber K. A multicellular systems biology model predicts epidermal morphology, kinetics and Ca2+ flow. Bioinformatics 2005;21(17):3541–7.
8. Farrell P. High resolution two-dimensional electrophoresis of proteins. J Biological Chem 1975;250(10):4007–21.
9. Fung E, Thulasiraman V, Weinberger S. Protein biochips for differential profiling. Curr Opin Biotech 2001;12(1):65–9.
10. Chaurand P, Sanders M, et al RJensen. Proteomics in diagnostic pathology: Profiling and imaging proteins directly in tissue sections. Am J Pathol 2004;165(4):1057–68.
11. Murphy R. Location proteomics: A systems approach to subcellular location. Biochem Soc 2005;33(3):535–8.

Tracking of Virus Particles in Time-Lapse Fluorescence Microscopy Image Sequences

W.J. Godinez[1], M. Lampe[2], S. Wörz[1], B. Müller[2], R. Eils[1] and K. Rohr[1]

[1]University of Heidelberg, IPMB, and DKFZ Heidelberg, Dept. Bioinformatics and
Functional Genomics, 69120 Heidelberg, Germany
[2]University of Heidelberg, Dept. of Virology, 69120 Heidelberg, Germany
Email: wgodinez@ieee.org

Abstract. Modern developments in time-lapse microscopy enable the
observation of a variety of processes exhibited by viruses. The dynamic
nature of these processes requires the tracking of viruses over time to
explore the spatio-temporal relationships. In this work, we developed
deterministic and probabilistic approaches for multiple virus tracking. A
quantitative comparison based on synthetic image sequences was carried
out to evaluate the performance of the different algorithms. We have
also applied the algorithms to real microscopy images of HIV-1 particles and have compared the tracking results with ground truth obtained
from manual tracking. It turns out that the probabilistic approach outperforms the deterministic schemes.

1 Introduction

Exploration of the spatio-temporal relationships of viruses advances the understanding of viral infections, e.g., HIV-1. Modern time-lapse microscopy of these
processes results in a large amount of visual data that, on the one hand, provides the basis for a solid statistical analysis, yet, on the other hand, requires
automatic image analysis methods. However, the task of virus tracking is ham-
pered by various issues. For instance, viruses are relatively small and exhibit a
complex motion behavior, in particular, abrupt changes in velocity and direction
are observable; this precludes the usage of motion constraints often employed in
other tracking applications. Another problem is the relatively large number of
viruses in the image sequences, which rules out the usage of algorithms that are
only applicable in the case of one or few objects. A further problem is the low
signal-to-noise ratio (SNR), which hinders the accurate localization of particles.

Only few approaches for virus tracking have been described in the literature.
Typically, a deterministic two-step approach is used consisting of: 1) virus detection, and 2) correspondence finding. For virus detection, most of the algorithms
employ some kind of maximum intensity search strategy, in which the position of viruses are associated with intensity peaks. Subsequently, thresholding
techniques or techniques based on the intensity moments of detected candidate
viruses (e.g., [1]) are employed for rejecting noise-induced maxima. The position
of the particles may be refined by model fitting (e.g., [2]). For correspondence

finding, a nearest-neighbor model, which assumes that a single virus carries out the smallest possible displacement between two consecutive time steps, is typically employed. However, in image regions with a high density of viruses, the search for correspondences becomes ambiguous, since several possibilities are plausible. To address this issue, approaches that consider the motion of all viruses between two consecutive time frames have been introduced. For instance, in [1] the total distance between all viruses is minimized.

We introduce deterministic and probabilistic algorithms for tracking multiple viruses in microscopy time-lapse images. For the first time, a particle filter approach has been employed for the task of virus tracking.

2   Tracking of Multiple Virus Particles

We have developed four two-step deterministic tracking approaches for virus particle tracking by combining two virus detection schemes and two correspondence finding techniques. The first virus detection scheme is comprised by the application of the spot-enhancing filter ("SEF") [3], based on the Laplacian-of-Gaussian filter, and a thresholding step, which yields a binarized image from which viruses can be detected. The second technique is an enhanced 2D Gaussian fitting algorithm ("Gauss") along with rejection criteria for noise-induced candidate viruses, such as minimum integrated intensity, and maximum ellipticity of the fitted 2D Gaussian function. For correspondence finding, we have investigated an algorithm based on a smooth motion model along with a greedy optimization step ("Smooth") [4], and an algorithm based on a nearest-neighbor scheme with an optimization step inspired by an algorithm for the transportation problem ("NNeigh") [1]. The first algorithm ("Smooth") assumes a gradual change in direction and displacement, and only considers the motion of one virus at a time to resolve correspondence conflicts. The second algorithm ("NNeigh") assumes small displacements between two consecutive time-frames, and minimizes the overall frame-to-frame displacement induced by all viruses.

We have also developed a probabilistic approach for multiple virus tracking, which formulates the task of tracking as a Bayesian sequential estimation problem. Such probabilistic approaches are relatively novel in the area of biological imaging. An initial effort in this direction is introduced in [5], in which a joint particle filter is utilized for a different tracking application, namely the tracking of growing microtubules. We have extended and applied this method for the tracking of multiple viruses. In our case, each virus is represented by a state vector $\mathbf{x}_t$ that includes the position, velocity, and intensity. This state evolves in time according to a predefined dynamic model $p(\mathbf{x}_t \mid \mathbf{x}_{t-1})$ (here we used Brownian dynamics) and is observed at discrete times t through measurement vectors $\mathbf{y}_t$. The predictions generated by the dynamic model are tested against the information provided by the measurement $\mathbf{y}_t$ via an observation model $p(\mathbf{y}_t \mid \mathbf{x}_t)$ (in our case, the probability that the predicted state $\mathbf{x}_t$ generated a Gaussian intensity distribution in the image, i.e., a virus). Inference on the true state is based on the posterior distribution $p(\mathbf{x}_t \mid \mathbf{y}_{1:t})$, which is conditioned on a sequence of observations $\mathbf{y}_{1:t-1}$, and which is obtained using Bayes' theorem:

Fig. 1. Tracking results for a synthetic image sequence

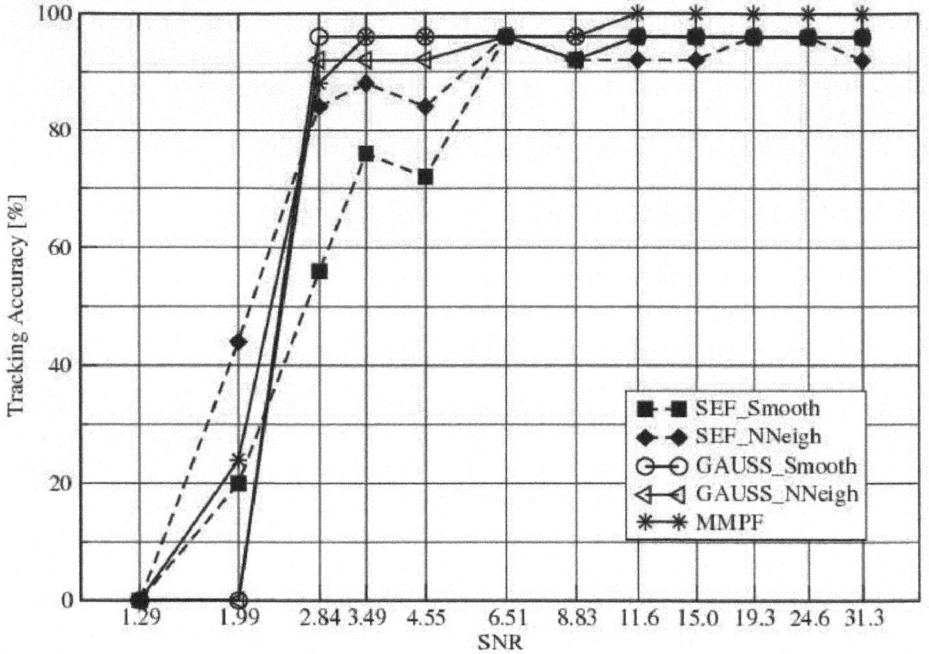

$$p(\mathbf{x}_t \mid \mathbf{y}_{1:t-1}) = \int p(\mathbf{x}_t \mid \mathbf{x}_{t-1})p(\mathbf{x}_{t-1} \mid \mathbf{y}_{1:t-1})d\mathbf{x}_{t-1} \qquad (1)$$

$$p(\mathbf{x}_t \mid \mathbf{y}_{1:t}) \propto p(\mathbf{y}_t \mid \mathbf{x}_t)p(\mathbf{x}_t \mid \mathbf{y}_{1:t-1}) \qquad (2)$$

The numeric implementation of these equations has been done via a joint particle filter. In contrast to [5], in which manual initialization is employed, in our algorithm we automatically initialize the tracking via one of the above-mentioned virus detection approaches. Furthermore, instead of using a fixed value for the σ parameter which defines the Gaussian intensity distribution in the observation model $p(\mathbf{y}_t \mid \mathbf{x}_t)$, we automatically compute this parameter based on the Gaussian fitting results; in this way, we can track virus particles with different apparent sizes.

3   Experimental Results

We have applied our algorithms to both synthetic as well as real microscopy image sequences. In total, we generated four synthetic image sequences, each consisting of 50 images (size 400×400 pixels) containing 25-40 simulated moving viruses using 12 different signal-to-noise ratio (SNR) levels. The noise model was assumed to be Poisson distributed. To measure the performance, we employed the tracking accuracy defined as $P_{\text{track}} = \frac{n_{\text{track,correct}}}{n_{\text{track,total}}}$, which reflects the ratio between the number of completely correctly computed trajectories $n_{\text{track,correct}}$

Table 1. Tracking results for a real microscopy image sequence

	SEF+Smooth	SEF+NNeigh	Gaussian+Smooth	Gaussian+NNeigh	MMPF
P_{track}	60.87%	73.91%	60.87%	69.57%	95.65%

Fig. 2. Sample image from a real microscopy image sequence (a) and results obtained by the MMPF (b). An enlarged section delineated with a black rectangle in (b) is shown in (c). The image intensities have been inverted for visualization purposes

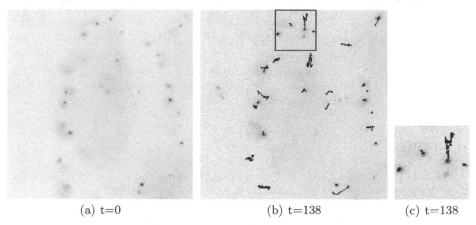

(a) t=0   (b) t=138   (c) t=138

and the number of all true trajectories $n_{track,total}$. $n_{track,correct}$ counts those trajectories that span the same time period as their true counterparts, and yield a mean-squared error (MSE) between the measured object displacement and the true object displacement lower than a certain threshold (in our case we used a threshold of 2). A statistical test (one-way ANOVA) for each of the synthetic sequences yielded no significant differences between the performance of the different algorithms (see Fig. 1). The reason for this result is probably the simplistic nature of the synthetic images (e.g., constant number of objects and constant intensity). We also validated the algorithms based on a real microscopy image sequence (see Fig. 2), consisting of 250 16-bit images (size 512×512 pixels) with 23 well-defined virus particles. In this sequence, fluorescently labeled HIV-1 particles [6] were imaged using a fluorescence widefield microscope; fluorophores were excited with their respective excitation wavelengths and movies were recorded with a frequency of 10Hz. Ground truth on the virus positions was obtained by manual tracking using the commercial software MetaMorph. The experimental results, which have been listed in Table 1, indicate that the probabilistic approach (MMPF=multimodal particle filter) outperforms the deterministic approaches (95.65% accuracy vs. 73.91% and 69.57% for the two best deterministic approaches, Fig. 2).

4 Discussion

We have developed deterministic and probabilistic approaches for the tracking of viruses in microscopy images sequences. Our quantitative comparison based on real microscopy image sequences shows that among all four deterministic approaches, the combinations of spot-enhancing filter (SEF) or Gaussian fitting with an enhanced nearest-neighbor motion model achieve the best results. Overall, the probabilistic approach based on a particle filter outperforms the deterministic schemes. The developed algorithms provide information on the displacements, sizes, and intensities of the virus particles. Nevertheless, there are still some open issues. For instance, in areas of high object density with fast changing dynamics all algorithms have difficulties in determining the correct correspondences. In future work, the performance of the algorithms should be further improved in this regard.

References

1. Sbalzarini IF, Koumoutsakos P. Feature point tracking and trajectory analysis for video imaging in cell biology. J Struct Biol 2005;151(2):182–195.
2. Seisenberger G, Ried MU, Endre T, Buning H, Hallek M, Bräuchle C. Real-time single-molecule imaging of the infection pathway of an adeno-associated virus. Science 2001;294(5548):1929–1932.
3. Sage D, Neumann FR, Hediger F, Gasser SM, Unser M. Automatic tracking of individual fluorescence particles: application to the study of chromosome dynamics. IEEE Trans Image Process 2005;14(9):1372–1382.
4. Chetverikov D, Verestoy J. Tracking feature points: a new algorithm. Int Conf Pattern Recognit 1998;02:1436.
5. Smal I, Niessen W, Meijering E. Bayesian tracking for fluorescence microscopic imaging. Procs ISBI 2006; 550–553.
6. Lampe M, Briggs JAG, Endress T, Glass B, Riegelsberger S, Kr"ausslich H, et al. Double-labelled HIV-1 particles for study of virus-cell interaction. Virology 2006;In Press.

Subcellular Localisation of Proteins in Living Cells Using a Genetic Algorithm and an Incremental Neural Network

Marko Tscherepanow and Franz Kummert

Applied Computer Science, Faculty of Technology,
Bielefeld University, P.O. Box 100 131, D-33501 Bielefeld
Email: {marko, franz}@techfak.uni-bielefeld.de

Abstract. The subcellular localisation of proteins in living cells is a crucial means for the determination of their function. We propose an approach to realise such a protein localisation based on microscope images. In order to reach this goal, appropriate features are selected. Then, the initial feature set is optimised by a genetic algorithm. The actual classification of possible protein localisations is accomplished by an incremental neural network which not only achieves a very high accuracy, but enables on-line learning, as well.

1 Introduction

Location Proteomics, i.e. the automatic subcellular localisation of many or all proteins of a cell, has made considerable progress during the last decade [1]. By investigating fluorescence images of tagged proteins in living cells, essential information about their functions can be obtained. This knowledge is applicable for the simulation of cell behaviour which might facilitate the investigation of diseases and the development of novel drugs.

2 State of the Art and New Contribution

In comparison to the direct application of pixel intensities, the usage of numerical features has proven advantageous for the classification of fluorescence images showing tagged proteins [1, 2]. The feature sets proposed in the literature comprise, for instance, morphological data of binary image structures, Zernike moments and edge information. Wide-field microscope images are usually preprocessed by digital deconvolution in order to enhance the contrast.

Since unnecessary features adversely influence the result of the classification if too small a number of training samples is available and increase the computational effort, they should be removed. Several methods have been applied in order to achieve this goal [3]. At this, stepwise discriminant analysis (SDA) and a genetic algorithm have attained particularly good results. As classifiers, multilayer perceptrons (MLPs) [4] and support vector machines (SVMs) [3] are utilised frequently.

We propose an approach to protein localisation in living *Spodoptera frugiper-da* cells (Sf9) which does not require digital deconvolution as a preprocessing step, thereby reducing the computational effort. In addition, we employ a classifier which has been developed for incremental learning. So, in principle, potential users can incorporate new data during the application. The relevance of features is determined by a genetic algorithm. In contrast to other approaches, here, no binary masking is performed (cf. [3, 5]). So, discontinuities in the optimisation function are avoided. Finally, the protein localisation is adapted for a cell recognition method introduced in [6]. Since automatic cell recognition constitutes a crucial precondition for performing an automated protein localisation, this connection enables a better collaboration enhancing the performance of the final complete system.

3   Methods

The protein localisations are classified based on three different types of features:

(i)   Zernike moments [7] which are sensitive to the position of tagged proteins with respect to the surrounding cell,
(ii) granulometries [8] enabling the investigation of the shape and the size of protein accumulations directly using the image intensities,
(iii) and fractal features [9] allowing for the determination of the granularity and self-similarity at different scales.

Instead of utilising classifiers which compute discrimination planes, we employ the simplified fuzzy ARTMAP (SFAM) [10], an incremental neural network. Its neurons span hyper-rectangular regions in the feature space – the categories. Their maximal size is determined by the vigilance parameter ρ. An input which is to be classified receives the label of the best-matching category enclosing it. Unknown inputs can easily be rejected, as they do not belong to an existing category. We have extended the subspace of known inputs by a small distance τ from each category so as to cope with slightly varying data.

In order to assess the importance of the n available features, each input $\underline{x}$ is multiplied by a weight vector $\underline{w}$. Its components w_i as well as the parameters ρ and τ are evolved by a genetic algorithm utilising rank-based selection in order to handle slight differences in the fitness values of the population. Furthermore, arithmetic cross-over and mutation for continuous-valued genes are employed [11]. The fitness $f(X)$ corresponds to the cross-validation accuracy $\mathrm{acc}(X)$ of the classifier X diminished by a punishment for large values of τ and high weights w_i. These punishments are scaled by the constants c_τ and c_w, respectively (see (1)).

$$f(X) = \mathrm{acc}(X) - c_\tau \cdot \tau - c_w \cdot \frac{1}{n} \sum_{i=0}^{n} w_i \qquad (1)$$

So, only the weights of features which are important for obtaining a good accuracy receive high values and the considered subspace is reduced. After a run

Fig. 1. Protein distributions in Sf9 cells: The white contours represent the surrounding cells which were manually extracted from corresponding bright-field images by biological experts

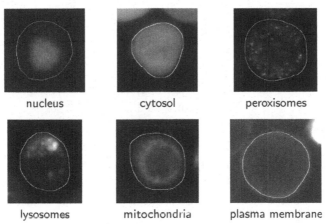

nucleus	cytosol	peroxisomes
lysosomes	mitochondria	plasma membrane

of the genetic algorithm, all weight vectors are normalised in such a way that the maximal component equals 1 in order to enable the usage of the possible input space $(\forall i \in \{1, \cdots, n\} : x_i \in [0, 1])$ and to avoid multiple solutions of the optimisation function resulting from scaling the occupied region of the feature space. By considering the weights of the final generation, conclusions about the relevance of features can be drawn, as these individuals are adapted to the task at hand.

4   Results

Our approach was evaluated on 972 images of single cells manually extracted from 99 bright-field micrographs taken in parallel with each fluorescence image. Here, six different protein locations were considered: nucleus (150 cells), cytosol (164 cells), peroxisomes (71 cells), lysosomes (222 cells), mitochondria (268 cells), and plasma membrane (97 cells). Protein distributions of these six classes are depicted in Fig. 1.

In addition to the manually segmented cells, 5368 cell images were generated automatically using an active contour approach [6]. This method yields segments which resemble the manually determined cells. As we plan to utilise it for cell recognition, the resulting segments are more likely to occur during an automated application of our protein localisation technique. In addition, the number of training samples is increased which alleviates the classification task.

After computing the features of every cell image, the resulting data set was split into ten disjoint parts. Five groups of eight data sets each were used for the determination of the input weights by our genetic algorithm. Here 100 generations with 100 individuals were applied after performing preliminary trials. Results from the literature confirm that these values are sufficiently high $\big(\text{cf. } [3]\big)$.

Table 1. Confusion matrix for manually segmented cells. The table entries represent the number of cells from a specific class i (row) which were recognised as class j (column). A correct classification is characterised by equal labels i and j

cell compartment	classification result						
	(a)	(b)	(c)	(d)	(e)	(f)	unknown
nucleus (a)	145	3	0	0	1	1	0
cytosol (b)	0	156	0	4	3	1	0
peroxisomes (c)	0	0	63	2	5	1	0
lysosomes (d)	1	5	0	195	18	3	0
mitochondria (e)	0	0	2	14	250	2	0
plasma membrane (f)	0	0	2	3	5	87	0

The parameters c_τ and c_w were chosen in such a way that the fitness is mainly determined by the accuracy ($c_\tau=0.02$ and $c_w=0.1$). At this, only slight variations of the fitness were intended, since the accuracy should not be decreased by the feature selection method.

The evaluation occurred based on the remaining groups of two data sets averaging the results (five-fold cross-validation). In order to determine the fitness value of a classifier, eight-fold cross-validation was applied in each group (see Section 3). During the evaluation, manually and automatically obtained samples were distinguished, since the manually segmented cells are more biologically relevant. At this, an accuracy of 92% was achieved. Table 1 shows the corresponding confusion matrix. For the automatically determined samples, accuracies up to 94% were reached.

In order to reduce the dimensionality of the feature space, a computation of the mean weight vector over all individuals of the final generation occurred. Then, inputs with mean weights smaller than a threshold τ_w were rejected (see Fig. 2). Using a value of $\tau_w=0.9$, the number of required features n could be decreased from 64 to 19.2 on average without impairing the classification results. Higher values of τ_w resulted in considerably reduced accuracies.

5   Discussion

We have proposed an approach to the localisation of proteins with a high accuracy. The number of the employed features, which were chosen with respect to the task at hand, was significantly reduced by means of a genetic algorithm. In contrast to known approaches, our method enables on-line learning and does not require optical deconvolution. Furthermore, it can be applied in an automated context, since it is adapted for an automatic cell recognition method.

References

1. Chen X, Velliste M, Murphy RF. Automated interpretation of subcellular patterns in fluorescence microscope images for location proteomics. Cytometry 2006;69A:631–640.

Fig. 2. Accuracy with respect to the manually segmented cells and number of required features n, which decreases if the threshold τ_w is rising or the accuracy remains high for values of τ_w up to 0.9

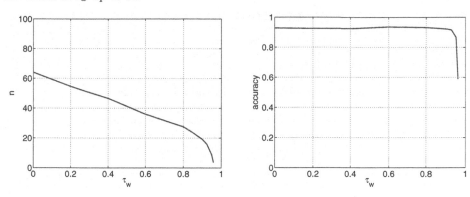

2. Murphy RF, Velliste M, Porreca G. Robust numerical features for description and classification of subcellular location patterns in fluorescence microscope images. Journal of VLSI Signal Processing 2003;35:311–321.

3. Huang K, Velliste M, Murphy RF. Feature reduction for improved recognition of subcellular location patterns in fluorescence microscope images. Procs SPIE 2003;4962:307–318.

4. Boland MV, Murphy RF. A neural network classifier capable of recognizing the patterns of all major subcellular structures in fluorescence microscope images of HeLa cells. Bioinformatics 2001;17(12):1213–1223.

5. Raymer ML, Punch WF, Goodman ED, Kuhn LA, Jain AK. Dimensionality reduction using genetic algorithms. IEEE Trans on Evolutionary Computation 2000;4(2):164–171.

6. Tscherepanow M, Zöllner F, Kummert F. Classification of segmented regions in brightfield microscope images. Procs ICPR 2006;3:972–975.

7. Khotanzad Alireza, Hong YawHua. Invariant Image Recognition by Zernike Moments. IEEE Trans on Pattern Analysis and Machine Intelligence 1990;12(5):489–497.

8. Soille P. Morphological Image Analysis: Principles and Applications. Springer; 2003.

9. Wu CM, Chen YC, Hsieh KS. Texture features for classification of ultrasonic liver images. IEEE Trans on Medical Imaging 1992;11(2):141–152.

10. Vakil-Baghmisheh MT, Pavešić N. A fast simplified fuzzy ARTMAP network. Neural Processing Letters 2003;17(3):273–316.

11. Engelbrecht AP. Fundamentals of Computational Swarm Intelligence. John Wiley & Sons; 2005.

Non-rigid Temporal Alignment of 2D and 3D Multi-channel Microscopy Image Sequences of Human Cells

I. Kim[1], S. Yang[1], P. Le Baccon[2], E. Heard[2], C. Kappel[1], R. Eils[1], K. Rohr[1]

[1]University of Heidelberg, IPMB, and DKFZ Heidelberg,
Dept. Bioinformatics and Functional Genomics, Biomedical Computer Vision Group,
Im Neuenheimer Feld 364, 69120 Heidelberg, Germany
[2]CNRS UMR 218, Curie Institute, 26 rue d'Ulm, 75248 Paris Cedex 05, France
Email: i.kim@dkfz-heidelberg.de

Abstract. The analysis of fluroescence tagged proteins in live cells from multi-channel microscopy image sequences requires a registration to a reference frame to decouple the movement and deformation of cells from the movement of proteins. We have developed an intensity-based approach for the registration of 2D and 3D multi-channel microscopy image sequences. This approach can be directly applied to the intensity images or to the segmented images. Also, we have performed a comparison using a direct registration scheme to the reference frame and an incremental scheme taking into account results from preceding time steps. We have evaluated our approach based on 3D synthetic images of a simulated spherical cell with known deformation which has been calculated based on an analytic solution of the Navier equation given certain boundary conditions. We have also successfully applied our approach to 2D and 3D real microscopy image sequences.

1 Introduction

Current time-lapse microscopy technology allows to analyze the location and movement of fluorescent tagged structures (proteins) within a living cell (see Fig. 1). Such an analysis is important to study subcellular processes. However, live cells change in position and shape over time. Therefore, when observing the tagged structures then only a superposition of the movement of proteins and that of the cell can be seen. To determine the real motion of proteins one has to compensate the movement and deformation of the cell. To this end it is necessary to register dynamic cell microscopy images w.r.t. a reference frame.

In previous work on the registration of microscopy images of moving cells mainly rigid registration approaches recovering translation and rotation have been used (e.g., [1]). However, rigid registration cannot cope with deformations of live cells. The assumption that the shape does not change only holds for certain applications. In applications where there are considerable shape changes, non-rigid registration schemes are required to decouple the global movement of cells from the movement of fluorescent tagged protein particles. So far, only few approaches for non-rigid registration of cell microscopy images have been described in the literature [2, 3]. The work in [2] is based on semi-automatic extraction of point landmarks and uses a thin-plate spline transformation model. 2D images of fixed cells are analyzed and the deformation between two images is due to different stainings. In [3] segmented images and an optic flow-based registration scheme are used to register 3D static images of different cells. A disadvantage of this approach is that a segmentation of the images is required.

In comparison to [2, 3], we here introduce an approach for the registration of multi-channel cell microscopy image sequences which directly uses the original intensities to utilize the full image information. Our approach is fully automatic and is applied for the registration of 2D and 3D temporal image sequences of moving cells. We have compared the results of our approach with results based on segmented images. In addition, we have studied two different schemes for registering the images of an image sequence to a reference frame. In the first scheme, each image is directly registered to the first frame of the sequence (the reference frame). In the second scheme, subsequent images are registered and concatenated to obtain a registration to the first frame. We have evaluated our approach based on 3D synthetic images of a simulated spherical cell with known deformation which has been calculated based on an analytic solution of the Navier equation. We have also successfully applied our approach to 2D and 3D real microscopy image sequences.

2   Non-rigid Temporal Registration of Cell Images

For the registration of 2D and 3D multi-channel microscopy image sequences we have developed an intensity-based approach combining rigid and non-rigid transformations. The implemented scheme for registering two successive images consists of three steps: Preprocessing of the images by Gaussian filtering, rigid registration, and non-rigid registration. For rigid registration of 3D images we use a quaternion-based registration scheme which minimizes the mean-squared intensity error by a gradient descent optimizer. For non-rigid registration we use a variant of the demons algorithm [4], which is driven by symmetric forces and also incorporates a multi-resolution scheme.

We have also implemented two different schemes for the registration of the images to a reference frame. In the first approach, each image of a sequence is directly registered to the first image, without considering results from preceding time steps. Instead, in the second approach, information from previous time steps is exploited by an incremental scheme. To this end two subsequent images g_1 and g_2 at time steps 1 and 2 are registered, which results in a rigid transformation $\mathbf{R}(g_2, g_1)$ and a non-rigid transformation $\mathbf{U}$. The combination of both transformations then gives $\mathbf{u}(g_2, g_1) = \mathbf{U}(\mathbf{R}(g_2, g_1), g_1)$. For the registration of the subsequent image at time step 3 we concatenate this result with the transformation $\mathbf{u}(g_3, g_2)$ between time steps 3 and 2 to obtain the registration to the reference frame $\mathbf{u}(g_3, g_1) = \mathbf{u}(g_3, g_2) \circ \mathbf{u}(g_2, g_1)$. Generally, an image at time

Fig. 1. Example of one slice of a 3D cell microscopy image at a certain time step: (Left) Channel 1 with labelled cell, (Middle) Channel 0 visualizing the tagged protein in z-slice 25, (Right) Registered channel 0 with the tagged protein in z-slice 35

step k can be registered to the reference frame by concatenating previously calculated transformations by $\mathbf{u}(g_k, g_1) = \mathbf{u}(g_k, g_{k-1}) \circ \mathbf{u}(g_{k-1}, g_{k-2}) \circ \cdots \circ \mathbf{u}(g_2, g_1)$. To regularize the resulting deformation fields over time, we use a Gaussian filter on the final concatenated field. Our approach is directly applied to the intensity images. For a comparison we have also applied the algorithm to segmented images of the original image sequences.

3   Experimental Results

To evaluate the developed approach we have generated 3D synthetic image sequences simulating the compression of a spherical cell. By solving the Navier equation $\mu\Delta\mathbf{u}(\mathbf{x}) + (\mu + \lambda)\nabla(\nabla\mathbf{u}(\mathbf{x})) = \mathbf{0}$, where $\mathbf{u}(\mathbf{x})$ denotes the deformation $\mathbf{u}$ at $\mathbf{x}$, and μ as well as λ are the Lamé coefficients, the deformation has been calculated analytically. The solution has been obtained by defining displacements at the border of the sphere, which act as boundary conditions.

The generated image sequences consist of 15 images with a resolution of $128{\times}128{\times}128$ pixels. The spherical cell consists of an inner sphere (radius of 20 pixels) with uniform intensity of 150 and an outer sphere (radius 20 to 40) with an intensity level of 200. The compression of the simulated cell is obtained by defining displacements of 1 pixel per time step at the border of the sphere. To evaluate the effects of the registration on a moving subcellular structure a second image sequence was generated, which acts as second channel. This second sequence shows a spherical spot with a radius of 5 pixels, which moves by 2 pixels per time step from the center to the border of the sphere.

Given these 3D image sequences the performance of our approach was determined by calculating the errors in angle and magnitude of the deformation vectors w.r.t. the correct vectors as well as calculating the error in the location of the spot. The angular error and the normalized magnitude error at each pixel $\mathbf{x}$ of the computed vector $(\mathbf{u}(\mathbf{x}), 1)$ w.r.t. the correct vector $(\mathbf{u}_{true}(\mathbf{x}), 1)$ using a temporal distance of 1 are given by:

$$\bar{e}_{\text{angle}} = \arccos\left[\frac{(\mathbf{u}(\mathbf{x}), 1)\cdot(\mathbf{u}_{\text{true}}(\mathbf{x}), 1)}{\sqrt{1 + |\mathbf{u}(\mathbf{x})|}\sqrt{1 + |\mathbf{u}_{\text{true}}(\mathbf{x})|}}\right], \quad \bar{e}_{\text{magn}} = \frac{(|\mathbf{u}(\mathbf{x})| - |\mathbf{u}_{\text{true}}(\mathbf{x})|)^2}{|\mathbf{u}(\mathbf{x})|^2 + |\mathbf{u}_{\text{true}}(\mathbf{x})|^2}$$

Table 1. Averaged angular and magnitude error of the deformation field as well as spot location error for segmentation- and intensity-based registration of the synthetic image sequences

	$\bar{e}_{\text{angle}}$ [°]	$\bar{e}_{\text{magn}}$	$\bar{e}_{\text{spot}}$ [pixel]
Segmentation, incremental	7.16	0.08	2.40
Segmentation, direct	6.25	0.10	2.04
Intensities, incremental	7.87	0.08	1.59
Intensities, direct	5.90	0.09	1.31

The direct registration scheme as well as the incremental scheme have been applied to the original intensity images as well as to the segmented images. The errors have been averaged over all 14 images that have been registered to the first image of the sequence. The error in the location of the spot $\bar{e}_{spot}$ is determined by calculating the Euclidian distance w.r.t. the ground truth position. For the non-registered images, the location error of the spot is up to 13.5 pixels for the last image of the sequence. In Table 1 the calculated errors have been listed. It can be seen that registration using the original intensities gives significantly better results for the location of the spot (right column). The angular and magnitude errors (averaged over the whole images) are comparable for intensity-based and segmentation-based registration. It can also be seen that direct registration to the first image gives slightly better results than the incremental approach. The reason is probably that the assumed uniform deformation over time allows a relatively good direct registration from each image of the sequence to the first image. Instead, with the incremental approach small errors between two subsequent images accumulate.

We have also applied our approach to 2D and 3D multi-channel microscopy image sequences of live cells. The 2D image sequences depict two cells over 150 images at a resolution of 512×512 pixels. The cells show relatively small deformations between subsequent time steps but high total deformations over the whole sequence as well as considerable motion of subcellular structures. The internal structure of the cells exhibits high intensity variations. Registration based on the original intensity images yields a more accurate result for the internal structures of the cells compared to using the segmented images. In the latter case a smoother deformation field is obtained.

The 3D image sequences consist of up to 15 images per sequence with xy-resolutions between 160×152 and 196×196 pixels and z-depths between 31 and 41, showing a single cell nucleus and, in a second channel, a tagged protein, see Fig. 1. The cell nucleus exhibits relatively low intensity variations, moderate deformations between subsequent time steps, but large rigid motion. Since the sequence consists of 15 images, the overall deformation for the whole sequence is relatively small compared to the 2D image sequences consisting of 150 images. Registration based on the original intensities gave similar results as using the segmented images (see Fig. 2 and Fig. 1 (right)). The reason is probably the comparably low intensity variation inside the cell. Since here the overall de-

Fig. 2. Example of one slice of the 3D cell microscopy images: Original reference image at time step 1 (left) and step 8 (middle left), Registered image based on segmentation with edge overlay of the reference image (middle right) and using intensities with edge overlay of the reference image (right)

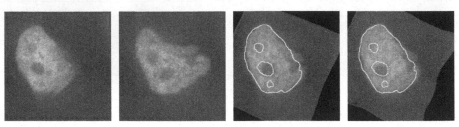

formations are moderate the direct registration scheme yielded more accurate results compared to the incremental scheme.

4   Discussion

We have presented an approach for the registration of 2D and 3D multi-channel temporal microscopy image sequences which utilizes the full image information. The approach has been applied to 3D synthetic image sequences as well as 2D and 3D real microscopy image sequences. It turned out that using directly the intensities gives more accurate registration results (compared to using segmented images) if the internal structure of the observed cells exhibits high intensity variations. We have also implemented and compared two different schemes for registering the images to a reference image. Here it turned out that the incremental scheme yields better results in case of large overall and non-uniform deformations. Future work will focus on analyzing a larger spectrum of 2D and 3D temporal microscopy image sequences in different applications.

References

1. Rieger B, Molenaar C, Dirks RW, Vliet IJVan. Alignment of the cell nucleus from labeled proteins only for 4D in vivo imaging. Microsc Res Tech 2004;64(2):142–150.
2. Mattes J, Nawroth J, Boukamp P, et al. Analyzing motion and deformation of the cell nucleus for studying co-localizations of nuclear structures; 2006.
3. Yang S, Köhler D, Teller K, et al. Non-rigid registration of 3D multi-channel microscopy images of cell nuclei. LNCS 2006;4190:907–914.
4. Thirion JP. Image matching as a diffusion process: An analogy with Maxwell's demons. Med Image Anal 1998;2(3):243–260.

Interactive Guidance System for C-Arm Repositioning Without Radiation

Visual Servoing for Camera Augmented Mobile C-Arm (CAMC)

Tassilo Klein[1], Selim Benhimane[1], Joerg Traub[1], Sandro M. Heining[2],
Ekkehard Euler[2], Nassir Navab[1]

[1]Chair for Computer Aided Medical Procedures (CAMP), TU Munich, Germany
[2]Trauma Surgery Department, Klinikum Innenstadt, LMU Munich, Germany
Email: tjklein@gmail.com

Abstract. The problem of repositioning mobile C-arms to defined target locations during surgical procedures currently requires not only time, but also skill and additional radiation exposure. This paper shows a guidance system based on the previously introduced camera augmented mobile C-arm (CAMC). Techniques of visual servoing are applied in order to present the repositioning task in the parameter space of the C-arm. Here we describe a representation for the estimated parameters in order to provide an easy to use interface that helps to speed up relocation procedure in the surgery room. The system which is based on an interactive 3D model, is controlled by tracking visible markers on the patient's skin using an optical camera attached to the X-ray housing. The visual servoing methods are used to guide the C-arm to target positions by the representation of the interactive visual guidance system. Addititionally, the system provides a number of tools for feedback to assess the required accuracy of the repositioning task. First tests for C-arm repositioning were performed in a laboratory environment.

1 Introduction

The mobile C-arm has become an essential tool in everyday trauma and orthopedic surgery. During the course of surgical interventions, the mobile C-arm frequently has to be moved by OR-staff. This results in the problem of finding the exact position again in order to compare the second image/sequence with the one acquired before the C-arm was (re)moved. In order to guarantee accurate and fast repositioning of the C-arm, a simple step-by-step approach is required. In addition, a system interacting with the OR-staff should be especially unambiguous and self-explaining as possible to avoid error and the need of training.

The camera augmented mobile C-arm (CAMC) [1, 2] has an attached optical camera mounted beside the X-ray housing which in combination with a navigation software allows to minimize the exposure to radiation. By using a double mirror system, X-ray images can be aligned and overlaid on real-time images for simultaneous display. This merely requires an one-time calibration step supposed the patient does not move. If the patient moves simply a new x-ray image has to be aquired and the modalities are aligned again. Additionally, CAMC supports repositioning tasks by using optical image-based visual servoing. This is achieved by tracking fiducals and comparing their locations to given target positions. Using this information visual servoing techniques, as described in [3], iteratively compute joint increments. Due to the manual manipulation nature of the mobile C-arm unit, this information is passed to the OR-staff, which adjusts the joints accordingly.

The previous introduced system [3] only provides the parameters in C-arm coordinates. However, the main contribution of the system described in this paper is to provide an easy to use interface. Thus the visual servoing procedure is extended by a user interface in order to make the repositioning task simple and unambiguous for the surgical staff in the OR. This contains the display of the isolated C-arm parameters as instructions on a 3D model of the C-arm and for the confirmation of the correct repositioning a visualization of a difference video image.

2   C-Arm Control and Motion Model

Visual servoing aims to control the C-arm using the visual information taken from the on-board camera observing the scene at the current position $\mathcal{F}$ such that it reaches the desired (or the reference) position $\mathcal{F}^*$. If we denote by $\mathbf{q}$ the vector containing the current positions of the joints, the objective of visual servoing is then to compute the direction and the amplitude of the increments of the joints, that correspond to $\dot{\mathbf{q}}$, in order to accomplish the positioning task. Consequently, we need to model the forward kinematics and the Jacobian of the C-arm.

The kinematic of the C-arm has five degrees of freedom : height, wigwag-movement, length, angular and orbital movement. We assigned a coordinate frame to each joint according to the Denavit-Hartenberg rules. Let $^{i}\mathbf{A}_{i+1}$ be the (4×4) transformation matrix from the coordinate system of the joint $i + 1$ to the coordinate system of the joint i. Multiplying the different transformation matrices makes it possible to obtain the camera pose wrt. the world reference frame: $^{0}\mathbf{A}_{6} = {}^{0}\mathbf{A}_{1}{}^{1}\mathbf{A}_{2}{}^{2}\mathbf{A}_{3}{}^{3}\mathbf{A}_{4}{}^{4}\mathbf{A}_{5}{}^{5}\mathbf{A}_{6}$ The transformation matrix $^{5}\mathbf{A}_{6}$ takes into account the rotation between the coordinate system of the last joint and the coordinate system of the camera.

To relate the motion of the camera to the motion of the C-arm joints, we have to compute the manipulator Jacobian $\mathbf{J}_{carm}$ of the C-arm. It converts the velocities of the single joints $\dot{\mathbf{q}}$ to the Cartesian velocity of the camera $\mathbf{v}_{c}$.

The C-arm consists of five joints so $\mathbf{J}_{carm} \in \mathbb{R}^{6 \times 5}$. Its entries can be derived from the forward kinematics. The rotation axis $\mathbf{z}_{i}$ of each joint is found in the 3rd column of the matrix $^{0}\mathbf{A}_{i} = {}^{0}\mathbf{A}_{1} \ldots {}^{i-1}\mathbf{A}_{i}$, where the origin $\mathbf{o}_{i}$ is found in the 4th column.. Equation 1 lists first the column of the manipulator Jacobian for a prismatic joint (like length and height of the C-arm) and second for a revolute joint (like wigwag, angular and orbital movement).

$$\mathbf{j}_i = \begin{pmatrix} \mathbf{z}_i \\ \mathbf{0} \end{pmatrix} \; ; \mathbf{j}_i = \begin{pmatrix} \mathbf{z}_i \times (\mathbf{o}_5 - \mathbf{o}_i) \\ \mathbf{z}_i \end{pmatrix} \tag{1}$$

2.1 Visual Servoing

At the desired position $\mathcal{F}^*$, a 3D point $\boldsymbol{\mathcal{X}}$ is projected on a virtual plane perpendicular to the optical axis of the camera into a 2D point $\mathbf{m}^*$:

$$\mathbf{m}^* = (x^*, y^*, 1) \propto \begin{bmatrix} \mathbf{I}_{3\times 3} \; \mathbf{0}_{3\times 1} \end{bmatrix} \boldsymbol{\mathcal{X}} \tag{2}$$

The same 3D point $\boldsymbol{\mathcal{X}}$ is projected into a 2D point $\mathbf{m}$ in the current camera position $\mathcal{F}$: $\mathbf{m} = (x, y, 1) \propto \begin{bmatrix} \mathbf{R} \, \mathbf{t} \end{bmatrix} \boldsymbol{\mathcal{X}}$ where $\mathbf{R}$ is the rotation matrix and $\mathbf{t}$ is the translation vector between the two coordinate systems $\mathcal{F}$ and $\mathcal{F}^*$. The information given by a pinhole camera, which performs a perspective projection of 3D points, is an image point $\mathbf{p} = (u, v, 1)$ verifying $\mathbf{p} = \mathbf{Km}$ where $\mathbf{K}$ is the camera internal parameter matrix.

Visual servoing using 2D target image can be accomplished by building a vector $\mathbf{s}$, containing visual information extracted from the current acquired image (at the current position $\mathcal{F}$), converging to a vector $\mathbf{s}^*$ containing visual information extracted from the reference image (at the reference position $\mathcal{F}^*$). In our case, the visual information are the image coordinates of the n markers:

$$\mathbf{s} = \begin{bmatrix} \mathbf{m}_1^\top \; \mathbf{m}_2^\top \; \dots \; \mathbf{m}_n^\top \end{bmatrix}^\top \tag{3}$$

An interaction matrix (also known as image jacobian) $\mathbf{L}$ is then defined in order to establish the relationship between the Cartesian velocity of the camera $\mathbf{v}_c$ and the derivative of the vector $\mathbf{s}$ wrt. time. This relationship can be written as: $\dot{\mathbf{s}} = \mathbf{L}\mathbf{v}_c$. The $(3n \times 6)$ interaction matrix $\mathbf{L}$ can be expressed with the following formula: $\mathbf{L} = \begin{bmatrix} \mathbf{L}_1^\top \; \mathbf{L}_2^\top \; \dots \; \mathbf{L}_n^\top \end{bmatrix}^\top$ where:

$$\mathbf{L}_i = \begin{bmatrix} \frac{1}{Z_i} & 0 & -\frac{x_i}{Z_i} & x_i y_i & -(1 + x_i^2) & y_i \\ 0 & \frac{1}{Z_i} & -\frac{y_i}{Z_i} & (1 + y_i^2) & -x_i y_i & -x_i \\ 0 & 0 & 0 & 0 & 0 & 0 \end{bmatrix}$$

Finally the vector $\mathbf{s}$ is servoed using the task function approach [4, 5] by minimizing iteratively the following vector $\mathbf{e} = \widehat{\mathbf{L}}^+(\mathbf{s} - \mathbf{s}^*)$, where $\widehat{\mathbf{L}}^+$ is an approximation of the pseudo-inverse of the true interaction matrix $\mathbf{L}^+ = (\mathbf{L}^\top \mathbf{L})^{-1}\mathbf{L}^\top$. If we differentiate this equation, we obtain:

$$\dot{\mathbf{e}} = \frac{d\widehat{\mathbf{L}}^+}{dt}(\mathbf{s} - \mathbf{s}^*) + \widehat{\mathbf{L}}^+ \dot{\mathbf{s}} = (\mathbf{O}(\mathbf{s} - \mathbf{s}^*) + \widehat{\mathbf{L}}^+ \mathbf{L})\mathbf{v}_c \tag{4}$$

where $\mathbf{O}(\mathbf{s} - \mathbf{s}^*)$ is a (6×6) matrix that can be neglected for $\mathbf{s} \approx \mathbf{s}^*$. Let's consider the control law: $\mathbf{v}_c = -\lambda \mathbf{e}$ where λ is a positive scalar. Plugging this equation into equation (4), we obtain the following closed-loop equation: $\dot{\mathbf{e}} = -\lambda(\mathbf{O}(\mathbf{s} - \mathbf{s}^*) + \widehat{\mathbf{L}}^+\mathbf{L})\mathbf{e}$. It is well known from the control theory that this non-linear system is locally asymptotically stable in a neighborhood of $\mathbf{s} = \mathbf{s}^*$, if and only if, the matrix $\widehat{\mathbf{L}}^+\mathbf{L}$ has eigenvalues with a positive real part $real(eig(\widehat{\mathbf{L}}^+\mathbf{L})) > 0$. Obviously, if the pseudo-inverse of the interaction matrix is well approximated, we have: $\widehat{\mathbf{L}}^+\mathbf{L} \approx \mathbf{I}$ and the control law is locally asymptotically stable. Then, using the camera Cartesian velocity $\mathbf{v}_c$, it is possible to compute the joints increments $\dot{\mathbf{q}}$ given the pseudo-inverse of the C-arm Jacobian:

$$\dot{\mathbf{q}} = \mathbf{J}^+_{carm}\mathbf{v}_c \qquad (5)$$

3   Reposition Guidance

During the reposition task, the joints of the C-arm have to be moved in a structured way by the OR-stuff to re-assume the correct target position. In order to achieve this goal an easy to use and unambiguous guidance system is presented to the staff in oder to fulfill the required motion $\dot{\mathbf{q}}$ estimated by the visual servoing algorithm. Given the numbers of the parameters in C-arm coordinate system are difficult to understand, misinterpretation can easily prolong the process of repositioning.

To cope with the problem of information representation several interfaces were created and tested. The main component of the guidance system is an interactive 3D model of the C-arm. The joints of the model can be moved independently featuring the same five degrees of freedom as the real mobile C-arm. Figure 1a shows a screenshot of the 3D model. Within the model the suggested movement estimated by the visual servoing algorithm is simulated to the OR-staff.

During the process of motion animation, the affected joint was displayed in its corresponding color while the inactive parts remained gray. However, to give a better impression of the motion, passively moved parts remained uncolored, but were displayed translucent just like the active joint. For simplicity of the user interface and interaction only one joint at a time was assumed to be moved and simulated accordingly. Considering the fact that the 3D model is impractical for conveying quantitative information, e.g. express the magnitude of motion, supplemantary indicators were added. For this purpose, a gauge in terms of a progress bar was used to display relative motion extent. Additionally, the proximity of the markers to the target position by means of the euclidean norm was color-coded to give an easy and fast visual impression of the progress made during the visual servoing steps.

For qualitative validation of the repositioning task checkerboard views, commonly used for registration verification purposes, for both the video and the x-ray were integrated into the guidance system. Therefore, the images of the video camera and x-ray at the target position are stored. The checkerboard difference image shows from the beginning of the visual servoing procedure, the current video overlayed with the stored reference image (Fig. 1).

Fig. 1. Visualization for the CAMC visual servoing task

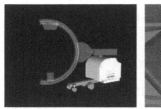 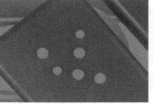 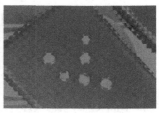

(a) 3D model of C-arm   (b) At target position   (c) Close to target position

4   Results and Conclusion

Tests for the visual servoing were performed on cadaver and published [3]. First tests on the usability of the representation for the visual servoing parameters were conducted on phantoms and showed the validity of the designed system. Even untrained persons could manipulate the C-arm to the indicated target position and orientation. Tests in real scenarios are subject for further work within this project.

The CAMC system and its extension for repositioning the C-arm by means of visual servoing can facilitate various applications in the domain of trauma and orthopedics surgery where the use of mobile C-arms is essential. Exemplary applications that can benefit from the proposed system are e.g. pedicle screw placement, im-nail locking, or other implant positioning procedures. An intuitive user interface and representation of available data is a crucial step towards the acceptance of this system in the OR.

Acknowledgments

The work was partially supported by Siemens Medical SP.

References

1. Navab N, Mitschke M, Bani-Hashemi A. Merging visible and invisible: Two camera-augmented mobile C-arm (CAMC) applications. In: Procs IWAR. San Francisco, CA, USA; 1999. 134–141.
2. Mitschke M, Bani-Hashemi A, Navab N. Interventions under video-augmented X-ray guidance: Application to needle placement. Procs MICCAI 2000; 858–868.
3. Navab N, Wiesner S, Benhimane S, Euler E, Heining S. Visual servoing for intra-operative positioning and repositioning of mobile C-arms. LNCS 2006.
4. Samson C, Le Borgne M, Espiau B. Robot Control: The Task Function Approach. Oxford Engineering Science Series. Oxford, UK: Clarendon Press; 1991.
5. Espiau B, Chaumette F, Rives P. A new approach to visual servoing in robotics. IEEE Trans Robot Automat 1992;8(3):313–326.

A New Approach to Ultrasound Guided Radio-Frequency Needle Placement

Claudio Alcérreca[1,2], Jakob Vogel[2], Marco Feuerstein[2] and Nassir Navab[2]

[1]Image Analysis a. Visualization Lab, CCADET UNAM, 04510 México City, México
[2]Chair for Computer Aided Medical Procedures (CAMP), TU München, Germany
Email: claudio@uxmcc2.iimas.unam.mx

Abstract. The transformation from an ultrasound (US) image plane to the coordinate system of a position sensor attached to the US transducer can be computed with US calibration algorithms. This knowledge can be used in many applications, including freehand 3D US and US guided surgical navigation. We present a software system assisting the surgeon to position a radio-frequency (RF) tumor ablation needle using augmented ultrasound, thus simplifying the treatment by (1) dividing it into two simple consecutive tasks, lesion finding and needle placement, and (2) relating the needle to the US plane at any time.

1 Introduction

Since their introduction into clinical practice, ultrasound (US) systems gained wide acceptance among physicians. With US images evolving in sharpness and overall quality, the combination of tracking with US systems allows the development of interactive navigation systems, which facilitate common minimally invasive treatments, for instance radio-frequency (RF) tumor ablation. The latter uses a high power and high frequency generator connected to electrodes in the tip of special needles. Electricity flows from these electrodes to a foil pad, usually attached to the patient's back or thighs [1], causing local necrosis in cells around the tip of the needles. This way, the tumor can be treated without the need of open surgery or other highly invasive procedures.

Currently, RF is used in every part of the body. In order to place the tip of the needle in the center of the lesion, US imaging is commonly used for guidance. In this case, the surgeon tries to visualize the tumor and the needle in the same US plane. The needle, however, is not visible in the US image before insertion, making it difficult to predict the tumor location relative to the needle tip and its orientation. Additionally, the surgeon needs to precisely handle the US transducer and the needle at the same time.

2 Related Work

Many authors have published articles on freehand US calibration. Prager et al. suggested the single wall method [2], where a tracked probe is used to scan the planar bottom of a water basin. This surface is clearly visible in the US image as a single line and may be recovered automatically using image processing algorithms. This approach has two major advantages over other procedures [3]. First, the calibration phantom does not need to be carefully manufactured. Secondly, US images containing a straight line can be processed automatically with high accuracy in real time. Langø enhanced this method by adding a nylon mesh to the setup, which produces even sharper features in the images [4].

Some surgical navigation systems have been developed to support needle placement procedures. BrainLAB[1] has a commercial system that can be used to guide a needle using preoperative 3D data (CT, MRI, or PET). The main problem with this approach is the need of a correct registration to match the preoperative studies with the anatomy of the patient. This is usually done by manually selecting corresponding points. In contrast to this solution, Ultraguide 1000 [5] relies on US data for guided needle placement, without the need for data registration. Using an electro-magnetic tracking system, it however requires additional cabling and is prone to distortions. Another approach proposed by Khamene et al. [6] uses a head mounted display with augmented reality capabilities. This method gives a very intuitive navigation, but requires specific and expensive hardware.

3   Methods

We developed a US calibration and needle placement system, which makes use of the CAMPAR framework [7]. We use an infrared based optical tracking system with four ARTtrack2 cameras, which defines the world coordinate system. For US image acquisition we use a Picker Computer Sonograph CS 9300 with a curvilinear 3.5-MHz transducer. After calibration of the US probe, needle tip, and an additional tracked camera, we are able to obtain all necessary transformations to relate every tracked object to the world coordinate system (Fig. 1, left). For testing, we first obtained a calibration transformation and applied it to our needle placement component. In the next sections, we describe our system in more detail.

3.1   Automatic Line Detection

Selecting a suitable water basin is a major factor for single wall US calibration, since many materials create reflections in the image and thus complicate the automatic detection of the basin's ground. We used a clay pot for our first experiments. Later on, as we required more space, we switched to a plastics box holding a planar nylon membrane stretched over an aluminum frame [4]. In both cases, our system is able to automatically detect the bottom plane using an algorithm proposed by Prager et al. [2]. Lines are detected in two separate steps: First, the algorithm attempts to find feature points along certain predefined vertical scan lines. These one-dimensional signals are smoothed using a Gaussian

---

[1] http://www.brainlab.com

filter kernel, then median-filtered, and finally differentiated. All positions above a predefined threshold are kept. In a second step, an implementation of the random sample consensus algorithm (RANSAC) attempts to match several candidate lines through these feature points [8]. The final line is chosen from these candidates taking into account the number of features supporting the respective line and the proximity to the line detected in the last frame.

3.2 Ultrasound Calibration Procedure

First, a temporal calibration can be performed. In principle, we adopted the protocol suggested by Treece et al. [9]. The full pose data of the probe is recorded and principal components analysis (PCA) is applied to find the major axis of movement independent from the orientation of the world coordinate system.

Next, we compute the spatial transformation from the US coordinate system to the probe system. The user therefor needs to perform a series of motions to cover all six degrees of freedom. At the same time, tracking data and line positions are stored. The calibration parameters are obtained using the Levenberg-Marquardt optimizer. We are using a second position matrix to relax the system. Originally, we recorded data continuously, thus working with about 2,000 to 3,000 samples. As the results were not as good as expected, we switched to the protocol proposed by Hsu et al. that requires human interaction to select suitable poses [10].

3.3 Needle Placement

The US guided needle placement application helps the surgeon to insert the tip of an RF needle into a precise region of interest, defined by the user, in a similar way as the Ultraguide system [5], which has been proven to have good accuracy. Unlike Ultraguide, our system provides the means to automatically calibrate an RF needle with high accuracy. Additionally, various 3D rendering techniques are utilized. It has four different views (Fig. 1, right):

- Ultrasound view: The user sees the US video, with the option to freeze an image and define a spherical target. Using the US calibration results, the system maps the defined target to the world coordinate system.
- World interactive view: The surgeon can see the needle and the sphere target in a virtual environment. This view allows to specify the point of view using translation, rotation, and scale primitives. The model includes a line extending the needle and a line from its tip to the center of the target. The needle should be set in the direction where these two lines meet. One problem with this view is the need of mouse interaction, which is usually not practical.
- Needle view: The user can see the needle and the target, in the direction of the needle. This is especially intuitive for directing the needle.
- Augmented camera view: This view includes a camera video. The camera, like the US probe and the needle, is tracked and calibrated, so it is possible to superimpose the virtual models on top of the video. This way, the point

Fig. 1. Coordinate systems and transformations (left), views of the needle placement system: ultrasound, world interactive, needle, augmented camera view (right)

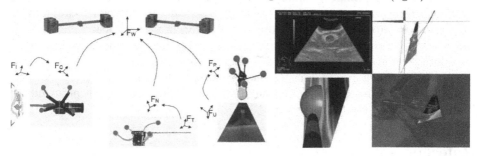

of view is defined by the camera. The main advantage of this view is the ability to integrate other, non tracked elements into the environment. It also helps to qualitatively evaluate the accuracy of the system.

4   Evaluation of the System

For testing the overall US navigation accuracy, we submerged the RF needle in water and scanned its tip with the US transducer. When the US image containing the tip was found, the image along with all tracking information was stored and the RF needle's tip was marked manually in the US image. US pixel coordinates were scaled back to millimeters. The needle tip's coordinates in the tracking coordinate frame were transformed into the US plane coordinate system, so both the marked and the tracked coordinates are in the same US plane coordinate system. The Euclidean distance from the marked tip to the tracked tip was calculated and considered as error. We repeated this experiment for 7 times to obtain a more significant error distribution.

5   Results

During US calibration we obtained a root mean square error of 1.96 mm for the needle tip reconstruction accuracy. However, it was difficult to find the needle tip in the US images due to US noise.

To apply the calibration results to a patient, speed of sound correction needs to be incorporated into the calibration procedure, since US machines are usually calibrated to the speed of ultrasound in tissue (1540 m/s) and not to its speed in water at room temperature of 21°C (ca. 1485 m/s) [11].

6   Conclusion

The surgical navigation system presented in this paper is stable and easy to use. It helps to simplify the RF needle placement by dividing it into two simple consecutive tasks: lesion finding and needle placement. The surgeon does not have to simultaneously navigate both the US probe and the RF needle. Additionally, the needle can always be visualized relatively to frozen or live US images.

Since the overall system accuracy mainly relies on an accurate US calibration, we will investigate in further development of an accurate evaluation phantom to validate the US reconstruction accuracy. The navigation system can be improved by adding features such as automatic registration with preoperative data and more complex target modeling, including deformable tissue and anatomic features. This way, the system would help not only to find the target point in the body but also to select a safe path.

References

1. Gazelle GS, Goldberg SN, Solbiati L, Livraghi T. Tumor ablation with radio frequency energy. Radiology 2000;217:633–646.
2. Prager RW, Rohling RN, Gee AH, Berman L. Rapid calibration for 3-D freehand ultrasound. Ultrasound in Medicine and Biology 1998;24(6):855–869.
3. Mercier L, Langø T, Lindseth F, Collins DL. A review of calibration techniques for freehand 3-D ultrasound systems. Ultrasound in Medicine and Biology 2005;31(4):449–471.
4. Langø T. Ultrasound Guided Surgery: Image Processing and Navigation. Ph.D. thesis. Norwegian University of Science and Technology; 2000.
5. Howard MH, Nelson RC, Paulson EK, Kliewer MA, Sheafor DH. An electronic device for needle placement during sonographically guided percutaneous intervention. Radiology 2001;218:905–911.
6. Khamene A, Vogt S, Azar F, Sielhorst T, Sauer F. Local 3D reconstruction and augmented reality visualization of freehand ultrasound for needle biopsy procedures. In: Procs MICCAI; 2003. 344–355.
7. Sielhorst T, Feuerstein M, Traub J, Kutter O, Navab N. CAMPAR: A software framework guaranteeing quality for medical augmented reality. Int J Comp Assist Radiol Surg 2006;1(Supplement 1):29–30.
8. Fischler MA, Bolles RC. Random sample consensus: A paradigm for model fitting with applications to image. Analysis and Automated Cartography, Commun ACM 1981;24(6).
9. Treece GM, Gee AH, Prager RW, Cash CJC, Berman LH. High-definition freehand 3-D ultrasound. Ultrasound in Medicine and Biology 2003;29(4):529–546.
10. Hsu PW, Prager RW, Gee AH, Treece GM. Rapid, easy and reliable calibration for freehand 3D ultrasound. University of Cambridge, Department of Engineering. Trumpington Street, Cambridge CB2 1PZ; 2005.
11. Marczak W. Water as a standard in the measurements of speed of sound in liquids. Acoustical Society of America Journal 1997;102:2776–2779.

Zur Genauigkeit der Vermessung von Hartgewebe-Landmarken mittels Ultraschall

Steffen H. Tretbar[1], Josef Kozak[2], Peter Keppler[3], Stefan Klein[4]

[1]Fraunhofer Institut für Biomedizinische Technik, 66386 St. Ingbert
[2]Aesculap AG & CO. KG, 78532 Tuttlingen
[3]Universitätsklinikum Ulm, Chirurgische Klinik und Poliklinik, 89075 Ulm
[4]Universitätsklinikum Ulm, Radiologische Klinik und Poliklinik, 89075 Ulm
Email: steffen.tretbar@ibmt.fraunhofer.de

Zusammenfassung. Zur prä-, intra- und postoperativen Vermessung von Körpergeometrien genügt es für bestimmte Applikationen nicht, eine Registrierung von Hartgewebestrukturen mittels Abtasten der Strukturen mit dem Pointer durchzuführen. Um die Anwendung nicht invasiv und damit patientenschonender zu gestalten, sollen zukünftig in Navigationssystemen Ultraschallsysteme integriert werden. Da die unterschiedlichen Schallausbreitungsgeschwindigkeiten die Genauigkeit einer Vermessung von Landmarken mittels Ultraschall limitieren, wird anhand dieser Studie der Einfluss der unterschiedlichen Schallgeschwindigkeiten in den verschiedenen Geweben auf die Genauigkeit einer Abstandsmessung mittels Ultraschall evaluiert.

1 Einleitung

Die Sonografie hat sich insbesondere in den letzten beiden Jahrzehnten zu einem diagnostischen Routineverfahren entwickelt, das für den niedergelassenen Arzt und für die klinischen Anwendungen gleichermaßen wichtig ist.

Aufgrund der starken Verbreitung von Ultraschallgeräten sollen die Bilddaten auch für die medizinische Navigation genutzt werden. Der intraoperative Informationszugewinn eines bildunterstützten Navigationssystems im Vergleich zur bildlosen Navigation ist nicht von der Hand zu weisen [1]. Der Vorteil des Einsatzes von Ultraschall für diese Bilddatengewinnung wird beim direkten Vergleich mit anderen Bild gebenden Verfahren, wie der CT oder der NMR ersichtlich. Dieser Vorteil lasst sich durch den Einsatz eines navigierten Ultraschallgeräts auch für die therapeutische Anwendungen nutzen [2].

Bei diagnostischen Ultraschallgeräten wird System bedingt mit einer mittleren Schallgeschwindigkeit von 1540 m/s gearbeitet. Die Ausbreitungsgeschwindigkeit des Ultraschalls ist allerdings vom Medium (d.h. Gewebe) abhängig. Dies hat zur Folge, dass bei einer Geometrievermessung im Ultraschallbild eines Gewebes mit abweichender Schallgeschwindigkeit Messfehler auftreten. Beispielsweise bei der Anwendung eines navigierten Ultraschallsystems zur Vermessung der Position eines Femurs werden unterschiedlich dicke Schichten von Fett und Muskelgewebe durchschallt. Hierbei zeigen die Literaturwerte schon die grundsätzlichen Unterschiede der Schallgeschwindigkeit zwischen Fett- und Muskelgewebe. So beträgt der Unterschied bei Lehmann/Johnson [3] zwischen Schweinefett (1454 m/s) und Muskelfleisch vom Schwein (1558 m/s) 104 m/s. Bei Frucht [4], der bei 24°C gemessen hat, beträgt der Unterschied 136 m/s. Dieser Unterschied würde einen Messfehler bei einer Abstands-Messung, unter Nutzung der Schallgeschwindigkeit vom Muskel, von 8,6% ergeben. In diesem Beitrag werden die Gewebegeschwindigkeiten beispielhaft evaluiert, als signifikant für den Einsatz in der medizinischen Navigation eingestuft und mögliche Lösungsansätze aufgezeigt.

2 Material und Methode

Um die Problematik, eines zu erwartenden Messfehlers bei Nutzung einer mittleren Schallgeschwindigkeit von 1540 m/s genauer zu betrachten, wurde eine Messreihe zur Bestimmung dieser Unterschiede beispielhaft für Fett- und Muskelgewebe durchgeführt.

Um der späteren Messsituation mit den Messreihen sehr nahe zu kommen, wurden Messungen im Puls-Echo-Mode durchgeführt. Der Messaufbau wurde dahingehend vereinfach, dass kein „klassischer" diagnostischer Ultraschallkopf sondern Einzel-Element-Ultraschallwandler eingesetzt wurden. Um etwaige Einflusse der Ultraschallfrequenz auszuschließen, wurden die Untersuchungen mit Ultraschallwandlern der Mittenfrequenzen von 1; 3,5; 5; 7,5 MHz (Fa. Panametrics) durchgeführt. Als Ultraschallsystem wurde das Einkanalige Labormesssystem SEM II des Fraunhofer IBMT eingesetzt, welches in einen PC integriert ist. Dieses vereint eine freiprogrammierbare Sendestufe und eine A/D –Wandlerkarte, mit der die empfangenen Ultraschallsignale mit 100 MHz Samplerate digitalisiert und als HF-Daten speichert werden. Als Sendecode wurde eine Burst-1-Sequenz entsprechend der Mittenfrequenz der Ultraschallwandler genutzt. Zur Vereinfachung des Probenhandlings und um die Messstrecke konstant zu halten, wurden die Messungen in speziell entwickelten Probengefäßen (Abb. 1) durchgeführt. Die Messstrecke betrug 50 mm (100 mm Puls-Echo). Da die Schallgeschwindigkeit einer Temperaturabhängigkeit unterliegt, wurde zusätzlich von jeder Probe die Temperatur gemessen.

Ca. eine Stunde nach den Ultraschallmessungen wurden die Proben im CT bezüglich der Dichteverteilung auf der zentralen Ultraschall-Messachse und zur Bestimmung der genauen Messstrecke mit einem CT der Firma Philips vom Typ Brilliance 40 vermessen.

2.1 Proben

Die von Dussik und Fritch [5], Frucht [4], Lehmann und Johnson [3] und Schwan [6] ermittelten Schallgeschwindigkeitswerte von Fett- bzw. Muskelgewebe des Schweins und des Menschen zeigen, dass es auf Grund der geringen Unterschiede zwischen Schwein und Mensch, sowohl bei Fett- als auch bei Muskelgewebe, plausibel ist, Schweinefleisch als Probenmaterial zu nutzen. Es standen einmal

Abb. 1. Messaufbau

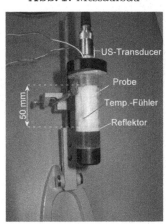

als Proben für Fett, Bauchspeck vom Schwein und als Proben für Muskelfleisch, Schweinerücken vom Schwein, zur Verfügung. Die Materialien waren nicht älter als ein Tag und wurden bei 8-10°C gelagert. Für die Messungen standen je 5 Proben mit Fett- und Muskelgewebe zur Verfügung.

3   Ergebnisse

Die durchgeführten Messungen ergaben im Mittel eine Schallgeschwindigkeit des Muskelgewebes von 1558 m/s (SD 12, 0,79%). Der Mittelwert der Schallgeschwindigkeit des Fettgewebes beträgt 1495 m/s (SD 12, 0,78%) (Abb. 2).

Da diese Messungen bei 17°C durchgeführt wurden und später am Patienten bei 37°C gemessen wird, wurden Messungen durchgeführt, die den Einfluss dieser Temperatursteigerung betrachten. Die Ergebnisse dieser Messungen sind in Abbildung 3 dargestellt. Es wird deutlich das Muskelgewebe und Fettgewebe gegenläufigen Effekten unterliegen. Im Muskelgewebe steigt die Schallgeschwindigkeit um 72 m/s und im Fettgewebe fällt sie um 37 m/s, bei einer Temperaturerhöhung auf 37°C.

Damit ergab sich eine korrigierte Schallgeschwindigkeit im Fettgewebe von 1458 m/s und in der Muskulatur von 1630 m/s. Die verschiedenen Ausbreitungsgeschwindigkeiten im Gewebe haben zur Folge, dass eine Geometrievermessung mit Standardultraschallgeräten (c=1540 m/s) in Muskel- und Fettgewebe potentiell fehlerhaft durchgeführt wird. Für die Abstandsmessung ist bei Nutzung einer fehlerhaften Schallgeschwindigkeit mit einem maximalen Messfehler von ± 15% bei einer Temperatur von 37°C zu rechnen. Der Bereich des relativen Fehlers beim Fettgewebe beträgt -15% und bei der Muskulatur +15%. Dies bedeutet, dass bei einer mit einem Standardsystem gemessenen Gewebeschicht von 100 mm Dicke, die tatsächliche Schichtdicke im Fett nur 85 mm und in der Muskulatur 115 mm beträgt.

Abb. 2. Schallgeschwindigkeit in Muskelgebewebe (a) in Fettgewebe (b)

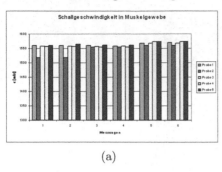 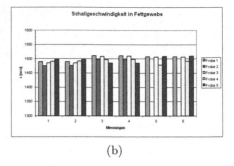

(a)   (b)

Abb. 3. Temperaturabhängigkeit der Schallgeschwindigkeit von Muskelgewebe (a) und Fettgewebe (b)

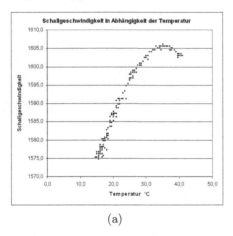 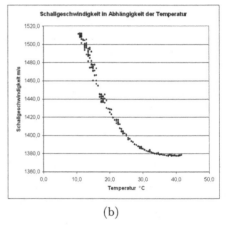

(a)   (b)

4 Diskussion und Ausblick

Die Evaluierung des Einflusses der unterschiedlichen Schallgeschwindigkeiten in den verschiedenen Geweben auf die Genauigkeit einer Abstandsmessung mittels Ultraschall hat einen Bereich des relativen Fehlers beim Fettgewebe -15% und bei der Muskulatur +15% gezeigt. Auf Grund der allgemeinen Anforderung an die Genauigkeit der Navigation, die bei einer Schichtdicke von 100 mm Länge maximal ±1 mm betragen soll, ist die Ultraschall-Bildverzerrung alleine ein Faktor, der die Navigation unbrauchbar macht. Zur Kompensation dieses Messfehlers sind zwei Verfahren denkbar:

1. Es werden für bestimmte Applikationen (Condylen, Spina, Femur, etc.) bei denen eine Vermessung mittels Ultraschall eingesetzt werden soll, in eine durchzuführende Studie applikationsspezifische Schallgeschwindigkeitswerte bestimmt. Diese können dann mit entsprechender statistischer Sicherheit,

welche sich aus der Studie ergibt; zur Korrektur des Messfehlers bei den unterschiedlichen Anwendungen genutzt werden.

2. Es werden für jede Messung patientenspezifischen Schallgeschwindigkeitswerte bestimmt und den Messungen entsprechend korrigiert.

Um diese patientenspezifischen Schallgeschwindigkeitswerte zu bestimmen, ist eine Differenzierung zwischen den unterschiedlichen Gewebearten nötig. Diese kann dadurch erfolgen, dass vor der eigentlichen Messung Ultraschall-HF-Daten von Zielbereich akquiriert werden. In diesen Daten werden nun gewebespezifische Parameter, wie die frequenzabhängige Dämpfung [7, 8, 9] oder die Rückstreuung [10, 11] in Abhängigkeit der Eindringtiefe betrachtet. An den Grenzschichten der unterschiedlichen Gewebe kommt es dann zu einer Änderung dieser Parameter. Diese können detektiert werden und lassen die Kalkulation einer angepassten Schallgeschwindigkeit entsprechend dem Verhältnis der Schichtdicken zu. Erfolgt nun eine Vermessung im Ultraschallbild mit der neu kalkulierten Schallgeschwindigkeit sollte es möglich sein, den Messfehler auf ca. 1 mm zu reduzieren.

Literaturverzeichnis

1. Eisenmann U, Schneider J, Quintus K, Helbig M, Dickhaus H. Ultraschallgestützte Navigation für die minimalinvasive HNO Chirurgie. In: Biomedizinische Technik; 2004. 876–877.
2. Hassenpflug P, et al. Generation of of attributed relational vessel graphs from three-dimensional freehand ultrasound for intraoperative registration in image-guided liver surgery. Procs SPIE 2003;5029:222–230.
3. Lehmann JF, Johnson EW. Some factors influencing the temperature distribution in thighs exposed to ultrasound. Arch Phys Med Rehab 1958;39:347–356.
4. Frucht AH. Die Schallgeschwindigkeit in menschlichen und tierischen Geweben. Z Gesamte Exp Med 1953;120:551–557.
5. Dussik KT, Fritch DJ. Determination of sound attenuation and sound velocity in the structure constituting the joints, and of the ultrasound field distribution within the joints on living tissues and anatomical preparations, both in normal and pathological conditions, Public Health Service. NIH; 1956.
6. Schwan HP, Carstensen EL, Li K. Heating of fat-muscle layers by electromagnetic and ultrasonic diathermy. IEEE Trans Commun Electron Pt I 1953;72:483–488.
7. Ophir J, Maklad NF, Bigelow RH. Ultrasonic attenuation measurement of in vivo human muscle. Ultrason Imag 1982;4:290–295.
8. Ophir J, Shawker TH, Maklad NF, et al. Attenuation estimation in reflection: progress and prospects. Ultrason Imag 1984;6:349–395.
9. Kuc R. Estimating the acoustic attenuation from reflected ultrasound signals: Comparison of spectral shift and spectral-difference approaches. IEEE Trans Acoust ASSP 1984;32:1–6.
10. Sehgal CM, Greenleaf JF. Scattering of ultrasound by tissues. Ultrason Imag 1984;6:60–80.
11. Roth SL, et al. Spectral analysis of demodulated ultrasound returns: Detection of scatterer periodicity and application to tissue classification. Ultrason Imag 1997;19:266–277.

Navigation in der minimal-invasiven Prostatachirurgie
Kamerapositionsbestimmung für eine Visualisierung mittels Augmented Reality

M. Baumhauer[1], T. Simpfendörfer[1], R. Schwarz[1],
M. Seitel[1], B.P. Müller-Stich[2], C.N. Gutt[2],
J. Rassweiler[3], H.-P. Meinzer[1], I. Wolf[1]

[1]Abteilung für Medizinische und Biologische Informatik,
Deutsches Krebsforschungszentrum (DKFZ), 69120 Heidelberg
[2]Chirurgische Klinik der Universität Heidelberg
[3]Urologische Klinik Heilbronn, SLK Kliniken,
Akademisches Lehrkrankenhaus der Universität Heidelberg
Email: m.baumhauer@dkfz.de

Zusammenfassung. Wir evaluieren ein Kernmodul eines Navigationssystems zur Unterstützung der minimal-invasiven Prostatektomie. Das
System nutzt transrektalen Ultraschall (TRUS) und nadelförmige Navigationshilfen um versteckte Strukturen via Augmented Reality zu visualisieren. Während des Eingriffs werden die Navigationshilfen einmalig
semi-automatisch in einem 3D TRUS Datensatz segmentiert und daraufhin von der Endoskopiekamera getrackt. Um die Position der Endoskopiekamera direkt in Relation zu den Navigationshilfen zu bestimmen
werden sogenannte Camera Pose Estimation Algorithmen verwendet.
Folglich sind für die Navigation mit unserem System keine zusätzlichen
Trackingverfahren und Geräte nötig, um die Daten des Kameraendoskops
mit denen des Ultraschallgeräts zu registrieren.
Neben einem präoperativen Planungsschritt besteht das System aus zwei
Vorgängen, welche beide während der Intervention durchgeführt werden:
Zum einen die Registrierung der präoperativen Operationsplanung mit
einem intraoperativ akquirierten Ultraschalldatensatz der Prostata ein-
schließlich Navigationshilfen, zum anderen der Bestimmung der Kame-
raposition und der Visualisierung der Planung.
Dieses Paper bezieht sich auf das für die Visualisierung erforderliche Ka-
meratracking. Hierfür wurden echtzeitfähige Algorithmen in das Open-
Source Toolkit MITK implementiert und in Bezug auf minimal-invasive
Navigationsszenarien evaluiert.

1 Einleitung

Prostatakrebs ist heute die am häufigsten diagnostizierte Tumorerkrankung des
Mannes. Obwohl die operative Entfernung der Prostata einschließlich der Sa-
menblasen (Prostatektomie) als eine der sichersten Behandlungsmethoden gilt,

kann dennoch in bis zu 29 Prozent aller Eingriffe ein Rezidiv des Prostatakrebses innerhalb von fünf Jahren beobachtet werden. Neuere Studien belegen eine Optimierung der Prostatektomie durch den Einsatz von intraoperativem, transrektalem Ultraschall [1, 2, 3]. Jedoch bringt diese Vorgehensweise auch Nachteile mit sich: Zunächst ist ein erheblicher Zeitwaufwand für die intraoperative Analyse der 3D Ultraschalldaten nötig. Auch können medizinisch relevante Strukturen, die im Rahmen einer Diagnose erhoben wurden nicht miteinbezogen werden. Darüberhinaus erschwert eine zeitverzögerte Visualisierung einzelner 2D Schichten eine Navigation und zeigt sich als fehleranfällig. Mit einem Navigationssystem soll diese Problematik gelöst werden.

2   Stand der Forschung

Computergestützte Planung und Therapie bei der Behandlung von Prostatakarzinomen ist Routine im Bereich der Strahlentherapie [4, 5]. Für chirurgische Eingriffe an der Prostata hingegen, sind uns keine Verfahren der computerunterstützten Intervention bekannt.

Pose Estimation ist ein klassisches Problem der Photogrammetrie [6] und wird heute oftmals bei Augmented Reality Anwendungen erfolgreich eingesetzt [7, 8, 9]. Mit diesem Beitrag werden Pose Estimation Algorithmen erstmals für die Bestimmung der extrinsischen Parameter einer Endoskopiekamera in der minimal-invasiven Chirurgie erprobt und evaluiert.

3   Methoden

3.1   Navigationskonzept

Dieses Navigationssystem wurde bereits unter [x] detailliert vorgestellt. Im Zuge der Krebsdiagnose wird gewöhnlich ein Ultraschalldatensatz akquiriert. Bereits erprobte Methoden der Strahlentherapie ermöglichen eine Registrierung mit zusätzlichen CT, MRT oder PET/CT (Abb. 1, i) Daten um die präoperative Planung zu erweitern. Während des Eingriffs bringt der Chirurg nach Freilegung des Organs sechs Navigationshilfen ein (ii). Obwohl die Platzierung hierbei frei gewählt werden kann, ist es wichtig, dass die Nadelköpfe direkt auf der Organoberfläche aufliegen. Eine auf Landmarken basierende, nicht-rigide Registrierung (iii) wird verwendet, um die präoperative Planung mit dem intraoperativen TRUS Datensatz zu registrieren. Für die Visualisierung der Planung muss der sichtbare Teil der Navigationshilfen getrackt werden (iv). Mit Hilfe der segmentierten Navigationshilfen im Ultraschall lässt sich die Position und Orientierung der Kamera bestimmen und medizinisch relevante Strukturen können in das Videobild eingeblendet werden (v). Die folgende Ausarbeitung bezieht sich auf das Tracking der Navigationshilfen und die Pose Estimation (iv).

Abb. 1. Illustration des Navigationskonzepts

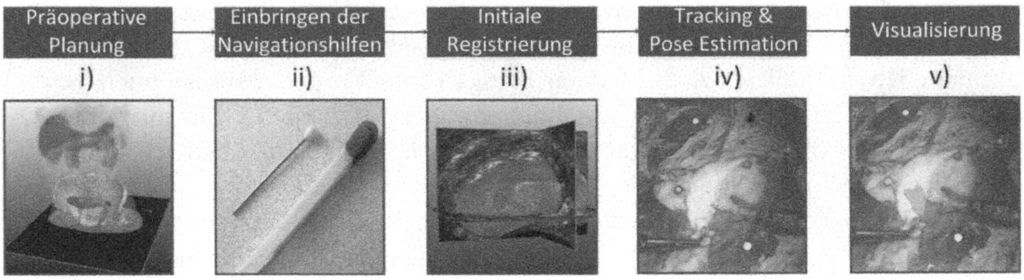

Präoperative Planung	Einbringen der Navigationshilfen	Initiale Registrierung	Tracking & Pose Estimation	Visualisierung
i)	ii)	iii)	iv)	v)

3.2   Segmentierung der Navigationshilfen aus den Endoskopiebildern

Aufgrund der bei Endoskopiekameras verwendeten Optik müssen die Bilder vor einer weiteren Verarbeitung entzerrt werden. Zum Einsatz kommt hierbei ein Modell, das sowohl die Kissen- bzw. Tonnenverzeichnung einer Linse (radial Distortion), als auch eine ungenaue Zentrierung einer Linse (tangential Distortion) miteinbezieht [10]. Nach einer Konvertierung in den HSV-Farbraum wird mit einem einfachen Region-Growing nach den farblich gekennzeichneten Nadelköpfen gesucht. Da für eine exakte Berechnung der Kameraposition der Mittelpunkt des kugelförmigen Nadelkopfes möglichst genau bestimmt werden muss, dient diese Vorsegmentierung lediglich zur Definition von Regions of interest (ROIs). Innerhalb jeder einzelnen ROI extrahiert ein Canny Filter die Objektkontouren, woraufhin eine Hough Transformation (Verfahren: 21HT,[11]) den wahrscheinlichsten Aufenthalt der jeweiligen Navigationshilfe ermittelt. Durch dieses Vorgehen kann auch bei teilweiser Verdeckung der Navigationshilfe der tatsächliche Mittelpunkt gefunden werden.

3.3   Camera Pose Estimation zur Positionsbestimmung der Endoskopiekamera

Pose Estimation Algorithmen nutzen die Korrespondenzen von 3D Objektpunkten und ihren 2D Abbildungen, welche durch eine kalibrierte Kamera vorgenommen wurden. Sie bestimmen aus diesen Korrespondenzen die Lage und Orientierung der Kamera in Relation zu den gegebenen Objektpunkten. Da die Navigationshilfen sowohl in den Ultraschalldaten, als auch in den Endoskopiebildern sichtbar sind, können die extrinischen Kameraparameter direkt im Koordinatensystem des Ultraschalldatensatzes errechnet werden. Wir implementierten mehrere numerische und iterative Algorithmen in das Open Source Toolkit MITK (www.mitk.org) [7, 12, 13]. Mit Hilfe einer virtuellen, auf OpenGL basierenden, Evaluationsumgebung konnten diese auf objektive Weise miteinander verglichen und ihre Parameter angepasst werden. Desweiteren wurde eine zusätzliche Evaluation an einer Trainingseinheit für minimal-invasive Chirurgie (sog. Pulsatile Organ Perfusion Trainer) durchgeführt. Hierfür wurden in Schweinenieren Navigationshilfen eingebracht und mittels einem hochauflösenden CT registriert.

4   Ergebnisse

Die Ergebnisse bezüglich der Segmentierung der Navigationshilfen aus den Endoskopiebildern hängen von vielen Faktoren, wie z.b. dem verwendeten Endoskop, den Navigationshilfen und deren Platzierung etc. ab. Bei Versuchen mit einem Karl Storz Endoskop (Tuttlingen) konnten unterschiedlich farbig gekennzeichnete Nadeln in über 90 % erfolgreich segmentiert und deren Mittelpunkt bestimmt werden.

Experimente zur Bestimmung der Camera Pose mit der OpenGL Evaluationsumgebung zeigten, dass die Kameraposition mit dem Verfahren von De-Menthon [12] bei sechs zufällig auf einer Organoberfläche verteilten Navigationshilfen über eintausend Pose Estimations mit einer Genauigkeit im Median von $\tilde{X} = 0.05\ mm$ (mit den Quantilen $Q_{0.05} = 0.01\ mm$ und $Q_{0.95} = 0.8\ mm$) bestimmt werden kann. Bei zusätzlicher Simulation von Meßfehlern auf den 2D Bildpunkten von $\epsilon_{2D} = \pm 2\ pixel$ je Bildpunkt und $\epsilon_{3D} = 1\ mm$ je Objektpunkt nahm die Genauigkeit auf $\tilde{X} = 2.2\ mm (Q_{0.05} = 0.9\ mm, Q_{0.95} = 13.9\ mm)$ deutlich ab.

Obwohl der von Lu vorgestellte Algorithmus [7] bei fehlerfreien Eingangswerten verleichbare Ergebnisse lieferte, konvergierte das Verfahren bei der Simulation von Meßfehlern in lediglich in ca. 30 % aller Versuche zu einer brauchbaren Camera Pose. Auch die von den Autoren zur Verfügung gestellte MatLab Implementierung zeigte dieses Verhalten. Wir haben aus diesem Grund mit den Autoren Kontakt aufgenommen, bislang ohne Antwort.

Das SoftPosit Verfahren von David [13] benötigt im Gegensatz zu den übrigen Methoden für die Berechnung einer Pose nicht zu jedem Objektpunkt den zugehörigen Bildpunkt als Eingangswert, sondern kann diese Zuordnung selbst rechnerisch ermitteln. Hierdurch könnte auf eine farbliche Kodierung der Navigationshilfen verzichtet werden. Bei Versuchen mit sechs Navigationshilfen konnten allerdings in lediglich 50 % der Versuche eine korrekte Zuordnung der Punktpaare und somit die Camera Pose errechnet werden.

Für den vorgestellten Einsatzzweck zeigten sich die Algorithmen in Bezug auf Ihre Laufzeit auf aktueller PC-Hardware (C++ Implementierung) als brauchbar $(t_{DeMenthon} = 0.05s,\ t_{Lu} = 0.12s,\ t_{David} = 0,20s)$.

5   Diskussion

Aufgrund ihrer Robustheit gegenüber Messfehlern sind Camera Pose Estimation Algorithmen eine brauchbare Möglichkeit zur Bestimmung von Kameraposition und -orientierung bei Augmented Reality Anwendungen. Ausschlaggebend für ihren Einsatz ist die einfache und möglichst exakte Definition von Landmarken im Navigationsraum, wie sie etwa bei diesem Navigationssystem durch die Verwendung von transrektalem Ultraschall möglich wird.

Problematisch zeigt sich die Bestimmung einer Camera Pose je nach Anzahl verwendeter Landmarken, falls ein oder mehrere der Landmarken verdeckt sind, oder sich außerhalb des Kamerabildes befinden. Derzeit werden deswegen Methoden entwickelt, die die Genauigkeit einer berechneten Camera Pose möglichst zuverlässig beurteilen und somit eine fehlerbehaftete Visualisierung verhindern.

6   Danksagung

Die vorliegende Arbeit wurde im Rahmen des von der Deutschen Forschungsgemeinschaft unterstüzten "Graduiertenkollegs 1126: Intelligente Chirurgie - Entwicklung neuer computerbasierter Methoden für den Arbeitsplatz der Zukunft in der Weichteilchirurgie" durchgeführt.

Literaturverzeichnis

1. Ukimura O, Gill IS. Real-time transrectal ultrasonography during laparoscopic radical prostatectomy. The Journal of Urology 2004;172:112–118.
2. Ukimura O, Gill IS. Real-time transrectal ultrasound guidance during laparoscopic radical prostatectomy: Impact on surgical margins. The Journal of Urology 2006;175:1304–1310.
3. Ukimura O, Gill IS. Real-time transrectal ultrasound guidance during nerve sparing laparoscopic radical prostatectomy: pictorial essay. The Journal of Urology 2006;175:1311–1319.
4. Wei Z, Ding M, Downey D, Fenster A. 3D TRUS guided robot assisted prostate brachytherapy. LNCS 2005;3750:17–24.
5. Wei Z, Fenster A. Oblique needle segmentation and tracking for 3D TRUS guided prostate brachytherapy. Med Phys 2005;32:2928–2941.
6. Hartley R, Zisserman A. Multiple View Geometry in Computer Vision. Cambridge University Press; 2000, 2003.
7. Lu CP, Hager GD, Mjolsness E. Fast and globally convergent pose estimation from video images. IEEE Trans PAMI 2000;22:610–622.
8. Schweighofer G, Pinz A. Robust Pose Estimation from a Planar Target. Graz University of Technology; 2005. Submitted to IEEE[PAMI] 05/2005.
9. Shi F, Zhang X. A new method of camera pose estimation using 2D 3D corner correspondence. Pattern Recognition Letters 2004;25:1155–1163.
10. Zhang Z. A flexible new technique for camera calibration. IEEE Trans PAMI 2000;22:1330–1334.
11. Yuen HK, Princen J, Illingworth J, Kittler J. Comparative study of Hough transform methods for circle finding. Image and Vision Computing 1990;8:71–77.
12. DeMenthon D, Davis LS. Model-based object pose in 25 lines of code. International Journal of Computer Vision 1995;15:123–141.
13. David P, DeMenthon D. SoftPOSIT: Simultaneous pose and correspondence determination. International Journal of Computer Vision 2004;59(3):259–284.

3D-Rekonstruktion aus DSA-Projektionsdaten mittels diskreter Tomographie

Christoph Bodensteiner[1], Volker Martens[1], Stefan Schlichting[2],
Norbert Binder[1], Rainer Burgkart[3], Achim Schweikard[1]

[1]Institut für Robotik und kognitive Systeme, Universität zu Lübeck
[2]Klinik für Chirurgie, Universitätsklinikum Schleswig Holstein, Campus Lübeck
[3]Klinik für Sportorthopädie, Klinikum rechts der Isar, TU München
Email: bodensteiner@rob.uni-luebeck.de

Zusammenfassung. Mit Hilfe der diskreten Tomographie können unter bestimmten Voraussetzungen hochwertige Rekonstruktionen aus sehr wenigen Projektionen, welche auch über einen eingeschränkten Winkelbereich aufgenommen worden sind, errechnet werden. Dadurch kann eine signifikante Reduktion der Strahlenbelastung für Patient und Personal erzielt werden. So konnten Lebergefäßbäume aus jeweils 3-5 simulierten Projektionen nahezu exakt rekonstruiert werden. Des Weiteren wurden erste Versuche mit real aufgenommen Projektionsdaten durchgeführt. Dabei wurde die Robustheit dieser Rekonstruktionstechnik durch eine Kombination mit einem iterativen Rekonstruktionsverfahren (ART) deutlich gesteigert. Auf diese Weise konnten in der Praxis auftretende Inkonsistenzen besser berücksichtigt werden.

1 Einleitung

Zur Rekonstruktion mit Hilfe der diskreten Tomographie sind Projektionsbilder nötig, welche nur auf der Abschwächung einer diskreten Menge an Objekten beruhen. In der medizinischen Bildgebung ist diese Voraussetzung beispielsweise bei der digitalen Subtraktionsangiographie erfüllt, bei der korrespondierende Projektionspaare vor und nach Kontrastmittelgabe zu einer Projektion verrechnet werden. Durch diese Informationsreduktion können nun hochwertige 3D-Rekonstruktionen aus sehr wenigen Projektionen, welche auch nur über einen eingeschränkten Winkelbereich aufgenommen werden müssen, errechnet werden. Dadurch kann eine signifikante Reduktion der Strahlenbelastung für Patient und Personal erzielt werden. Es ist geplant diese Technik in Kombination mit einem roboterisierten C-Bogen [1, 2] zur intra-operativen Bildgebung und Navigation von Gefäßstrukturen zu benutzen.

2 Stand der Forschung und Fortschritt durch den Beitrag

Diskrete Tomographie mittels linearer Programmierung betrachtet analog zu algebraischen Rekonstruktionsmethoden das Rekonstruktionsproblem als Lösung eines linearen (Un-)Gleichungssystems unter bestimmten Optimalitätskriterien. Hierbei wurden u.a. folgende Ansätze mittels linearer Optimierung vorgeschlagen [3, 4].

$$(\text{FSSV}) \min_{x \in \Re^n} 0^T x, Ax = b, 0 \leqslant xi \leqslant 1, \forall i \tag{1}$$

$$(\text{BIF}) \min_{x \in \Re^n} -e^T x, Ax \leqslant b, 0 \leqslant xi \leqslant 1, \forall i \tag{2}$$

Die Arbeiten von Weber et al. [5] erweitern diese Ansätze unter anderem um eine Regularisierung (3) zur Bevorzugung zusammenhängender Rekonstruktionsregionen als auch mit einer automatischen Bestimmung eines Binarisierungsschwellwertes.

$$(\text{R-BIF}) \min_{x \in \Re^n} -e^T x + \frac{\alpha}{2} \sum_{<j,k>} |xj - xk|, Ax \leqslant b, 0 \leqslant xi \leqslant 1, \forall i \tag{3}$$

In der Praxis treten auf Grund von Messfehlern jedoch oft stark inkonsistente Rekonstruktionsprobleme auf. Aus diesem Grund führten wir vor der eigentlichen linearen Optimierung ART-Iterationen bis zur Konvergenz durch und berechneten anschließend Projektionsdaten mit gleicher Projektionsgeometrie aus der Least-Squares-Lösung des Rekonstruktionsgleichungssystems $Ax = b$. Auf diese Weise konnten auch mit unseren real akquirierten Daten gute Rekonstruktionsergebnisse erzielt werden, was mit herkömmlichen Methoden nicht möglich war. Darüber hinaus wurden die Algorithmen so angepasst, dass eine Aufsplittung mit einer senkrecht zur Rotationsachse und auf dem Isozentrum liegenden Ebene möglich ist. So kann bei entsprechenden Aufnahmen die Problemgröße reduziert werden.

3 Methoden

Für die Evaluation der Implementierungen wurden sowohl synthetisch erzeugte als auch real aufgenommene Röntgenbilder verwendet. Bei den simulierten Röntgenbildern (568x568) handelte es sich um MR- und CT-Aufnahmen der Leber von verschiedenen Patienten, in denen einzelne Gefäßbäume zur Planung von Leberresektionen heraussegmentiert worden waren (MeVis, Bremen). Aus den segmentierten Gefäßbäumen wurden 3-5 elementige Projektionsdatensätze generiert und der zugrunde liegende Gefäßbaum rekonstruiert.

Für die Versuche mit realen Projektionsdaten diente ein roboterisierter C-Bogen der Firma Ziehm Imaging. Aufgrund der bekannten Kinematik kann hier die Projektionsgeometrie aus Gelenkwinkeln bestimmt und auch für die nötigen Subtraktionsbilder wieder exakt angefahren werden.

So wurde ein Gefäß mit Schachfiguren aus verschiedenen Positionen vor und nach Kontrastmittelbefüllung (Imeron 300) aufgenommen (Abb. 1) und die logarithmierten Bilder voneinander abgezogen.

Abb. 1. Versuchsaufbau für den roboterisierten C-Bogen: Projektion ohne (links) und mit (Mitte) Kontrastmittel sowie Subtraktionsbild (rechts)

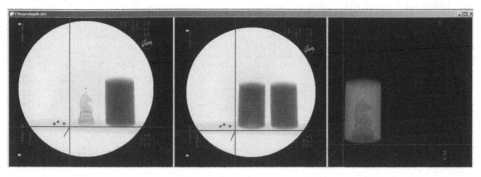

Abb. 2. Verzeichnungskorrektur mit Hilfe bivariater Polynome 5. Grades: Originalaufnahme (links unten), entzerrte Projektion (links oben) sowie Kalibrierphantomprojektionen

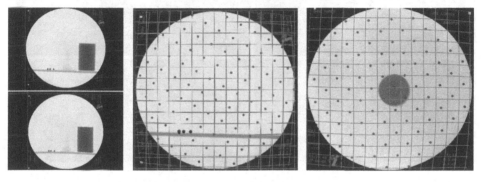

Um möglichst viele Fehlereinflüsse auszuschliessen, wurden die geometrischen Verzeichnungen in einem vorher durchgeführten Lauf mit einem am Bildverstärker angebrachten Kalibrierkörper bestimmt (Abb. 2) und mittels bivariater Polynome 5.Grades herausgerechnet [6].

4   Ergebnisse

Da bei den simulierten Projektionen das ursprüngliche Volumen die Grundwahrheit darstellt, liess sich hier die Qualität der 3D-Rekonstruktion mit einem einfachen voxelweisen Vergleich evaluieren. Dabei konnten die Gefäßstrukturen (Rekonstruktionsvolumen der Größe 128^3) nahezu exakt rekonstruiert werden (Abb. 3). Die Rekonstruktionszeiten (Tab. 1) lagen je nach verwendetem Algorithmus und in Abhängigkeit der Gefäßbaumkomplexität, hinsichtlich der aufgetretenen Okklusionen, zwischen 15s und 28 min (CPLEX 10.0 - Barrier Opt - Dual Xeon 5160 - 3GHz, 16GB Ram).

Tabelle 1. Rekonstruktionsergebnisse mit synthetischen Projektionsdaten (3er-Teilmengen-Gefäßbaum aus Fig. 3a/b mit 4 Threads. Fehlermaße [7]: relative mean (R), misplaced voxel (MV), shape error (SE), volume error (VE)

Datensatz / Optimierungsfkt.	max/min/med # Voxelfehler	R [%]	MV [%]	SE [%]	VE [%]	Rek.-Zeit [s] max/min/med	#
3a) / BIF (2)	567 / 1 / 35	1,12	0,56	1,15	0,46	200 / 15 / 51	179
3a) / R-BIF (3)	198 / 1 / 6	0,18	0,09	0,18	0,10	900 / 37 / 161	179
3b) / BIF (2)	657 / 154 / 248	3,49	1,75	3,54	2,52	471 / 132 / 194	175
3b) / R-BIF (3)	375 / 154 / 198	2,79	1,39	2,83	2,51	1636 / 391 / 609	175

Abb. 3. Rekonstruktionsergebnisse mit synthetischen Projektionen (DRRs): Projektionsdaten (links), rekonstruiertes 3D-Volumen (rechts)

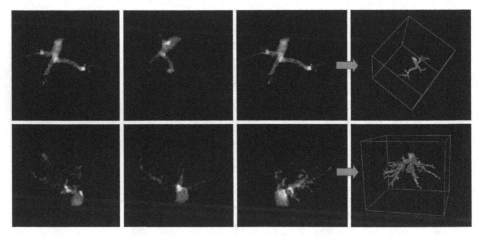

Bei real aufgenommen Daten konnten erst mit Hilfe des kombinierten ART-Verfahrens gute Rekonstruktionsergebnisse erzielt werden, da aufgrund der Bauweise von mobilen C-Bögen ein Positionsfehler aufgrund von Verwindung auftritt. Auch ist der Fehlereinfluss durch Digitalisierung und Quantisierung der Projektionsdaten erheblich, was sich wiederum in Rekonstruktionsartefakten bemerkbar macht.

5   Diskussion

Obwohl das Problem der diskreten Tomographie schon sehr genau untersucht wurde, existieren immer noch sehr wenige praxistaugliche medizinische Anwendungen [7], was auf die fehlende Robustheit und die Berechnungskomplexität der einzelnen Verfahren zurückzuführen ist. So erwiesen sich auch hier die implementierten Algorithmen als sehr sensitiv im Bezug auf Positionierfehler und Rauschen in den Bildern. Aus diesem Grunde wird der Fokus unserer zukünftigen Arbeit vor allem auf der weiteren Verbesserung von Algorithmen im Bezug auf

Abb. 4. Rekonstruktionsergebnisse in Graustufen (ungerundet) [5]

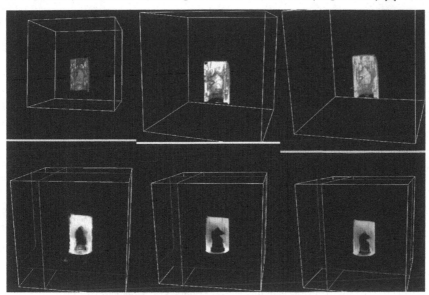

Robustheit und Geschwindigkeit durch Parallelisierung liegen. So skalierten die verwendeten Algorithmen durch die Verwendung von mehreren Prozessorkernen sehr gut, was im Bezug auf kommende Multi-Core-Architekturen auf eine entsprechende Reduktion der Rekonstruktionszeit hoffen lässt.

Literaturverzeichnis

1. Binder N, Bodensteiner C, Matthäus L. Image guided positioning for an interactive C-arm fluoroscope. In: CARS. Springer, Osaka; 2006. 5–7.
2. Binder N, Matthäus L, Burgkart R, et al. A robotic C-arm fluoroscope. Int Journal on Medical Robotics and Computer Assisted Surgery 2005;1(3):108–116.
3. Fishburn P, Schwander P, Shepp L, et al. The discrete radon transform and its approximate inversion via linear programming. Discr Appl Math 1997;(75):39–61.
4. Gritzmann P, de Vries S, Wiegelmann M. Approximating binary images from discrete X-Rays. SIAM J Optimization 2000;11:522–546.
5. Weber S, Schüle T, Hornegger J, et al. Binary tomography by iterating linear programs from noisy projections. In: IWCIA. Springer, Auckland; 2004.
6. Dötter M. Flouroskopiebasierte Navigation zur intraoperativen Unterstützung orthopädischer Eingriffe. Ph.D. thesis. Technische Universität München; 2006.
7. Herman GT, Kuba A. Discrete tomography in medical imaging. Proceedings of the IEEE 2003;91(10):1612–1626.

Beam Hardening Correction with an Iterative Scheme Using an Exact Backward Projector and a Polychromatic Forward Projector

Rüdiger Bock, Stefan Hoppe, Holger Scherl, Joachim Hornegger

Institute of Pattern Recognition
Martensstraße 3, University of Erlangen-Nuremberg, 91058 Erlangen
Email: ruediger.bock@informatik.uni-erlangen.de

Abstract. In computed tomography (CT), reconstructions from cone-beam (CB) data acquired with a polychromatic X-ray device show so called beam hardening artifacts. Beam hardening artifacts are highly undesirable for a medical diagnosis, because details in the reconstructed image are severely disturbed or completely lost. In this work, we demonstrate the significant reduction of beam hardening artifacts by using an iterative reconstruction scheme which consists of a backward and a forward projector. For the backward projector, an exact reconstruction approach was used. The forward projector was extended by a polychromatic model to mimic a realistic X-ray device. The presented experiments use simulated CB data to restrict the evaluation to beam hardening artifacts. The discussion is focused on CB data acquired along a helical trajectory.

1 Introduction

Real CT systems are equipped with X-ray beams which emit photons of different energy and frequency. However, most reconstruction approaches do not properly consider the non-linear nature of the polychromatic X-rays. This leads to severe beam hardening artifacts with streaks, flares and inhomogenities in the vicinity of high contrast structures which makes a medical diagnosis difficult or even impossible.

In this work, we present an iterative scheme which significantly reduces beam hardening artifacts. The algorithm consists of two components: (i) The backward projector and (ii) the forward projector. For the backward projector, an exact reconstruction method is used. The forward projector is extended by a polychromatic model which mimics the nature of a realistic X-ray device. We restrict the evaluation to beam hardening artifacts by using simulated CB data, acquired along a helical trajectory.

The organisation of the paper is as follows. Section II gives an overview of the state of the art and discusses advances of our approach. In Section III, the iteration process together with the backward and forward projector are explained. Experiments and results are presented in Section IV. Section V gives a final discussion and describes future directions.

Fig. 1. The iterative reconstruction process (see also [7])

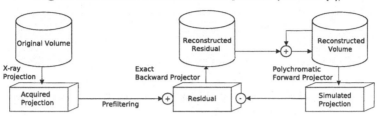

2   State of the Art and New Contribution

Approaches to correct beam hardening artifacts can be divided into three categories: (i) Dual-energy, (ii) preprocessing and (iii) postprocessing methods.

Dual-energy approaches are theoretically elegant, but they require CB data from two different X-ray beam spectra to calculate the complete energy dependency needed for beam hardening correction [1]. Thus, the amount of CB data and consequently the radiation dose is doubled compared to the other approaches. Preprocessing approaches mostly assume that soft tissues have a similar energy dependency as water. This presumption allows the mapping between monochromatic and polychromatic projection values [2]. Postprocessing correction methods are based on the assumption that every material attenuation coefficient of the volume can be described as a linear combination of two known substances like bone and water. They are mostly used in iterative algorithms which estimate the coefficients of the linear combination for each voxel under consideration [3, 4, 5, 6].

The presented approach can be classified into category (iii). The iteration shows similarities with the approach proposed in [7]. However, instead of using an approximate backward projector we combined the iteration process with an exact backward projector [8, 9]. This has the advantage that the so called cone-beam artifacts, arising from an incompletely filled Radon space, are already compensated by the backward projector and therefore do not influence the iteration process. Moreover, the forward projector is extended by a polychromatic model to significantly reduce beam hardening artifacts.

3   Methods

3.1   Iterative Reconstruction

The general structure of iterative reconstruction is shown in Fig. 1. It consists of four steps: (i) The acquired X-ray projections are prefiltered. (ii) The residual is computed between the filtered X-ray projections and the simulated X-ray projections. (iii) The residual is backprojected by using the exact backward projector and added to the reconstructed volume of the previous iteration. (iv) The reconstructed volume is forward projected by using the polychromatic forward projector. The resulting simulated projections are used to compute the residual in the next iteration. Before the iteration begins, the reconstructed residual, the reconstructed volume and the simulated X-ray projections are initialized with zeros.

Prefiltering of Projection Data The prefiltering of the acquired X-ray projections is necessary to stabilize the iteration process [10]. The acquired X-ray projections contain the whole range of representable frequencies. However, the backward projector and the forward projector involve interpolation steps which act like a low pass filter to the simulated projection data. Consequently, the residual contains high frequencies which accumulate in the reconstructed volume. To avoid this, the acquired X-ray projections have to be low pass filtered prior to the iteration process.

Exact Backward Projector For the backward projector, an exact reconstruction approach according to [9] was used. Exact approaches are based on a completely filled Radon space and provide excellent image quality without cone-beam artifacts in a monochromatic setup. However, they are not immune to beam hardening artifacts when polychromatic X-ray projections are involved.

Polychromatic Forward Projector In real CT systems, the X-ray beam is polychromatic and consists of photons of different energy. The beam is defined by its bremsstrahlung spectrum $S_{in}(E)$. The material attenuation $\mu(\boldsymbol{x}, E)$ depends on the location $\boldsymbol{x}$ and on the energy E of the photons. Low energy photons are more attenuated than high energy photons. The polychromatic projection value $p_\lambda(\boldsymbol{\theta})$ of each X-ray with direction $\boldsymbol{\theta}$, emitted from an X-ray source at position $\mathbf{a}(\lambda)$ can be computed with the non-linear attenuation law [11]:

$$p_\lambda(\boldsymbol{\theta}) = -\ln \frac{n_{out}}{n_{in}} = -\ln \frac{\int_0^\infty S_{in}(E) \exp\left(-\int_0^\infty \mu(\boldsymbol{a}(\lambda) + t\boldsymbol{\theta}, E)\, dt\right) dE}{\int_0^\infty S_{in}(E)\, dE} \quad (1)$$

While the bremsstrahlung spectrum of the X-ray beam $S_{in}(E)$ is usually known, the material attenuation $\mu(\boldsymbol{x}, E)$ of the traversed material is lost after the backward projection because the backward projector interprets the polychromatic projection values in a monochromatic sense without considering the energy dependency. Thus, the reconstructed volume consists of attenuation values which correspond to unknown energies. To compute the unknown material attenuation $\mu(\boldsymbol{x}, E)$, the effective energy E_{eff} can be used. The effective energy describes the monochromatic energy at which a given material produces the same projection value as if a polychromatic X-ray beam was used [11]. We assume, that the effective energy E_{eff} equals the energy of the X-ray beam. The material attenuation $\mu(\boldsymbol{x}, E)$ is then computed as a linear combination of soft tissue and bone, for which the material attenuation spectra are known (see also [4]):

$$\mu(\boldsymbol{x}, E) = v \cdot \mu_{bone}(E) + (1 - v) \cdot \mu_{soft}(E) \quad (2)$$

For each voxel $\mathbf{x}$, the linear combination coefficient can be computed by solving Eq. (2) for v while setting $E = E_{eff}$.

Fig. 2. Iterative reconstruction of a phantom of different materials: (a) monochromatic case after 1 iteration (40.61 keV), (b) - (d) polychromatic case (80 kV) after 1 (b), 4 (c) and 10 iterations (c)

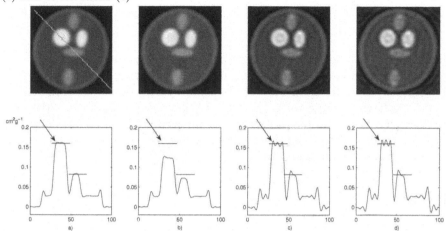

4   Results

The effectiveness of the proposed iterative approach is shown based on a water phantom with inlays of varying shape and density. A helical source trajectory was chosen to provide a complete set of CB data for the exact backward projector. The projections were created with an analytical forward projector (DRASIM, Siemens AG, Medical Solutions, Forchheim, Germany). Two cases are evaluated: (i) In the monochromatic case, the corresponding effective energy $E_{eff} = 40.61$ keV was estimated by using a water phantom. (ii) In the polychromatic case, the tube acceleration voltage was set to 80 kV. For both experiments, volumes of 128^3 voxels were reconstructed.

Fig. 2 shows the reconstruction results. In the top of the figure, the volume slices are shown while in the bottom, the corresponding profiles are depicted. The profiles are determined along the line which is plotted in the top left volume slice. As a reference, Fig. 2a shows the reconstruction result after the first iteration for the monochromatic case. The first iteration corresponds to an application of the exact backward projector without involving the forward projector. Because the charge of the X-ray quanta is known, the attenuation coefficients can be used to determine the phantom material. The hardest material shows the desired attenuation coefficient $\mu_{silicon}(E_{eff}) = 1.59$ cm^{2}g^{-1}. These attenuation coefficients should also be achieved for the polychromatic case. Fig. 2b shows the result after the first iteration for the polychromatic case. Here, the characteristic beam hardening artifacts like inhomogeneities and too low attenuation coefficients in comparison to the monochromatic case can be clearly seen. Fig. 2c and 2d show the result after the 4th and 10th iteration respectively for the polychromatic case. After the 4th iteration, the preferred attenuation coefficients are already reached and the beam hardening artifacts are completely compensated while the iteration converges to the result of Fig. 2a. The overshoots can be blamed on the prefiltering of the acquired X-ray projections and on the Gibbs phenomenon.

5 Discussion

We have shown that beam hardening artifacts are significantly reduced by our approach. The exact backward projector and a polychromatic forward projector nicely complement each other. While the backward projector is free of cone-beam artifacts, the forward projector is used to get rid of beam hardening artifacts. We believe that it is possible to extend the forward projector to model other physical effects like scatter and noise and to reduce salting image artifacts in a similar manner as demonstrated here.

References

1. Alvarez RE, Macovski A. Energy-selective reconstruction in X-ray computerized tomography. Phys Med Biol 1976;21(5):733–744.
2. Herman GT. Correction for beam Hardening in computed tomography. Phys Med Biol 1979;24(1):81–106.
3. Hsieh J, Molthen RC, Dawson CA, Johnson RH. An iterative approach to beam hardening correction in cone beam CT. Med Phys 2000;27(1):23–29.
4. Yan CH, Whalen RT, Beaupre GS, Yen SY, Napel S. Reconstruction algorithm for polychromatic CT maging: Application to beam hardening correction. IEEE Trans Med Imaging 2000;19:1–11.
5. de Man B. Iterative Reconstruction for Reduction of Metal Artifacts in Computed Tomography. Ph.D. thesis. Katholieke Universiteit Leuven; 2001.
6. Van de Casteele E. Model-based Approach for Beam Hardening Correction and Resolution Measurement in Microtomography. Ph.D. thesis. Universiteit Antwerpen; 2004.
7. Danielsson PE, Magnusson M. Combining Fourier and Iterative Methods in Computer Tomography. Analysis of an Iterative Scheme. The 2-D Case; 2004. Report No. LiTH-ISY-R-2634, Linköping University.
8. Katsevich A. Theoretically exact FBP-type inversion algorithm for spiral CT. SIAM Journal on Applied Mathematics 2002;62(6):2012–2026.
9. Noo F, Pack J, Heuscher D. Exact helical reconstruction using native cone-beam geometries. Phys Med Biol 2003;48:3787–3818.
10. Kunze H, Stierstorfer K, Härer W. Pre-processing of Projections for Iterative Reconstruction. In: The Eighth International Meeting on Fully Three-dimensional Image Reconstruction in Radiology and Nuclear Medicine; 2005. 84–87.
11. Kak AC, Slaney M. Principles of Computerized Tomographic Imaging. IEEE Press; 1999.

A New Approach for Motion Correction in SPECT Imaging

Hanno Schumacher and Bernd Fischer

University of Lübeck, Institute of Mathematics,
Wallstraße 40, 23560 Lübeck, Germany
Email: schumaha@math.uni-luebeck.de

Abstract. Due to the long imaging times in SPECT, patient motion is inevitable and constitutes a serious problem for any reconstruction algorithm. The measured inconsistent projection data lead to reconstruction artifacts which can significantly affect the diagnostic accuracy of SPECT if not corrected. Among the most promising attempts for addressing this cause of artifacts is the so-called data-driven motion correction methodology. But even this algorithm is restricted to the correction of abrupt rigid patient motion and exclusive correction of gradual motion, which may lead to unsatisfactory results. In this note we present for the first time a motion correction approach which overcomes the mentioned restrictions. The new approach is based on the super-resolution methodology. To demonstrate the performance of the proposed scheme, corrections of abrupt and gradual motion are presented.

1 Introduction

In Single Photon Emission Computed Tomography (SPECT), the imaging time is typically in the range of 5-30 minutes. Here, patient movement, which has frequently been reported in clinical applications [1], constitutes a serious problem for any reconstruction scheme. The movements cause misalignment of the projection frames, which degrades the reconstructed image and may introduce artefacts. These motion artefacts may significantly affect the diagnostic accuracy [2, 3, 4]. Different methods have been proposed for the correction of motion in SPECT studies. These methods may be divided into three categories. The first two approaches do produce motion corrected projections and thus may be used in conjunction with any reconstruction method. The first approach is purely hardware based, like, for example the triple scan [5] or dual scan [6] protocol. The second approach corrects for the patient motion by using a computational method applied within the projection-space [7, 8]. It should be noted, that due to the projection geometry the latter method is not able to compensate for rotational movement. In this paper, we are concerned with the third methodology. Here the correction is performed in the image space. A widely used member out of this class is the so-called data driven motion correction (DDMC) approach [9, 10]. It can handle full rigid-body motion. To start the scheme, it is assumed that the point in time of the rigid-body motion of the patient during the SPECT imaging is known. Once the point in time of the motion is known it needs to be corrected. The idea is to subdivide the projection data into subsets or motion-sets where no motion has been detected and to estimate the motion in between these subsets accordingly by using a partial reconstruction of the subset containing the largest number of projections and calculate a suitable transformation in order to fit it to the other subsets. To this end the rigid-body parameters after the ith movement of the patient are stored in the vector T_i. Furthermore, all projections that were measured between the ith and the $i + 1$st movement are collected in the projection set $\mathbf{P}_i$. The image, which has been in the course of the algorithm reconstructed up to the ith step, is denoted by $\mathbf{f}^{(i)}$. This image has to be corrected with respect to the next object position T_{i+1}. The result is denoted by $\mathbf{f}^{(i)}(T_{i+1})$. Next the partial reconstruction $\mathbf{f}^{(i)}(T_{i+1})$ is updated with the help of measured projections $\mathbf{P}_{i+1}$ via

$$\mathbf{f}^{(i+1)} = \mathbf{R}[\mathbf{P}_{i+1}, \mathbf{f}^{(i)}(T_{i+1})] \tag{1}$$

where $\mathbf{R}$ denotes a reconstruction algorithm. Ideally, the resulting image $\mathbf{f}^{(m)}$ should contain less motion artefacts. But this approach has two main disadvantages. The first is the needed information about the point in time of the patient motion during the SPECT imaging, and the second is the motion estimation using partial reconstructions. Due to this the quality of the motion estimation depends on the quality of the partial reconstruction, which is only of good quality if $\frac{1}{3}$ of all projections are in one subset. To overcome these disadvantages we present a new approach for motion correction in SPECT imaging that combines reconstruction and motion correction.

2   State of the Art and New Contribution

The data-driven approach, as outlined in the introduction, constitutes the state of the art in motion correction approaches. Nevertheless, it does produce non-satisfactory results if the time of movement is not correctly estimated and if there are too many movements such that the set projections without movement does not contain enough information to produce a meaningful partial reconstruction. Here, we present a motion correction approach which does combine reconstruction and motion correction in using the super-resolution methodology to advantage. To our best knowledge, this has not been conducted before. Moreover, the novel approach does overcome the just mentioned shortcomings of schemes working solely on the raw data.

3   Methods

Let us now describe the main idea of combining reconstruction and motion correction within SPECT imaging. Given SPECT raw data $\mathbf{g}$, we are searching for a reconstructed image $\mathbf{f}$ and for possible motion parameters γ. The whole problem may be formulated as an optimization problem

$$J \begin{pmatrix} \mathbf{f} \\ \gamma \end{pmatrix} = \frac{1}{2} \sum_{i=1}^{K} \| \mathbf{A}_i \mathbf{f}(\gamma_i) - \mathbf{g}_i \|_2^2 + R(\mathbf{f}) \rightarrow \min \quad s.t. \, \mathbf{f} \geq 0 \qquad (2)$$

Some comments are in order. Here, K denotes the number of motion-sets. As it will be shown in the result section, the actual value of K is not critical and may be overestimated. Note, that K just denotes the number and not the precise time of motion. Furthermore, $\mathbf{A}_i$ denotes the i-th part of projection operator $\mathbf{A}$, simulating a SPECT imaging. At least γ_i denotes the motion parameters and $\mathbf{g}_i$ the measured data of motion-set i. It is well-known that the optimization problem is illposed and does need some regularization. Here, we have chosen as regularizer R the TV functional, which is widely used in image processing [11]. Furthermore, the image $\mathbf{f}$ has only non-negative values, which is explicitly formulated in the constraint. To find a minimum of equation (2), we first resolve the constrain $\mathbf{f} \geq 0$, following [12], by the substitution $\mathbf{f} = e^{\mathbf{z}}$. Afterwards we use a Newton method [13] to minimise iterative equation (2) by solving

$$\nabla^2 J \begin{pmatrix} \mathbf{z} \\ \gamma \end{pmatrix} \begin{pmatrix} \mathbf{z}_u \\ \gamma_u \end{pmatrix} = -\nabla J \begin{pmatrix} \mathbf{z} \\ \gamma \end{pmatrix}$$

in every iteration to update the actual solution $(\mathbf{z}, \gamma)^T$ with $(\mathbf{z}_u, \gamma_u)^T$

4   Results

To clarify the power of our new approach we are choosing in a first step γ as a rigid motion model and compare it to the DDMC approach. Therefor three 2D academic examples were created (Fig. 1). Every image is of size 64×64 pixels and perturbed with noise. For every image we simulate a SPECT imaging with 60 projections and two abrupt rigid movements, one after projection 20, the other after projection 40. Due to the fact that the DDMC approach need to know when motion occur we also use this information in our approach, so we can set $K = 3$ in equation (2). Fig. 1 presents the results for all three tests. It shows that the results of our new approach are comparable to the quality of DDMC. To demonstrate that our approach is more powerful than DDMC we are calculating the same tests with $K = \#\text{projections} = 60$. This means we use no information after which projection motion occurs. The DDMC approach can not be started without this information but our approach handle this situation (Fig. 2) only with the restriction that the method has no information about the original position of the object, resulting in a rotated or shifted position. Additionally we present a test for gradual motion in Fig. 3, simulating a SPECT imaging with a translation of the object after every projection. So each projection belongs to a different object position. Due to this the DDMC approach has not enough information for the needed partial reconstruction and can not calculate a motion corrected reconstruction. From the presented results one can see that our approach can not only correct abrupt motion without any information after which projection motion occurs, it can also correct gradual motion. Due to this it overcomes all restrictions of all other motion correction approaches working only with the raw data of a SPECT imaging.

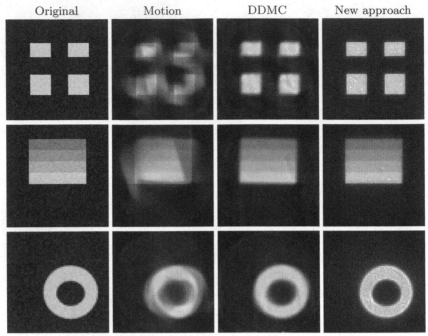

Original   Motion   DDMC   New approach

Fig. 1. The SPECT imaging of three academic examples (Original) are perturbed with abrupt rigid motion and reconstructed (Motion). Using the DDMC or the new approach the motion can be corrected

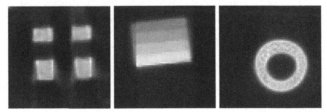

Fig. 2. Motion correction with the new approach of the examples known from Fig. 1 with $K = 60$

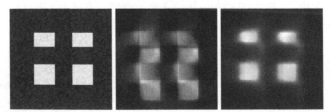

Fig. 3. A SPECT imaging of an academic example (left) is perturbed with gradual motion and reconstructed (middle). Using the new approach this motion can be corrected (right)

5   Discussion

We presented a new approach for motion correction in SPECT imaging, which can correct abrupt and gradual rigid object motion. The power of this approach was clarified with some academic 2D examples. Our next step will be a 3D implementation and further tests with academic examples. Afterwards tests with real patient data are planed.

References

1. Wheat JM, Currie GM. Incidence and characterization of patient motion in myocardial perfusion SPECT: Part 1. J Nucl Med Technol 2004;32(2):60–65.
2. Botvinick EH, Zhu YY, O'Connell WJ, Dae MW. A quantitative assessment of patient motion and its effect on myocardial perfusion SPECT images. J Nucl Med 1993;34(2):303–310.
3. Cooper JA, Neumann PH, McCandless BK. Effect of patient motion on tomographic myocardial perfusion imaging. J Nucl Med 1992;33(8):1566–1571.
4. Friedman J, van Train K, Maddahi J, Rozanski A, Prigent F, Bietendorf J, et al. "Upward creep" of the heart: A frequent source of false-positive reversible defects during thallium-201 stress-redistribution SPECT. J Nucl Med 1989;30(10):1718–1722.
5. Pellot-Barakat C, Ivanovic M, Weber DA, Herment A, Shelton DK. Motion detection in triple scan SPECT imaging. IEEE Trans Nucl Sci 1998;45(4):2238–2244.
6. Passalaqua AM, Narayanaswamy R. Patient motion correction of SPECT images: dual scan approach. IEEE Proc NSSS'94, Norfolk, VA 1995;3:1270–1274.
7. Lee KJ, Barber DC. Use of forward projection to correct patient motion during SPECT imaging. Phys Med Biol 1998;43:171–187.
8. Chen QS, Franken PR, Defrise M, Jonckheer MH, Deconinck F. Detection and correction of patient motion in SPECT imaging. J Nucl Med Technol 1993;21(4):198–205.
9. Fulton RR, Eberl S, Meikle SR, Hutton BF, Braun M. A practical 3D tomographic method for correcting patient head motion in clinical SPECT. IEEE Trans Nucl Sci 1999;46(3):667–672.
10. Kyme AZ, Hutton BF, Hatton RL, Skerrett DW, Barnden LR. Practical aspects of a data-driven motion correction approach for brain SPECT. IEEE Trans Med Imag 2003;22(6):722–729.
11. Vogel CR, Oman ME. Fast numerical methods for total variation minimization in image reconstruction. Procs SPIE 1995.
12. Hanke M, Nagy JG, Vogel C. Quasi-Newton approach to nonnegative image restoration. Linear Algebra and its Applications 2000;316:223–236.
13. Nocedal J, Wright SJ. Numerical Optimization. Springer; 1999.

An Unified Approach for fMRI-Measurements Used by a New Real-Time fMRI Analysis System

Maurice Hollmann[1], Tobias Moench[1], Claus Tempelmann[2], Johannes Bernarding[1]

[1]Institute for Biometry and Medical Informatics, University Magdeburg
[2]Clinic for Neurology II, University Magdeburg
Email: maurice.hollmann@medizin.uni-magdeburg.de

Abstract. Real-time functional MRI (rfMRI) offers new experimental paradigms, such as biofeedback and interactive experiments. Usually, several separated software systems are used to control the MRI measuring sequence, the stimulus presentation, and the statistical analysis, which leads to problems concerning the user communication and synchronisation and interaction of the different software systems. Here, an approach is developed which helps to overcome those difficulties by utilising a uniform parameter management using a flexible parameter description that can be used simultaneously by different separated software systems. This approach is used to control two modules: a realtime fMRI application which extracts the current activation, and an analysis-system which evaluates the current brain activation to influence the stimulus presentation and provide feedback to the volunteer.

1 Introduction

The real-time analysis of brain activation using functional MRI data offers a wide range of new experiments such as investigating self-regulation, bio-feedback or learning strategies [1]. However, besides special data acquisition and real-time data analysing techniques such examination requires dynamic and adaptive stimulus paradigms and selfoptimising MRI-sequences. This paper presents an approach that enables the unified handling of parameters influencing the different software systems involved in the acquisition and analysis process. By developing a custom made Experiment Description Language (EDL) this concept is used for a fast and flexible software environment which treats aspects like extraction and analysis of activation as well as the modification of the stimulus presentation. Furthermore we describe how activation is extracted in real-time using the EDL-approach. The results showed that the developed system in combination with EDL is able to reliably detect and evaluate activation patterns in real-time. With a processing time for data analysis of about one second the approach is only limited by the natural time course of the hemodynamic response function of the brain activation.

Fig. 1. EDL is the central information repository, which controls the fMRI experiment

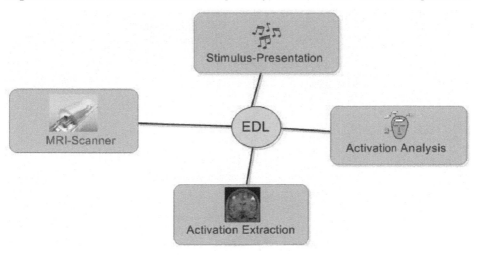

2   State of the Art and New Contribution

Compared to the vast fMRI literature only few experiments were reported for rfMRI [2, 3, 4]. The presented analysis-systems are using no external parameter-descriptions. As usual in fMRI-Experiments the user has to enter all necessary experiment information (e.g. the used stimulus-paradigm) separately for the involved sub-systems, like the MRI acquisition, the stimulus presentation, the activation-extraction and activation analysis. The described disconnected structure leads to an error-proneness concerning input-errors of the user and it complicates the interaction between the different systems. As figure 1 clarifies, the custom made description-language EDL permits a new way to provide essential information to all experimental subsystems. Furthermore the information can be validated and checked for comprehensive consistency. The implemented activation-extraction and -analysis is using the new approach. The whole system is able to perform a fast and unified analysis and classification of real-time fMRI-data.

3   Methods

3.1   System Overview

An EDL-File contains information about the paradigm, which is used to control real-time activation-extraction and -analysis. It may also contain parameters affecting the scan-process. This file is parsed (either in the analysis-system or in the scanner sequence) and the parameters are extracted. More details on the used experiment-description can be found in section "Experiment Description".

Fig. 2. Structure of an EDL-document: Section *statistic*

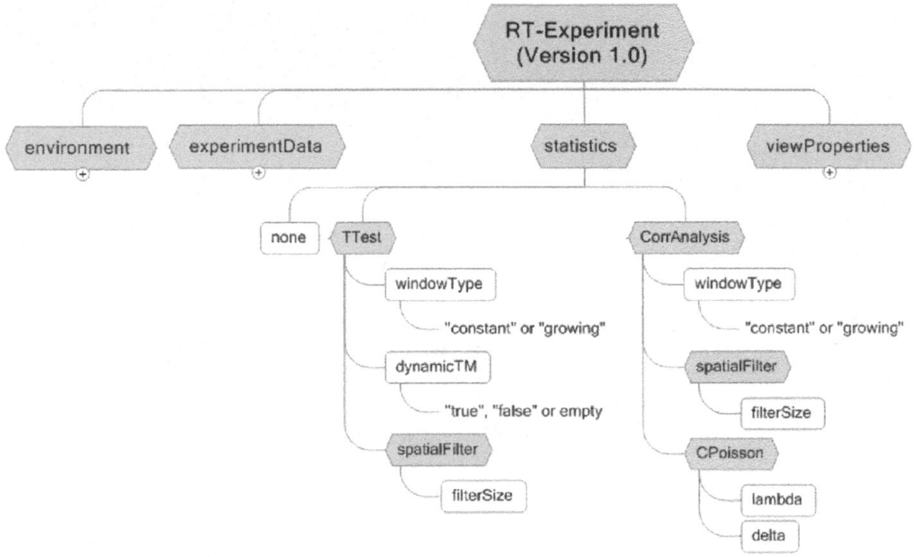

For the realtime-analysis an application was developed, that allows flexible integration of different statistical methods. The developed software modules for activation extraction and activation analysis are implemented in MATLAB, as functions in different packages.The statistical methods of the activation extraction comprehend students t-test and correlation analysis. The visualisation of the statistical results is realised using a maximum-intensity projection on three orthogonal slices (Fig. 3).

3.2   Experiment Description with EDL

The basis for the description-language EDL is XML. Therefore EDL-forms can be validated using predefined structural information. This structural information is saved as ".xsd"and describes the internal hierarchy as well as parameter limits of the defined elements. As mentioned an EDL-document contains different objects in a hierarchical manner. At the moment an experiment contains four sections:

- *environment* (environment parameters like data-folders etc.)
- *experimentData* (paradigm description and functional image modalities)
- *statistics* (statistical method that should be used and its parameters)
- *viewProperties* (parameters concerning visualisation)

A representative part of an EDL-document is depicted in figure 2. With the document definition given in a xsd-file, an EDL-document can be validated. For this purpose several tools are available (e.g. OXYGEN, http://www.oxygenxml.com). The validation ensures, that all parameters are within their defined limits, and that the document is syntactically correct.

3.3 Scanner Sequence and Experiments

The experiments using this approach were performed on a 3 Tesla scanner and a 7 Tesla Scanner (Siemens Medical Systems, Erlangen) at the University of Magdeburg. For the real-time export of the functional data, the sequences on the scanner had to be adapted. The standard *epi*-sequence and the corresponding reconstruction program (ICE-Program) of Siemens were modified to export every single 3D dataset during the measurement. The sequence parameters were optimized following [5].

Subjects Volunteers were two healthy right-handed males (25 and 28 years). Both gave written consent in participation in our experiments. The study was approved by the ethic committee of the Medical faculty of the University of Magdeburg.

Paradigm and Measurement The volunteers performed right- and left hand finger tapping. The orders for the required action (start, stop, right, left etc.) were given verbally using scanner-compatible headphones and predefined wav-files. After a preparation phase of 40 images ([5 images baseline, 5 images right tapping, 5 images left tapping]*2) the templates for the activation of the left and the right motor-cortex were derived. These templates were used as input for the activation analysis. The experimental paradigm consisted of a constant block of 20 images: [10 images baseline, 10 images tapping], which was repeated several times in an experimental run. In the experiments the software extracts the activation, analyses the resulting activation maps and automatically classifies which hand was moved by the subject. During the sessions the volunteer was able to explore the visualisation of the activation as well as the result of the activation analysis. The used scan parameters were: TR= 2000ms, TE= 29ms(3T Scanner) / 20ms(7T Scanner), Resolution= 64x64x31(3T Scanner) / 64x64x16(7T Scanner).

4 Results

All experiment parameters were stored in an EDL-document, including the paradigm, preparing-phases and parameters for the activation extraction and -analysis. In that way the experiments were easy and conveniently to plan and to conduct. The activated areas in the presented examples were determined using t-test analysis. Figure 3 shows the statistical result of the 12th image of the constant window (second one after stimulus onset and 4 seconds after beginning of tapping respectively). The subject moved the left hand. Even if the activation could not clearly be identified visually in the MIP-projection, the activation classifier was able to identify correctly which hand had performed the motor action. The software displayed the classification with a string ('Left Hand').

5 Discussion

In known studies concerning rfMRI no unified concept connecting the involved systems was used. The new approach of storing parameters for different systems

60   M. Hollmann et al.

Fig. 3. Result of the activation analysis with left hand tapping

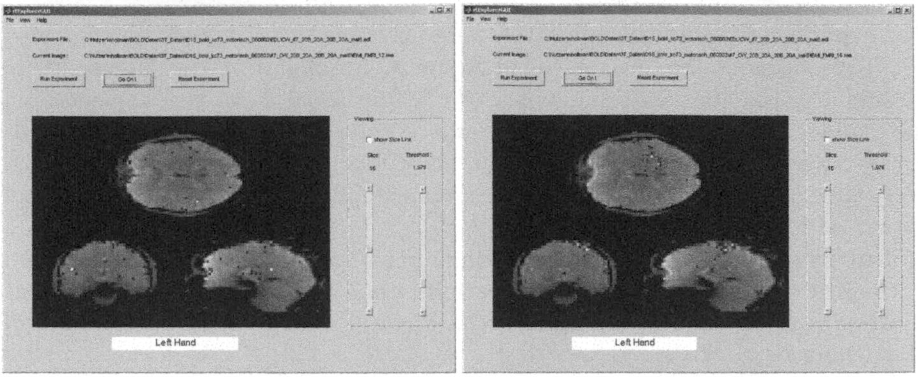

(a) 4s after stimulus-onset   (b) 12s after stimulus-onset

that are involved in real-time fMRI studies in EDL helps to simplify the whole
working process. Furthermore it prevents from errors in the parameter design of
experiments, because parameter dependencies can be checked automatically. The
introduced software system proved to be usable for real-time fMRI studies and integrated control of other applications like activation analysis. The demonstrated
influence on stimulus presentation may for example be used to control attention
effects in fMRI studies. For further refining the interaction within complex 3D
scenes and with the scanner sequence the introduced system can be adapted
easily and fast. New methods of activation extraction and the implementation
of scan-parameter management trough EDL will serve this process.

References

1. Weiskopf N, Scharnowski F, Veit R, et al. Physiological self-regulation of regional
   brain activity using real-time functional magnetic resonance imaging (fMRI). J
   Physiol 2004;98:357–373.
2. Yoo SS, Fairneny T, Chen NK, et al. Brain-computer interface using fMRI: Spatial
   navigation by thoughts. Neuroreport 2004;15:1591–1595.
3. Posse S, Binkofski F, Gao K, et al. Real-time fMRI of temporolimbic regions
   detects amygdala activation during single-trial self-induced sadness. NeuroImage
   2003;18:760–768.
4. de Charms RC, Christoff K, Glover GH, et al. Learned regulation of spatially
   localized brain activation using real-time fMRI. NeuroImage 2004;21:436–443.
5. Posse S, Binkofski F, Schneider F, et al. A new approach to measure single-event
   related brain activity using real-rime fMRI: feasibility of sensory, motor, and higher
   cognitive tasks. Human Brain Mapping 2001;12:25–41.

Neuroimaging: SPM als verteilte Komponente in Grid- und Cluster-Architekturen

Michael Luchtmann, Sebastian Baecke, Johannes Bernarding, Lama Naji

Institut für Biometrie und Medizinische Informatik
Medizinische Fakultät der Otto-von-Guericke-Universität Magdeburg
Email: luchtmann@googlemail.com

Zusammenfassung. Statistical parametric mapping (SPM) ist ein umfangreiches, auf Matlab basierendes Softwarepaket zur bildgestützten Analyse in der funktionellen Hirnbildgebung. Es dient zum Nachweis von Aktivitätsänderungen in Hirnarealen bei Durchführung definierter Aufgaben und Wahrnehmung sensorischer Stimuli mittels fMRT, SPECT oder PET. Je nach Datenmodalität sind unterschiedliche, zeitintensive Vorverarbeitungsschritte erforderlich. Im vorgestellten Projekt wurde eine Infrastruktur zur Parallelverarbeitung der Daten mittels SPM entwickelt, die außer Matlab keine weitere Software benötigt. Es konnte eine signifikante Reduktion der Auswertezeit entwickelt werden. Das Konzept ist skalierbar und erlaubt somit in Rechnerclustern eine weitere Reduktion der Auswertezeit.

1 Einleitung

SPM baut auf den Modulen der Vorverarbeitung, der statistische Analyse und der visuellen Darstellung auf. Die einzelnen Bausteine stellen unterschiedliche Anforderungen: während die visuelle Darstellung technisch sehr rudimentär ist und wenig Rechenzeit benötigt, ist die Vorverarbeitung, abhängig von der Anzahl der auszuwertenden Bilddaten, der verwendeten Interpolationsverfahren und der definierten Iterationsschritte, sehr zeitintensiv. Allerdings können die Vorverarbeitungsschritte Registrierung, Normalisierung auf ein Standard-Template und Glättung auf Untermengen der Bilddaten ausgeführt und somit parallelisiert werden. Das Modul Realign dient der Elimination von Bewegungen während der Aufnahme durch Registrierung auf eine Referenzbild der Zeitserie[1]. Mit dem Modul Normalise werden die Strukturen der gemessenen Hirnbilddaten auf ein ideales „Durchschnitts"-Gehirn (MNI-Template) [2] transformiert. Dies dient zum Vergleich der Ergebnisse verschiedener Probanden und ermöglicht eine Gruppenanalyse [1]. Das Modul Smooth dient der Glättung der Original-Bilddaten, wodurch das Rauschen minimiert und die statistische Analyse unabhängiger von der genauen Lage und Ausdehnung der aktivierten Hirnareale verschiedener Probanden ist [1].

Abb. 1. Auswahl und Transfer eines Referenzdatensatzes (hier beispielhaft Bildserie 4) auf einen Cluster. Zur Vereinfachung ist die minimale Clustergröße mit zwei Rechnern gewählt. Die Referenz wird allen aufgeteilten Untermengen als erste fMRI-Aufnahme vorangestellt. Image i entspricht dem Volumendatensatz zum Zeitpunkt i

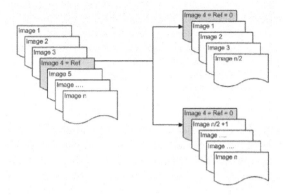

2   Stand der Forschung und Fortschritt durch den Beitrag

Nur wenige Arbeiten haben sich der genannten Thematik gewidmet und interessante Lösungen erarbeitet [3]. Aufgrund der Verwendung sehr komplexer Technologien, wie MPI und CORBA, sind diese Verfahren nicht uneingeschränkt geeignet, um sie in bestehende Cluster- oder Grid-Architekturen zu integrieren. Der vorliegende Beitrag stellt einen Ansatz vor, welcher unabhängig von der existierenden Netzwerk-Architektur eine parallele Berechnung von funktionellen Hirnbilddaten realisiert. Das Konzept verzichtet dabei bewusst auf die Verwendung einer zusätzlichen proprietären Middleware, um das gezeigte Design für alle Umgebungen offen zu gestalten.

3   Methoden

Das Gesamtkonzept beruht darauf, die Bilddaten in Untermengen aufzuteilen, die auf den einzelnen Rechnern unabhängig vorverarbeitet werden können. Da SPM unter Matlab läuft, ist hierzu nur die Installation von Matlab auf den einzelnen Rechnern erforderlich. Nach der Vorverarbeitung werden die Bilddaten zusammengeführt und statistisch ausgewertet. Da hierzu alle Daten vorliegen müssen, kann dieser Schritt nicht parallelisiert werden. Zur Aufteilung, zum bidirektionalen Datentransfer und zur Remote-Steuerung der Auswertung wurde ein Prototyp entwickelt, welcher das vorliegende Konzept realisiert.

Für die Bewegungskorrektur wird ein Volumendatensatz der Zeitserie ausgewählt, welcher für alle Untermengen als Referenz dient. Anschließend wird im Cluster über externe Matlabschnittstellen eine Batchroutine verteilt, welche die Prozesse Registrierung, Normalisierung und Glättung auf jedem der Remote-Rechner initialisiert und ausführt.

Zur Auswertung wurden verschiedene funktionelle Bilddatensätze mit folgenden Parametern verwendet: 64x64x32 Voxel bei 16 Bit Farbtiefe und bis zu 400 Bilder in einer Zeitserie. Die Daten wurden zur Vorverarbeitung von DICOM in das Analyze-Format überführt.

4 Ergebnisse

Im Rahmen des Projektes MediGRID (http://www.medigrid.de) wurde ein erster Prototyp für die Evaluierung des vorgestellten Konzeptes realisiert. Ziel war die Prüfung der Integrierbarkeit der parallelisierten Vorverarbeitung in bestehende Grid-Architekturen [4].

4.1 Realisierung Prototyp

Als Grundlage für die Umsetzung eines Prototypen wurde ein einfacher Cluster mit vier Computern auf Basis von Windows XP verwendet(Intel Pentium D, 2GB RAM). Auf den Einzelrechnern wurde Matlab 7 und SPM2 installiert. Alle Knoten im Cluster wurden per Hub über ein 100 MBit Ethernet verbunden. Es wurde mit Microsoft Visual Studio eine Applikation erstellt, welche die Verteilung der Images auf die gegebenen Ressourcen koordiniert und gleichzeitig auch per DCOM den externen Kommandozeileninterpreter von Matlab zur Verfügung stellt. Das Konzept erlaubt es, dass die beschriebene Schnittstelle im Rahmen eines Unix/Linux-Clusters oder innerhalb einer Grid-Architektur auch durch andere Methoden, wie Web Services oder RPC, ersetzt werden kann.

4.2 Validierung

Abbildung 2 veranschaulicht den Geschwindigkeitsvorteil bei der Nutzung eines Clusters im Gegensatz zur Einzelplatzlösung. So benötigt die Vorverarbeitung eines Datensatzes von 400 Bilder in einem Cluster mit vier Knoten inklusive aller Kopiervorgänge nur noch knapp ein Drittel der ursprünglich auf einem Rechner verwendeten Zeit. Die Messungen umfassten dabei den vollständigen Prozess der Vorverarbeitung inklusive aller notwendigen Verteilungen der Daten. Dies beinhaltete sowohl das divergente Kopieren der Ausgangsdaten auf die verschiedenen Knoten des Clusters, als auch die konvergente Rückführung der berechneten Images.

Zu jeder Messung wurde der gleiche Satz an Images verwendet. Die Verteilung auf die einzelnen Knoten im Cluster erfolgte bei einem Messdurchgang von einem vorher definierten Knoten. Die Ergebnisse wurden durch Wiederholen bestätigt. Dabei dauerte die vollständige Vorverarbeitung für eine Messung von 400 Bildserien unter Verwendung von vier Knoten im Durchschnitt 280 Se-

Abb. 2. Prozentuale Entwicklung der Dauer der Vorverarbeitung abhängig von der Zahl der Knoten und Bildserien im Cluster

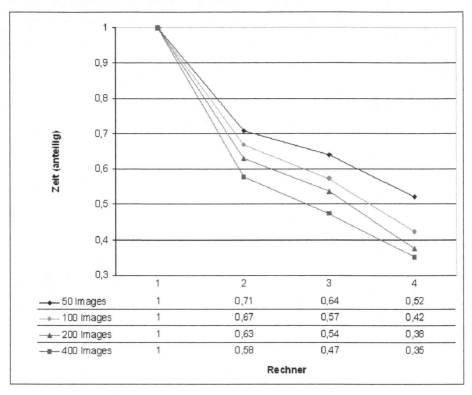

kunden[1]. Innerhalb der Prozedur fielen dabei für das Transferieren[2] der Images 28 Sekunden an. Das reine Preprocessing benötigte dementsprechend 252 Sekunden. Der gleiche Vorverarbeitungsschritt auf einem einzelnen Rechner, ohne das Kopieren von Bildinformationen, dauerte für 400 Images durchschnittlich 799 Sekunden. Es wird deutlich, dass zeitlich fixe Prozeduren, wie z.B. die Berechnung der Transformationsmatrix für die Überführung des Referenzbildes in den Talairach-Raum, mit steigender Zahl zu berechnender Images an Bedeutung verlieren, d.h. je höher die Zahl der MRT-Daten desto größer ist auch der Geschwindigkeitsvorteil bei deren Vorverarbeitung.

---

[1] Die Messung wurde durch den langsamsten Rechner im Cluster(Bottleneck) terminiert. Nach 280 Sekunden, war dementsprechend der letzte Knoten im Cluster mit der Berechnung und Transferierung fertig.

[2] Im Rahmen der Transferierung wurden die originären Bilddaten auf den Remote-Host und die vorverarbeiteten Images wieder auf den Quellknoten kopiert.

5 Diskussion

Die Berechnungen zur Auswertung von funktionellen Hirnbilddaten nehmen trotz aller technologischer Fortschritte, abhängig von der jeweiligen Stichprobe, immer noch zu viel Zeit ein. Aufgrund der Verwendung von immer höher aufgelösten Hirnbilddaten, wird sich an diesem Zustand bei der Verwendung einer Einzelplatzlösung nicht viel ändern. Mit pSPM existiert ein auf MPI basierendes Modul, welches bereits parallele Vorverarbeitung ermöglicht. Allerdings bieten nicht alle Grid-Architekturen und -Konzepte eine Unterstützung für Applikationen auf Basis von MPI. Im Gegensatz dazu ist unser Konzept aufgrund seiner offenen Struktur in herkömmliche Grid-Architekturen integrierbar. Darüberhinaus publizierte keine der genannten Arbeiten verwertbare Benchmarkergebnisse [3]. Unsere Resultate zeigen, dass das Verfahren realisierbar ist und es bei gleichbleibender Qualität einen signifikanten Geschwindigkeitsvorteil mitbringt. Der Ansatz ist einfach skalierbar und plattformunabhängig. Bei Verwendung größerer Cluster ist eine weitere signifikante Reduktion der Rechenzeit zu erwarten.

Literaturverzeichnis

1. Huettel SA, Song AW, McCarthy G. Functional Magnetic Resonance Imaging. 1st ed. Sinauer Associates, Inc; 2004.
2. Talairach J, Tournoux P. Co-Planar Stereotaxic Atlas of the Human Brain: 3-Dimensional Proportional System: An Approach to Cerebral Imaging. 1st ed. Thieme Medical Publishers; 1988.
3. May M, Munz F, Ludwig T. CORBA-basierte verteilte Berechnung medizinischer Bilddaten mit 1118-9. Procs BVM 2000; 213–217.
4. Foster I. The grid: Computing without bounds. Scientific American 2003;288:78–85.

Method for Projecting Functional 3D Information onto Anatomic Surfaces
Accuracy Improvement for Navigated 3D Beta-Probes

Oleg Kishenkov[1], Thomas Wendler[2], Jörg Traub[2],
Sibylle I. Ziegler [3] and Nassir Navab [2]

[1] Faculty of Molecular and Biological Physics,
Moscow Institute of Physics and Technology, Moscow, Russia
[2] Chair of Computer Aided Medical Procedures (CAMP), TU Munich, Germany
[3] Nuclear Medicine Department, Klinikum rechts der Isar, TU Munich, Germany
E-mail: oleg_kishenkov@mail.ru

Abstract. Today the main challenge in cancer surgery is increasing the
accuracy in tumor resections. Malignant cells must be completely removed, while harm to the surrounding healthy tissue must be minimized.
An interesting idea to solve this problem is the use of nuclear-labeled
cancer tracers and intraoperative navigated nuclear probes for residual
control after minimal tumor resection. The idea is to produce an activity encoded surface, which localizes the radioactively marked residual
malignant cells. The thus created surface map is consequently used to
direct the surgeon during resection by means of augmented reality or by
simulating a count-rate at the tip of a surgeon's instrument improving
the accuracy. However, there is a certain distance between the surface
and the probe's tip during the scan procedure. Moreover, the nuclear
probe is not always positioned perpendicular to the surface. The main
contribution of this work is to develop a data post-processing procedure
that takes into account these factors, aiming to increase the accuracy
of the nuclear probe navigation system and thus contribute to a more
accurate tumor resection procedure.

1 Introduction

The main trend in today's surgery is toward a minimally invasive treatment. In
cancer resection, this means that malignant cells must be completely removed
with minimal invasion to normal tissue. Beta-probes have been developed to
aid the surgeon in this process by detecting residual cancer on the resection
borders. This can be achieved by marking cancer with beta-emitting tracers.
Since beta-particles are emitted almost exclusively from malignant cells and do
not penetrate far into tissue, such a device allows accurate detection of residuals
[1, 2].

Navigated 3D beta-probe imaging increases the accuracy of cancer resection
by detecting and applying therapy simultaneously. In that case, the nuclear probe
is tracked and based on its synchronized position and reading, a 3D activity

surface map is generated. This can be used to direct the surgeon by augmented reality or by simulating the count-rate at the tip of surgeon's instrument [3]. However, in order to have high accuracy in navigated 3D beta-probe imaging, it is important to visualize the readings as accurate as possible on the activity encoded surface. Therefore a crucial aspect of the navigated 3D beta-probe is data post-processing.

The current work on navigated 3D beta-probe imaging has been limited to generation of activity maps based on the synchronized position and reading of the probe [3]. Since the probe is not necessarily directly touching the surface nor perpendicular to it, the there introduced visualization could be improved in terms of accuracy. No methods for the projection of the data onto preoperative anatomic images have been considered in the past.

A similar problem arises in functional brain imaging where the functional information is acquired in 3D. Here, the information has to be projected onto the anatomy of the brain to analyze the cortical structure that is active. The state of art for that projection restricts to the use of interpolation for the activity of each surface element based on the closest volume element or the closest one in direction of the normal of the surface element [4, 5]. The inverted approach, i.e. the projection of the data onto the surface, is not known to us.

2   Methods

We have two sets of input data: a 3D CT scan and a 7D set of navigated beta-probe data (position of the tip of the probe, position of the tail of the probe and beta-radiation intensity). As an output we need a surface with activity levels at its points– activity encoded surface (4D set of data). In order to get the desirable result we need

- to create a vector image of the surface on the basis of its image (segmentation);
- to transform the acquired vector image of the surface into the coordinate system of the beta-probe data (registration);
- to project the beta-probe data to the surface for data representation (visualization).

The latter was done for a phantom data-set shown in figure 1.

2.1   Segmentation

In the first step we extracted the surface of the phantom from the CT scan of dimension $512 \times 512 \times 159$ [$voxels$] and resolution $0.98 \times 0.98 \times 1$ [mm^3].

For the extraction of phantom's volume we used a graph cut algorithm as proposed in [6]. Two thresholds were used to segment only the phantom volume. Furthermore a seed point was chosen manually inside the phantom.

In order to acquire the surface of the phantom we used the matching cube algorithm. The result was saved in an Open Inventor (.iv) file and used for visualization with surface rendering techniques.

Fig. 1. The phantom with the CT spots

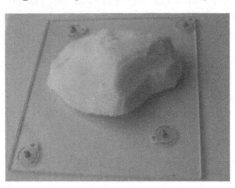

2.2   Registration

To do a proper projection, it is necessary to have both data-sets in the same
coordinate system (here the phantom coordinate system in the tracking space).
In order to correspond the coordinate system of the CT scan and the coordinate
system of the phantom in the tracking space four fiducial points (CT spots)
were attached to the phantom before the examination. For the acquisition of the
coordinates of the spots in the CT scan we used a threshold algorithm, since
they have unique and high Hounsfield units in the CT data. The correspondence
of points between the fiducial points in the phantom coordinate system "P"and
the CT coordinate system "CT"was established fully automatically [7]. Based
in the point correspondences the transformation matrix $T_{CT \to P}$ was calculated
according to [8]. After the estimation or the registration matrix the entire surface
of the phantom in CT coordinates was transformed into the phantom coordinate
system: $p_P = T_{CT \to P} \ p_{CT}$.

2.3   Projection and Visualization

The final step and major contribution of this work is the projection of the data
onto the previous extracted anatomic surface. The standard approach is to find
the closest point on the surface to each of the beta-probe data-points and to
attach the beta-probe activity level to the found point. A considerable disadvantage of this approach is that an activity level acquired at a certain distance
from the surfaces is attached to a point determined by the distribution of the
vertices in the surface rendering procedure rather than to a point of the surface
which affected the beta-radiation level at beta-probe's tip.

In this work the orientation of the beta-probe was taken into account. The
activity level at the beta-probe's tip was attached to the point of intersection of
the beta-probe axis with the closest facet to the tip.

According to the .iv file data the points on the surface form facets in triplets.
To determine the projection the axis of the probe was extended and intersected
with the surface. The closest facet to the tip was chosen as facet where the

Fig. 2. (a) The activity level at the tip of the probe P_0 is attached to the point Q of intersection of the axis of the probe and the facet. (b) The activity encoded surface, blue (dark) points determine the surface, red (light) points show high activity zones and thus localize the malignant cells

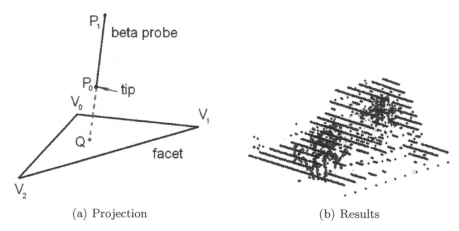

(a) Projection   (b) Results

activity was originated. As final output of our implementation a matrix with the correspondence between points in the beta-probe data-set and facets on the surface was created. As a result the set of original points of the surface is extended by the points with activity levels. This result is visualized in a 3D plot with a color encoded surface (fig. 2a).

3   Results

The described procedures in the previous section were performed for a phantom data-set. The activity encoded surface was visualized by Matlab graphs and is shown in figure 2b. Each original surface point was shown in blue color (dark points), each point with activity level was shown in red color (light points) in size according to its activity level (higher activity level means bigger point).

4   Discussion

In the present work a first step toward an improved accuracy by means of post-processing for a navigated beta-probe imaging system was made. The algorithms proposed showed to work well on the available data-set. The chosen segmentation and registration steps managed to generate a proper 3D dimensional surface to project the data onto. The projection algorithms here introduced were also applicable to the problem and allowed a qualitatively adequate solution for the task set in the introduction. However, there are still steps ahead.

In particular the first problem to be addressed is efficiency. The current projection algorithm is rather time-consuming. Using our Matlab implementation, it took approximately 30 hours to correspond a beta-probe data-set of approximately 2000 points with a surface data-set of approximately 7500 points in a Pentium 4 $1.6[GHz]$ PC. However, this can be easily improved by an implementation based on efficient algorithms and data structures and implementations in C++. This is however not an issue and out of scope for a first prove of concept for the system.

To complete this work a thorough comparison of the original system and the said with the proposed algorithms is needed. In order to do so, we already scheduled a row of ex-vivo experiments for the evaluation of the overall system performance in minimal tumor resection.

We strongly believe that this extension will allow a better visualization and a better user-interface and a more precise detection of residual malignancy. As a consequence we hope to contribute with another 'grain' toward a less-invasive and yet higher-efficacy therapy for cancer.

5   Acknowledgment

The authors would like to thank Dr. Farhad Daghighian for providing the beta-probe for the experiments, as well as, the personnel at the Klinikum rechts der Isar, in particular, Helga Fernolendt and Ralph Bundschuh, for helping to acquire the data here used.

References

1. Daghighian F, Mazziotta JC, Hoffman EJ, et al. Intraoperative beta probe: A device for detecting tissue labeled with positron or electron emitting isotopes during surgery. Med Phys 1994;21(1):153–157.
2. Raylman RR, Hyder A. A dual surface barrier detector unit for beta-sensitive endoscopic probes. IEEE Trans Nucl Sci 2004;51(1):117–122.
3. Wendler T, Traub J, Ziegler SI, Navab N. Navigated three-dimensional beta probe for optimal cancer resection. LNCS 2006;4190:561–569.
4. Saad Z, Reynolds C, Argall B, Japee S, Cox RW. Suma: An interface for surface-based intra- and inter-subject analysis with afni. In: Procs IEEE IISBI; 2004. 1510.
5. Andrade A, Kherif F, Mangin JF, et al. Detection of fMRI activation using cortical surface mapping. Hum Brain Mapp 2001;12:79–93.
6. Boykov Y, Jolly MP. Interactive graph cuts for optimal boundary and region segmentation of objects in N-D images. Procs ICCV 2001;1:105–112.
7. Wang MY, Jr CRMaurer, Fitzpatrick JM, Maciunas RJ. An automatic technique for finding and localizing externally attached markers in CT and MR volume images of the head. IEEE Trans Biomed Eng 1996;43(6):627–637.
8. Umeyama S. Least-squares estimation of transformation parameters between two point patterns. IEEE PAMI 1991;13(4):376–380.

Variation der Fokusebenen zur 3D-Rekonstruktion weißer Blutkörperchen

Andrea Fürsich[1,2], Sebastian Mues-Hinterwäller[1], Thorsten Zerfaß[1],
Thomas Wittenberg[1]

[1]Fraunhofer-Institut für Integrierte Schaltungen IIS, Erlangen
[2]Institut für Computervisualistik, Universität Koblenz-Landau
Email: fuersich@uni-koblenz.de

Zusammenfassung. Für die Rekonstruktion mikroskopisch beobacht-
barer Objekte sind aus der Literatur Verfahren bekannt, die aus mehreren lichtmikroskopischen Aufnahmen unterschiedlicher Fokussierung die
Objektoberfläche rekonstruieren. Das sog. Shape-from-Focus-Verfahren
berechnet dazu durch Maximierung eines Schärfemaßes für jede Pixelposition einen Höhenindex. Während diese Maximierung bei diffusen Oberflächen gute Ergebnisse liefert, sind bei teilweise transparenten Objekten, wie beispielsweise weißen Blutkörperchen, Erweiterungen notwendig.
Dieser Beitrag beschreibt Ansätze zur Verbesserung der Höhenkarte für
diesen Anwendungsfall, die zum einen auf einer Median-Maximierung
und zum anderen auf einem Differenzbildverfahren basieren. Zudem beschränkt sich die Rekonstruktion bisher meist ausschließlich auf den Re-
konstruktionsvorgang. Dieser Beitrag befasst sich zusätzlich mit der Verbesserung des Rekonstruktionsergebnisses durch gezielte Festlegung der
Fokusserie. Die berechnete Höhenkarte wird schließlich als Punktwolke
dreidimensional visualisiert.

1 Einleitung

Die Untersuchung des Blutes spielt für die Diagnosefindung im Bereich der inneren Medizin eine bedeutende Rolle. Mit dem durchflusszytometrischen Automa-
ten steht eine Analysemethode zur automatischen Erstellung eines Differentialblutbildes zur Verfügung. Bei Abnormalitäten im Differentialblutbild ist jedoch
immer noch die Betrachtung einzelner Zellen unter dem Lichtmikroskop mittels
manuellem Durchfokussieren notwendig. Um den Hämatologen bei der objektiven Beurteilung der Blutproben bzw. spezieller Einzelzellen zu unterstützen,
bietet die Auswertung digitaler Blutausstriche am Computer Möglichkeiten einer
räumlichen Darstellung der Zelle, wodurch zusätzliche strukturelle Informationen sichtbar und reproduzierbar gemacht werden können. Verfahren, die auf
einer Variation der Fokusebene basieren, stellen einen Ansatz zur dreidimensionalen Rekonstruktion von Zellen dar. Bekannte Anwendungen dieses Ansatzes
existieren hauptsächlich für diffuse Objekte aus der Industrie oder Geologie [1].
Bei den weißen Blutkörperchen (Leukozyten) als zu rekonstruierende Objekte,
handelt es sich dagegen um partiell transparente Objekte mit einem Durchmesser
von wenigen Mikrometern.

2   Stand der Forschung

Grundsätzlich nutzen Verfahren zur 3D-Rekonstruktion, die auf einer Änderung der Fokuseinstellung beruhen, den Effekt der Unschärfe bei defokussierter Abbildung.

Shape-from-Defocus Verfahren schätzen durch Vergleich der Unschärfe zweier korrespondierender lokaler Bildbereiche die Höheninformation des beobachteten Objektes ab [2]. Voraussetzung dafür ist jedoch eine präzise Kamerakalibrierung.

Das sogenannte *Shape-from-Focus* Verfahren dagegen verwendet eine Serie von Bildern vom zu rekonstruierenden Objekt, die durch sukzessive Veränderung der Fokusebene mit einer konstanten Schrittweite Δz aufgenommen werden. Für jeden Bildpunkt wird die Bildschärfe mittels eines lokalen Schärfemaßes ermittelt. In der Literatur werden eine Vielzahl von Schärfemaßen vorgeschlagen, wie z.B. die Varianz, der Laplace-Operator oder der Gradientenbetrag. Anhand der Betrachtung des Verlaufs der Schärfemaßwerte für einen bestimmten Bildpunkt $p(x, y)$ über alle Ebenen z kann der Maximalwert bestimmt werden. Die Zuordnung des jeweiligen Höhenindex z zu dieser Pixelposition liefert eine Höhenkarte, die zur dreidimensionalen Visualisierung des Objektes herangezogen werden kann [1].

3   Fortschritt durch den Beitrag

Im vorliegenden Beitrag dient das *Shape-from-Focus* Verfahren als Grundlage für die Rekonstruktion von weißen Blutkörperchen. Aufgrund der Morphologie der Leukozyten wird die einfache Maximierung eines Schärfemaßes durch eine Median-Maximierung ersetzt. Durch die Verwendung eines Differenzbildverfahrens kann die Höhenkarte zusätzlich verbessert werden. Außerdem wird neben dem eigentlichen Rekonstruktionsprozess die zur Rekonstruktion verwendete Fokusserie eigens festgelegt, wodurch mögliche Fehlerquellen bei der Maximierung und zusätzlicher Rechenaufwand vermieden werden.

4   Methoden

4.1   Festlegung der Fokusserie

Die Festlegung der Fokusserie beruht zum einen auf der Bestimmung der axialen Ausdehnung einer weißen Blutzelle und zum anderen auf der Ermittlung der optimalen Schrittweite Δz für die Aufnahme der Fokusserie.

Ist die Höhe des betrachteten Objektes bekannt, kann vermieden werden, dass Bilder oberhalb und unterhalb der Zellgrenze verarbeitet werden. Die Verarbeitungsschritte können somit auf Schichtbilder reduziert werden, die für die Rekonstruktion relevante Informationen enthalten. Da es sich bei den Leukozyten um verformbare Gebilde handelt, von denen nicht genau bekannt ist, wie sie auf dem Objektträger liegen, wird ihre axiale Ausdehnung durch Aufsummierung der Gradientenbeträge über einem bestimmten Schwellwert innerhalb des segmentierten Zellbereichs bestimmt. Anhand der Steigung im Verlauf der Kurve über alle z-Positionen lässt sich der relevante Bereich festlegen, in dem die Zelle liegt.

Neben der Festlegung des gesamten zu betrachtenden Bereichs ist die Bestimmung der Schrittweite, mit der die Mikroskopbühne verfahren wird, ein weiterer wichtiger Gesichtspunkt. Ein bestimmter Bereich um die fokussierte Ebene wird als Schärfentiefebereich bezeichnet und stellt ein Maß für die Auflösung entlang der optischen Achse dar. Objektpunkte, die innerhalb dieses Bereichs liegen, werden mit der gleichen Auflösung abgebildet. Eine Aufnahme im Schärfentiefebereich ist daher ausreichend, um die gesamte darstellbare Information zu erhalten. Werden die Abstände zwischen den einzelnen Aufnahmeebenen verringert, führt das nicht zu einem zusätzlichen Informationsgewinn, sondern die Abbildung eines Punktes kann über alle z-Positionen nicht mehr eindeutig einer Ebene zugeordnet werden. Werden dagegen die Abstände zwischen den Aufnahmen größer als der Schärfentiefebereich gewählt, wird die mögliche Auflösung nicht ausgenutzt. Der optimale Abstand zwischen den Aufnahmepositionen entspricht somit dem Schärfentiefebereich.

4.2 Bestimmung der Höhenkarte

Das Verfahren zur Maximierung des Schärfemaßes basiert auf der Annahme, dass das Schärfemaß einen charakteristischen, parabelähnlichen axialen Verlauf aufweist. Da die Leukozyten auch nach der Färbung zum Teil transparent sind, kann es passieren, dass mehrere Objektpunkte unterschiedlicher Entfernung auf ein und dieselbe Position im Bild abgebildet werden und somit mehrere Maxima im Verlauf des Schärfemaßes auftreten [3]. Aufgrund experimenteller Untersuchungen wird aber angenommen, dass für die Mehrzahl der Punkte das Hauptmaximum entweder am Zellkern oder der Zellhülle gefunden wird, so dass in der Höhenkarte zwischen benachbarten Positionen keine extrem unterschiedlichen Höhenwerte auftreten. Um auftretende Ausreißer zu beseitigen, wird die Höhenkarte anhand einer Median-Maximierung ermittelt, wobei ein lokaler Bereich um die aktuelle Position Einfluss auf die Maximumfindung nimmt. Durch Anwendung des Median-Filters auf die Schärfemaßbilder werden Werte mit großer Abweichung in der lokalen Umgebung eliminiert. Dabei wird in Abhängigkeit von der verwendeten Maskengröße die Ortsauflösung gesenkt. Die Bestimmung der Höhenkarte findet im Anschluss daran durch Maximierung der Werte aus den auflösungsreduzierten Schärfemaßbildern statt.

Die erzeugte Höhenkarte wird anschließend nochmals auf Plausibilität hin untersucht und die entsprechenden Werte gegebenenfalls ersetzt. Dazu wird auf der berechneten Höhenkarte zunächst eine Median-Filterung ausgeführt. Die Differenz zwischen der originalen und der gefilterten Höhenkarte liefert diejenigen Stellen, an denen durch die Filterung „Rauschen" entfernt wurde [4]. Während große Differenzwerte auf unerwünschte Ausreißer hinweisen, wird eine geringe Variation der Werte in der Maske aber nicht als Fehlerwert angesehen, sondern spiegelt die Struktur des Objektes wieder. Es wird deshalb ein Schwellwert verwendet, der den Teil der Differenzwerte als Fehlerwerte ausschließt, die

Abb. 1. Beispielbild aus der Fokusserie eines Leukozyten (a) und die dazugehörige Höhenkarte (b)

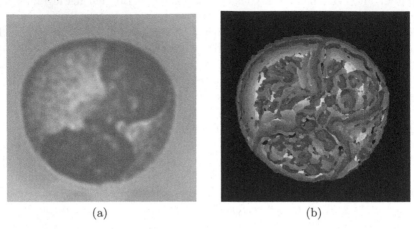

(a)   (b)

einen Schwellwert nicht überschreiten. Für die ermittelten Fehlerpunkte wird der Höhenwert durch Mittelung in einer lokalen Umgebung neu berechnet. Dabei fließt der mittlere Wert, der als Ausreißer erkannt wurde, nicht mehr mit ein, um die Höhe dieses Pixels besser an die umgebenden Werte anzugleichen.

5   Ergebnisse

Die beschriebenen Methoden wurden an Fokusserien von unterschiedlichen Leukozyten, sowie an der Fokusserie eines Kalibiermusters getestet. Für die Aufnahme wurde ein Durchlichtmikroskop der Firma Zeiss mit einem 1000-fachen Gesamtvergrößerungsfaktor verwendet. Das verwendete Objektiv ist für die Anwendung in Immersionsöl vorgesehen und besitzt eine numerische Apertur von 1.3.

Die berechneten Höhenkarten wurden anhand von Grauwertbildern dargestellt. Abb. 1 zeigt ein Bild aus der Fokusserie eines Leukozyten und die dazugehörige Höhenkarte. Für die dreidimensionale Visualisierung der Rekonstruktionsergebnisse wurde aus der Höhenkarte eine Punktwolke erstellt (siehe Abb. 2). Die Herstellung des korrekten Abbildungsverhältnis zwischen lateraler Ausdehung und Höhe des Objektes geschieht dabei über einen konstanten Höhenfaktor, der mit dem Bildindex z multipliziert wird [1].

6   Diskussion

Die Anwendung des *Shape-from-Focus* Verfahrens zur Rekonstruktion von Leukozyten, insbesondere die Adaptionen bei der Bestimmung der Höhenkarte und die eigens dafür festgelegte Fokusserie liefern eine dreidimensionale Darstellung, bei der deutlich die Struktur der unterschiedlichen Zellbestandteile erkennbar wird. Experimentelle Untersuchungen zeigen, dass die im Verlauf des

Abb. 2. Ansicht der dreidimensionalen Punktwolke eines Leukozyten

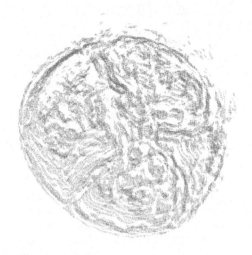

Schärfemaßes auftretenden Maxima unterschiedlichen Zellstrukturen zugeordnet werden können. Somit ist es denkbar, dass zukünftig verschiedene Oberflächenstrukturen, wie Kern und Plasma getrennt voneinander darstellbar werden.

Literaturverzeichnis

1. Niederoest M, Niederoest J, Scucka J. Automatic 3D reconstruction and visualization of microscopic objects from a monoscopic multifocus image sequence. International Archives of the Photogrammetry 2003;(XXXXIV-5).
2. Ens J, Lawrence P. An investigation of methods for determing depth from focus. IEEE PAMI 1993;15(2):97–108.
3. Dierig T. Gewinnung von Tiefenkarten aus Fokusserien. Ph.D. thesis. Ruprecht-Karls-Universität Heidelberg; 2002.
4. Scheurmann T. Berührungslose Gestaltvermessung von Mikrostrukturen durch Fokussuche. Wissenschaftliche Schriftreihe des ICT 1997;13.

Shape Analysis for Ultrasound Breast Lesion Evaluation

Miguel Alemán-Flores[1], Patricia Alemán-Flores[2], Luis Álvarez-Leén[1],
Rafael Fuentes-Pavón[2], José M. Santana-Montesdeoca[2]

[1]Departamento de Informática y Sistemas
Universidad de Las Palmas de Gran Canaria, 35017, Las Palmas, Spain
[2]Sección de Ecografía, Servicio de Radiodiagnóstico
Hospital Universitario Insular de Gran Canaria, 35016, Las Palmas, Spain
Email: maleman@dis.ulpgc.es

Abstract. This work presents a new approach for a wide analysis of the shape of breast tumors in ultrasound images. We have developed an environment for the filtering of the images, the segmentation of the nodules and the extraction of a series of measurements which describe the shape of the nodules. This will help in the computer-aided evaluation of the tumors and the distinction of benign and malignant nodules. The results extracted for the different features are coherent with the assessment of the specialists and represent a great help for the examination of the images and the decision making process.

1 Introduction

Ultrasonography is widely used for the detection and evaluation of many diseases. In the case of breast cancer, it is a very useful complementary imaging technique to mammography. Not only does it provide a different assessment of the lesion, but it also allows detecting very small lesions and analyzing dense breasts, which is quite difficult using mammography. Furthermore, a series of features related to the shape of the nodule, the regularity of the contour and the intensity and contrast between different regions have been described to characterize the lesions and help distinguish benign from malignant nodules [1]. In this work, we present a common framework which, by means of several computer vision and image processing techniques, allows extracting some measurements of the shape of a nodule. These include the roundness of its shape, the size of ramifications, the number of microlobulations and angular margins, the presence of spiculation or a taller-than-wide shape.

In order to accelerate and simplify this task, a semi-automatic segmentation of the lesion is performed, so that it is no necessary to delineate the lesion manually. This is carried out by filtering the image using a speckle noise reducing filter, obtaining a presegmentation using a region-growing algorithm, and refining the presegmentation using active contours.

Due to the difficulties that speckle characteristic noise represents for the automatic analysis of ultrasound images, little work has been done in this filed, and the results are usually moderate. Some previous works try to adjust the parameters of the ultrasound systems to help in the decision making process [2], segment the tissues [3], or deal with certain particular aspects of the nodules, such as their texture [4]. Other works deal with the detection of the lesions [5] or a general description of the nodules [6]. However, we intend to obtain a more detailed description of the shape of the nodules, so that their benignity or malignancy can be determined in a more accurate way.

2 Methods

In this section, we present the methods we have used for the segmentation of the nodules and for the shape analysis, according to the diagnostic criteria described by the specialists.

2.1 Filtering and Segmentation

Before analyzing the shape of the tumor, it must be segmented from the surrounding tissues. Due to the characteristic speckle noise of ultrasound images, a noise reducing filter must first be applied. We use the truncated median filter, which, in a few iterations, progressively reduces the speckles and provides quite satisfactory results [7]. From an inner point, which is the only interaction asked to the physician, a region-growing algorithm is used to extract an initial presegmentation. This technique is very fast, but does not provide accurate enough results. However, it can be used to obtain an initial contour for the active contour technique [8][9], which generates very precise segmentations if it is initialized with a close approximation. For the implementation we apply a level set approach [10]. Once the segmentation is obtained, we proceed to analyze the shape of the nodule.

2.2 Shape Analysis

The main features which allow discriminating benign from malignant tumors, thus avoiding performing the biopsy, are related to the shape of the nodules and the regularity of their contours. When analyzing the general shape of the tumor, an ellipsoid shape or the presence of a few gentle and well circumscribed lobulations are considered as benignity findings. On the other hand, ramifications or a taller-than-wide shape are considered as malignancy findings. Moreover, when examining the smoothness of the contour, if it presents microlobulations, angular margins or spiculation, they are interpreted as malignancy findings, as opposite to a rounded and well defined contour. In this work, we analyze both, the global and the local features of the contours, so that some robust, reproducible and accurate measurements can be provided to the specialists in order to perform a more reliable distinction between benign and malignant nodules.

The ideal benign nodule has a well defined ellipsoid shape. We not only intend to binary decide whether a nodule is ellipsoidal or not, but we also try to measure how ellipsoidal it is. In order to automatically determine it, we extract the ellipse which best fits the contour of the nodule. We apply a gradient descent technique in which the five parameters of the ellipse (two coordinates for the center, two dimensions for the axes and an angle for the orientation) are iteratively adjusted. Since we need some initial values, we roughly estimate them from the position, the dimensions and the orientation of the segmentation. The distance from the contour to the final ellipse, with respect to the size of the nodule, measures how ellipsoidal the lesion is. If it is not enough, we search for two or three gentle lobulations by splitting the contour at the closest points to the center.

Once the minimum distance ellipse (or ellipses) has been found, the regions where it clearly differs from the contour allow locating the eventual ramifications of the nodule. Their relative size with respect to the total size indicates their relevance. To decide whether a nodule is likely to invade different tissues, we consider the ratio between its dimensions, since the different tissue layers are supposed to be approximately horizontal.

The local variations of the contour require a detailed analysis of its regularity. Angular margins are identified by searching for pseudo-corners on the contour of the nodule. Microlobulations are extracted using a similar approach to that used for ellipse extraction, but, in this case, we search for small arcs of ellipses which fit certain parts of the contour. Spiculation is measured through the variance of the orientation of the gradient along the contour, for which the structure tensor is used.

3   Results

Figure 1 shows some examples of nodules which have been segmented on the ultrasound images. As observed, the segmentations are quite satisfactory and allow a precise analysis of the shape of the nodules.

Table 1 shows the values of the different measurements for the set of nodules shown in figure 1. For every feature, we show the numerical measurement provided by the system (sys), as well as the assessment performed by three specialists (phy). As observed, not only is it coherent with the appearance of the nodule, but it also allows setting a threshold for each feature if the values are compared with the binary assessment of the physicians. Only isolated cases differ and, in most cases, they are due to a reduction of the specificity produced by trying to adjust the parameters and thresholds to increase the sensitivity, since it is better to perform a biopsy of a benign nodule than overlooking a malignant one.

4   Discussion

In this paper we have presented a common framework for the assessment of a set of parameters regarding the shape of a breast lesion in an ultrasound image. These measurements allow analyzing the shape of the nodule in a robust and accurate way and provide numerical values which describe the contour in terms

Fig. 1. Examples of breast nodules in ultrasound images and their corresponding automatic segmentations

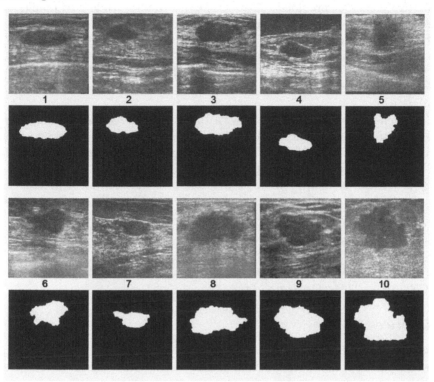

Table 1. Numerical measurements obtained by the system (sys) and assessment of the specialist physicians (phy) for the nodules in fig. 1 regarding the features related to the shape of the nodules: ellipsoid shape (ES), gentle lobulations (GL), ramifications (RM), taller-than-wide shape (TW), angular margins (AM), microlobulations (ML) and spiculation (SP). In the values of the specialists, 0 means that a malignant factor has not been found or a benignant finding has been found, and 1 means the opposite

Nodule	ES sys	ES phy	GL sys	GL phy	RM sys	RM phy	TW sys	TW phy	AM sys	AM phy	ML sys	ML phy	SP sys	SP phy
1	1.9	0	2.2	0	0.0	0	0.36	0	3.9	0	1.8	0	0.8	0
2	6.1	1	3.9	0	7.6	0	0.53	0	5.1	1	2.4	0	0.0	0
3	3.4	0	5.2	1	5.7	0	0.47	0	5.2	1	1.8	0	1.7	0
4	7.3	1	3.2	0	9.4	0	0.50	0	3.3	0	0.6	0	0.9	0
5	10.7	1	10.5	1	13.4	1	1.24	1	6.5	1	3.1	1	0.0	0
6	10.3	1	9.4	1	12.5	1	0.65	0	4.8	1	3.7	1	1.4	0
7	7.0	1	12.4	1	13.6	1	0.45	0	4.3	1	3.1	1	1.2	0
8	10.6	1	12.5	1	7.1	0	0.66	0	5.0	1	3.1	1	0.8	0
9	7.0	1	8.9	0	4.7	0	0.50	0	5.5	1	2.4	1	2.5	1
10	19.9	1	12.4	1	8.7	0	0.78	0	5.0	1	6.8	1	1.4	0

of global and local regularity. Prior to the analysis of the shape, the segmentation, performed using a noise reduction filter, a region growing presegmentation and active contours, provides quite satisfactory results, while it simplifies and accelerates the process of delimiting the nodules.

The numerical techniques we have applied allow examining global features, such as how ellipsoidal a nodule is, whether it has two or three gentle lobulations and whether it has ramifications. On the other hand, the local variations in the contour help determine whether it has angular margins, microlobulations or spiculation.

The measurements are coherent with the assessment of the specialists and, instead of providing a binary evaluation, they generate scalar values which permit determining in what degree each factor is present and what the probability is of being a benign or malignant tumor. Our results confirm the usefulness of image processing techniques in the evaluation of ultrasound for a precise early detection of breast cancer.

Acknowledgements

This work was partially supported by project TIN 2005 02004, Ministerio de Educación y Ciencia, Spain.

References

1. Stavros AT, Thickman D, Rapp CL, et al. Solid breast nodules: Use of sonography to distinguish between benign and malignant lesions. Radiology 1995;196(1):123–134.
2. Kuo WJ, Chang RF, Moon WK, et al. Computer-aided diagnosis of breast tumors with different US systems. Acad Radiol 2002;9(1):793–799.
3. Kaufhold J, Chan R, Karl WC, Castanon DA. Ultrasound tissue analysis and characterization. Procs of SPIE 1999; 73–83.
4. Chen DR, Chang RF, Juang YL. Computer-aided diagnosis applied to US of solid breast nodules by using neural networks. Radiology 1999;213(1):407–412.
5. Drukker K, Giger ML, et al KHorsch. Computerized lesion detection on breast ultrasound. Medical Physics 2002;29(7):1438–1446.
6. Revell J, Mirmehdi M, McNally D. Applied review of ultrasound image feature extraction methods. In: Procs. of The 6th Medical Image Understanding and Analysis Conference; 2002. 173–176.
7. Davis ER. On the noise suppression and image enhancement characteristics of the median, truncated median and mode filters. Pattern Recognition Letters 1988;7:87–97.
8. Caselles V, Kimmel R, Sapiro G. Geodesic active contours. International Journal of Computer Vision 1997;22(1):61–79.
9. Kass M, Witkin A, Terzopoulos D. Active Contour Models. In: Procs. of 1st International Conference on Computer Vision; 1987. 259–268.
10. Osher S, Sethian J. Fronts propagating with curvature dependent speed: algorithms based on the Hamilton-Jacobi formulation. Journal of Computational Physics 1988;79:12–49.

Automatische Erkennung von Ischämien mit Bolus Harmonic Imaging

Adam Maciak[1], Christian Kier[1], Günter Seidel[2], Karsten Meyer-Wiethe[2],
Ulrich G. Hofmann[1]

[1]Institut für Signalverarbeitung, Universität zu Lübeck
[2]Klinik für Neurologie, Universitätskrankenhaus Schleswig–Holsteinn
Email: am@avallia.com

Zusammenfassung. Mit dem ultraschallbasierten Harmonic Imaging Verfahren ist die Darstellung der Gehirnperfusion möglich. Die Auswertung geschieht bisher manuell durch klinische Experten. Basierend auf dem Bolus Harmonic Imaging Verfahren wird eine neue Methode zur automatischen Erkennung von ischämischen Gehirnregionen vorgestellt und somit die Grundlage für ein Computer Aided Diagnosis (CAD) System geschaffen. Das Verfahren erkennt perfusionsgestörte Gehirnregionen, löscht Streifenartefakte und das abgebildete kontralaterale Gehirnareal, vermisst die Perfusionsstörungen und generiert ein binäres Aussagenbild. Basierend auf diesem Bild wird eine Aussage über das Vorhandensein von Ischämien erstellt.

1 Einleitung

Die erfolgreiche Behandlung zerebraler Gefäßerkrankungen basiert hauptsächlich auf der frühen und sicheren Erkennung von minderperfundierten Gehirnarealen. Die Darstellung der Hirnperfusion geschieht überwiegend mit verschiedenen Schnittbildverfahren. Die transkranielle Perfusionsbildgebung des Gehirns, basierend auf dem Einsatz von Ultraschall (US), hat sich bereits etabliert. Als Bedside–Verfahren ist es einfach zu handhaben, wenig belastend, wiederholbar und sicher in der diagnostischen Aussagekraft [1, 2, 3, 4].

Ultraschallgestützte Verfahren basieren größtenteils auf dem Einsatz eines Ultraschallkontrastmittels (UKM), welches Mikrobläschen enthält. Diese Mikrobläschen dienen zur Steigerung der Echogenität, da sie harmonische Schwingungen emittieren, wenn sie US–Wellen ausgesetzt werden. Diese harmonischen Schwingungen können gemessen werden und ermöglichen Rückschlüsse über die Perfusion des Gewebes.

Eine verbreitete Methode ist das Bolus Harmonic Imaging (BHI). Dem Patienten wird das UKM als Bolusinjektion appliziert. Während dessen wird die Schallsonde an den Temporalknochen der Schädelkalotte angelegt. Es werden hierbei im Abstand von 1.5s Bilder aufgezeichnet, welche die Ausbreitung des UKM im Gehirn wiedergeben. Die Signalintensität des perfundierten Gewebes beschreibt hierbei einen charakteristischen Verlauf. Erst wird das UKM im Blutstrom eingewaschen, verbleibt kurz auf einem Peak und wird langsam verdünnt und ausgewaschen. Minderperfundiertes Gewebe und abgeschattete Regionen, wie Streifenartefakte, weisen derlei charakteristische Kurven nicht auf.

2   Stand der Forschung und Fortschritt durch den Beitrag

Es werden grundsätzlich zwei Arten der Kontrastmittelbeigaben unterschieden, die in verschiedenen Prinzipien der Perfusionsbildgebung resultieren. Eine Übersicht findet sich in [4]. Hierbei ist neben dem BHI das Contrast Burst Depletion Imaging ein vielversprechender Ansatz [5]. Allen Verfahren ist gemein, dass die Perfusion durch geübte klinische Experten ermittelt werden muss. Hierzu kann zum Einen eine Aussage über die Stärke der Gehirnperfusion, die zur Signalintensität des perfundierten Gewebes korreliert, direkt aus der aufgezeichneten Bildsequenz gewonnen werden. Zum Anderen können Parameterbilder (PI, TTP, AUC, SLOPE) aus der Bildsequenz extrahiert werden, die die Perfusion beschreiben [6, 7]. Die Extraktion von Parameterbildern stellt hierbei einen Ansatz für ein Semi–Automatisches Expertensystem dar. Die automatische Befundung wird durch die unterschiedliche und zum Teil schwache Korrelation der Parameter zur tatsächlichen Perfusion erschwert. Nachfolgend wird ein Verfahren vorgestellt, welches automatisch ischämische Gehirnregionen erkennt ohne Parameterbilder extrahieren zu müssen. Dieses System kann zur automatischen Erstellung von Diagnosen (Computer Aided Diagnosis) herangezogen werden.

3   Methoden

Das hier vorgestellte Verfahren wird in folgende Teilschritte unterteilt (Abb. 1):

1. Erkennung von perfusionsgestörten Gehirnregionen
2. Erkennung von Streifenartefakten
3. Löschung von Streifenartefakten
4. Löschung des kontralateralen Gehirnteils
5. Generierung des binären Aussagenbildes

Die Erkennung von perfusionsgestörten Gehirnarealen basiert auf dem in [8] vorgestellten Verfahren der Analyse der Zeit–Intensitätskurven des Einwasch– und Auswaschvorgangs des UKM. Hierbei wird der gesamte Zeit–Intensitätsverlauf einer Region als ein Merkmalsvektor aufgefasst. Dieser Merkmalsraum wird mit dem K–Means Verfahren unüberwacht partitioniert. Experimentell ergibt sich eine optimale Clusterzahl von 5. Anschließend erfolgt eine Zusammenfassung von perfusionsgestörten Gehirnarealen. Dieses erfolgt über die Verschmelzung charakteristischer Cluster. Die Merkmalsvektoren von Perfusionsstörungen oder Artefakt–Arealen liegen hierbei in zwei a–priori bekannten Clustern, während Merkmalsvektoren von normal perfundiertem Gehirngewebe sich auf die restl-chen drei Cluster verteilt. Das bedeutet, dass Regionen mit Ähnlichem Zeit–Intensitätsverlauf in gleichen Clustern liegen. Diese Verschmelzung resultiert in einem Binärbild.

Im zweiten Schritt werden Streifenartefakte erkannt. Streifenartefakte sind Abschattungen der Signalintensität entlang der Schallrichtung. Ihr Signalverlauf ähnelt denen von ischämischen Gehirnregionen. Die Ursachen für diese Abschattungen liegen nah an der Schallsonde, z.B. eingeschlossene Luftbläschen, Knochenunregelmäßigkeiten, Haare. Diese Abschattungen erstrecken sich somit über die volle Eindringtiefe des Ultraschalls und haben eine charakteristische Form. Sie sind lang und oftmals schmal und haben somit eine hohe Exzentrizität.

Zur Erkennung von runden oder exzentrischen Objekten eignet sich die Exzentrizität [9]. Diese wird über die zentralen Momente 2.ter Ordnung ($m_{0,2}$, $m_{2,0}$, $m_{1,1}$) definiert als

$$\varepsilon = \frac{(m_{2,0} - m_{0,2})^2 - 4m_{1,1}^2}{(m_{2,0} - m_{0,2})^2}. \tag{1}$$

Die Exzentrizität liefert Werte zwischen 0 für rundliche und 1 für längliche Objekte [9]. Da Streifenartefakte unterschiedlich breit sein können, wird das Eingabebild in 32 gleichbreite Segmente aufgeteilt. Dadurch ergeben sich bei Streifenartefakten Werte bei 1 für die Formel (1). Jedes dieser Segmente wird anschließend einzeln untersucht. Ein Segment wird als Streifenartefakt markiert, wenn die Exzentrizität den experimentell ermittelten Wert von 0.9 für die optimale Erkennung von Streifenartefakten überschreitet. Somit ergibt sich eine Maske, die Auskunft über Streifenartefakte im Binärbild gibt. Diese Maske wird mit dem Binärbild pixelweise multipiziert, sodass Streifenartefakte ausgeblendet werden.

Im Anschluss wird der kontralaterale Gehirnteil ausgeblendet, in dem falsch positive Flächen geschwärzt werden. Als kontralateraler Gehirnteil werden die unteren 2cm des Bildes angenommen. Somit entsteht ein binäres Bild, in welchem nur noch ischämische Gehirnregionen weiß und nicht–ischämische Bereiche schwarz markiert sind.

Nun werden alle weißen, zusammenhängenden Regionen durchnummeriert und die jeweiligen Flächen berechnet. Die Regionen mit der größten Fläche wird markiert und bei Überschreiten des experimentell ermittelten Schwellwertes von 6 cm^2 als ischämisch klassifiziert. Experimentell wird die Länge und Breite eines Pixels auf 0.15 cm gemittelt, obwohl die longitudinale Auflösung des Ultraschalls nicht der axialen Auflösung entspricht. Somit sind mindestens 267 zusammenhängende Pixel nötig um eine Fläche als positives Ergebnis zu markieren. Die erkannten Ischämien werden im Bild eingefärbt, alle anderen zusammenhängenden Objekte verbleiben weiß. Somit ergibt sich für den Arzt auch eine Information darüber, ob es mehrere minderperfundierte Gehirnareale gibt.

4   Ergebnisse

Es wurden Datensätze zweier Patientenkollektive mit insgesamt 26 Ultraschallbildsequenzen zur Validierung des Verfahrens herangezogen. Diese Daten wurden in den Kliniken für Neurologie und Neurochirurgie der Universität zu Lübeck gewonnen. Das Untersuchungsziel ist hierbei, in wie weit das binäre Aussagenbild

Abb. 1. (a) Ergebnis des KMeans Verfahrens. Das Bild ist in 5 Grautönen eingefärbt. Es folgt die Verschmelzung charakteristischer Cluster nach [8]. (b) Resultierendes Binärbild mit Ischämien und Artefakten in einem Cluster und perfundierten und vom US–Kegel nicht erfasstem Gewebe im anderen Cluster. (c) Erkannte Streifenartefakte (weiß). (d) Resultierendes Perfusionsbild, nachdem die Streifenartefakte entfernt wurden. Weiße Flächen repräsentieren Perfusionsstörungen. (e) Die Linie symbolisiert die Grenze zwischen ipsilateralem und kontralateralem Gehirnteil. Der kontralaterale Teil wurde entfernt. (f) Das Ergebnis ist in einem MRT–Bild des Gehirn dargestellt. Die gefundene Ischämie liegt im Mediateritorium

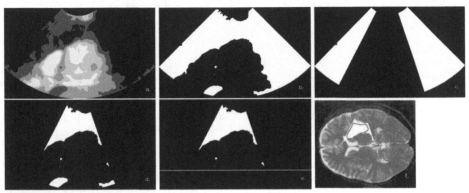

mit ischämischen Regionen übereinstimmt. Die Kontrolluntersuchung erfolgte CT– bzw. MRT–basiert.

Die 26 Patientendatensätze stammen von 16 unterschiedlichen Patienten. Als Ultraschallkontrastmittel wurde Sonovue^{TM} (2.4 ml als Bolusinjektion) eingesetzt. Die Anzahl der Patientendatensätze, bei denen keine ischämischen Gehirnregionen vorlagen, belief sich auf 10. Bei 16 Bilddatensätzen wurden ischämische Gehirnregionen durch die Kontrolluntersuchung identifiziert (Tab. 1).

In den Kontrollbildern wurden ischämische Gebiete durch klinische Experten markiert, indem die Ischämien umrandet wurden. Dann wurden die Ergebnisbilder des Verfahrens mit den Kontrollbildern verglichen. Hierbei wurden die segmentierten Flächen miteinander übereinander gelegt. Wenn diese Überdeckung mindestens 67% der Summe beider Flächen entsprach, wurde die Ischämie durch das automatische Verfahren korrekt erkannt. Dabei wurde angenommen, dass keine Ischämie vorlag, wenn das Ergebnis der automatischen Erkennung eine Fläche von weniger als 3cm^2 hervorbrachte. Dies konnte auf Rauscheinflüsse oder Bewegungsartefakte zurückgeführt werden.

5   Diskussion

Falls keine Minderperfusionen vorhanden sind, segmentiert die Erkennung von Perfusionsstörungen immer die Streifenartefakte und den kontralateralen Gehirnteil, so dass die Nachverarbeitungsschritte (Streifenartefakterkennung, Entfernung des kontralateralen Gehirnteils) notwendig sind. Die Erkennung von

Tabelle 1. Vierfeldertafel der Erkennung von ischämischen Gehirngebieten

Verfahren	Kontrolle	
	ischämisch	nicht ischämisch
ischämisch	13	1
nicht ischämisch	3	9

Streifenartefakten funktioniert auch für andere ultraschallbasierte Perfusions-messmethoden, wie das Diminution Harmonic Imaging (DHI).

Die schnelle Prüfung auf ischämische Gehirnregionen bietet offensichtliche Vorteile. Das hier vorgestellte Verfahren ist gegenüber Rauschen robust und im Vergleich zur manuellen oder Parameterbild–gestützten Auswertung schnell. Insgesamt stellt diese Methode einen wesentlichen Schritt dar, um mit ultraschallbasiertem Harmonic Imaging ischämische Gehirnregionen vollautomatisch zu erkennen und somit die Arbeit des Arztes zu unterstützen.

Eine deutliche Verbesserung der Erkennungsleistung verspricht die Registrierung der B–Bilder. Da Bewegung den dynamische Verlauf der Zeit–Intensitätskurve erheblich stört, wird eine Reduktion von Bewegungsartefakten zu einer verbesserten Detektion von ischämischen Gehirnregionen führen. Die Reduktion von Bewegungsartefakten wird das Ziel weiterer Untersuchungen sein.

Literaturverzeichnis

1. Burns PN. Harmonic imaging with ultrasound contrast agents. Clinical Radiology 1996;51:50.
2. Seidel G, Meyer-Wiethe K. Harmonic Imaging: Eine neue Methode zur sonographischen Darstellung der Hirnperfusion. Nervenarzt 2001;72(1):600–610.
3. Meves S, Wilkening W, Thies T, Eyding J, Ermert H, Postert T. Comparison between echo contrast agent-specific imaging modes and perfusion-weighted magnetic resonance imaging for assessment of brain perfusion. Stroke 2002;33(1):2433–2437.
4. Martina AD, Seidel G, Meyer-Wiethe K, Allemann E. Ultrasound contrast agents for brain perfusion imaging and ischemic stroke therapy - instrumentation in practice. Journal of Neuroimaging 2005;33(1):1530–1537.
5. Eyding J, Wilkening W, Reckhard M. Contrast burst depletion imaging: A new imaging procedure and analysis method for semiquantitative ultrasonic perfusion imaging. Stroke 2002;34(1):77–83.
6. Kier C, Toth D, Schindler LA, Meyer-Wiethe K, Cangür H, Seidel G, et al. Cerebral perfusion imaging with bolus harmonic imaging. Procs SPIE 2005;5750:437–446.
7. Metzler V, Seidel G, Meyer-Wiethe K, Wiesmann M, Aach T. perfusion harmonic imaging of the human brain. Procs SPIE 2003;5035:337–348.
8. Maciak A, Kier C, Seidel G, Meyer-Wiethe K, Aach T. Parameterfreie Erkennung von Ischämien mit ultraschallbasiertem Harmonic Imaging. In: Proceedings BMT 6.–9. September 2006. vol. 1. Zürich; 2006.
9. Jähne B. Digital Image Processing. 6th ed. Berlin Heidelberg: Springer–Verlag; 2005.

Vollautomatisierte Tumordiagnose in der dynamischen MRT der weiblichen Brust

Dirk Mayer[1], Adam Maciak[1], Thomas Rösler[1], Tim Keszler[1],
Heiner Faber[1], Massimo Buscema[2], Marco Mattiuzzi[3], T.W. Vomweg[1]

[1]CADMEI GmbH, Otto-Hahn-Straße 6, 55218 Ingelheim, Deutschland
[2]Semeion Research Centre of Sciences of Communication, Rom, Italien
[3]Bracco Imaging, Via E. Folli 50, Mailand, Italien
Email: dmayer@cadmei.com

Zusammenfassung. Es wird eine automatisierte Prototypensoftware
zur Diagnose von Läsionen in der Kontrastmittel gestützten funktionalen
MRT der weiblichen Brust vorgestellt. Die Software führt auf 4D-Daten
eine Bildverarbeitungspipeline bestehend aus Bewegungskorrektur, Segmentierung, Berechnung von dynamischen und morphologischen Merkmalen sowie Klassifizierung der Merkmale durch Neuronale Netze aus.
Das CAD-System detektiert gut- oder bösartige Läsionen ohne jegliche
Benutzerinteraktion und ist damit als Zweitmeinung verwendbar.

1 Einleitung

Die Diagnose von Brustkrebs in der Kontrastmittel (KM) gestützten MRT ist eine anspruchsvolle und zeitintensive Aufgabe. Die Auswertung wird durch Bewegungsartefakte, falsch-positive Kontrastanreicherungen und der großen Anzahl
an Bildern erschwert. Um eine Diagnose treffen zu können, muss der Radiologe zunächst verschiedene morphologische und dynamische Merkmale aus jeder
verdächtigen Läsion identifizieren und abschließend bewerten. Die Qualität der
Befundung variiert dabei sehr stark mit der Vorgehensweise und Erfahrung des
Radiologen. Um die Auswertung zu standardisieren und die Qualität der Diagnose zu verbessern, wurde ein Prototyp zur vollautomatisierten Erkennung und
Diagnose von Brustläsionen entwickelt.

Einzelne Gruppen haben von unterschiedlichen Bildregistrierungen zur Reduktion von Bewegungsartefakten in der KM gestützten MRT der Brust berich-
tet [1]. Unabhängig davon wurden verschiedene Arten Neuronaler Netze (NN)
zur Erkennung von Läsionen [2, 3] sowie zur Charakterisierung der dynamischen
Merkmale eingesetzt [4, 5]. In einer vorhergehenden Studie unserer Arbeitsgrup-
pe wurde gezeigt, dass NN in der Bewertung dynamischer und morphologischer
Merkmale von kontrastanreichernden Läsionen statistischen Mitteln gegenüber
überlegen sind [6]. Bis heute ist kein anderes System bekannt, das eine Diagnose
durch die Kombination verschiedener Bildverarbeitungsverfahren vollautomatisch generieren kann.

2 Methoden

Alle Untersuchungen der weiblichen Brust wurden auf einem 1,5 Tesla MR-Scanner durchgeführt. Nach einer nativen Aufnahme werden nach der intravenösen Gabe von KM vier weitere Serien in je 72 Sekunden Abstand gemessen [7]. Die unterschiedlich starke Anreicherung des KM im Gewebe kann anhand des Intensitätsverlauf des MR-Signals nachvollzogen werden. Jedes 3D-Volumen besteht aus 512 x 256 x 80 Voxeln mit einer Ortsauflösung von 0,65 x 0,65 x 1,8mm. Die Subtraktion der nativen von den KM angereicherten Bildserien eliminiert Gewebeareale ohne Signalveränderung hebt anreicherndes Gewebe oder potentielle Läsionen hervor.

2.1 Bewegungskorrektur

Während der Untersuchung ergeben sich zwangsläufig Bewegungen durch Herzschlag, Atmung, Vibration des Scanners und späterer Entspannung der Patientin. Diese Bewegungen bewirken Bildartefakte, die zu falsch-positiv detektierten Läsionen führen können. Die Registrierung der weiblichen Brust ist durch den Mangel an starren und kontrastreichen biologischen Landmarken im MR-Bild schwierig. Die Bewegungen können in den verschiedenen Bereichen der Brust unterschiedlich stark sein, benachbarte Regionen können sich in unterschiedliche Richtungen verschieben. Angesichts dieser Aspekte wurde ein nicht-rigides, mono-modales 3D-Registierungsverfahren entwickelt, das speziell an die Bedürfnisse KM-gestützter funktionaler MRT-Bilder der Brust angepasst ist.

Zunächst müssen korrespondierende Landmarken innerhalb zweier Serien, die zu verschiedenen Zeitpunkten aufgenommen wurden, gefunden werden. Die Selektion und das Verfolgen der Landmarken basiert auf einer dreidimensionalen Verallgemeinerung des 2D Kanade-Lucas-Tomasi-Feature-Tracker (KLT) [8]. Die Merkmale werden, nachdem sie einmal in der ersten, nativen Bildserie identifiziert worden sind, fortlaufend in jeder folgenden Serie gesucht, beginnend mit der ursprünglichen Position in der vorhergehenden Serie. Da ein einzelnes Bildvoxel zur Charakterisierung einer wiederauffindbaren Landmarke unzureichend ist, wird ein auf das Merkmalsvoxel positioniertes 3D-Fenster verwendet. Das Tracken eines Merkmals ist nur dann erfolgversprechend, wenn sich innerhalb des Fensters eine charakteristische Struktur zeigt, so dass der Tracking-Algorithmus nur für solche Positionen gestartet wird. Der Algorithmus geht davon aus, dass sich die Charaktereigenschaft innerhalb des Fensters nur geringfügig zwischen den aufeinander folgenden Bilderserien ändert. Die resultierende Liste an Translations-Vektoren ist unregelmäßig über das ganze Bildvolumen verstreut.

Für das Transformieren der Bildinformation der getrackten Bildserien auf das native Volumenbild müssen die Translations-Vektoren der ausgewählten Positionen für jedes Voxel einer Bildserie interpoliert werden. Diese muss dabei sowohl die lokale als auch globale Verschiebungen des Brustgewebes verarbeiten können. Ein schneller Interpolations-Algorithmus für unregelmäßig verteilte Datenmengen wie unter [9] beschrieben wurde zu folgendem 3D-Ansatz erweitert. Ein in einheitlichen Abständen aufgebautes 3D-Raster bestehend aus Kontrollpunkten wird erzeugt und die Translations-Vektoren mittels einer B-Spline Funktion auf seine Kontrollpunkte verteilt. Jeder Translations-Vektor beeinflusst dabei einen Satz von 4x4x4 benachbarten Kontrollpunkten. Die Genauigkeit der Interpolation durch die B-Spline Funktion hängt von der Dichte des Rasters ab. Während ein grobes Raster den globalen Einfluss der Translations-Vektoren widerspiegelt, führt die Verteilung der Vektoren auf einem feineren Raster zu einer größeren lokalen Genauigkeit. Ein Beginnen mit einem groben Raster und immer weiterer Verfeinerung steigert die Genauigkeit, die Werte der Kontrollpunkte nähern sich immer weiter den gegebenen Vektoren an. Abschließend wird eine trilineare Interpolationsfunktion eingesetzt, um die Grauwerte der getrackten Bildserien anhand der Interpolationsergebnisse auf das native Volumenbild abzubilden.

2.2 Segmentierung der Anreicherungen

Zunächst wird jede Anreicherung von Signalintensität (SI) als potentielle Läsion betrachtet. Segmentierungsverfahren mit globalem Schwellwert führen jedoch zu keinem optimalen Ergebnis. Wir verwenden daher eine lokal adaptive Schwellwertsegmentierung, welche den Schwellwert für jede Läsion automatisch bestimmt. Ein iteratives Vorgehen verwendet zusätzliche Regeln um Läsionen vom ebenfalls anreichernden Gewebe zu trennen. Das Verfahren nimmt an, dass der Bereich innerhalb der Subtraktionsserie mit der höchsten SI einer Läsion angehört. Anhand der SI des Hotspots wird ein optimaler Schwellwert zur Segmentierung der Läsion ermittelt. Eine einfache Division durch zwei ist bereits zufriedenstellend.

Nachfolgend wird ein Schwellwert-Seeding auf dem Volumendatensatz gestartet. Das 3D-Seeding resultiert in einer segmentierten Läsion. Die Iteration fährt mit dem Voxel der nächst höchsten Intensität fort und endet, wenn die betrachtete SI unter eine bestimmte Schranke fällt. Eine Regel trennt während der iterativen Segmentierung Läsionen von umgebenden Gewebe: Wenn ein neu segmentiertes Objekt ein oder mehr bereits segmentierte Objekte berührt, wird das zuletzt segmentierte Objekt von der Ergebnisliste der erfolgreich segmentierten Objekte wieder entfernt.

2.3 Morphologie

Zur Bewertung der potentiellen Läsionen und zur Beschreibung von Artefakten (falsch-positiv segmentierten Objekten) extrahiert der Prototyp zunächst in Nachahmung der Bildinterpretation durch einen Radiologen verschiedene morphologische Merkmale.

Neben der Größe der Läsion wird ihr minimaler sowie ihr maximaler Durchmesser berechnet. Die Form eines Objektes ist ein wichtiges Merkmal, da z.B. gutartige Läsionen einer eher rundliche Form zeigen, bösartige Läsionen spikuliert sind und Artefakte oder Gefäße eher länglich erscheinen. Das Verhältnis von Oberfläche zu Volumen der Objekte liefert dafür eine Formbeschreibung, wohingegen die fraktale Dimension in der Lage ist, die Kompaktheit von größeren

Objekten genauer zu beschreiben. Ein Skelettierungs-Algorithmus wird verwendet um vorhandene Spikulationen oder Gefäße zu erfassen. Bösartige Läsionen können zentrale Nekrosen beinhalten, die sich als eingeschlossene Hohlräume in der Segmentierung bestimmen lassen. Während gutartige Läsionen einen scharfen Rand zu dem umliegenden Gewebe bilden, zeigen bösartige Läsionen einen weichen Übergang. Aus diesem Grund werden die angrenzenden Voxel durch einen Dilatations-Algorithmus bestimmt und ihre durchschnittliche SI als ein Maß der Randschärfe berechnet. Abschließend wird die Homogenität der SI innerhalb der Läsion berechnet. Insgesamt wird ein Merkmalsvektor bestehend aus 13 morphologischen Werten zusammengestellt.

Darüber hinaus liefert die Analyse der Dynamik der KM-Anreicherung weitere Informationen: Die durchschnittliche SI der gesamten Läsion wird auf allen Bildserien bestimmt und in einer Zeit-SI-Kurve zusammengestellt. Während die meisten bösartigen Läsionen zu einem schnellen Anstieg aufgrund einer intensiven KM-Aufnahme neigen und ein „Wash-out" infolge eines ebenso schnellen Wiederabgebens des KMs zeigen, tendieren gutartige Läsionen zu einem langsamen aber kontinuierlichen Anreichern. Zusätzlich wird eine zweite Zeit-SI-Kurve der gemittelten SI einer Region um den Hotspot herum bestimmt. Der Verlauf beider Kurven wird anhand von vier fest vorgegebenen Zeitpunkten erfasst, es resultieren weitere acht dynamische Merkmale [10].

2.4 Klassifzierung

Jede segmentierte Läsion wird von einem Vektor aus 21 morphologischen und dynamischen Merkmalen beschrieben. Weil die einzelnen Merkmale nur schwach mit der Bösartigkeit einer Läsion korrelieren [6], setzen wir selbst-reflexive „Feed-Forward" Netze ein, die mit einer modifizierten back-propagation Lernregel trainiert wurden. Ein unabhängiger Trainings-Datensatz von Läsionen mit bekannten histologischen Befunden (nach Biopsie oder durch follow-up MRT-Untersuchungen über mehr als einem Jahr) wurde benutzt um zwei NN zu trainieren. Das erste NN wurde trainiert um Läsionen von Artefakten zu unterscheiden, ein zweites NN lernte Läsionen als gut- oder bösartig zu klassifizieren. Beide Netze sind auf demselben Merkmalsvektor mit 21 morphologischen Werten trainiert worden.

3 Ergebnisse

Das Leistungsverhalten der Prototypsoftware wurde anhand von 71 MRT Untersuchungen, die insgesamt 89 Läsionen mit bekannter Histologie enthielten, von einem Radiologen bewertet. Die durchschnittliche SI der Brust der Subtraktionsserie vor und nach der Bewegungskorrektur wurde um 32% reduziert. Durchschnittlich wurden pro Untersuchung ca. 2500 Objekte segmentiert. Dieser Übersegmentierung wird mit einem einfachen Klassifikator entgegengewirkt, der auf den berechneten Morphologie-Werten basierend zu kleine oder längliche

Objekte verwirft. Die Liste der Läsionen wurde dadurch drastisch auf durchschnittlich ca. 8,6 Objekten pro Untersuchung reduziert. Das erste NN schloss durchschnittlich weitere 6,2 Objekte pro Untersuchung als Artefakte aus. Das zweite NN klassifizierte die verbliebenen 2,4 Läsionen in durchschnittlich 1,5 bösartige und 0,9 gutartigen Befunde pro Untersuchung. Insgesamt wurden 37 der 39 histologisch geprüften, bösartigen Läsionen detektiert und korrekt als bösartig eingestuft. Die zwei verbliebenen Läsionen sind während der Segmentierung verloren gegangen. Die Performance der Detektion und Klassifikation bezogen auf die bösartigen Läsionen beläuft sich auf 95% Sensitivität and 92% Spezifität.

4   Schlussfolgerung

Eine geschickte Kombination unterschiedlicher Methoden der Bildverarbeitung, nämlich der nicht rigiden 3D-Bildregistierung, adaptive Schwellwertsegmentierung, morphologischen Merkmalsbestimmungen und künstlicher NN führen zu einem leistungsstarken Softwareprototyp für eine vollautomatisierte Computerdiagnose. Weitere Untersuchungen an größeren und heterogeneren Patientenkollektiven werden benötigt, um diesen Softwareprototyp als zuverlässige Zweitmeinung zu festigen.

Literaturverzeichnis

1. Sivaramakrishna R. 3D breast image registration: A review. Technol Cancer Res Treat 2005;4:39–48.
2. Middleton I, Damper RI. Segmentation of magnetic resonance images using a combination of neural networks and active contour models. Med Eng Phys 2004;26:71–86.
3. el Kwae EA, et al. Detection of suspected malignant patterns in three-dimensional magnetic resonance breast images. J Digit Imaging 1998;11:83–93.
4. Lucht RE, Knopp MV, Brix G. Classification of signal-time curves from dynamic MR mammography by neural networks. Magn Reson Imaging 2001;19:51–57.
5. Vergnaghi D, Monti A, Setti E, Musumeci R. A use of a neural network to evaluate contrast enhancement curves in breast magnetic resonance images. J Digit Imaging 2001;14:58–59.
6. Vomweg TW, Buscema M. Improved artificial neural networks in prediction of malignancy of lesions in contrast-enhanced MR-mammography. Med Phys 2003;30:2350–2359.
7. Vomweg TW, Teifke A, Kunz RP, et al. Combination of low and high resolution sequences in two orientations for dynamic contrast-enhanced MRI of the breast: more than a compromise. Eur Radiol 2004;14:1732–1742.
8. Shi J, Tomasi C. Good features to track. IEEE Comp Vis Pattern Recognition 1994; 593–600.
9. Lee S, Wolberg G, Shin SY. Scattered data interpolation with multilevel B-splines. IEEE Vis Comp Graphics 1997;3(3):228–244.
10. Heywang-Koebrunner S, Bick U, Bradley WG, et al. International investigation of breast MRI: results of a multicentre study. Eur Radiol 2001;11(4):531–46.

Complete Digital Iconic and Textual Annotation for Mammography

Thomas Wittenberg[1], Matthias Elter[1] and Rüdiger Schulz-Wendtland[2]

[1]Fraunhofer Institute for Integrated Circuits IIS, Erlangen
[2]Dept. of Gynecological Radiology, University Hospital Erlangen
E-mail: thomas.wittenberg@iis.fraunhofer.de

Abstract. This work aims to propose an interactive method for a iconic and textual annotation of digital mammograms. The suggested annotation tool consists of a semantic network to represent all information about a set of mammograms obtained from experts in a structured manner based on the BIRADS standard, a correlated XML file system for persistence, data exchange and storage, and a graphical user interface, allowing a combination of iconic and textual annotation. This approach allows a complete annotation of all findings in a set of mammograms in a structured way, which is also machine readable and interpretable. Thus, systematically annotated image data sets can be used for structured information retrieval as well as case based reasoning systems for computer assisted diagnosis (CAD). Furthermore, such a digital annotation system can be used to replace paper reports and hence avoid unnecessary media breaks during the process of the examination and documentation.

1 Introduction

In the past years, direct digital mammography (DDM) systems have entered clinical routine and have replaced conventional screen film systems (SFS) for the acquisition of mammograms [1] in the context of screening and diagnostic processes. Nevertheless, currently in clinics worldwide, the steps to analyze the acquired digital mammograms with the goal to detect lesions such as calcifications or spiculated masses, remain the same as before. Thus, the chain of steps used to analyze the mammograms properly is related to a series of breaks between different types of media. Such breaks occur, when the digital mammogram is released on analogue film, the analogue film is viewed on a light-screen, an optical magnifying glass is used to analyze details in the detected lesions, all detected lesions are marked, noted and documented on a structured paper report, and finally the information from the paper reports are transferred back to a digital database. Along this chain of media breaks from digital images to paper reports and back to digital case databases, loss of information has to be considered. Such loss is related to information depicted in the mammograms and not recorded on the paper reports, or to information marked on the reports and not transferred completely to the digital database. Especially iconic markers on the paper formular denoting the relative positions of lesions with respect to the viewing angle cannot be transferred into the standard case databases at all.

2   State of the Art and New Contribution

Currently, some PACS systems allow the annotation of overlay masks and markers directly into the radiographic images, which can be stored into the DICOM image files in the context of building structured reports. The drawback of this solution is, that only the iconic part of the mammogram is stored in the DICOM file, while most parts of the BIRADS documentation sheet are left undocumented. An approach collecting all information screening has been introduced by [2]. While we focus on the annotation of mammograms only, this work takes a much broader view and tries to organize the complete screening process, including ultrasound images.

One new notion of our work is the avoidance of the named media breaks during the diagnostic process between the image acquisition and the documentation. Secondly, using one single and common medium for image acquisition, annotation and storage, a consistent and complete description and documentation of a mammography examination can be obtained. Finally, such a unified and standardized documentation and annotation of mammography examinations and cases can be used to build consistent reference image data-sets.

3   Methods

To overcome these restrictions and media breaks, we propose the use of a digital annotation tool, which simultaneously allows the iconic annotation of regions in the images as well as a structured textual report. Such an annotation has the purpose to describe the contents of the images with respect to certain applications in a machine readable manner. For a proper documentation of mammograms, this means that all findings of lesions have to be marked and described properly. Our annotation tool consists of major components: For the representation of knowledge and facts a semantic network model is applied, implemented as a hierarchical, multi-dimensional data structure, cf. Sec. 3.1. Within a certain problem domain, this data structure organizes all related image views, the objects depicted in the images and delineated or marked by the user, as well as their individual parts and features. Secondly, a graphical user interface allows interactive annotation of image data and acquisition of application related knowledge, cf. Sec. 3.2. Finally, a XML-data structure is used for persistence, archiving and communication.

3.1   Knowledge Representation

A possible model to organize application knowledge needed to analyse the content of images applying image processing methods as well as to represent and structure information acquired and obtained from image analysis procedures are *semantic networks* [3]. A semantic network can be defined as a labeled, directed and acyclic graph $\mathcal{G} = (\mathcal{V}, \mathcal{E})$. The set $\mathcal{V} = \{v_1, v_2, \ldots, v_n\}$ is a set of vertices (nodes) representing concepts, ideas, physical or conceptual objects, or features of objects. $\mathcal{E} = \{e_1, e_2, \ldots, e_m\}$ is a subset of $\mathcal{V} \times \mathcal{V}$ and denotes edges (or arcs) connecting *ordered* pairs of vertecis $(v_i, v_j) \in \mathcal{V}$. Edges denote relations between objects. The most important types of relations used within semantical networks are relations between classes and subclasses of objects such as *is a, has a* or *has feature*, and instance-relations between object-instances and object-classes. Within the scope of our activities — the image-based computer-assisted detection (CAD) of conspicuous regions and lesions and their pre-classification — a semantic network $\mathcal{N} = (\mathcal{I}, \mathcal{V}, \mathcal{E}, \mathcal{O})$ is applied to represent knowledge depicted in and obtained from a set of images $\mathcal{I} = \{I_1, I_2, \ldots, I_n\}$. Since the images are usually related to a distinct imaging modality (mammography), a certain organ system (breast) and a special problem domain (mamma cancer diagnosis), a standardized *ontology* $\mathcal{O}$ is used to describe the corresponding image contents. For the classification of lesions depicted in mammograms, the BI-RADS (Breast Imaging - Reporting And Data System) standard of the ACR [4] is applied. Two different types of views onto a semantic network can be considered. With respect to the annotation of mammograms, where an expert describes the image contents, a knowledge-based view on the semantic network has to be taken. In this case, the vertices v_i in the network correlate to physical objects or entities, such as the breasts, landmarks on the breast (e.g. mammilla), as well as any lesions, speculae, calcifications, clusters of micro-calcifications, etc. depicted in the images. Regarding the images from a machine vision – data-driven – point of view, the vertices represent single pixels or features, groups of pixels, sub-regions or regions, higher-level and semantic meaningful objects, as well as images or hyper-images, depicting the objects from different views. Even though different views can be taken, on a practical level the vertices of both views can be projected onto each other.

The edges e_i denote logical or physical relations between different objects as well as relations to features of an object. In the context of mammogram annotation, the edges represent relations between different objects such as 'micro-calcification M_i belongs to calcification cluster C_i', 'breast B_{left} has mamilla M_{left}', 'lesion L_i is of type B', or 'lesion L_i has textural features c_j'.

Fig. 1 depicts two different views of the semantic network used to represent knowledge acquired from mammograms by the annotation process. The left side represents the data-driven approach, starting at the bottom with pixels and features, which are combined to form regions and objects and finally construct complete images. On the right side, the corresponding knowledge-driven approach is shown, starting with views (*cc* and *mlo*) of a breast, describing its quadrants and landmarks, and finally any depicted lesions and their features.

3.2 User Interfaces

To annotate image objects with a certain form and class, they have to be marked on the screen to provide the iconic annotation. By drawing the contours of the objects, and flood-filling them with a pre-defined class colour, each image object is annotated. In the internal data structure, the object is represented either by a binary pixel mask, or as a chain code. Both can be saved in standard image file

Fig. 1. Overview of the organisation of the hierarchical semantic network used to describe the image contents in digital mammograms

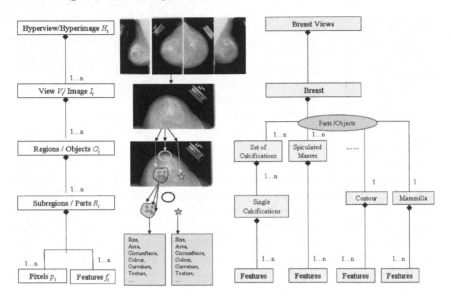

formats. If an object is depicted as several parts (e.g. a cluster of calcifications), all parts can individually be marked and then be grouped to a higher level object. If more than one image is in the data set, one physical object may have several image entities, meaning the same object can be seen from different views. E.g., usually the mammilla or a lesion are depicted from different observation angles (*cc* and *mlo*). Such connections between different entities can also be tagged and visualized. Furthermore, for each annotated lesion as well as for the complete set of images (usually 2 views of each breast), the most important parts of the BIRADS standard can be annotated using pre-defined check-boxes and radio-buttons. This part of the digital annotation mimics completely the mammography documentation sheet.

Fig. 2 shows a view of the user interface for the annotation of mammograms. The left window pane (usually depicted on an upright monitor) shows the images and the iconic annotation. The right window pane (on a second monitor) depicts the textual part of the BIRADS documentation sheet as well as the demographic data of the patient.

4   Results

The proposed annotation tool for digital mammograms is currently applied in the Department for Gynaecological Radiology of the University Hospital Erlangen with several goals: First, the annotation tool is used to obtain a complete and machine-readable description of the image contents of mammograms with respect to any diagnostic findings, in the context of building a *reference image*

Fig. 2. User interface for the iconic and textual annotations of mammograms

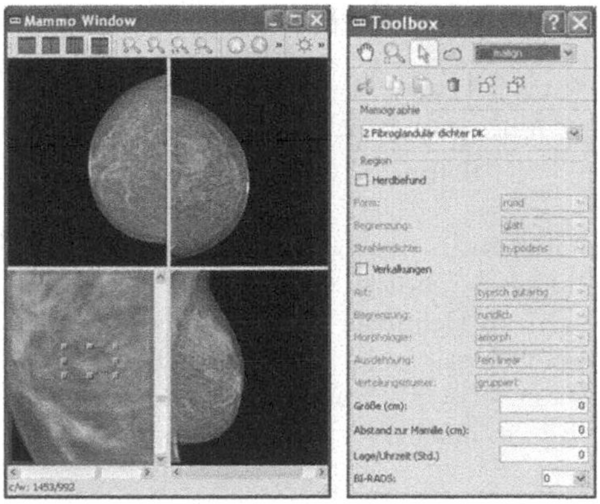

database (RID). Secondly, the thus obtained formal annotated RID will be used as a reference (gold-standard, ground truth) for the evaluation of image analysis algorithms for the automatic detection of lesions in the context of computer assisted diagnosis of mammograms. Furthermore, the RID will used for automatic information retrieval in the context of a case-based reasoning system. Currently, about 250 complete image data sets have been entered in the data base. Additionally, the annotation of each RID-set has been cross-checked and validated with the corresponding histological findings.

5   Discussion

The use of a complete and unified digital annotation mechanism is capable to support and enhance the process of mammography examinations and screening by unifying the interfaces between the different steps, such as image acquisition, image analysis, description of findings and documentation. Furthermore, using the described annotation tool, a complete, formal and machine-readable reference database for mammography can be obtained.

References

1. Krug B, et al. Vergleich der digitalen direkten Flachdetektor- und der analogen Film-Folien-Technik in der Darstellung normaler anatomischer Strukturen der weiblichen Brust. Geburtsh Frauenheilk 2006;66:171–178.
2. Dashmahapatra S, et al. Facilitating multi-disciplinary knowledge-based support for breast cancer screening. Int J Healthc Tech Management 2006;7(5):403–20.
3. Niemann H, Sagerer G, Schröder S, Kummert F. ERNEST: A semantic network system for pattern understanding. IEEE PAMI 1990;12(9):883 – 905.
4. American College of Radiology. Breast Imaging Reporting and Data System (BI-RADS©) Atlas; 2006.

Referenzdaten für die computerassistierte Diagnose in der Mammographie

M. Elter[1], A. Horsch[2], R. Schulz-Wendtland[3], H. Sittek[5], M. Athelogou[4], G. Schmidt[4], T. Wittenberg[1]

[1]Fraunhofer-Institut für Integrierte Schaltungen IIS, Erlangen
[2]Inst. für Medizinische Statistik und Epidemiologie, TU München
[3]Definiens AG, München
[4]Radiologisches Institut der Universität Erlangen-Nürnberg
[5]Diagnostisches Mammazentrum München
Email: matthias.elter@iis.fraunhofer.de

Zusammenfassung. Die Computerassistierte Diagnose (CAD) in der Mammographie hat durch den europaweiten Aufbau von nationalen Screeningprogrammen in den letzten Jahren stark an Bedeutung gewonnen. Für die Evaluierung und vor allem für den Vergleich von CAD Algorithmen sind öffentlich zugängliche Referenzdaten nötig. Am Fraunhofer IIS wird derzeit eine Referenzdatenbank für die Mammographie aufgebaut, die die veralteten bestehenden Datenbanken ersetzen bzw. ergänzen soll. Dabei wurde auf dem Stand der Gerätetechnik entsprechende Bildqualität und zeitgemäße ikonische und textuelle Annotation geachtet. Die Veröffentlichung dieser Referenzdaten wird es Forschungsgruppen erlauben, CAD Algorithmen für die Mammographie auf umfangreichen und aktuellen Referenzdaten zu evaluieren und ihre Leistungsfähigkeit miteinander zu vergleichen.

1 Einleitung

Am Fraunhofer Institut für Integrierte Schaltungen (IIS) wird im Kontext eines mehrjährigen Projektes zur Computerassistierten Diagnose für die Mammographie eine Referenzdatenbank von digitalen Mammographien mit ikonischer und textueller Annotation aufgebaut. Die öffentliche Verfügbarkeit dieser Referenzdaten wird es Forschungsgruppen aus aller Welt erlauben, CAD Algorithmen für die Mammographie auf umfangreichen und aktuellen Referenzdaten zu evaluieren und ihre Leistungsfähigkeit miteinander zu vergleichen. Die Referenzdaten werden derzeit im Radiologischen Institut der Universität Erlangen-Nürnberg und im Diagnostischen Mammazentrum München erfasst, annotiert und kreuzvalidiert. Über die Projektlaufzeit von drei Jahren soll die Datenbank von derzeit 250 auf insgesamt 1000 Fälle erweitert werden.

2 Stand der Forschung und Fortschritt durch den Beitrag

Seit der Erstbeschreibung eines Systems zur computerassistierten Analyse von Mammographien durch Winsberg im Jahr 1967 [1] haben sich zahlreiche Arbeitsgruppen mit dieser Problematik beschäftigt. Obwohl seither unzählige Lösungsansätze für diese Problemstellung veröffentlicht wurden (z.B. [2, 3, 4]), stehen weltweit nur zwei öffentliche Referenzdatenbanken zur Evaluation und zum Vergleich der verschiedenen Ansätze zur Verfügung. So hat die *Mammographic Image Analysis Society* bereits 1994 eine 320 Fälle umfassende Referenzdatenbank für die Mammographie veröffentlicht [5]. Die zweite Referenzdatenbank stammt von der University of South Florida [6] und umfasst zrika 2.500 Fälle. Beide Referenzdatenbanken stammen aus den frühen neunziger Jahren. Durch die rasante Weiterentwicklung der Akquisitionsgeräte und vor allem durch den Wechsel von analoger auf digitale Technik gilt die Bildqualität der enthaltenden Mammographien mittlerweile als veraltet. De facto steht derzeit weltweit keine Referenzdatenbank mit Mammographien, die dem aktuellen Stand der Gerätetechnik entsprechen, zur Verfügung.

Neben der, aus heutiger Sicht, unzureichenden Bildqualität der bestehenden Referenzdaten, ist auch der Umfang und die Qualität der Annotation der Daten nicht mehr zeitgemäß. So hat das *American College of Radiology* (ACR) mit dem *Breast Imaging Reporting and Data System* (BI-RADS) [7] in der Zwischenzeit einen weltweit angewandten Standard für die Befundung und damit auch Annotation von Mammographien entwickelt bzw. weiterentwickelt. Dieser umfasst neben der Klassifizierung von Läsionen wie Herdbefunden und Mikrokalzifizierungen auch eine standardisierte Beschreibung ihrer konkreten Eigenschaften wie der Form, Verteilung oder Begrenzung.

Um mögliche Risikofaktoren und Symptome des Mammakarzinoms zu erfassen, lassen Radiologen umfangreiche Anamnesedaten, wie zum Beispiel Angaben zu Krebserkrankungen in der Familie, in ihre Diagnose miteinfließen. Um eine höhere Erkennungsrate zu erzielen werden derartige Zusatzinformationen zunehmend auch von CAD Systemen berücksichtigt. Die beiden bestehenden Referenzdatenbanken enthalten aber leider keine bzw. nur sehr wenig Anamnesedaten.

Eine zeitgemäße Referenzdatenbank sollte also neben einer ikonischen Annotation von Läsionen auch eine auf der BI-RADS Nomenklatur basierende textuelle Annotation der Eigenschaften dieser Läsionen sowie textuelle Anamnesedaten enthalten. Daher wird am Fraunhofer IIS eine Referenzdatenbank für die Mammographie aufgebaut. Sie enthält im Gegensatz zu den bestehenden Referenzdatenbanken ausschließlich mit modernen volldigitalen Geräten gewonnenes Bildmaterial. Die Annotation enthält neben BI-RADS konformen und kreuzvalidierten Diagnosen auch umfangreiche Anamnesedaten.

3   Methoden

Die im Aufbau befindliche Referenzdatenbank enthält Mammographien die im Radiologischen Institut der Universität Erlangen-Nürnberg und im Diagnostischen Mammazentrum München erfasst werden. Jeder Datensatz umfasst in der Regel zwei Mammographien (die Standardansichten medio-lateral oblique und cranio caudal) je Brust. Am Radiologischen Institut der Universität Erlangen-

Abb. 1. Ikonisch und textuell annotierte Mammographie (rechte Brust medio-lateral oblique) aus einem typischen Datensatz der Referenzdatenbank

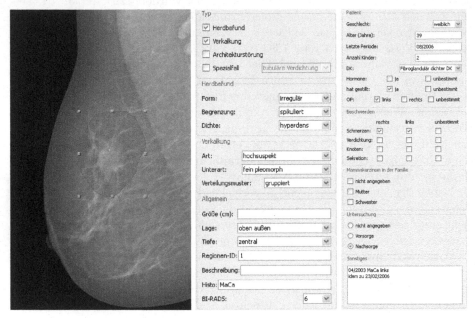

Nürnberg kommen dazu zwei volldigitale Geräte (Siemens Mammomat Novation DR) und am Diagnostischen Mammazentrum München ein Speicherfoliengerät von Agfa zum Einsatz. Neben den Mammographien im DICOM Format enthält jeder Datensatz textuelle sowie ikonische Annotation. Zur einfachen Weiterverarbeitung ist die gesamte Annotation im XML Format gespeichert.

3.1   Ikonische Annotation

Die ikonische Annotation von Läsionen erfolgt mittels einer Annotationssoftware die am Fraunhofer IIS speziell für die Annotation von Mammographien entwickelt wurde. Läsionen werden dazu vom Befunder mit der Maus bzw. am Touchscreen eingezeichnet. Diese eingezeichneten Regionen dienen zusammen mit einer zugeordneten Klassifizierung nach BI-RADS als Ground-Truth Daten. Sie werden in den XML basierten Annotationsdateien sowohl vektoriell als Polygonzug, wie auch rasterorientiert mittels einer Binärmaske gespeichert.

3.2   Textuelle Annotation

Jede ikonische Annotation einer Läsion ergänzen zusätzliche, der BI-RADS Nomenklatur entsprechende, textuelle Annotationen. Diese umfassen bei Mikrokalzifizierungen die Art, Unterart und das Verteilungsmuster des Kalks und bei

Herdbefunden die Form, Begrenzung sowie Dichte des Herdes. Sowohl bei Mikrokalzifizierungen als auch bei Herden umfasst die textuelle Annotation zusätzlich die Größe und Lage der Läsion sowie den histologischen Befund.

Neben der textuellen Beschreibung von Läsionen umfasst ein Referenzdatensatz auch textuelle Anamnesedaten. Diese beinhalten das Alter, Geschlecht und Gewicht des Patienten, sowie das Datum der letzten Periode, die Anzahl der Kinder, Angaben über verabreichte Hormonpräparate und frühere Brustoperationen. Dazu kommen Angaben zu Beschwerden wie Schmerzen, tastbaren Knoten oder Sekretion der Brust sowie Angaben zu Mammakarzinomen in der Familie.

3.3 Pseudonymisierung

Um die persönlichen Daten der Patienten zu schützen ist es erforderlich alle personenbezogenen Daten, die Rückschlüsse auf die Identität der Patienten liefern können, aus den Mammographiedaten zu entfernen (Anonymisierung). Um einzelne Patientengeschichten langfristig (mehrere Mammographiekontrollen über Monate oder Jahre verteilt) verfolgen zu können, ist es aber gleichzeitig wichtig, Mammographiedatensätze ein und desselben Patienten, die zu verschiedenen Zeitpunkten erstellt wurden, einander zuordnen zu können. Daher werden die Patientendaten für die Referenzdatenbank pseudonymisiert.

Bei der Pseudonymisierung wird der Name oder ein anderes Identifikationsmerkmal durch ein eindeutiges Pseudonym ersetzt, um die Identifizierung des Betroffenen auszuschließen. Im Gegensatz zur Anonymisierung bleiben bei der Pseudonymisierung Bezüge verschiedener Datensätze, die auf dieselbe Art pseudonymisiert wurden, erhalten. Konkret wird für die Mammographiereferenzdatenbank aus dem Patientennamen und dem Geburtsdatum mittels der MD5 (Message Digest Algorithm 5) [8] Hashfunktion ein Hashwert gebildet und als Pseudonym verwendet. Auf diese Weise können Mammographiedatensätze ein und desselben Patienten sicher einander zugeordnet werden ohne die Annonymität der Patienten zu gefährden.

4 Ergebnisse

Am Fraunhofer IIS wird zur Zeit eine umfangreiche Referenzdatenbank für die Mammographie aufgebaut und anschließend öffentlich verfügbar gemacht. Die Datenbank umfasst derzeit 250 Fälle. Für die textuelle und ikonische Annotation der Daten wurde eine Annotationssoftware entwickelt, die eine Annotation von Mammographien anhand der Nomenklatur des BI-RADS Standards erlaubt. Art und Umfang der Annotation richtet sich neben den Vorgaben des BI-RADS Standards vor allem nach den Anforderungen moderner CAD Systeme für die Mammographie. Das Problem der Anonymisierung von Patientendaten wurde mittels eines Pseudonymisierungsansatzes gelöst. Ein typischer Datensatz der Referenzdatenbank ist in Abb. 1 dargestellt.

5 Diskussion

Die neue Referenzdatenbank für die Mammographie ist eine Alternative zu den beiden bestehenden aber veralteten frei zugänglichen Datenbanken. Durch den Einsatz von modernen volldigitalen Akquisitionsgeräten ist die Bildqualität deutlich höher als die der bisher verfügbaren Referenzdaten. Neben den Bilddaten und der ikonischen Annotation von relevanten Bildbereichen besteht ein Datensatz auch aus textueller Annotation der Eigenschaften von Läsionen sowie der Patientengeschichte. Die Referenzdaten zeichnen sich daher auch durch einen größeren Umfang an Zusatzinformationen aus. Diese Informationen können vor allem in wissensbasierten Systemen oder für das fallbasierte Schließen verwendet werden. Neben dem Einsatz zum Training, zur Evaluation und zum Vergleich von CAD Systemen für die Mammographie eignen sich die annotierten Daten auch als Fallbeispiele für die medizinische Aus- und Weiterbildung.

Danksagung

Diese Arbeit wurde von der Bayerischen Forschungsstiftung im Rahmen des Projektes Mammo-iCAD gefördert.

Literaturverzeichnis

1. Winsberg F, Elkin M, Marcy J, Bordaz V, Weymouth W. Detection of radiographic abnormalities in mammograms by means of optical scanning and computer analysis. Radiology 1967;89:211–215.
2. Yu Songyang, Guan Ling. A CAD system for the automatic detection of clustered microcalcifications in digitized mammogram films. IEEE Transactions on medical imaging 2000; 115–126.
3. Peitgen ThomasNetsch*andHeinzOtto. Scale-Space signatures for the detection of clustered Microcalcifications in digital mammograms. IEEE Transactions on medical imaging 1999;18(9).
4. Linda J Warren Burhenne,Susan A Wood, et al. Potential contribution of computer-aided detection to the sensitivity of screening mammography. Radiology 2000;215(2):554–562.
5. Suckling J, Parker J, Dance D, Astley S, Hutt I, Boggis C, et al. The mammographic images analysis society digital mammogram databases. Exerpta Medica International Congress Series 1069 1994; 375–378.
6. Heath M, Bowyer K, Kopans D, Moore R, Jr PKegelmeyer. The Digital Database for Screening Mammography. In: The Proceedings of the 5th International Workshop on Digital Mammography. Madison, WI, USA: Medical Physics Publishing; 2000.
7. American College of Radiology. Breast Imaging Reporting and Data System (BI-RADS©) Atlas; 2006.
8. Rivest R. Request for comments (RFC) 1321 - The MD5 message-digest algorithm. http://www.ietf.org/rfc/rfc1321.txt; 1992.

A New Class of Distance Measures for Registration of Tubular Models to Image Data

Thomas Lange[1], Hans Lamecker[2], Michael Hünerbein[1], Sebastian Eulenstein[1], Siegfried Beller[1], Peter M. Schlag[1]

[1]Klinik für Chirurgie und Chirurgische Onkologie,
Charité - Universitätsmedizin Berlin, 13125 Berlin
[2]Zuse-Institut Berlin, 14195 Berlin
Email: thomas.lange@charite.de

Abstract. In some registration applications additional user knowledge is available, which can improve and accelerate the registration process, especially for non-rigid registration. This is particularly important in the transfer of pre-operative plans to the operating room, e.g. for navigation. In case of tubular structures, such as vessels, a geometric representation can be extracted via segmentation and skeletonization. We present a new class of distance measures based on global filter kernels to compare such models efficiently with image data. The approach is validated in a non-rigid registration application with Powerdoppler ultrasound data.

1 Introduction

The importance and clinical use of 3D planning systems [1] in liver surgery is increasing. First navigation systems based on intra-operative 3D ultrasound have been developed and clinically applied [2]. Until now the transfer of pre-operative models and plans to the patient in the operating room (OR) is mentally performed by the surgeon. Robust and fast methods are needed for a precise multimodal non-rigid registration of the pre-operative data and the intra-operative 3D ultrasound image volume.

Although efficient implementations of parametric (multilevel B-splines) [3] as well as non-parametric [4] non-rigid image-based registration methods have been developed they are still very time-consuming for the intra-operative use. Only few papers and only for rigid transformations have been published regarding multi-modal registration of ultrasound with CT/MR data [5].

One of the main building blocks of a registration method is a suitable distance measure. The focus of this paper is on the definition of a new distance measure. Different distance measures for multi-modal registration have been published. These measures assume a functional (Correlation Ratio) [5], statistical (Mutual Information) [6] or locally affine relationship (Local Correlation Coefficient) [7] between the template and reference intensity values of corresponding image points. On the contrary Haber et al. [8] (Normalized Gradient Field) and Droske et al. [9] used measures based on the morphology of the image data to be independent of the actual intensity values.

The incorporation of previous knowledge about the characteristics of the imaging modality or the geometry of relevant anatomical structures potentially leads to a more robust and efficient registration process. Henn et el. [10] suppress a known unwanted area (a lesion) in their distance measure. A more general formulation of weighted distance measures based on user-defined masks is presented by Schumacher et al. [11].

The idea of our approach is to incorporate previous knowledge in terms of extracted vessel models from pre-operative data and their special tube-like structure. In a typical computer-assisted liver surgery planning process the vessels are segmented from CT/MR data and the one-dimensional set of vessel center lines $C \subset \mathbb{R}^3$ are explicitly extracted via skeletonization. A hybrid distance measure comparing this data directly with intra-operative intensity data is proposed. It is based on the work of Aylward et al. [12], where a measure is presented which evaluates the response of a local Gaussian filter at each point on vessel center lines. The sum of all these filter responses is maximized assuming a high response in the presence of a vessel in the intra-operative data. However, this approach fails for non-rigid registration. Therefore, we reformulate the presented measure (section 2) and improve it by using a more appropriate vessel detecting filter class (section 3). The approach is validated in a non-rigid registration application with Powerdoppler ultrasound data (section 4).

2   Variational Reformulation of Aylward's Distance Measure

The new distance measure is formulated in the parametric variational registration framework, but it is equally suitable for non-parametric approaches. We reformulate Aylward's measure in this framework to illustrate similarities and differences to the new measure.

Let $\Omega \subset \mathbb{R}^3$ be the image domain. For a reference image $\mathbf{R} : \Omega \to \mathbb{R}$ and a template image $\mathbf{T} : \Omega \to \mathbb{R}$ a parametric transformation $\varphi_{\mathbf{a}} : \mathbb{R}^3 \to \mathbb{R}^3$ is sought, which minimizes the following functional by deforming $\mathbf{T}$:

$$J(\mathbf{R}, \mathbf{T}; \mathbf{a}) = D(\mathbf{R}, \mathbf{T}(\varphi_{\mathbf{a}}(\mathbf{x}))) \to min \qquad (1)$$

In the case of the well-known B-spline approach [3], the parameters $\mathbf{a}$ are the positions of the control grid points. The distance measure D determines the similarity between $\mathbf{R}$ and $\mathbf{T}$. In the following the abbreviation $\mathbf{T_a}(\mathbf{x}) := \mathbf{T}(\varphi_{\mathbf{a}}(\mathbf{x}))$ is used. For efficiency reasons, the pre-operative CT/MR data is chosen as reference $\mathbf{R}$ and the intra-operative Powerdoppler ultrasound data as template $\mathbf{T}$. The clinically relevant deformation from $\mathbf{T}$ to $\mathbf{R}$ is computed subsequently by inverting $\varphi_{\mathbf{a}}$.

Let $r : C \to \mathbb{R}^+$ denote the radius and $\mathbf{t} : C \to \mathbb{R}^3$ the tangential direction of the pre-operatively generated vessel center lines C. The idea of Aylward et al. is to determine a filter response at each point of the center lines and to integrate all those filter responses: the image data is locally convolved with a Gaussian kernel adapted to the radius r at this point. The presented distance measure can be formulated essentially (neglecting additional weighting) as:

$$D_G[C(\mathbf{R}), r(\mathbf{R}), \mathbf{T}; \mathbf{a}] = -\int_C \int_\Omega G(\mathbf{x} - \mathbf{y}, r(\mathbf{y})) \mathbf{T_a}(\mathbf{x}) \, d\mathbf{x} \, d\mathbf{y} \qquad (2)$$

with $G(\mathbf{x}, \sigma) = e^{-\frac{\mathbf{x}^T \mathbf{x}}{2\sigma^2}}$.

The order of integration can be exchanged. Instead of convolving all points $\mathbf{y} \in C$ on the vessel center lines with a local kernel G all local kernels can be integrated first and then the resulting global kernel

$$\mathbf{P}_G(\mathbf{x}) = \int_C G(\mathbf{x} - \mathbf{y}, r(\mathbf{y})) \, d\mathbf{y} \qquad (3)$$

can be multiplied with the template $\mathbf{T}$. Thus, we may re-parameterize the distance measure D_G in terms of a global kernel P_G

$$D(\mathbf{P}_G, \mathbf{T}; \mathbf{a}) = -\int_\Omega \mathbf{T_a}(\mathbf{x}) \mathbf{P}_G(\mathbf{x}) \, d\mathbf{x} \qquad (4)$$

such that the expressions $D_G[\cdot]$ of (2) and $D(\cdot)$ of (4) are equal. This implies that the global kernel $\mathbf{P}_G$ can be computed pre-operatively and only the cross correlation of $\mathbf{P}_G$ and the template image $\mathbf{T}$ has to be determined intra-operatively in each iteration of the registration.

Although the Gaussian filter G not only gives high responses to tube-like structures but also to other bright structures, the measure is shown to work quite well on the data of Aylward et al. However, the distance measure is inappropriate for non-rigid registration. Optimizing the deformation of the data leads to an enlargement of the vessels and thus in an increase of bright voxels until, after few optimization steps, the image is completely bright.

3   New Distance Measure Based on Vesselness Filter

To overcome the drawback of the approach of Aylward et al. we propose to use filter kernels, which give high responses for tube-like structures of similar radius and direction. A similar kind of vesselness filter was published for example by Frangi et al. [13]. They analyze the eigenvalues $|\lambda_1| \le |\lambda_2| \le |\lambda_3|$ of the Hessian matrix $\mathbf{H}$ for each voxel. The eigenvector $\mathbf{v}_1$ corresponding to λ_1 points in the direction of the vessel. For bright vessels on a dark background the eigenvalues have the property: $\lambda_1 \approx 0$ and $\lambda_1 \ll \lambda_2 \approx \lambda_3$. Frangi et al. define a scalar valued vesselness function depending on this property. Because the radii of the vessels are unknown, the vesselness response is calculated at multiple scales by computing the Hessian with Gaussian derivatives at multiple scales. At every voxel the vesselness value with the highest response is selected and the corresponding scale represents the radius of the vessel.

Since the vessels are parameterized explicitly by their radius and direction, so is the filter kernel. Let us define a local coordinate system at each center line point $\mathbf{y}$ by two normal directions $\mathbf{n}_1, \mathbf{n}_2 : C \mapsto \mathbb{R}^3$, $\mathbf{n}_1(\mathbf{y}) \perp \mathbf{n}_2(\mathbf{y})$, perpendicular to $\mathbf{t}(\mathbf{y})$. Motivated by the vesselness filters we define a filter kernel based on the sum of the second Gaussian derivatives in the two normal directions. This results in a Laplacian filter in the normal plane which is Gaussian weighted in the vessel direction. These second Gaussian derivatives

$$G_{\mathbf{xx}}(\mathbf{x}, \sigma) = \left(\frac{x^2}{\sigma^4} - \frac{1}{\sigma^2} \right) G(\mathbf{x}, \sigma) \qquad (5)$$

are defined for $\sigma = \sqrt{2}r$, such that the zero crossings of the kernel are located at the vessel radius. The kernel has to be transformed to the position of a center line point $\mathbf{y}$ and orientation of the local coordinate system $\mathbf{z} = [\mathbf{t}, \mathbf{n}_1, \mathbf{n}_2] (\mathbf{x} - \mathbf{y})$. This yields the following filter kernel:

$$L(\mathbf{x}, \mathbf{y}, r, \mathbf{t}, \mathbf{n}_1, \mathbf{n}_2)) = G_{\mathbf{z}_2\mathbf{z}_2}(\mathbf{z}, r) + G_{\mathbf{z}_3\mathbf{z}_3}(\mathbf{z}, r) \qquad (6)$$

and subsequently the global kernel

$$\mathbf{P}_L(\mathbf{x}) = \int_C L(\mathbf{x}, \mathbf{y}, r, \mathbf{t}, \mathbf{n}_1, \mathbf{n}_2) \, d\mathbf{y} \qquad (7)$$

which replaces $\mathbf{P}_G$ in equation (4).

4   Results

In order to qualitatively validate the proposed distance measure we use the measure in a multilevel B-Spline scheme (without effective multi-resolution strategy) to register artificially deformed data. Vessel center lines are extracted with radii from real intra-operative 3D Powerdoppler ultrasound data. These center lines are deformed by a realistic B-spline deformation. The global kernel $\mathbf{P}_L$ is determined on the deformed center lines (Fig. 1a) and rigidly (Fig. 1b) resp. non-rigidly (Fig. 1c) registered. The deformation is substantially reduced and the original state is recovered well from a visual point of view. It cannot be expected that the original state can be perfectly reproduced by the registration algorithm, since segmentation, skeletonization and as well as radius computation introduce certain inaccuracies.

5   Discussion

We have re-parameterized the distance measure of Aylward et al. using a global kernel function. The latter can be computed pre-operatively and thus the distance measure can then be evaluated efficiently intra-operatively. This is an important aspect for non-rigid registration applications with tight time constraints. Furthermore we have derived a new distance measure suitable for comparing geometric representations of tubular structure with image data, as we have shown in a preliminary validation. Extended validation in more registration applications is in progress. Although we apply our method to tube-like features, the framework is general and we expect it to work also for other (e.g. plate-like) features. Such investigations are subject to future work.

Fig. 1. Powerdoppler ultrasound data of liver vessels with a) artificially deformed, b) rigidly and c) non-rigidly registered vessels

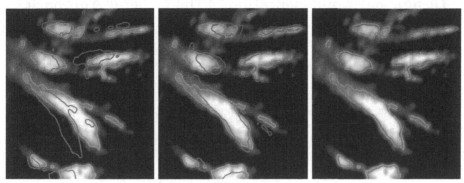

References

1. Selle D, Preim B, Schenk A, Peitgen HO. Analysis of vasculature for liver surgical planning. IEEE Trans Med Imag 2002;21(11):1344–1357.
2. Beller S, Hünerbein M, Lange T, Eulenstein S, Gebauer B, Schlag PM. Image-guided surgery of liver metastases by 3D ultrasound-based optoelectronic navigation. Brit J Surg accepted.
3. Kybic J, Unser M. Fast parametric elastic image registration. IEEE Trans Med Imag 2003;12(11):1427–1441.
4. Modersitzki J. Numerical Methods for Image Registration. Oxford University Press; 2004.
5. Roche A, Pennec X, Malandain G, Ayache N. Rigid registration of 3-D ultrasound with MR images: A new approach combining intensity and gradient information. IEEE Trans Med Imag 2001;20(10):1038–1049.
6. Viola PA, III WMWells. Alignment by maximization of mutual information. Procs ICCV 1995; 16–23.
7. Weese J, Rösch P, Netsch T, Blaffert T, Quist M. Gray-value based registration of CT and MR images by maximization of local correlation. In: MICCAI; 1999. 656–663.
8. Haber E, Modersitzki J. Intensity gradient-based registration and fusion of multimodal images. Procs MICCAI 2006; 726–733.
9. Droske M, Rumpf M. A variational approach to non-rigid morphological registration. SIAM Appl Math 2004;64(2):668–687.
10. Henn S, Hömke L, Witsch K. Lesion preserving image registration with applications to human brains. In: Procs DAGM; 2004. 143–154.
11. Schumacher H, Franz A, Fischer B. Weighted medical image registration with automatic mask generation. Procs SPIE 2006; in print.
12. Aylward SR, JJomier, Weeks S, Bullitt E. Registration and analysis of vascular images. Int J Comput Vision 2003;55(2-3):123–138.
13. Frangi AF, Niessen WJ, Vincken KL, Viergever MA. Multiscale vessel enhancement filtering. Procs MICCAI 1998; 130–137.

A Fast and Flexible Image Registration Toolbox
Design and Implementation of the General Approach

Nils Papenberg[1], Hanno Schumacher[1], Stefan Heldmann[2], Stefan Wirtz[3],
Silke Bommersheim[1], Konstantin Ens[1], Jan Modersitzki[1], Bernd Fischer[1]

[1]University of Lübeck, Institute of Mathematics, Lübeck, Germany
[2]Department of Mathematics and Computer Science, Emory University, USA
[3]MeVis Research GmbH, Universitätsallee 29, 28359 Bremen, Germany
Email: papenber@math.uni-luebeck.de

Abstract. In the last decades there has been tremendous research towards the design of fully automatic non-rigid registration schemes. However, apart from the ITK based implementation of Rueckerts B-spline oriented approach, there is a lack of sound publicly available implementations of the modern schemes. The Flexible Image Registration Toolbox (FLIRT) is an attempt to close this gap. It focuses on non-parametric schemes as popularized in the book by Modersitzki [1]. To be successful, it is crucial for any registration scheme to reflect the special properties of the underlying registration problem. Consequently, FLIRT has an open object-oriented architecture which allows for the incorporation of user prescribed building blocks. In its present form, most of the prominent blocks are already implemented. They may be arranged in a consistent way and cover a wide range of applications. Apart from the flexibility issue, great care has been taken towards fast execution times. The most computationally intensive part, the solution of the underlying linear systems, is implemented by state-of-the-art solution techniques.

The FLIRT package is publicly available, it comes with a user guide and a collection of example problems. It is the purpose of this note, to describe some of the features of the toolbox.

1 Introduction

Registration of medical images is an active field of current research and still constitutes one of today's most challenging image processing problems [1, 2, 3, 4]. In basic terms, registration is the process of finding a geometric transformation between two or more images such that corresponding image structures correctly align. These images may have been acquired with the same or different imaging modalities, at the same or different times, from one or several patients. Accurate image registration is a necessary prerequisite for many diagnostic and therapy planning procedures where complementary information from different images has to be combined. All existing registration schemes can be divided in two approaches, a parametric approach, describing the transformation as a linear combination of pre-selected basis functions, and a non-parametric approach, describing the transformation as the solution of an associated partial differential equation [1]. The Flexible Image Registration Toolbox (FLIRT) focusses on non-parametric non-rigid registration techniques. This registration strategy is one of the most promising non-linear approaches currently used in medical imaging. The approach attempts to minimize an appropriate functional. It typically consists of two building blocks. The first is responsible for external forces, which are computed from the reference image R and the template image T, whereas the second computes the internal forces, which are defined for the wanted displacement field u itself. The internal forces are designed to keep the displacement field smooth during deformation, while the external forces are defined to obtain the desired registration result. The registration problem may be phrased as

$$\mathcal{J}[u] := \mathcal{D}[R, T; u] + \alpha \mathcal{S}[u] = \min, \tag{1}$$

with some additional boundary conditions. Here, $\mathcal{D}$ represents a *distance measure* (external force), whereas $\mathcal{S}$ denotes a *smoother* for u (internal force). The parameter α may be used to control the strength of the smoothness of the displacement versus the similarity of the images. The most common choices for distance measures in image registration are the *sum of squared differences* (SSD), *cross correlation* (CC), and mutual information (MI) [1]. The smoother $\mathcal{S}$ is also called *regularizing* term. This term is unavoidable. Arbitrary transformations may lead to cracks, foldings, or other unwanted deformations. With an appropriate smoother it becomes possible to distinguish particular transformations which seem to be more likely than others. Typical regularizer are the *elastic* [5], *diffusive* [6] and *curvature* [7] smoother.

2   State of the Art and New Contribution

In contrast to the wealth of literature, surprisingly only a few publicly non-rigid image registration software packages are available. Possibly the most well-known is the one designed by Rueckert [8], which is part of the software library ITK (www.itk.org). In non-rigid registration one distinguishes between parametric and non-parametric approaches. The just mentioned package belongs to the class of parameter-dependent schemes. That is, the thought after transformation is prescribed with respect to a given space, like, e.g. B-splines. To our best knowledge, there exists no publicly available software package for parameter-free non-rigid image registration.

The FLIRT package consists of a variety of non-parametric, non-rigid registration routines, written in C/C++. The toolbox realizes the concept outlined in a paper by Fischer and Modersitzki [9]. It is designed for easy use and its versatile concept allows for the application to a wide range of registration problems. In addition, the object-oriented architecture does permit a straightforward implementation of further building blocks. Great care has been taken in the design of solution strategies for the underlying optimization problem. The outcome is a highly competitive implementation both in terms of reliability and computing time.

3 Methods

Our software design is highly related to the structure of the energy functional $\mathcal{J}$, see (1). At this point we give only a short repetition to motivate our design, for more details we refer to the literature, for example [1, 9]. Using an optimize-discretize approach and the calculus of variations we arrive at the so called Euler-Lagrange equations

$$f(x, u(x)) + \alpha A[u](x) = 0, \tag{2}$$

which constitute a necessary condition for u being a minimizer of (1). Its summands are directly related to the used distance-measure and regularizer, i.e. the so-called force f corresponds to the measure $\mathcal{D}$ and the smoothness operator A to the regularizer S. To solve these non-linear equations, it is common to linearize them by means of a fixed-point type iteration or by introducing an artificial time and employing a time-marching scheme. Discretizing the force f and the operator A leads to an iteration process, where at each step a large linear system has to be solved. Here, the structure of the system matrix depends only on the chosen regularizer, the force constitutes the right hand side of the system. To arrive at an efficient algorithm, special care has to be taken for the solution of the linear system. Therefore, for each smoother in FLIRT a highly specialized solver has been designed and implemented, resulting in very competitve running times.

Our software design deals with two main aspects:

1. the variability of the approach, i.e. the interchangeability of distance measure, regularizer etc
2. the necessity for fast numerical algorithms, i.e. solvers for linear systems, interpolation.

First of all we have chosen an object oriented software design. This allows us to compose abstract classes, which are used to define interfaces between the convertible components. In the following we list the regarded components, give an overview about their functionality and in brackets a list of possible derived classes, that implement the interfaces:

- **distance-measure**, evaluation of the functional, providing the derivative of the functional, i.e. the force f (sum of squared differences (SSD), mutual information, normalized gradient field)
- **regularizer**, evaluation of the functional, providing the derivative of the functional, i.e. the smoothness operator A (elastic regularizer, curvature regularizer, diffusive regularizer)
- **optimizer**, the way the nonlinear Euler-Lagrange equation is linearized (fixed-point iteration, time-marching iteration)
- **stopping criteria**, condition for stopping the iteration (stopping criteria from Gill, Murray and Wright [10])

Fig. 1. Example. *left:* reference image, *middle:* deformed template image after registration, *right:* template image

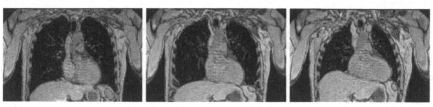

Furthermore we have composed abstract classes for images and displacement-fields, dealing with parameters like image size, voxel size and managing storage. These classes can be concretized for $2D$ or $3D$.

All of this is implemented using C/C++.

Embedded into the object oriented part we have developed a machine oriented library. This is associated with the second aspect of our design: the necessity for fast algorithms. The library provides fast codes for solving the arising linear systems as described above. For each regularizer a special solver is implemented. For more details on the the underlying numerics, we refer to [11, 1]. Since two of these solvers depend on fast Fourier transformation techniques, the fftw-library (www.fftw.org) is included. Beside the solvers we have implemented interpolation and gradient calculation schemes. This machine oriented part of our library is written in the C-language, so it cooperates easy with other software, like, for example, MATLAB using its `mex`-interface.

The software can be downloaded from the homepage of the SAFIR (solutions and algorithms for image registration) group
`http://www.math.uni-luebeck.de/safir/FLIRT-Download`. It is available for Linux and - in future - for the Windows platform. Furthermore it is planned to include the toolbox as an additional part of MeVisLab.

4 Results

For lack of space this paper contains only one example to illustrate the efficiency and capability of the implemented software. We use CT-images of the lunge, showing two different states of the respiration cycle. These images are provided by Thomas Netsch, Philips, Hamburg. The image size is 256×171. We restrict to $2D$-data for better visualization. The calculation was performed on an AMD 64 3000+ with 1 GB RAM using the SSD distancemeasure, the elastic regularizer and fixed-point optimizer with 25 iterations. The overall computation time was approximatly 2 seconds. The energy $\mathcal{J}$ was reduced to 30%. The results are illustrated in figure 1.

5 Discussion

An object-oriented toolbox for non-parametric and non-linear registration problems is presented. To our best knowledge, the discussed toolbox is the first publicly available package out of this class. In its present state, the most well-known smoothers are incorporated. However, due to its versatile style, an extension to additional smoothers or distance measures is straightforward and it is part of the project to enhance the package step by step. The toolbox is publicly available and everybody is highly welcome to test its performance and to report any flames or praises to the SAFIR group.

References

1. Modersitzki J. Numerical Methods for Image Registration. Oxford University Press; 2003.
2. Hajnal JV, Hill DLG, Hawkes DJ. Medical Image Registration. CRC Press, Boca Raton; 2001.
3. Maintz JBA, Viergever MA. A survey of medical image registration. Med Image Anal 1998;2(1):1–36.
4. Zitová B, Flusser J. Image registration methods: A survey. Image Vis Comp 2003;21(11):977–1000.
5. Bajcsy R, Kovačič S. Multiresolution elastic matching. Comp Vis Graph Image Process 1989;46:1–21.
6. Fischer B, Modersitzki J. Fast diffusion registration. In AMS contemporary mathematics, inverse problems, image analysis, and medical maging 2002;313:117–129.
7. Fischer B, Modersitzki J. A unified approach to fast image registration and a new curvature based registration technique. Linear Algebra and its Applications 2004;380:107–124.
8. Schnabel JA, Rueckert D, Quist M, et al. A generic framework for non-rigid registration based on non-uniform multi-level free-form deformations. Procs MICCAI 2001; 573–581.
9. Fischer B, Modersitzki J. FLIRT: A flexible image registration toolbox. LNCS 2003;2717:261–270.
10. Gill PE, Murray W, Whright MH. Practical Optimization for Non-linear Approximation. Academic Press; 1981.
11. Fischer B, Modersitzki J. Fast inversion of matrices arising in image processing. Numerical Algorithms 1999;22:1–11.

On Validation of Non-physical Techniques for Elastic Image Registration

Evgeny Gladilin, Karl Rohr and Roland Eils

University Heidelberg, IPMB, and German Cancer Research Center, TBI,
Im Neuenheimer Feld 580, 69120 Heidelberg
Email: e.gladilin@dkfz.de

Abstract. Non-physical techniques for elastic image registration such as different spline-based optimization methods are often applied in biomedical applications for image normalization w.r.t. non-rigid transformations. Since mechanical properties of biological structures to be registered are usually unknown, a "ground truth" validation of the results of image registration is not possible. This article presents a framework for the validation of elastic image registration techniques by a direct comparison of displacement fields vs analytical or numerical reference solutions of customizable boundary value problems. The proposed procedure enables an easy handling of material parameters, domain shapes and boundary conditions, and provides a flexible benchmark-tool for quantitative validation of elastic image registration algorithms.

1   Introduction

Elastic registration techniques are widely used for normalization of biomedical images with respect to non-rigid transformations (deformations). Depending on core principles utilized for computation of object deformations, these techniques can be formally subdivided into two major groups: physical and non-physical approaches. Low number of required image correspondences, straightforward implementation, computational efficiency and robustness make non-physical registration techniques, such as numerous spline- or optical flow-based methods [1], appear more advantageous for automatic and routine application compared to extensive physical approaches which are based on numerical solving partial differential equations of continuum mechanics. On the other hand, non-physical methods are still expected to produce realistic deformations of biological tissues. Since mechanical properties of biological tissues are highly complex and variable, an exact quantitative validation of the results of image registration by a direct proof of the "ground truth" is usually not possible. In practice, the accuracy of non-rigid registration methods can be benchmarked by exemplary comparison of a non-physical method with (i) physical methods, e.g. finite element methods, or (ii) experimentally assessed deformation fields for some biological or surrogate tissue samples, e.g. the "truth-cube" [2]. However, the results of such validation are firstly limited to that particular BVP which was used for benchmarking or training of an algorithm, and can not be generalized to the cases with different material constants, domain shapes, boundary conditions, etc. Further comparative tests with a strongly differing combination of parameters are required to show the ability of a particular method to cope with a more general class of non-rigid registration problems and to prove its accuracy. In this article, a framework for validation of non-physical image registration techniques vs exact analytical or numerical solutions of elastostatic boundary value problems BVPs is presented, which enables a flexible handling of canonical material parameters, boundary conditions and domain shapes for constructing different benchmark-tests.

2   Methods

2.1   Analytical Solutions of Linear Elasticity

Analytical solution of partial differential equations of elasticity theory is possible only for particularly simple domain shapes and boundary conditions, such as spheric, cylindric, cubic domains or infinite elastic medium. Nevertheless, a boundary value problem for an arbitrarily shaped 3D domain can be constructed using these special closed-form solutions. To demonstrate the idea of this approach, we focus on the fundamental solution of linear elasticity, which describes the response of an infinite 3D elastic medium Ω_∞ with the stiffness E and compressibility ν to the impact of a point-force $\mathbf{f}(r) = \mathbf{f}\delta(r)$ [3]

$$\mathbf{u}(\mathbf{f}, \mathbf{r}) = \frac{1 + \nu}{8\pi E(1 - \nu)r} \left((3 - 4\nu)\mathbf{f} + \frac{(\mathbf{f}\,\mathbf{r})\,\mathbf{r}}{r^2} \right) \tag{1}$$

where $\mathbf{r}$ is the radial vector from the force application point to an arbitrary observation point. Assume a compact subset $\Omega \subset \Omega_\infty$ with the boundary Γ_Ω, see Fig. 1. In accordance with the Somigliana identity [4], the displacement field $\mathbf{u}_p$ for all inner points $p \in \Omega$ of a homogeneous elastic domain (e.g. particular image region) can be computed from the displacements $\mathbf{u}_q$ and tractions $\mathbf{t}_q$ of the boundary points $q \in \Gamma_\Omega$ only [5]

$$\mathbf{u}_p = \int_\Gamma \mathbf{G}_{pq}\mathbf{t}_q ds - \int_\Gamma \mathbf{T}_{pq}\mathbf{u}_q ds \tag{2}$$

whereas $\mathbf{G}_{pq}$ and $\mathbf{T}_{pq}$ are the fundamental solutions for displacements and tractions, respectively. Typically, non-rigid registration is applied for computation of displacements of domain deformations for some predefined boundary correspondences. Thus, we can formulate following procedure for benchmarking a non-rigid registration technique:

- define an arbitrarily shaped spatial domain Ω with the boundary Γ_Ω,
- calculate displacements for all points of Ω and Γ_Ω using (1),
- apply your method to compute displacements of inner points $\mathbf{u}_\Omega$ for boundary conditions given by the displacements of boundary points $\mathbf{u}_\Gamma$,
- compare displacements of inner points obtained with your method vs. reference displacements from (1).

2.2   Numerical Solutions of Elastostatic BVPs

Following the same basic steps as described above, numerical solutions of arbitrary elastomechanical BVPs obtained for a finite number of mesh nodes can be used for benchmarking a non-rigid image registration algorithm. Using numerical solving techniques such as the finite element method, more complex boundary conditions and material properties can be simulated. We apply the FEM on tetrahedral grids for computation of deformations of of a cubic domain modeled as a St. Venant-Kirchhoff material [6]. Such BVPs resemble the experiments carried out with the "truth cube"and can be seen as its virtual counterpart with homogeneous, isotropic and non-linear elastic material properties.

2.3   Correlation of Vector Fields

For quantification of similarity/dissimilarity between two displacement fields, the normalized scalar product (NSP) can be used

$$NSP(\mathbf{u}_1, \mathbf{u}_2) = \frac{\mathbf{u}_1\,\mathbf{u}_2}{|\mathbf{u}_1|\,|\mathbf{u}_2|} \tag{3}$$

(3) serves as a descriptor of the relative spatial orientation for each pair of vectors, whereas $NSP = 1, 0, -1$ stands for correlated, uncorrelated and anti-correlated pairs of vectors, respectively.

2.4   Topology Preservation

A natural requirement on a realistic material deformation is the preservation of local topology of the registered spatial domain. Violation of the topology preservation by elastic image registration algorithms often occurs when the registration problem is associated with computation of large deformations, and is expressed in penetration of boundaries, distortion of mesh elements, crossing of field lines, etc. Monitoring of the local topology preservation on FE meshes can be done by computing the determinant of the deformation gradient

$$C = \det(\mathbf{I} + \nabla\mathbf{u}) \tag{4}$$

Topology preservation corresponds to positive $C > 0$, while small or negative values $C \leq 0$ indicate extremely deformed or corrupted elements with violated local topology.

3   Experimental Results

In this section we present some examples of benchmark-tests based on analytical and numerical solutions of elastostatic BVPs, which can be used for the validation of elastic image registration algorithms.

Fig. 1. Fundamental solution of linear elasticity (1) describes a global displacement field **u** in an infinite elastic continuum Ω_∞ induced by a point-force **f**

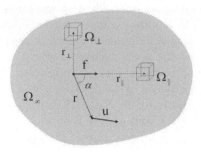

3.1   Construction of a BVP Using the Fundamental Solution

Consider a cubic subdomain Ω of an unloaded infinite elastic medium Ω_∞ with material parameters $E = 1$ and $\nu = 0.45$. According to (1), a point-force generates a global displacement field in Ω_∞ including boundary and inner points of $\Omega \in \Omega_\infty$. Fig. 2 shows the resulting deformation of Ω for two different cases of its relative orientation w.r.t. the point-force vector, namely $\alpha(\mathbf{r}, \mathbf{f}) = \pi$ and $\alpha(\mathbf{r}, \mathbf{f}) = \frac{\pi}{2}$. The displacements of boundary points $\mathbf{u}_\Gamma$ yield boundary conditions for computation of the displacements of inner points $\mathbf{u}_\Omega$ with the subsequent validation of the result vs the reference solution (1). By varying E and ν in (1), different material properties can be simulated. In order to avoid unnatural effects of the r^{-1} singularity of the Green function, the test-domain Ω should be placed sufficiently far away from the source point, i.e. $r >> 0$. The orientation of Ω relatively to the force vector $\alpha(\mathbf{r}, \mathbf{f}) \in [0, \pi]$ can be varied to study cross-contraction effects for different values of the Poisson ratio $\nu \in [0, 0.5]$.

3.2   FEM Benchmark-Tests

An advantage of numerical solving techniques such as the finite element method is that non-linear material properties and arbitrary complex boundary conditions can be simulated. Smooth displacement fields resulting from closed-form solutions of elasticity theory can, in fact, be approximated by almost any sufficiently smooth spline function. However, non-smooth distributions of deformation energy, which can arise due to geometrical or physical constraints, such as material inhomogeneities in multicomposite biological structures, are more difficult to "mime" with non-physical registration methods. Alternatively to the above described BVPs with the fixed outer boundaries and homogenous one-material model, we suggest FEM benchmark-tests with mixed boundary conditions, including partially-free and -fixed outer and inner boundaries, as well as non-homogenous material properties.

Fig. 2. Deformation of a cubic subdomain of an infinite elastic medium Ω_∞ for two different cases of its relative orientation w.r.t. the point-force vector: $\alpha(\mathbf{r}, \mathbf{f}) = \pi$ (left) and $\alpha(\mathbf{r}, \mathbf{f}) = \frac{\pi}{2}$ (right), respectively

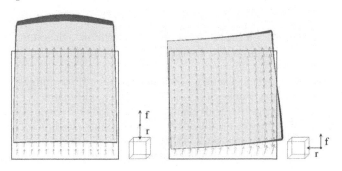

4   Conclusion

We have presented a framework for validation of non-rigid image registration techniques using analytical and numerical solutions of customizable elastostatic boundary value problems (BVPs). The proposed validation procedure is based on comparison between theoretically-predicted and simulated displacements of inner domain points computed for predefined boundary displacements. The modeling scheme enables a flexible handling of material properties, domain geometries and boundary conditions for benchmarking non-rigid registration algorithms or fitting free modeling parameters. Numerical criterions for quantification of degree of similarity/dissimilarity between simulated and reference displacements as well as monitoring of local domain topology have been proposed. The presented approach is straightforward in implementation and intends to put the validation of non-rigid registration algorithms vs theoretical solutions of elasticity theory on a more accurate and quantifiable platform.

References

1. Zitova B, Flusser J. Image registration methods: a survey. Image and Vision Computing 2003;21:977–1000.
2. Kerdok AE, Cotin SM, Ottenmeyer MP, Galea A, Howe RD, Dawson SL. Truth cube: Establishing physical standards for soft tissue simulation. Medical Image Analysis 2003;7:283–291.
3. Landau LD, Lifschitz EM. Theory of Elasticity. Oxford: Pergamon Press; 1986.
4. Beskos DE. Boundary Element Methods in Mechanics. Amsterdam: North-Holland; 1987.
5. Gladilin E, Pekar V, Rohr K, Stiehl S. A comparison between BEM and FEM for elastic registration of medical images. Image Vision Computing 2006;24(4):375–379.
6. Ciarlet PG. Mathematical Elasticity. Volume I: Three-Dimensional Elasticity. vol. 20 of Studies in Mathematics and its Applications. Amsterdam: North-Holland; 1988.

Matching von Baumstrukturen
Zuordnung von Gefäßsystemen aus Leber und Lunge

Jan Hendrik Metzen[1], Tim Kröger[2], Andrea Schenk[2], Stephan Zidowitz[2],
Heinz-Otto Peitgen[2], Xiaoyi Jiang[3]

[1]University of Bremen, Faculty of Mathematics and Computer Science,
Robert Hooke Str. 5, 28359 Bremen, Germany
[2]MeVis Research GmbH, Universitätsallee 29, 28359 Bremen, Germany
[3]University of Münster, Faculty of Mathematics and Computer Science,
Einsteinstraße 62, 48149 Münster, Germany
Email: jhm@informatik.uni-bremen.de

Zusammenfassung. In vielen medizinischen Anwendungen ist eine Registrierung verschiedener Bilddatensätze desselben Organs sinnvoll. Häufig geschieht eine solche Registrierung mit Hilfe manuell in den Bilddatensätzen platzierter Landmarken. In dieser Arbeit wird ein Verfahren vorgestellt, mit dem automatisiert sinnvolle Landmarken bestimmt werden können. Dazu werden Knoten der zuvor mittels eines Segmentierungsverfahrens extrahierten Gefäßbäume mit Hilfe des Assoziationsgraph-Verfahrens einander zugeordnet und die Koordinaten der so zugeordneten Knoten als Landmarken benutzt. Das vorgestellte Verfahren wurde in der *MeVisLab* Entwicklungsumgebung realisiert und getestet.

1 Einleitung

Sowohl von der Leber als auch von der Lunge können mit bildgebenden Verfahren wie Computertomographie (CT) oder Magnetresonanztomographie (MRT) dreidimensionale, digitale Abbilder erstellt werden. In vielen medizinischen Anwendungen existieren mehrere Aufnahmen desselben Organs. Beispiele sind Aufnahmen einer Lunge sowohl im eingeatmeten Zustand als auch im ausgeatmeten Zustand sowie CT und MRT Aufnahmen desselben Organs. Häufig muss für solche Aufnahmen eine *Registrierung* durchgeführt werden, d. h. es müssen Stellen, die denselben Bereich eines Organs in den Bildern repräsentieren, identifiziert werden.

Klassische volumenbasierte Registrierungsmethoden schlagen aufgrund von Lageveränderungen und Deformationen der jeweiligen Organe – verursacht vor allem durch Atmung und Herzschlag – häufig fehl. Um eine Registrierung der Datensätze automatisiert zu ermöglichen, gilt es, nach Eigenschaften der Organe zu suchen, die unter den oben genannten Bedingungen vergleichsweise invariant sind. Ein geeigneter Ansatzpunkt sind hierfür die verschiedenen Gefäßsysteme innerhalb der Organe. Diese verändern zwar ebenfalls Lage und Ausdehnung, jedoch bleibt ihre Struktur nahezu unverändert. Gelingt es, korrespondierende

Verzweigungen innerhalb dieser Strukturen zu identifizieren, so können die Koordinaten dieser Zuordnungen als Landmarken verwendet werden. Somit können auch landmarkenbasierte Registrierungsmethoden eingesetzt werden, die in diesem Anwendungskontext vielversprechender sind.

Bei den Gefäß- und Versorgungssystemen aus Lunge und Leber (Bronchien, Portalvene der Leber etc.) handelt es sich stets um baumförmige Strukturen mit einer ausgezeichneten Wurzel; es existieren Algorithmen, mit denen diese Gefäßsysteme automatisiert extrahiert werden können[1]. Daher sind verschiedene Verfahren aus der strukturellen Mustererkennung zum Matching von Bäumen anwendbar.

2   Stand der Forschung und Fortschritt durch den Beitrag

Ein Ansatz zum Matching von Baumstrukturen ist das so genannte Assoziationsgraph-Verfahren. In diesem wird basierend auf den Gefäßbäumen ein Assoziationsgraph gebildet, der wie folgt definiert ist:

Definition 1 (Baum - Assoziationsgraph). *Seien $T_1 = (V_1, E_1, w_1)$ und $T_2 = (V_2, E_2, w_2)$ zwei Bäume mit ausgezeichneten Wurzeln. Dann definieren wir den* Assoziationsgraphen $G_A = (V_A, E_A)$ *von T_1 und T_2 wie folgt:*

1. $V_A = V_1 \times V_2$
2. $E_A = \{e = (v_a, v_b) \in V_A \times V_A \mid g(v_a, v_b) = true\}$

Jeder Knoten $v_a = (v_{a1}, v_{a2}) \in V_A$ korrespondiert zu einer Zuordnung der Knoten $v_{a1} \leftrightarrow v_{a2}$. Sind zwei Knoten des Assoziationsgraphen verbunden, so bedeutet dies, dass die beiden korrespondierenden Zuordnungen zueinander konsistent sind. Ob zwei Knoten des Assoziationsgraphen zueinander konsistent sind, wird durch die Bedingung $g(v_a, v_b)$ festgelegt. Pellilo et al.[2, 3] geben je nach Anwendungskontext verschiedene Bedingungen g an. Durch Variation dieser Bedingungen (im Weiteren *binäre Constraints* genannt) wird das Verfahren jeweils an eine neue Anwendungssituation (zum Beispiel Finden von Subgraph-Isomorphismen, Many-to-Many Matching etc.) angepasst.

Ziel des Machingverfahrens ist es, eine möglichst große Menge von Knotenzuordnungen zu finden, die paarweise konsistent sind. Eine Clique[1] maximaler Knotenkardinaltität im Graphen G_A induziert genau eine solche maximale Menge konsistenter Knotenzuordnungen: Ist der Knoten $v_a = (v_{a1}, v_{a2})$ in der Clique C, so wird die Zuordnung $v_{a1} \leftrightarrow v_{a2}$ in das Matching aufgenommen.

Das von Pellilo vorgestellte Verfahren hat als Zielsetzung u. a. das Finden von Teilbaum-Isomorphismen maximaler Größe zwischen zwei Bäumen. Aufgrund von Rauschen in den Aufnahmen und daraus resultierenden Fehlern in den segmentierten Gefäßbäumen ist eine Bedingung wie die Isomorphie zweier Bäume für das Matching von Gefäßbäumen zu strikt. Diese Striktheit liegt in den jeweiligen binären Constraints g begründet. In Abschnitt 3 wird eine Modifikation des Assoziationsgraph-Verfahrens beschrieben, die weniger strikte

---

[1] Bei einer Clique handelt es sich um einen vollständig verbundenen Teilgraphen.

binäre Constraints einsetzt und das Verfahren somit erheblich unempfindlicher gegenüber Rauschen und Fehlsegmentierungen macht.

3 Methoden

Während von Pelillo et al.[2, 3] für jede Anwendungssituation nur ein binärer Constraint definiert wird, wird im Weiteren eine Variante des Assoziationsgraph-Verfahrens eingeführt, die eine Menge C_G von binären Constraints berücksichtigen kann. Jeder solche Constraint kann auf zwei Knoten des Assoziationsgraphen angewendet werden und gibt eine Bewertung im Intervall $[0, 1]$ zurück. Im Gegensatz zu einer reinen Ja/Nein Antwort wie in Definition 1 kann ein Constraint somit auch zu einem gewissen Grad erfüllt sein. Zudem wird jeder Constraint mit einem Faktor ω_i gewichtet, der seine Relevanz für die jeweilige Anwendungssituation bestimmt. Analog wird eine Menge C_F unärer Constraints definiert, die festlegen, ob ein Knoten in den Assoziationsgraphen aufgenommen wird.

Definition 2 (Baum - Assoziationsgraph). *Seien* $T_1 = (V_1, E_1, w_1)$ *und* $T_2 = (V_2, E_2, w_2)$ *zwei Bäume mit ausgezeichneten Wurzeln. Dann definieren wir den Assoziationsgraphen* $G = (V_A, E_A)$ *von* T_1 *und* T_2 *unter den unären Constrains* C_F *und den binären Constraints* C_G *wie folgt:*

1. $V_A = \{v_a \in V_1 \times V_2 | \sum_{f_i \in C_F} \omega_i f_i(v_a) \geq 0.5\}$ *mit* $\omega_i \in [0, 1]$, $\sum_i \omega_i = 1$
2. $E_A = \{(v_a, v_b) \in V_A \times V_A | \sum_{g_j \in C_G} v_j g_j(v_a, v_b) \geq 0.5\}$ *mit* $v_i \in [0, 1]$, $\sum_j v_j = 1$

Durch die Einführung der unären Constraints kann die Knotenkardinalität des Assoziationsgraph erheblich verringert werden. Das ist insbesondere deswegen wünschenswert, weil es sich bei dem Auffinden einer maximalen Clique in einem Graph um ein $\mathcal{NP}$-vollständiges Problem handelt. Das Bilden einer gewichteten Summe aller Constraints ermöglicht es, dass eine fehlerhafte Bewertung durch einen Constraint durch eine korrekte Bewertung einer Mehrheit der anderen Constraints (bzw. durch einen höher gewichteten Constraint) korrigiert werden kann.

3.1 Constraints

Unäre Constraints haben das Ziel, frühzeitig Knoten in den beiden Bäumen mit ähnlichen Eigenschaften zu identifizieren, da nur diese als Kandidaten für sinnvolle Zuordnungen in Frage kommen. Eigenschaften von Knoten sind zum Beispiel ihr Level[2] im Baum, die Länge des eingehenden Gefäßes, das Volumen des an ihnen wurzelnden Teilbaums oder ihre räumlichen Koordinaten. Es hat sich jedoch erwiesen, dass jede der obigen Eigenschaften starken Schwankungen unterliegen kann. Ursachen sind beispielsweise unterschiedliche Auflösungen der

---

[2] Unter dem Level eines Knotens versteht man die Anzahl Kanten, die auf dem eindeutigen Weg von diesem Knoten zur Wurzel traversiert werden müssen.

Tabelle 1. Ergebnisse des Matchingverfahrens: Für die Portalvenen-Bäume konnte das Verfahren die Hälfte der Zuordnungen erzielen ohne dabei eine Fehlzuordnung zu treffen. Für die Bronchialbäume wurden 21 Zuordnungen korrekt ermittelt, jedoch auch 4 falsche Zuordnungen. Bei diesen Fehlern verrutschte die Zuordnung jedoch meist nur um ein Level nach oben oder unten in der Baumhierarchie, d. h. der fehlerhaft zugeordnete Knoten war ein Nachbar des eigentlich zuzuordnenden Knotens

Datensatz	Portalvene	Bronchialbaum
Korrekt	17	21
Fehler	0	4
Laufzeit [sec.]	202	369

bildgebenden Verfahren oder Rauschen in den Aufnahmen. Ersteres kann die Größe eines Teilbaums erheblich verändern, letzteres durch fehlerhaft segmentierte Äste unter anderem die Länge einer Kante verändern.

Eine Eigenschaft, die vergleichsweise unempfindlich gegen solche Störfaktoren ist, ist der räumlich Verlauf des Gefäßes von der jeweiligen Wurzel zu dem jeweiligen Knoten. Diese räumliche Kurve wird durch einen dreidimensionalen Streckenzug beschrieben. Es wurde ein Maß entwickelt, dass die Ähnlichkeit zweier solcher Streckenzüge bewertet[4]. Für binäre Constraints wurde ebenfalls festgestellt, dass naheliegende Ähnlichkeitsmaße - wie zum Beispiel die topologische Distanz zweier Knoten - sehr anfällig gegenüber Rauschen sind. Auch hier hat sich erwiesen, dass der räumlicher Verlauf des zwei Knoten verbindenden Pfades ein besserer Ansatzpunkt ist.

4 Ergebnisse

Als Grundlage für die Bewertung der Güte des vom Assoziationsgraph-Verfahren gelieferten Matchings lag für zwei Baumpaare ein per Hand erstelltes Matching als *Ground Truth* vor. Bei diesen Datensätzen handelte es sich um ein Paar von Bronchialbäumen (im eingeatmeten und ausgeatmeten Zustand) und ein Paar von Portalvenen-Bäume (mittels MRT und mittels CT aufgenommen). Die Bäume besaßen jeweils circa 200 Knoten, und die Ground-Truths ordneten jeweils 34 dieser Knoten zu.

In einem ersten Schritt wurde eine Teilmenge der Constraints ausgewählt, die für den Portalvenen-Datensatz gute Ergebnisse lieferte. Für diese Constraints wurde daraufhin ein Parametersatz bestimmt, der optimale Ergebnisse lieferte. Derselbe Satz an Constraints wurde daraufhin auch an dem Bronchialbaum-Datensatz getestet. Die Qualität des Ergebnisses ist im Falle der Portalvenen-Bäume besser als im Falle der Bronchialbäume (Tab. 1, Abb. 1). Die Ursache hierfür ist die Dichotomie der Bronchialbäume, die dazu führt, dass sich viele Bereiche innerhalb eines Baumes sehr ähneln. Ein Beispiel für ähnliche Teilbäume sind die rechte und die linke Hälfte des Bronchialbaum, die sich am ersten Hauptverzweigungspunkt trennen.

Abb. 1. Dargestellt sind zwei Portalvenen-Bäume sowie das ermittelte Matching. Hierbei sind einander zugeordnete Knoten mit derselben Farbe gefärbt. Sofern durch die Knotenzuordnung ein Isomorphismus zweier Teilbäume induziert wird, so wurden diese Teilbäume mit derselben Farbe gefärbt

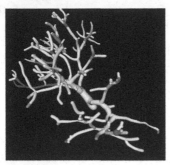 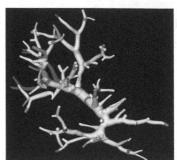

5 Diskussion

Die Ergebnisse zeigen, dass das implementierte Verfahren für typische Beispiele von Gefäßbäumen aus Leber und Lunge in der Lage ist, gute Ergebnisse zu liefern: Es wird ein signifikanter Anteil der Baumknoten mit einem akzeptablen Zeitaufwand sinnvoll zugeordnet. Das Verfahren liefert dabei ein Matching, das keine bzw. nur wenige Fehlzuordnungen beinhaltet und die meisten Teilbereiche der Bäume abdeckt. Zu untersuchen bleibt, inwiefern mit diesem Verfahren ähnliche Ergebnisse auch für schwierigere Anwendungsfälle zu erreichen sind. Als Beispiele seien hierfür die Aufnahme eines Organs mit verschiedenen bildgebenden Modalitäten mit deutlich verschiedenen Auflösungen sowie das Matching von Regenerationsdaten der Leber genannt. Auch eine Verringerung der Laufzeit durch eine hierarchische Zerlegung der Bäume wie von Tschirren et al.[5] beschrieben, wäre wünschenswert.

Literaturverzeichnis

1. Selle D. Analyse von Gefäßtrukturen in medizinischen Schichtdatensätzen für die computergestützte Operationsplanung. Shaker, Aachen; 2000.
2. Pelillo M, Siddiqi K, Zucker SW. Many-to-many Matching of Attributed Trees Using Association Graphs and Game Dynamics. In: Proceedings of the 4th International Workshop on Visual Form. Springer-Verlag, London; 2001. 583–593.
3. Pelillo M. Matching free trees, maximal cliques, and monotone game dynamics. IEEE Trans Pattern Anal Mach Intell 2002;24(11):1535–1541.
4. Metzen JH. Matching von Baumstrukturen in der medizinischen Bildverarbeitung. Diploma Thesis. Universität Münster; 2006.
5. Tschirren J, Mclennan G, Palagyi K, et al. Matching and anatomical labeling of human airway tree. IEEE Trans Med Imaging 2005;24(12):1540–1547.

Vergleich von CT- mit C-Bogen-Segmentierungen für eine navigiert kontrollierte Fräse in der Neurochirurgie

M. Dengl[1], R. Grunert[2], C. Trantakis[1,2], W. Korb[2],
E. Jank[3], J. Krüger[3], T. Lueth[4], J. Meixensberger[1,2]

[1]Klinik und Poliklinik für Neurochirurgie, Universität Leipzig
[2]Innovationszentrum Computerassistierte Chirurgie (ICCAS), Universität Leipzig
[3]Fraunhofer-Institut für Produktionsanlagen und Konstruktionstechnik IPK, Berlin
[4]Dep. of Micro Technology and Medical Device Technology (MIMED), Uni München
Email: markus.dengl@medizin.uni-leipzig.de

Zusammenfassung. Intraoperative Bildgebung im Rahmen der minimal invasiven Chirurgie an der Wirbelsäule nimmt einen zunehmenden Stellenwert ein. Deswegen war es Ziel der vorliegenden Studie Arbeitraumplanungen durch 2D-Bilder des C-Bogens mit der Segmentierungen von analogen CT-Datensätzen zu evaluieren. An unterschiedlich erfahrenen Chirurgen wurde Genauigkeit und Zeitaufwand der Segmentierung an einem Wirbelsäulenphantom analysiert. Insgesamt war die CT-Segmentierung der 2D-Segmentierung überlegen. Jedoch zeigte sich, dass bei Einhalten eines Sicherheitsabstandes von 1,5mm die 2D-Segmentierung mittels aufgenommener Bilder eines C-Bogens eine hinreichende Genauigkeit in der klinischen Praxis zulässt. Der durchschnittliche Zeitaufwand für die intraoperative Segmentierung ist mit ca. 3 Minuten für den Alltagsgebrauch vertretbar. Eine Lernkurve wurde bei allen unterschiedlich erfahrenen Chirurgen verifiziert.

1 Einleitung

Operative Eingriffe mit Unterstützung von Computern und Navigation nehmen einen immer größer werdenden Stellenwert ein. Damit wird auch der Wunsch nach einer erhöhten Automatisation und eine Vereinfachung des Arbeitsablaufes unter Einsatz eines Navigationssystems nachvollziehbar. Bisherige Systeme haben sowohl den Nachteil eines niedrigen Automatisationsgrades als auch oft den einer nicht unerhebliche Anzahl an zusätzlichen Arbeitsschritten, die durch präoperative Datenakquisition entstehen.

Dem Konzept navigiert kontrollierter chirurgischer Instrumente („navigated control") folgt zum Einen ein höherer Automatisationsgrad – die Funktion des Instrumentes ist direkt an die Navigation gekoppelt –, als zum Anderen die Integration der Datenakquisition in den bereits etablierten Arbeitsablauf und damit die Optimierung dessen.

2   Stand der Forschung

Bisher etabliert ist die 3D-gestützte Navigation an der Wirbelsäule über CT, MRT oder 3D-C-Bogen. Jedoch ergeben sich daraus einige Nachteile: zunächst ist die nicht unerhebliche Strahlenbelastung durch die Datenakquisition für den Patienten zu benennen. Weiterhin sind die Wirbel untereinander mobil, d.h. die CT muss entweder in der Position aufgenommen werden, in der der Patient operiert wird (intraoperatives CT) oder man muss eine mögliche Ungenauigkeit mit einkalkulieren. Schließlich haben alle diese Verfahren den Nachteil großer Kosten und eines wesentlich erhöhten Zeitaufwands. Vor kurzem wurde ein System mit einer Knochenfräse 2D-basierter Navigation eingeführt und evaluiert [1]. Dieses basiert auf einen C-Bogen (Vario 3D, Ziehm Imaging), einem optischen Navigationssystem (NaviBase, RoboDent GmbH) und einer Fräse (Aesculap GmbH). Dabei soll durch intraoperative Bildakquisition von sechs Röntgenprojektionen mit verschiedenen Winkeln in der Transversalebene ein Arbeitsraum segmentiert werden. Die Fräse kann dann nur innerhalb dieses Arbeitsraumes fräsen und somit können wichtige Strukturen geschützt werden („Gating"-Funktion).

Ziel der vorliegenden Arbeit ist es, die Arbeitsraumplanungen durch 2D-Bilder des C-Bogens zu evaluieren und mit Segmentierungen anhand von CT-Datensätzen zu vergleichen.

3   Material und Methoden

Ein lumbales Wirbelsäulenphantom aus mit Polyurethan infiltriertem Gips wurde für die Studie verwendet. Dieses wurde mit einem Rapid Prototyping Technology 3D-Drucker hergestellt. Die CT-Daten für dieses Phantom stammen aus dem Visible Human Project[1]. Ferner wird dieses Wirbelsäulenmodell mit einem Tracker für die Navigation versetzt.

Die Bildakquisition erfolgte mit dem C-Bogen im Isozentermodus. Es wurden sechs Röntgen-Projektionen angefertigt, deren Strahlengang mit der transversalen Achse folgende Winkel einschlossen: $0°$, $15°$, $30°$, $45°$, $55°$ und $90°$. Anschließend fanden an der NaviBase die Segmentierungen statt. Segmentiert werden sollte ein Volumen am Wirbelbogen, der üblicherweise bei einem Zugang zum Duralsack entfernt werden muss (Hemilaminektomie). Als Risikostruktur wurde die angrenzende Dura im Spinal-Kanal definiert. Die Teilnehmer wurden in drei Gruppen eingeteilt: fünf Nicht-Chirurgen (Gruppe A) , fünf unerfahrene Chirurgen (Gruppe B) und ein erfahrener Chirurg (Gruppe C). Jeder absolvierte zwanzig Segmentierungen, jeweils zehn an einer anatomischen Höhe im Modell und weitere Zehn an einer anderen Höhe. Alle Teilnehmer erhielten zuvor eine schriftliche Anleitung, in dem das genaue Segmentierungsvorgehen erläutert wurde. Nach jeder Segmentierung wurde jedem Teilnehmer die Möglichkeit gegeben seine Segmentierung als Überlagerung auf CT-Schnittbildern visuell zu überprüfen. Um eine Vergleichbarkeit zum Goldstandard, der Segmentierung

---

[1] http://www.nlm.nih.gov/research/visible/visible_human.html

Abb. 1. Segmentierter Arbeitsraum in einem CT-Bild. Der Spinal-Kanal ist die Risikostruktur, die geschützt werden muss

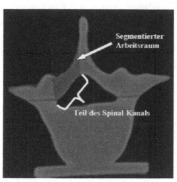

am CT, herzustellen, führten alle Teilnehmer die Segmentierung der gleichen Arbeitsräume am selben Phantom an CT-Schnittbildern durch (Abb. 1).

Der Arbeitsraum in der C-Bogen-Segmentierung (Patientenkoordinatensystem) wurde als STL-Datei vom Navigationsgerät NaviBase exportiert und im Programm Polyworks (InnovMetric) in ein DICOM-Koordinatensystem Koordinatensystem der CT-Segmentierung) überführt. Dazu wurde eine Transformationsmatrix wie folgt berechnet: aus der 0° und 90° Projektion wurden vier einfache Strukturen des Phantoms segmentiert. Diese STL-Dateien wurden zusammen mit der STL-Datei des Phantoms aus dem CT-Datensatz im Programm „PolyWorks" ausgerichtet (Methode „best fit"). Diese Prozedur wurde 10 Mal wiederholt um den mittleren Registrierfehler zu bestimmen.

Evaluiert wurden die Zeiten pro Segmentierungsvorgang im CT und am C-Bogen, und mit Hilfe des Programms „PolyWorks" wurde die Genauigkeit der Segmentierung berechnet und evaluiert. Gemessen wurde nur an der Fläche, die zum Wirbelkanal angrenzt, andere Grenzflächen wurden außer Betracht gelassen. Diese Fläche wurde jeweils vom gleichen Untersucher festgelegt. Das Programm wählte an dieser Fläche ca. 4000 Oberflächenpunkte pro Segmentierung aus und errechnete aus den Abständen der Überlagerung des segmentierten Randes (Oberflächenpunkt) zum Knochenrand den Mittelwert, die Standardabweichung und die maximale Überschreitung hin zum Spinal-Kanal.

4   Ergebnisse

Für die Genauigkeit der Segmentierung wurden drei Parameter herangezogen:

1. der Mittelwert der Abweichung Knochengrenze – Segmentierungsgrenze
2. die Standardabweichung vom Mittelwert
3. das Maximum der Abweichung Knochengrenze – Segmentierungsgrenze (positive Werte, Max)

Tabelle 1. Genauigkeit der Segmentierungen in den einzelnen Gruppen. Angegeben sind die Mittelwerte, deren Standardabweichungen und die Maxima der Abstände der Segmentierungsgrenze zur Knochengrenze nach Überlagerung in mm. Für die C-Bogen-Segmentierungen wurden jeweils die ersten fünf und letzten fünf Segmentierungen gemittelt. Die Werte für CT-Segmentierungen wurden über alle zwanzig Segmentierungen gemittelt. *Gruppe A* Nicht-Chirurgen, *Gruppe B* unerfahrene Chirurgen, *Gruppe C* erfahrener Chirurg, *n* Anzahl der Probanden in der Gruppe.

Gruppe	Mittelwert ± Standardabweichung (maximaler Wert)		
	CT	C-Bogen (Segmentnummern)	
	(20 Segmente)	zu Beginn (1.–5.)	Am Ende (16.–20.)
A (n = 5)	-0,37 ± 0,16 (0,75)	-1,75 ± 0,67 (3,43)	-1,60 ± 0,59 (3,03)
B (n = 5)	-0,24 ± 0,18 (0,99)	-1,44 ± 0,72 (2,57)	-1,53 ± 0,41 (1,40)
C (n = 1)	-0,30 ± 0,40 (0,64)	-0,82 ± 1,56 (3,20)	-0,85 ± 0,88 (0,90)

Für die Überführung der Daten vom Patientenkoordinatensystem in das DICOM-Koordinatensystem wurde ein Registrierfehler von -0,103 ± 0,328mm festgestellt mit einem Maximum von 1,010mm und einem Minimum -0,994mm.

Es zeigten sich keine signifikanten Lernkurven im Bereich der CT-Segmentierung für alle drei Gruppen in Hinblick auf die Genauigkeit (Tab. 1).

Für das Maximum der Abweichung konnte in der C-Bogen-Segmentierung entlang der Versuche festgestellt werden, dass die unerfahrenen Chirurgen und der erfahrene Chirurg sich unterschiedlich darstellen: So reduzierte sich das Maximum von 2,57mm auf 1,40mm für unerfahrene Chirurgen bzw. von 3,20mm auf 0,90mm beim erfahrenen Chirurgen. Für Nicht-Chirurgen zeigte sich keine eindeutige Tendenz. Die Maxima waren allesamt größer in der C-Bogen-Segmentierung als bei CT-Segmentierung, hielten sich aber bei den chirurgischen Gruppen in der gleichen Größenordnung.

Für den Mittelwert konnte keine Tendenz für alle drei Gruppen festgestellt werden.

Für die unerfahrenen Chirurgen zeigte sich eine Verkleinerung der Standardabweichung vom Mittelwert von Anfangs ± 0,72mm auf ± 0,41mm. Auch für den erfahrenen Chirurgen zeigte sich diese Tendenz (von ± 1,56mm auf ± 0,88mm), jedoch nicht für Nicht-Chirurgen. Auch hier zeigten sich sowohl für den Mittelwert als auch für die Standardabweichung bessere Werte in der CT-Segmentierung als in der C-Bogen-Segmentierung. Abb. 4 zeigt ein Beispiel für beide Segmentierungen im direkten Vergleich.

Es zeigten sich Lernkurven bezüglich der Zeit in allen drei Gruppen, die Zeiten für eine Segmentierung betrugen am Ende der zwanzig Versuche 317s, 228s bzw. 226s für Segmentierungen am CT für die Gruppen A, B bzw. C und 354s bzw. 136s am C-Bogen für Nicht-Chirurgen bzw. Chirurgen.

Abb. 2. Vergleich des Arbeitsraumes eines Segmentierungsbeispiels der a) C-Bogen-Segmentierung mit der b) CT-Segmentierung, die im CT-Bild dargestellt ist. Der segmentierte Arbeitsraum ist rot umrandet

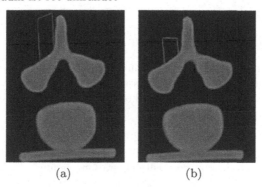

(a)   (b)

5   Diskussion

Anhand der Studie ist zu schlussfolgern, dass Segmentierungen mit dem 3D-C-Bogen in den 2D-Bildern technisch durchführbar sind und eine hinreichende Genauigkeit [2] liefern.

Lernkurven bezüglich der Genauigkeit bei Nicht-Chirurgen fanden sich für die C-Bogen-Segmentierung nicht. Ein Grund dafür könnte die mangelnde Vertrautheit mit den entsprechenden anatomischen Gegebenheiten sein. Der Mittelwert der Segmentierung scheint keiner Lernkurve zu folgen. Allerdings zeigten sich in den chirurgischen Gruppen deutliche Verbesserungen der Standardabweichung, also eine Verbesserung der Anpassung an die Knochgrenze und damit ein deutlicher Lerneffekt. Auch die Werte der maximalen Überschreitung reduzierten sich im Verlauf der durchgeführten Segmentierungen deutlich für die chirurgischen Gruppen. Rechnet man diesen Sicherheitsabstand bei der Arbeitsraumplanung mit ein, ist eine sichere Segmentierung möglich.

Die Vertrautheit mit dem System resultiert mit in einer Beschleunigung der Arbeitszeit. Am Ende der Lernkurve war der Zeitaufwand der C-Bogen-Segmentierung sogar geringer als bei der CT-Segmentierung für Chirurgen. Mit einem Zeitaufwand von unter 3 min ist dieser Teil des Arbeitsschnittes akzeptabel für die klinische Praxis.

Literaturverzeichnis

1. Jank E, Rose A, Huth S, et al. A new fluoroscopic based navigation system for milling procedures in spine surgery. In: Procs CARS; 2006. 196–198.
2. Rose A, Jank E, Huth S, et al. Experimental comparison of fluoroscopy and CT-based segmentation for spine application. In: Procs CARS; 2006. 194–196.

Segmentierung tubulärer Strukturen mittels Modell-zu-Bild-Registrierung

Nicolas Byl, Ingmar Wegner, Ivo Wolf und Hans-Peter Meinzer

Abteilung für Medzinische und Biologische Informatik
Deutsches Krebsforschungszentrum, 69120 Heidelberg
Email: n.byl@dkfz-heidelberg.de

Zusammenfassung. Die Segmentierung tubulärer Strukturen ist für vielerart Anwendungen essentiell (Operationsplanung, Navigation, Simulation etc.). Die zugrunde liegenden Originaldaten bilden die Strukturen in unterschiedlicher Qualität ab. Am Beispiel der Segmentierung des Tracheobronchialbaums bilden CT-Aufnahmen mit hinreichend guter Auflösung die feinen Strukturen der Segmentbronchien mit hinreichender Auflösung ab. Jedoch scheitern die gängigen Segmentierungsverfahren an der feinen Wanddicke der Bronchien. In MRT-Bilddaten wird bisher lediglich die zentrale Struktur des Bronchialbaums abgebildet. Aber auch hier versagen die herkömmlichen Segmentierungsansätze. Dieser Beitrag stellt einen neuartigen Ansatz für die Segmentierung tubulärer Strukturen vor. Der Ansatz sieht eine Modell-zu-Bild-Registrierung vor und soll insbesondere in verrauschten oder unkenntlichen Bilddaten seinen Einsatz finden.

1 Einleitung

Im Rahmen eines Forschungsprojekts der DFG, Forschungsschwerpunkt "Protektive Beatmungssysteme", sollen die instationären Strömungsvorgänge in den oberen und unteren Atemwegen untersucht werden. Dazu ist es nötig, aus vorgegebenen Datensätzen den Brochialbaum zu extrahieren, um somit entsprechende Strömungssimulationen durchführen zu können.

Hierzu wurde zunächst ein Anforderungskatalog erstellt, welcher alle nötigen Eigenschaften für die zu verwendeten Techniken beihaltet. Innerhalb des Projekts sollen sowohl CT- als auch MRT-Aufnahmen segmentiert werden können. Für eine weitere Analyse sollen zudem temporal aufgelöste Serien von MRT-Aufnahmen segmentiert werden. Daher wäre es hier nützlich, bereits auf einem Zeitschritt gewonnene Informationen auf andere Zeitschritte propagieren zu können, um sie dann zu verfeinern. Zudem soll das Verfahren besonders in der Peripherie der Lunge zu guten Ergebnisse führen. Dies gilt auch für Teile der Bronchien, deren Wände stellenweise nicht vollständig abgebildet worden sind, da ihre Dicke unterhalb des Auflösungsvermögens der Modalität liegt. Desweiteren sollte das Verfahren automatisiert ablaufen, um eine große Anzahl von Datensätzen segmentieren zu können.

2 Stand der Forschung und Fortschritt durch den Beitrag

Klassische Methoden, wie das Bereichswachstum, sind bei der Segmentierung des Bronchialbaums sehr problematisch, da sie bei feinen, nicht komplett abgebildeten Strukturen die Tendenz haben in das Lungenparenchym auszulaufen. Tschirren et al. arbeiteten daher in [1] mit dem Verfahren einer beweglichen Region zur schrittweisen Segmentierung. Auf verrauschten Bildern treten allerdings auch hier die bekannten Probleme auf.

Deschamps et al. stellen in [2] eine Methode zur Extraktion tubulärer Strukturen mittels Fast-Marching-Methoden vor, welche ebenfalls anfällig gegen Auslaufen sind. Hier wurde allerdings eine Segmentierung von kontrastierten Blutgefäßen in MRT-Aufnahmen vorgenommen.

Woerz et al. beschreiben in [3] die Segmentierung von tubulärer Strukturen mit Hilfe von Intensitätsmodellen. Diese beschreiben mathematisch den Grauwertübergang am Rande von Blutgefäßen. Der Übergang erfolgt vom Maximum innerhalb zu kleineren Werten ausserhalb, was den Bronchien im Parenchym nicht mehr gerecht wird.

Durch den in diesem Beitrag beschriebenen Algorithmus ist eine Segmentierung tubulärer Strukturen möglich. Durch die iterative Positionierung eines starren, frei wählbaren Modells an die am besten geeignete Stelle im Bild sollen Unterbrechungen in den tubulären Strukturen überwunden werden. Eine schnelle Anpassung an neue Bilder oder Modalitäten kann durch eine Generierung eines veränderten Modells erfolgen.

3 Methoden

Für den Algorithmus wird die Modellannahme getroffen, dass der Bronchialbaum aus einer Menge von Kreiszylindern aufgebaut ist. Ein Modell, welches in das Bild an einer definierten Stelle registriert werden soll, besteht aus einer Vielzahl an Punkten, die zusammen mehrere Ringe bilden. Jedem Punkt eines Rings wird ein Intensitätswert zugeordnet. Dieser Wert wird innerhalb des Registrierungsalgorithmus für den Vergleich zwischen Modell und Bild herangezogen. Zusätzlich wird jedem Modell ein Start- und ein Endpunkt, an denen weitere Modelle in folgenden Registrierungsschritten angehängt werden können, zugewiesen. Das Ergebnis ist eine Zusammensetzung von Modellen, die anhand von Mittelpunkten und Durchmesserb die Topologie des Bronchialbaums widerspiegeln. In einem Nachverarbeitungsschritt kann, durch diese Informationen unterstützt, die Oberfläche des Bronchialbaums segmentiert werden.

Der iterative Ablauf des Algorithmus sieht als erstes eine Detektion einer Verzweigung (Bifurkation) oder eines Endes vor. Wenn die Fortsetzung einer oder mehrerer tubulärer Strukturen erkannt wurde, wird eine Registrierung des Modells an der Stelle durchgeführt. Über das Ergebnis der Registrierung (Transformation) kann der optimale Mittelpunkt und die Dicke des Abschnitts errechnet und abgespeichert werden. Hiernach startet der Detektionsvorgang am Endpunkt des Modells erneut. Im Falle einer erkannten Bifurkation werden neue Registrierungsprozesse in den Richtungen der Teiläste angestoßen.

3.1 Detektion

Eine Verzweigungsdetektion erfolgt über die Erstellung und anschließende Analyse einer kugelförmigen Region. Hierzu werden mittels geeignetem Detektionsverfahren erstellte Hyperebenen, welche die Ein- und Austrittspunkte der tubulären Struktur darstellen, auf der Kugeloberfläche der Region berechnet (s. Abb. 2(a)). Unbedeutend klein erscheinende Hyperebenen werden gelöscht, so dass das Ergebnis eine Eintrittsebene und eine oder mehrere Austrittsebenen darstellen. Die Eintrittsebene wird über den Startpunkt der lokalen Segmentierung sowie vorhandene vorherige Modelle bestimmt. Alle weiteren Ebenen werden als Austrittsebenen charakterisiert. Wird keine weitere Ebene gefunden, wird das verwendete lokale Detektionsverfahren angepasst, oder es wird das Ende der tubulären Struktur angenommen. Wird eine zu große Hyperebene berechnet, erfolgt die Annahme, dass das lokale Detektionsverfahren in das Parenchym ausgelaufen ist. In diesem Fall wird die Berechnung der Hyperebenen mit einem weiteren Detektionsverfahren durchgeführt. Folgende lokale Detektionsverfahren können ihrer Laufzeit entsprechend zur Erstellung der Hyperebenen herangezogen werden:

Bereichswachstum Vom Startpunkt ausgehend erfolgt ein 3D-Bereichswachstum. Als Einschlusskriterium wird dabei ein oberer und unterer Grenzwert aus einer Statistik der Nachbarpixel des Betrachtunspunkts ermittelt. Nach Abschluss der Segmentierung erfolgt ein Schnitt des segmentierten Volumens mit der Kugeloberfläche der betrachteten Region um die Hyperebenen zu erzeugen. Abschließend wird der gefundene Bereich, sowie die Ein- und Austritte auf Plausibilität untersucht, um ein eventuelles Auslaufen zu vermeiden.

Adaptives Bereichswachstum Analog zum in [1] beschriebenen Verfahren werden bei einem Detektionsfehler die Parameter für das Bereichswachstums angepasst und ein erneuter Versuch gestartet. Die Anpassung erfolgt iterativ, bis die Detektion erfolgreich war, oder eine maximale Anzahl von Iterationen erreicht worden ist.

Partikelsystem Es wird mit Hilfe eines einfachen Partikelsystems der Weg der Luftmoleküle im Bronchus simuliert. Hierzu wird zunächst eine Schwellwertoperation durchgeführt und für die erzeugten Volumen jeweils Oberflächen mit Hilfe des Marching Cubes Algorithmus [4] erzeugt. Desweiteren wird ein Zielbild mit den selben Maßen wie die betrachtete Region angelegt. Dieses Zielbild wird vor dem Beginn der Partikelsimulation mit Grauwert 0 initialisiert. Vom Eintrittspunkt aus werden nun Partikel in zufälliger Richtung ausgesandt. Diese reflektieren an der zuvor berechneten Oberfläche. Wenn ein Partikel die Kugeloberfläche verläßt, wird an der Austrittstelle der Grauwert um einen definierten Wert erhöht. Aus der Summe aller Austrittsstellen von Partikeln ergeben sich Hyperebenen, die nach Filterung über die Größe der Ebenen die Austrittsstellen der tubulären Struktur darstellen.

Abb. 1. Detektion des Ein- und Austritts mittels Hyperebenen (Schnitt) (links) und Segmentierungs-Ergebnisse einer Trachea incl. Lappensegmente (CT-Datum) (rechts)

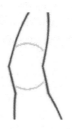
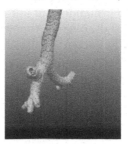

3.2 Registrierung

Nach der Detektion von Verzweigungs- oder Endpunkten wird das Modell in die Richtung des Austrittspunktes ausgerichtet und anhand des vorhergehenden Registrierungsergebnisses in der Größe angepaßt. Anschließend erfolgt die Registrierung des Modells mit dem Bild unter Verwendung des ITK-Registrierungsframeworks [5]. Als Komponenten werden hier eine affine Transformation, die quadrierte Differenz als Distanzwert und eine lineare Interpolation verwendet. Das Ergebnis der Registrierung ist eine Transformation, die den Endpunkt des Modells an eine neue Position verschiebt. Die neue Position wird zur erneuten Detektion von Bifurkations- bzw. Endpunkt mit anschließender Registrierung verwendet. So ähnelt der gesamte Algorithmus bildlich einem lokalen Entlangklettern and der tubulären Struktur.

4   Ergebnisse

Unter Verwendung des Insight Toolkits (ITK)[5] wurde ein Komandozeilenprogramm entwickelt, mit dessen Hilfe einzelne Modelle erstellt und in einem XML-Format gespeichert werden können. Ebenfalls kann hiermit der Segmentierungsvorgang initial eingestellt und gestartet werden. Ferner wurde im Medical Imaging Interaction Toolkit (MITK) [6] eine grafische Benutzeroberfläche zur interaktiven Definition der Ausgangsposition und Ansicht der Ergebnisse erstellt.

Der Algorithmus wurde initial an einem Ausschnitt der zentralen Geometrie des Bronchialbaums getestet (CT-Bilddatum, 512 x 512 Pixel, 376 Schichten). Dabei erwies sich der vollautomatische Algorithmus als sehr rechenaufwändig. Die zentrale Struktur des Bronchialbaums (6 Generationen) wurde erfolgreich bei einer Berechnungszeit von 8 Stunden mit einem Dual Xeon Prozessor PC mit 4 GB Hauptspeicher abgebildet. Bifurkationen wurden richtig erkannt und die anschliessenden Bronchien weiter verfolgt. Der Vergleich mit einem Segmentierungsergebnis eines Bereichwachstumsverfahren wurde hier nicht erstellt, da der hier vorgestellte Algorithmus weniger die Oberfläche als die Topologie extrahiert.

Die Qualität der Segmentierung erwies sich als vielversprechend für eine weitere Entwicklung. Da eine affine Transformation verwendet wird, kann der Algorithmus nicht jede Formänderung auf die zu registrierenden Modelle abbilden. Dies gilt vor allem für die oberen Atemwege, wo Knorpelspangen für eine Verminderung der Elastizität sorgen, so dass die Geometrie hier von der kreisförmigen Röhre abweicht.

5   Diskussion

Es wurde ein Algorithmus erstellt, der erfolgreich tubuläre Strukturen mittels Modell-zu-Bild-Registrierung erkennen kann. Durch eine Optimierung der Registrierungsparameter und eine Spezialisierung der einzelnen Registrierungskommponenten erwarten wir eine Minderung der Berechnungszeit auf unter eine Stunde. Dies erscheint ausreichend für die automatische Segmentierung von Bronchien im nicht-klinischen Bereich. Ferner wird die Entwicklung von Mehrkernprozessoren hier eine Unterstützung bieten. Zukünftige Pläne sehen eine Implementierung eines hybriden Segmentierungsansatzes, in dem der Registrierungsansatz nur in der bisher nicht segmentierbaren Peripherie der Lunge eingesetzt wird, vor. Desweiteren soll in zeitlich aufgelösten Bilddaten untersucht werden, inwiefern die Übernahme von Registrierungsergebnissen eines Zeitschritts zum nächsten die Gesamtlaufzeit beeinflußt.

Danksagung

Diese Arbeit wurde von der DFG im Rahmen des Projektes "Protektive Beatmungssysteme" (ME 833/11-1) gefördert.

Literaturverzeichnis

1. Tschirren J, Hoffman EA, McLennan G, Sonka M. Airway tree segmentation using adaptive regions of interest. Procs SPIE 2004.
2. Deschamps T, Cohen LD. Fast extraction of tubular and tree 3D surfaces with front propagation methods. In: Procs 16th International Conference on Pattern Recognition, ICPR'02. Quebec, Canada: IEEE Computer Society; 2002.
3. Wörz S, Rohr K. 3D parametric intesity models for accurate segmentaion and quantification of human arteries. Procs BVM 2004.
4. Lorensen WE, Cline HE. Marching cubes: A high resolution 3D surface construction algorithm. Procs SIGGRAPH '87 1987;21(4):163–169.
5. Ibanez L, Schroeder W, Ng L, Cates J. The ITK Software Guide. Kitware, Inc.; 2005. ISBN 1-930934-15-7.
6. Wolf I, Vetter M, Wegner I, Boettger T, Nolden M, Schoebinger M, et al. The medical imaging interaction toolkit. Med Image Anal 2005;9(6):594–604.

Segmentierung von Biopsienadeln in transrektalen Ultraschallaufnahmen der Prostata

Barbara Haupt, Dagmar Krefting, Thomas Tolxdorff

Institut für Medizinische Informatik,
Charité - Universitätsmedizin Berlin, 12200 Berlin
Email: haupt@inf.fu-berlin.de

Zusammenfassung. Die möglichst genaue Lokalisierung von Gewebe-proben im Prostatavolumen ist wichtig für die Diagnose und Therapie-planung von Prostatakarzinomen. In diesem Artikel wird ein Segmen-tierungsverfahren zur Erkennung der Biopsienadel in klinischen TRUS-Aufnahmen vorgestellt. Das Verfahren basiert auf einer multivarianten statistischen Klassifikation und konnte in 94% der 1835 Bilder aus 30 Bi-opsien unterschiedlicher Prostataregionen erfolgreich angewandt werden.

1 Einleitung

Prostatakarzinome gehören zu den häufigsten Tumoren bei Männern [1]. Der Goldstandard zur Diagnose ist die histologische Untersuchung von an bestimm-ten verschiedenen Stellen entnommenem Gewebe [2]. Dabei werden zur Führung der Biopsienadeln üblicherweise transrektale Ultraschallaufnahmen (TRUS) ver-wendet. In der bisherigen Praxis beschränkt sich die Positionsangabe der Gewe-beprobe auf die Angabe der Prostataregion, eine genauere Lokalisierung des ent-nommenen Gewebes wäre jedoch sowohl für eine verbesserte Diagnose als auch die Therapieplanung von großer Bedeutung. Das hier vorgestellte Verfahren ver-wendet dazu das während der Untersuchung aufgenommene Bildmaterial, so dass sich für die behandelnden Ärzte der Mehraufwand darauf beschränkt, nach jeder Biopsie die TRUS-Sequenz abzuspeichern. Da üblicherweise die Halterung der Biopsienadel am Schallkopf fixiert ist, ist die Orientierung und die Position der Nadel innerhalb der TRUS - Bilder auf einen festen Bereich beschränkt. Jedoch variieren Länge und Sichtbarkeit der Nadel stark. Zum einen kann die Nadel unterschiedlich weit ausgefahren werden, zum anderen liegt sie oft nicht exakt in der Bildebene, so dass sie nur unvollständig oder mit schwachem Kontrast abgebildet wird. Zusätzlich erschweren vom Hersteller des Gerätes eingeblende-te Markierungen, Gewebeinhomogenitäten und Artefakte, die durch Reflexionen entstehen, die korrekte Segmentierung. Einfache intensitätsbasierte Gradienten-methoden sind aufgrund des schlechten Signal-Rausch-Verhältnisses sowie der oft inhomogenen Intensitätsverteilung entlang der Nadel nur bedingt anwend-bar. Die Kombination von dynamisch varriierendem Schwellwert und einem mul-tivarianten statischen Klassifikator stellt hier eine Möglichkeit dar, die Nadel zu detektieren und segmentieren [3]. Der Merkmalsraum wird dabei durch Stan-dardmerkmale von Binärobjekten wie Fläche und Exzentrizität, sowie durch bildabhängige Merkmale wie die Distanz und die Orientierung relativ zu der Markierungslinie aufgespannt.

2   Stand der Forschung

Für die Segmentierung von Biopsie-Nadeln in zweidimensionalen Ultraschallbildern wird die Verwendung der Hough-Transformation vorgeschlagen [4]. Das vorgeschlagene Verfahren wurde anhand von Phantomen sowie einer Brust-Biopsie getestet. Dabei erweist es sich bei schlechtem Signal-Rausch-Verhältnis als unzuverlässig, außerdem muss zusätzlich die ungefähre Lage der Biopsienadel von der die Biopsie ausführenden Person angegeben werden. Zur Binarisierung der Bilder wurde ein histogrammbasiertes Schwellwertverfahren vewendet, dass eine feste Anzahl von "Objektpunkten", das heißt Pixel mit Intensitäten oberhalb des Schwellwertes, erzeugt. Dieses Verfahren ließ sich nur schlecht auf unser Datenmaterial anwenden: Da bei der Untersuchung unterschiedlicher Prostataregionen die Längen der auf dem Bild sichtbaren Biopsie-Nadeln stark variieren, und zudem starke, sehr helle Artefakte auftreten können, lässt sich ein globaler Wert für die Anzahl der "Objektpunkte" nicht einsetzen. Weitere Methoden zur Segmentierung von Nadeln in TRUS-Bildern beziehen sich auf 3D-Daten, in denen die Nadel voll enthalten und kontrastreich abgebildet ist [5]. Dies gilt, wie in der Einleitung erläutert, nicht für die klinischen 2D-TRUS-Aufnahmen. Das hier vorgestellte statistische Modell bietet die Möglichkeit, Informationen wie die erwartete Lage, Länge und Orientierung zu implementieren sowie die Abweichungen vom idealen Abbild der Nadel zu berücksichtigen. Damit kann zum einen aus einer Sequenz von Bildern der Zeitpunkt der Gewebeprobe als auch die Position der Biopsienadel automatisch bestimmt werden.

3   Methoden

Sämtliche TRUS-Aufnahmen wurden in der urologischen Poliklinik der Charité aufgenommen. Die Bildsequenzen werden verlustfrei digital gespeichert, wobei jede Sequenz aus 165 Bildern besteht und einen Zeitraum von 10s umfasst. Der Segmentierungsalgorithmus ist in *matlab* implementiert und umfasst folgende Schritte:

1. **Einschränkung des Suchraumes:** Da die ungefähre Lage der Nadel bekannt ist, wird eine Region of Interest (ROI) automatisch durch Detektion der Markierungslinie mittels Houghtransformation bestimmt (Abb. 1). Die Distanz der Markierungspunkte entspricht 5mm und wird als interne Einheit verwendet.
2. **Vorverarbeitung:** Innerhalb der ROI werden die Markierungspunkte durch die Intensitäten der benachbarten Pixel in einer 8-Nachbarschaft ersetzt. Anschließend wird das Bild mit einem Gaußfilter geglättet.
3. **Binarisierung:** Nadelkandidaten werden durch Binarisierung des Bildes mit verschiedenen Intensitätsschwellwerten gefunden. Objekte, die weniger als zehn Pixel umfassen, werden nicht berücksichtigt.

Tabelle 1. Objektmerkmale des Modells

Merkmal	Mittelwert	Standardabweichung
Fläche (pxl)	147.70	80.00
Länge der 1. Hauptachse	37.60	14.50
Länge der 2. Hauptachse	6.90	2.00
Exzentrizität	0.97	0.01
Abstand zur Markierungslinie	2.08	1.65
Winkeldifferenz zur Markierunslinie	4.06	3.02

4. **Bestimmung der Objektmerkmale:** Die folgenden Objektmerkmale werden für jedes Objekt bestimmt: Fläche, Exzentrizität, Länge der Hauptachsen, Position und Orientierung relativ zur Markierungslinie. Das Merkmalsmodell wird mittels einer Testmenge von per Hand segmentierten Nadeln gebildet (Tab. 1).

5. **Bestimmung des besten Objektes pro Bild:** Für jeden Frame und Intensitätsschwellwert wird das beste Objekt hinsichtlich der Mahalanobisdistanz ausgewählt [6]. Das beste Objekt innerhalb der verschiedenen Schwellwerte wird für jeden Frame ausgewählt, die Objekteigenschaften und ein Bild, das die segmentierte Region beinhaltet, werden zurückgegeben.

6. **Bestimmung des besten Objektes pro Bildsequenz:** Das Objekt mit der kleinsten Mahalanobisdistanz innerhalb einer Bildsequenz wird als Segmentierungsergebnis ausgewählt.

Der Algorithmus wurde auf vier Datensätzen, die jeweils eine komplette Untersuchung beinhalten, angewendet. Die Untersuchung wurde nach dem 10-Biopsie-Protokoll durchgeführt [7], so dass jeweils zehn Bildsequenzen aus unterschiedlichen Prostataregionen erzeugt werden. Ein Datensatz wurde als Trainingsmenge verwendet, wobei für jede Biopsie per Hand drei Nadeln segmentiert wurden. Die anderen drei Datensätze wurden als Testmenge verwendet. In den 1835 Bildern der Testmenge ist bekannt, dass Biopsienadeln sichtbar sind. Das Segmentierungsergebnis wurde in Abb. 2 im Originalbild dargestellt. Alle Bilder wurden

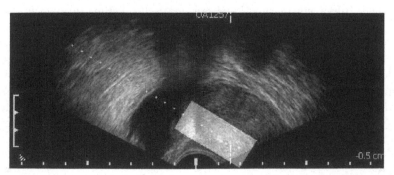

Abb. 1. Ergebnis der automatischen Bestimmung der Region of Interest, dargestellt als helle Fläche

Abb. 2. Erfolgreiches Segmentierungsergebnis, als weiße Fläche innerhalb des ursprünglinchen TRUS-Bildes dargestellt

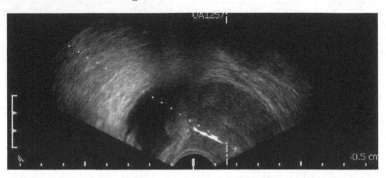

Abb. 3. Unvollständiges Segmentierungsergebnis der Biopsienadel. Die weiße Fläche überdeckt die Biopsienadel nur zum Teil

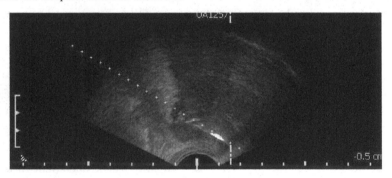

per Hand bewertet, ob das gefundene Objekt tatsächlich eine Biopsienadel darstellt.

4   Ergebnisse

In 94% aller Bilder wurde die Nadel automatisch erkannt, in allen Fällen wurde die Nadel als insgesamt bestes Objekt einer Sequenz gefunden (Abb. 2). Liegt die Nadel jedoch nicht exakt in der TRUS-Bildebene, treten starke Intensitätsgradienten entlang der Nadel auf. In diesen Fällen führt die Binarisierung des Bildes mit einem Intensitätsschwellwert zu unvollständiger Nadelsegmentierung (Abb. 3). In 104 Bildern (6%) schlug die Segmentierung fehl und das ausgewählte Objekt gehörte nicht zu einer Nadel. Die meisten dieser Bilder lagen am Anfang oder am Ende einer Probenentnahme, wo die zu sehende Nadel auf dem Bild nur sehr kurz ist (Abb. 4).

Abb. 4. Fehlgeschlagene Segmentierung. Das Segmentierungsergebnis ist als weiße Fläche dargestellt, der Pfeil zeigt auf die Biopsienadel

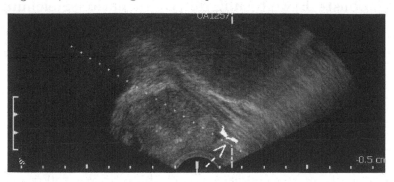

5 Diskussion

Die vorgestellte Arbeit stellt eine robuste, automatische Methode für die Erkennung von Biopsienadeln und deren Segmentierung dar. In 94% der Testbilder wurde die Nadel korrekt erkannt, in allen Fällen konnte die Nadel als insgesamt bestes Objekt bestimmt werden. Eine Schwierigkeit besteht darin, dass aufgrund von Intensitätsgradienten nicht die vollständige Nadel segmentiert wird. Eine kleinere Schrittweite der Schwellwerte, eine Kombination von aufeinanderfolgenden Nadelobjekten in der Bildsequenz und/oder ein nachfolgender Regiongrowing-Algorithmus, der die unvollständig segmentierte Nadel als Seed verwendet, könnten dieses Problem beheben.

Literaturverzeichnis

1. Gesellschaft der epidemologischen Krebsregister in Deutschland eV (GEKID) und RKI. Krebs in Deutschland, Häufigkeiten und Trends. http://www.rki.de; 2006.
2. Loch T, Eppelmann U, Lehmann J, et al. Transrectal ultrasound guided biopsy of the prostate: Random sextant versus biopsies of sono-morphologically suspicious lesions. World J Urol 2004;22:357–60.
3. Duda RO, Hart PE, Stork DG. Pattern Classification. Wiley; 2001.
4. Ding M, Fenster A. A real-time biopsy needle segmentation technique using Hough transform. Med Phys 2003;30(8):2222–33.
5. Wei Z, Gardi L, Downey DB, et al. Oblique needle segmentation and tracking for 3D TRUS guided prostate brachytherapy. Med Phys 2005;32(9):2928–41.
6. Mahalanobis PC. On the generalized distance in statistics. Proc Nat Inst Sci 1936;12:49–55.
7. Egevad L, Frimmel H, Norberg M, et al. Three dimensional computer reconstruction of prostate cancer from radical prostatectomy specimens: Evaluation of the model by core biopsy simulation. Adult Urology 1999;53(1):192–98.

Freiheit für Formmodelle!

Eine robuste Erweiterung der Deformationsgleichungen

Tobias Heimann, Sascha Münzing, Ivo Wolf und Hans-Peter Meinzer

Abteilung für Medizinische und Biologische Informatik,
Deutsches Krebsforschungszentrum, 69120 Heidelberg
Email: t.heimann@dkfz.de

Zusammenfassung. Wir stellen eine neuartige Methode zur Segmentierung volumetrischer Bilddaten vor, die Techniken von statistischen Formmodellen mit deformierbaren Oberflächen kombiniert. Die internen Kräfte der deformierbaren Oberfläche berechnen sich dabei aus einem mitlaufenden Formmodell, während die externen Kräfte aus einem graph-basierten Verfahren zur optimalen Oberflächenerkennung gewonnen werden. Testsegmentierungen der Leber auf über 50 CT-Datensätzen zeigen eine mittlere Oberflächenabweichung von 1.6 ± 0.7mm zu manuellen Referenzsegmentierungen und machen deutlich, dass mehr Freiheit für Formmodelle die Ergebnisse oft signifikant verbessern kann.

1 Einleitung

Die automatische Segmentierung dreidimensionaler Datensäze ist in der medizinischen Bildverarbeitung nach wie vor ein drängendes – und weitgehend ungelöstes – Problem. Aufgrund ihrer Robustheit auch bei verrauschten und artefaktbehafteten Bilddaten erfreuen sich statistische Formmodelle [1] in letzten Jahren steigender Beliebtheit. Aus einer Menge von Trainingsdaten wird bei diesem Verfahren eine Durchschnittsform und mögliche Variationsrichtungen berechnet, welche den Segmentierungsvorgang leiten. Da die Anzahl verfügbarer Trainingsdaten stets limitiert ist, sind die resultierenden Modelle allerdings oft nicht umfassend genug: Die erlaubten Deformationen sind zu stark eingeschränkt und die Bilddaten können nicht optimal segmentiert werden.

2 Stand der Forschung und Fortschritt durch den Beitrag

Neben der Einführung einer beschränkten Anzahl von künstlichen Freiheitsgraden in das Modell [2] (was die grundsätzliche Problematik nicht ändert), gibt es zwei Möglichkeiten, die Segmentierungsergebnisse besser an die Daten anzupassen: Entweder die Adaptierung findet als Nachbearbeitungsschritt statt (wie in [3]) oder die Segmentierung erfolgt über ein frei deformierbares Modell, das seine internen Kräfte an einem gleichzeit mitlaufenden Formmodell ausrichtet [4]. In diesem Artikel stellen wir eine robuste Methode vor, die dem zweiten Ansatz folgt. Hauptunterschied zu den bisherigen Arbeiten ist die Definition der externen Kräfte, die auf einem graph-basierten Algorithmus zur optimalen Oberflächenerkennung basiert. Zusammen mit den stabilisierenden internen Kräften, die längen- und winkelgetrieben sind, ergibt sich ein neues Segmentierungsmodell für 3D-Daten, das bisherigen Ansätzen deutlich überlegen ist.

3 Methoden

Das deformierbare Modell ist ein trianguliertes Gitternetzmodell (Mesh) des Objekts und stimmt topologisch mit dem korrespondierenden Formmodell (SSM) überein. Für jeden Knoten p_i im Mesh gibt es somit einen entsprechenden Punkt $\tilde{p}_i$ im SSM. Nach einer benutzerbasierten Initialisierung wird die Evolution des deformierbaren Modells über regularisierende (interne) ud datengetriebene (externe) Kräfte gesteuert. In diskreter Form ergibt sich für jeden Knoten p_i des triangulierten Meshes:

$$p_i^{t+1} = p_i^t + F_{\text{int}}(p_i^t) + F_{\text{ext}}(p_i^t) \tag{1}$$

Analog zu den klassischen Snakes [5] wird die interne Energie als Kombination von Spannung und Rigidität realisiert. Die Spannungskraft wirkt auf alle Kanten des Meshes und treibt sie auf die Länge der entsprechenden Kante im aktuellen Formmodell:

$$F_T(p,q) = \alpha \left(1 - \frac{|\tilde{p} - \tilde{q}|}{|p - q|}\right)(p - q) \tag{2}$$

mit α als Stärke der Spannungskraft. Die Rigiditätskraft wirkt auf die Winkel zwischen benachbarten Dreiecken und treibt sie auf die entsprechenden Winkel im Formmodell zu (Abb. 1):

$$F_R(q, [p_1, p_2]) = T(q, [p_1, p_2], \beta\delta) - q \tag{3}$$

Hierbei ist $T(q, [p_1, p_2], \delta)$ eine Rotation von Punkt q um die Kante $[p_1, p_2]$ um δ Grad und β die Stärke der Rigiditätskraft. Da die durchschnittlichen Positionen der betroffenen Punkte durch die internen Kräfte nicht verändert werden dürfen, muss eine entsprechende Gegenkraft auf alle Punkte der Gruppe wirken:

$$F_N([p_1, p_2]) = -\frac{1}{4}(F_R(q_1, [p_1, p_2]) + F_R(q_2, [p_1, p_2])) \tag{4}$$

Die interne Kraft F_{int} ergibt sich dann aus einer Summe aus F_T, F_R und F_N.

Die externen Kräfte werden aus Effizienzgründen nur alle 10 Iterationen aktualisiert: Für jede Landmarke wird dann entlang der Oberflächennormale an mehreren Stellen (nach innen und außen) eine Kostenfunktion ausgewertet, die den Übereinstimmungsgrad der Position mit einem zuvor berechneten Erscheinungsmodell berechnet. In dieser Arbeit verwenden wir dafür ein nichtlineares Grauwertmodell, das auf einem kNN-Klassifikator basiert und auf Kantenprofilen und zusätzlichen Umgebungsprofilen (von der echten Position verschoben) trainiert wurde [6]. Anstatt nun für jede Landmarke individuell die Position mit den jeweils minimalen Kosten als besten Kandidaten zu wählen, berechnen wir die

Abb. 1. Zwei angrenzende Dreiecke formen den Winkel θ. Die interne Rigiditätskraft (die im gezeigten Fall den Winkel vergrößert) wirkt nicht nur auf die äußeren Punkte q_1 and q_2, sondern auch auf die Kantenpunkte p_1 und p_2, um das Gleichgewicht der Gruppe zu halten

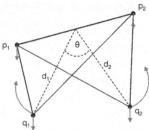

Abb. 2. Optimale Oberflächensuche für triangulierte Meshes: Links ist ein Ausschnitt aus dem Mesh abgebildet; die unterschiedlichen Testpositionen für jeden Punkt sind als graue Linien eingezeichnet. Auf der rechten Seite wird gezeigt, wie zwei benachbarte Testlinien im Graphen repräsentiert sind

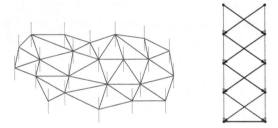

Oberfläche, die unter festgeschriebenen Stetigkeitskriterien global (d.h. über alle Landmarken summiert) die minimalen Kosten erreicht. Dazu wird das Problem der optimalen Oberflächensuche in das in polynomialer Laufzeit lösbare Problem des maximalen Flusses in einem Graphen überführt, wie in [7] beschrieben wird. Der verwendete Graph wird aus dem Mesh erstellt und verbindet sämtliche Testpositionen mit ihren direkten Nachbarn und der Mesh-Topologie (Abb. 2). Die berechneten Kosten werden als Kantengewichte zu speziellen Quell- und Senkknoten eingefügt. Durch den minimalen Schnitt zwischen Quelle und Senke (der sich aus dem maximalen Fluss ergibt) können die Punkte der optimalen Oberfläche gewonnen werden. Der Unterschied zwischen diesen Punkten und den entsprechenden Positionen im aktuellen Mesh ergibt nach einer Multiplikation mit dem Faktor γ die externe Kraft F_{ext}.

Die Parameter des SSM werden nun wie in [1] beschrieben auf die Punkte der optimalen Oberfläche angepasst. Für die folgenden 10 Iterationen werden die internen Kräfte versuchen, den Mesh zu dieser Form hin zu deformieren, während die externen Kräft die als optimal erkannten Punkte ansteuern. Durch eine Verschiebung der Gewichte α, β, γ von externen zu internen Kräften wird im Verlauf der Segmentierung der Schwerpunkt von Formerhaltung auf Datenanpassung verlagert.

4   Ergebnisse

Das beschriebene deformierbare Modell wurde auf über 50 abdominalen (zum Großteil pathologischen, d.h. mit Tumoren durchsetzten) CT-Datensätzen für die Segmentierung der Leber ausgewertet. Das für die internen Kräfte genutzte Formmodell wurde zuvor aus 32 anderen Lebersegmentierungen erstellt, ebenso wie die Erscheinungsmodelle für die externen Kräfte. Die zur Datenakquisition verwendeten Protokolle variieren sowohl in der Trainings- als auch in der Testgruppe bezüglich Auflösung, Voxelgrößen, genutztem Kontrastmittel und weiteren internen Parametern, was die Auswertung für das klinische Umfeld als realistisch erscheinen lässt. Nach einer kurzen benutzergesteuerten Initialisierung (d.h. grobe Anpassung von Position, Rotation und Größe des Modells auf den aktuellen Datensatz) lief die Segmentierung vollautomatisch. Die durchschnittliche Oberflächenabweichung von manuellen Referenzsegmentierungen betrug insgesamt 1.6 ± 0.7mm. Abb. 3 zeigt das Ergebnis für den Datensatz, der den Median der Oberflächenabweichungen markiert.

5   Diskussion

Die erzielte Genauigkeit bei der Lebersegmentierung ist deutlich besser als bisher veröffentlichte Werte anderer Methoden: So erreichten Soler et al. eine mittlere Oberflächenabweichung von 2mm mit frei deformierbaren Modellen [8] und Lamecker et al. 2.3 ± 0.3mm mit klassischen Formmodellen [9]. Hauptvorteil des vorgestellten Verfahrens im Gegensatz zu den klassischen Formmodellen ist, dass sich die Segmentierung besser an die Daten anpassen kann, was auch in Abb. 3 zu sehen ist. Die zusätzliche Freiheit in der Deformation zahlt sich hier direkt aus. Im Vergleich zu anderen deformierbaren Modellen sind die externen Kräfte des vorgestellten Verfahrens stabiler, da sie sich auf eine global optimale Oberfläche für den jeweiligen Iterationsschritt stützen, anstatt auf individuelle beste Positionen für jeden Punkt. Ausreißer können so völlig vermieden werden.

Probleme gibt es noch bei der Anpassung an spitz zulaufende Formen, da die Auflösung des verwendeten Meshes (ca. 2500 Punkte) an diesen Stellen nicht hoch genug ist. Neben der Lösung dieser Aufgabe werden wir den Algorithmus auch auf andere Objekte und Modalitäten anwenden. Wir hoffen, mit dem vorgestellten Verfahren den Großteil der anfallenden Segmentierungen in Zukunft weitgehend automatisch lösen zu können.

Literaturverzeichnis

1. Cootes TF, Taylor CJ, Cooper DH, Graham J. Active shape models: Their training and application. Comp Vis Image Underst 1995;61(1):38–59.

140   T. Heimann et al.

Abb. 3. Transversale, sagittale and frontale Schicht für eine durchschnittliche Leber-segmentierung. Oben: Die manuelle Referenzsegmentierung. Unten: Das Ergebnis für das Standard SSM in dunkelgrau, für das vorgestellte deformierbare Modell in weiss

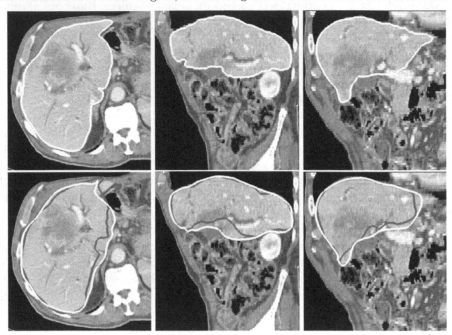

2. Tölli T, Koikkalainen J, Lauerma K, Lötjönen J. Artificially enlarged training set in image segmentation. LNCS 2006;4190:75–82.
3. Li B, Reinhardt JM. Automatic generation of object shape models and their application to tomographic image segmentation. In: Procs SPIE; 2001. 311–322.
4. Weese J, Kaus M, Lorenz C, Lobregt S, et al. Shape constrained deformable models for 3D medical image segmentation. In: Proc IPMI. Springer; 2001. 380–387.
5. Kass M, Witkin A, Terzopoulos D. Snakes: Active countour models. Int Journal Comp Vis 1988;1(4):321–331.
6. Münzing S, Heimann T, Wolf I, Meinzer HP. Evaluierung von Erscheinungsmodellen für die Segmentierung mit Statistischen Formmodellen. In: Proc BVM; 2007.
7. Li K, Millington S, Wu XD, Chen DZ, Sonka M. Simultaneous segmentation of multiple closed surfaces using optimal graph searching. In: Proc IPMI. Springer; 2005. 406–417.
8. Soler L, Delingette H, Malandain G, Montagnat J, Ayache N, et al. Fully automatic anatomical, pathological, and functional segmentation from CT scans for hepatic surgery. Procs SPIE 2000; 246–255.
9. Lamecker H, Lange T, Seebass M. Segmentation of the Liver using a 3D Statistical Shape Model. Zuse Institute. Berlin; 2004.

Fusion of Intracardiac Ultrasound with 3D Cardiac C-Arm CT from Animal Data for Electrophysiology

Matthias John[1], Yiyong Sun[2], Samuel Kadoury[2], Wolfgang Wein[2],
Yong Li[2], Jeff Resnick[3], Gerry Plambeck[3], Ann Dempsey[3],
Amin Al-Ahmad[4], Rebecca Fahrig[4], Frank Sauer[2]

[1]Siemens Medical Solutions, Erlangen, Germany
[2]Siemens Corporate Research, Princeton, NJ, USA
[3]Siemens Medical Solutions, Mountain View, CA, USA
[4]Stanford University Medical School, Stanford, CA, USA
Email: matthias.mj.john@siemens.com

Abstract. In electrophysiology catheter ablation is an established treatment for cardiac arrhythmias. Nevertheless, complicated ablation procedures such as pulmonary vein isolation for atrial fibrillation treatment are difficult to learn. This can be improved by a better integration of the image modalities available today and in the future electrophysiology lab. In this paper, we present a method to register ultrasound images from an ICE catheter and 3D cardiac C-arm CT images, which can both be obtained during the intervention. This is the first step required to display the ICE images relative to the complex anatomy of the left atrium.

1 Introduction

Atrial fibrillation is the most common heart arrhythmia and the major cause of stroke. Over 2 million people are affected in the U.S. alone. Cardiac CT and MR can deliver high resolution 3D images of the individual heart anatomy. In the future, this pre-interventional imaging could be replaced by a rotational C-arm technique, that is able to produce such images immediately before or during the intervention [1]. An imaging modality that is already used today in many electrophysiology (EP) labs is intracardiac echo (ICE) – a steerable catheter that contains an ultrasound transducer in its tip. By placing the catheter tip into the right atrium the physician is able to image the whole left atrium and some neighboring structures in real time. Therefore it has become an excellent tool for visualization of anatomical structures and instruments, and to monitor critical events.

The combination of 3D cardiac rotational C-arm imaging with ICE and a future integration in the EP lab could help the electrophysiologists to guide ICE and the ablation catheter. It could improve the learning curve for the use of ICE and therefore the whole pulmonary vein isolation procedure.

2   State of the Art and New Contribution

Several approaches have been suggested for the registration of ultrasound with MR and conventional CT, e.g. in [2] for kidney images from ultrasound and CT. There the ultrasound images are preprocessed by reducing speckle noise and shadows. In [3] a similarity measure is presented that consists of skin surface clamping (not necessary for ICE), edge correlation and Mutual Information. CT intensities, gradients and edge features are used for the computation.

Also for electrophysiological applications ultrasound was fused with CT data. In [4] a registration between conventional cardiac CT data and ICE is described. A point-to-surface registration, by first extracting surface point sets of the left atrium from the ICE images, is used. As far as we know, our results are the first on fusing the two image modalities ICE and cardiac C-arm CT.

3   Methods

3.1   System

In our system 3D images are acquired on a Angiographic C-arm system (AXIOM Artis, Siemens Medical Solutions). To image the left atrium of a patient we acquire images during 4 consecutive rotational 190° C-arm runs. Therefore we get enough images to reconstruct a 3D image of one cardiac phase. The images are reconstructed and processed on a PC workstation. The left atrium and other heart structures can be segmented using dedicated software.

The images acquired by the ICE catheter (AcuNav, Siemens Medical Solutions) are transferred via a frame grabber card into the PC. To track the position of the ICE catheter tip we used a magnetic tracking system (Microbird, Ascension). Its position sensor has been integrated in the same tubing with the ultrasound transducer. The transmitter is installed under the table of the C-arm system, such that an ICE catheter above the table can be tracked during an intervention.

During ICE imaging we record the ECG signal of the patient, and track the position of the ICE position sensor and a position sensor at the patient's chest (for correcting respiratory motion) synchronously.

3.2   Experimental Animal Data

In an animal experiment a 3D cardiac C-arm CT data set from a pig was taken. We additionally took various ICE image sequences from the pig's heart. The catheter was inserted by the physician into the right atrium of the pig. All image sequences were taken from this position by rotating and slightly moving the catheter tip. As mentioned above we also recorded the ECG signal and the coordinates of the two position sensors at catheter tip and chest. Based on these images we performed the following preprocessing and registration procedure offline.

Fig. 1. Preprocessing of a pig heart cardiac C-arm CT image: original image (left), gradient magnitude image (middle), and thresholding of 67 (right)

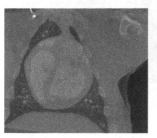 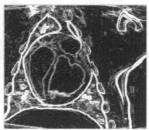 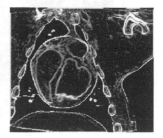

3.3   Motion Gating for ICE Images

The main difficulty of a good registration is the cardiac motion from the beating heart and the motion due to respiration in the ICE images. Therefore we need a good pre-selection of useful ICE images.

If we ignore patient movement we can observe the cyclic respiration motion in the graph of the vertical dimension of the 3D position sensor at the chest. This graph has regular peaks separated by long plateaus. The plateaus are of nearly constant height. We compute for every image the variation of this image and its previous images for a fixed time frame. For images with a low variation we can assume that these images were taken in a respiratory phase corresponding to a plateau. So we select those 'low variation' images from the whole sequence.

To compensate for cardiac motion we further select those images with a fixed time distance to the previous R-wave in the ECG signal.

3.4   Registration

For an initial registration the user has to select a point in the 3D data set that is close to the position of the catheter tip of the ultrasound image sequence. This gives an initial translation. For an initial rotation we assume that the tracking device is installed under the C-arm table in a fixed and given direction.

This initial registration is followed by an automatic local optimization step to find a good rigid body transformation. First we preprocess the C-arm CT data. We extract the magnitudes of the local gradients by applying a 3D Sobel filter [5]. Because there are many regions outside the heart with strong gradients that can worsen the registration quality, we apply a mask based on the grey values of the original volume to focus on the edges representing the heart walls (see Fig. 1). The ultrasound images are downsized by a factor of 4 in each dimension to improve the runtime.

We optimize the transformation according to the following similarity measure: We re-slice the C-arm CT gradient magnitude data in the ultrasound image planes using tri-linear interpolation. Now the similarity measure is computed using a normalized cross-correlation (NCC) [5]

Fig. 2. Registration using a sequence of 12 gated ICE images

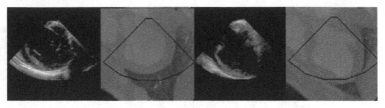

$$\text{Similarity}_T = \sum_{i=1}^{n} \text{NCC}(\text{US}_i, \text{CT}_{T,i}) \qquad (1)$$

where US_i is the ith ICE image from the gated sequence of n images. $\text{CT}_{T,i}$ is the resliced plane from the cardiac C-arm CT gradient magnitude data corresponding to US_i and a given transformation T. Observe that we take the measure only for those pixels located inside the fan shape of the ultrasound image.

The optimization is done using a best neighbor method. For an initial step size all transformation parameters are changed in turn with the step size and the resulting value of the similarity measure is computed. The change with the best improvement is taken and the step is repeated until there is no further improvement. Then the step size is decreased and the whole procedure starts again. We use an initial step size of 5.5mm and 5.5°. Both are reduced by a factor of 2 repeatedly until we reach a step size of 0.1mm or 0.1°.

4   Results

The registration was done offline with the cardiac C-arm CT and ICE data obtained from the animal experiment. A visual comparison of the registration can be obtained by aligning the ICE images side by side with their corresponding cardiac C-arm CT cut planes (see Fig. 2).

For a quantitative validation of the registration results we compared segmentations of cardiac chambers. For the 3D segmentation of the C-arm CT data set we used a semi-automatic tool developed for cardiac CT data. The segmentation of the ICE data was done manually by an expert.

We generated registrations and segmentations of 29 pairs of ICE images and their corresponding C-arm CT cut planes. For visual assessment we compared the contour of the ultrasound segmentation and the registered C-arm CT segmentation contour (see Fig. 3). For quantitative assessment we computed the shortest distance from each contour pixel of the C-arm CT segmentation to the registered ultrasound contour. The mean error was 3.14±3.13mm.

The whole registration procedure implemented in C++ took less than a minute on a system with an Intel P4 processor with 2.8GHz and 2GB DDR memory.

Fig. 3. Contour of a cardiac chamber manually segmented from ultrasound (left). The contour of the same chamber segmented from the cardiac C-arm CT image and projected to the registered ultrasound image (middle). A fusion of an ICE image with segmented cardiac chambers from the 3D cardiac C-arm CT image (right)

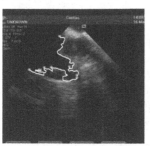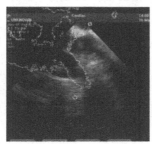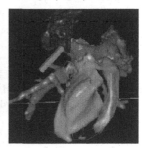

5 Discussion

The results show a good alignment of ICE images and their registered cardiac C-arm CT planes. Nevertheless, the quantitative analysis of registration accuracy shows some variation. The question is, whether this is related to the registration algorithm. A non-negligible additional source of registration and fusion errors that we currently ignore might be patient movement. Furthermore the registration algorithm is based on grey values, whereas the validation of these results is based on segmentations. Some segmented anatomical details and their contour lines might be different in both image modalities. In particular, a precise manual segmentation of the ultrasound images is difficult to achieve.

In the future our proposed methods can be used to build a system that makes it easy to integrate and fuse 3D cardiac rotational C-arm imaging and ICE in the EP suite. Both image modalities will be available during the EP procedure, in contrast with MR and CT which are acquired pre-intervention. A further step could be the fusion with Electro-anatomical mapping data. We believe that these image integrations make it much easier for physicians to learn and perform complex EP ablation procedures.

References

1. Lautisch G, et al. Towards cardiac c-arm computed tomography. IEEE Trans Med Imaging 2006;25(7):922–934.
2. Leroy A, et al. Rigid registration of freehand 3D ultrasound and CT-scan kidney images. Procs MICCAI 2004; 837–844.
3. Wein W, Roper B, Navab N. Automatic registration and fusion of ultrasound with CT for radiotherapy. Procs MICCAI 2005; 303–311.
4. Zhong H, Kanade T, Schwartzman D. Virtual touch: An efficient registration method for catheter navigation in left atrium. Procs MICCAI 2006; 437–444.
5. Gonzales RC, Woods RE. Digital Image Processing. Prentice Hall; 2002.

Wahl eines gewichteten Distanzmaßes für monomodale Bilder in der nicht-parametrischen Registrierung

Hanno Schumacher[1], Konstantin Ens[1,2], Astrid Franz[2], Bernd Fischer[2]

[1]Universität zu Lübeck, Institut für Mathematik, Wallstraße 40, 23560 Lübeck
[2]Philips Technologie GmbH Forschungslaboratorien, Röntgenstr. 24, 22335 Hamburg
Email: schumaha@math.uni-luebeck.de

Zusammenfassung. In der Bildregistrierung ist es häufig notwendig, die Methoden den speziellen Problemanforderungen der zu bearbeitenden Bilder anzupassen. Ein Weg, um zusätzliches Wissen in eine Registrierung einzubringen, ist die Nutzung gewichteter Distanzmaße, um damit die Bedeutung ausgewählter Bildbereiche zu verstärken, abzuschwächen oder auszublenden. Im Fall der parameterfreien Registrierung sind zwei gewichtete Distanzmaße, SSD^{mix} und MI^{add}, bekannt. Diese beiden Distanzmaße werden hier gegenübergestellt und ihre Wirkung auf monomodalen Bildern verglichen. Zusätzlich wird SSD^{mix} mit ungewichtetem MI verglichen. Die Ergebnisse verdeutlichen, dass SSD^{mix} und MI^{add} bessere Ergebnisse als SSD und MI liefern. Weiterhin zeigt sich, dass SSD^{mix} und MI^{add} für monomodale Bilder gleichmächtig sind.

1 Einleitung

Medizinische Bildregistrierung bestimmt eine Transformation zwischen zwei oder mehreren Bildern, um korrespondierende Strukturen abzugleichen [1, 2, 3]. Die gesuchte Transformation $\mathbf{u}$, auch Verrückungsfeld genannt, kann dabei durch eine Linearkombination von vorgewählten Basisfunktionen beschrieben werden. Dies wird als parametrischer Ansatz betrachtet. Eine weitere Möglichkeit ist es, das Verrückungsfeld als Lösung einer zugehörigen partiellen Differenzialgleichung zu bestimmen. Dieser parameterfreie Ansatz wird hier verwendet. Dabei wird für ein Referenzbild $\mathbf{R}$ und ein zu transformierendes Templatebild $\mathbf{T}$ das Funktional

$$J(\mathbf{u}; \mathbf{R}, \mathbf{T}) = \alpha S(\mathbf{u}) + D(\mathbf{u}; \mathbf{R}, \mathbf{T}) \qquad (1)$$

minimiert, wobei S als Glätter oder Regularisierer bezeichnet wird, D ein Distanzmaß ist und α als Steuerungsparameter zur Regelung des Einflusses von Glätter und Distanzmaß dient. Der Glätter gibt dabei vor, welche Art von Deformation zulässig ist, während das Distanzmaß die Ähnlichkeit von $\mathbf{R}$ und $\mathbf{T}$ misst. Die Wahl von S und D ist dabei von der Aufgabenstellung und den zugrunde liegenden Bildern abhängig. Eine typische Wahl für S ist ein elastischer, diffusiver oder auf Krümmung basierender Glätter [1]. Beispiele für das Distanzmaß D sind die Summe der quadrierten Grauwertdifferenzen (SSD) für monomodale oder Mutual Information (MI) [4] für multimodale Bilder. In einigen Anwendungen reichen diese Distanzmaße nicht aus, um gute Ergebnisse zu erzielen. Ein Beispiel sind CT-Aufnahmen des Abdominalbereichs des Menschen. Durch eine unterschiedliche Lage zu verschiedenen Aufnahmezeitpunkten müssen Gewebeübergänge angepasst werden, die sich nur gering im Grauwert unterscheiden (Abb. 2). Solche Fälle erfordern die Einbindung zusätzlichen externen Wissens. Eine Möglichkeit, Vorwissen zu integrieren, sind gewichtete Distanzmaße. Bekannt sind dabei zwei Ansätze, eine gewichtete Summe der quadrierten Grauwertdifferenzen (SSD^{mix}) [5], und eine gewichtete Mutual Information (MI^{add}) [6]. In dieser Arbeit werden diese gewichteten Maße gegenübergestellt und gleichzeitig mit ihren ungewichteten Varianten verglichen, wobei im Fokus monomodale Bilder stehen. Die Verfahren werden hinsichtlich der Verbesserung des Ergebnisses und dem dazu benötigten Aufwand bewertet.

2 Stand der Forschung und Fortschritt durch den Beitrag

Distanzmaße in einer Registrierung, die nicht speziell auf die Problematik angepasst sind, liefern oft ungenügende Ergebnisse. Dies motivierte die Entwicklung verschiedene Ansätze zur Integration von Vorwissen in eine parameterfreie Registrierung [5, 6]. Hier werden nun zum ersten Mal unterschiedliche gewichtete Distanzmaße gegenübergestellt und hinsichtlich der Verbesserung des Ergebnisses und des dazu benötigten Aufwands verglichen. Die so gewonnen Erkenntnisse helfen bei der Auswahl eines Distanzmaßes für die Registrierung.

3 Methoden

Wir beschränken uns hier auf die Wahl des elastischen Glätters

$$S(\mathbf{u}) = \int_\Omega \frac{\mu}{4} \sum_{j,k=1}^{2} (\partial_j u_k(\mathbf{x}) + \partial_k u_j(\mathbf{x}))^2 + \frac{\lambda}{2}(\text{div } \mathbf{u}(\mathbf{x}))^2 \mathrm{d}\mathbf{x} \qquad (2)$$

mit den materialabhängigen Lamé-Parametern λ und μ und dem zu untersuchenden Gebiet Ω. Um nun das Funktional (1) mit dem elastischen Glätter zu minimieren, betrachten wir die Gâteaux-Ableitung. Dies führt zu einer partiellen Differentialgleichung

$$\alpha(\mu\Delta\mathbf{u}(\mathbf{x}) + (\lambda + \mu)\nabla\text{div } \mathbf{u}(\mathbf{x})) = \mathbf{f}(\mathbf{x}, \mathbf{u}(\mathbf{x})) \qquad (3)$$

die zu lösen ist, wobei der Term $\mathbf{f}$ allein durch die Ableitung des Distanzmaßes bestimmt wird. Als Distanzmaße werden SSD, MI und die beiden gewichteten Maße SSD^{mix} und MI^{add} benutzt, auf die hier im folgenden näher eingegangen wird. Das Distanzmaß

$$\text{SSD}^{\text{mix}}(\mathbf{u}) = \frac{1}{2}\int_\Omega [(\mathbf{T}(\varphi(\mathbf{x})) - \mathbf{R}(\mathbf{x}))(\mathbf{M_T}(\varphi(\mathbf{x})) - \mathbf{M_R}(\mathbf{x}))\mathbf{M_A}(\mathbf{x})]^2 \mathrm{d}\mathbf{x} \qquad (4)$$

mit $\varphi(\mathbf{x}) = \mathbf{x} - \mathbf{u}(\mathbf{x})$ gewichtet die Differenz zwischen Referenz und Template. Die Gewichtungsfaktoren werden dabei durch die Masken $\mathbf{M_T}$, $\mathbf{M_R}$ und $\mathbf{M_A}$ festgelegt, deren Informationen durch Subtraktion zusätzlich kombiniert werden. Die Masken sind wie folgt definiert: Seien $B_{\mathbf{T}}^{(i)}, B_{\mathbf{R}}^{(i)} \subset \Omega, i = 1, 2, \ldots, m$ korrespondierende zusammenhängende Gebiete in $\mathbf{T}$ und $\mathbf{R}$ mit $B_{\mathbf{T}}^{(i)} \cap B_{\mathbf{R}}^{(j)} = \emptyset$ für $i \neq j$. Weiterhin sei $b_i \geq 0$ der Gewichtungsfaktor für $B_{\mathbf{T}}^{(i)}$ und $B_{\mathbf{R}}^{(i)}$. Somit folgt die Definition

$$\mathbf{M_T}(\mathbf{x}) = \begin{cases} b_i & : \quad \mathbf{x} \in B_{\mathbf{T}}^{(i)} \\ 1 & : \quad \text{sonst} \end{cases} , \quad \mathbf{M_R}(\mathbf{x}) = \begin{cases} b_i + 1 & : \quad \mathbf{x} \in B_{\mathbf{R}}^{(i)} \\ 0 & : \quad \text{sonst} \end{cases}$$

und

$$\mathbf{M_A}(\mathbf{x}) = \begin{cases} 0 & : \quad \mathbf{x} \in B_{\mathbf{R}}^{(i)} \wedge b_i = 0 \\ 1 & : \quad \text{sonst} \end{cases}$$

Die Gewichtungsfaktoren werden dabei dem Registrierungsproblem angepasst gewählt. Allgemein können die Masken für SSD^{mix} nach einem einfachen Schema gewählt werden: Ein Bereich wird durch den Faktor 0 ausgeblendet. Für eine Gewichtung wird die Höhe der Grauwertdifferenz zwischen einem zu gewichtenden Bereich und seiner Umgebung mit einem Faktor multipliziert. Somit geht dieser Bereich im Vergleich zu anderen Bildstrukturen stärker oder schwächer in die externen Kräfte der Registrierung ein. Im Unterschied zu SSD^{mix} gewichtet das Distanzmaß

$$\text{MI}^{\text{add}}(\mathbf{u}) = - \int_{\mathbb{R}^2} \rho(\mathbf{r}, \mathbf{t}) \log \frac{\rho(\mathbf{r}, \mathbf{t})}{(p_{\mathbf{R}}(\mathbf{r}) + p_{\mathbf{m_R}}(\mathbf{r}))(p_{\mathbf{T}}(\mathbf{t}) + p_{\mathbf{m_T}}(\mathbf{t}))} \mathrm{dr} \ \mathrm{dt} \quad (5)$$

die Kullback-Leibler-Distanz zwischen den Bildern [4] mit $\rho(\cdot, \cdot) := p_{\mathbf{RT}}(\cdot, \cdot) + p_{m_{\mathbf{RT}}}(\cdot, \cdot)$. Dabei sind $p_{\mathbf{R}}(\cdot)$ und $p_{\mathbf{T}}(\cdot)$ Histogramme (Verteilungsdichten der Grauwertintensitäten) der Bilder $\mathbf{R}$ und $\mathbf{T}$, $p_{\mathbf{RT}}(\cdot, \cdot)$ das gemeinsame Histogramm (Verbundverteilungsdichte der Grauwertintensitäten) der Bilder $\mathbf{R}$ und $\mathbf{T}$ und $p_{m_{\mathbf{R}}}(\cdot)$, $p_{m_{\mathbf{T}}}(\cdot)$ und $p_{m_{\mathbf{RT}}}(\cdot, \cdot)$ spezielle Gewichtungsfunktionen oder Masken. Die Masken sind in MI^{add} wie folgt definiert. Sei $\mathbf{I}$ ein Bild auf Ω und n die maximale mögliche Anzahl der Grauwerte in Ω. Die Gewichtungsmaske für $\mathbf{I}$ ist dann $p_{m_{\mathbf{I}}} : \mathbb{R}^n \longrightarrow \mathbb{R}^n$. Die Maske wird in diesem Fall auf das Histogramm des Bildes angewendet. Da die additive Masken in Histogrammbereich mit den additiven Masken im Bildbereich gleichmächtig sind [6], können die Masken im Histogrammbereich durch entsprechend nachgebildeten Masken im Bildbereich dargestellt werden. Dadurch wird ein visueller Vergleich mit den SSD^{mix}-Masken ermöglicht. Die Anwendung der Maske ist hier rein additiver Natur. Man beachte, dass die Resultate nach Anwendung einer Gewichtungsmaske die Normierung der Verteilungsdichte sowie der Verbundsverteilungsdichte nicht verletzen dürfen

$$\int_{\mathbb{R}^2} p_{m_{\mathbf{RT}}}(\mathbf{r}, \mathbf{t}) \ \mathrm{drdt} = \int_{\mathbb{R}} p_{m_{\mathbf{R}}}(\mathbf{r}) \mathrm{dr} = \int_{\mathbb{R}} p_{m_{\mathbf{T}}}(\mathbf{t}) \mathrm{dt} = 0 \ \text{ und}$$
$$\int_{\mathbb{R}^2} |p_{m_{\mathbf{RT}}}(\mathbf{r}, \mathbf{t})| \mathrm{drdt}, \int_{\mathbb{R}} |p_{m_{\mathbf{R}}}(\mathbf{r})| \mathrm{dr}, \int_{\mathbb{R}} |p_{m_{\mathbf{T}}}(\mathbf{t})| \mathrm{dt} \leq 1$$

Abb. 1. CT Aufnahme des Abdomen. Das Referenzbild (a) beinhalten im Vergleich zum Template (b) große Differenzen in Bereichen mit geringen Grauwertunterschieden. Die notwendigen Masken sind in (c) und (d) zu sehen. Durch die Masken werden die Bereiche mit geringem Kontrast verstärkt

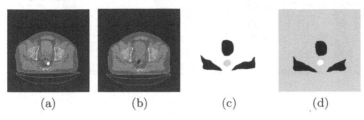

(a)   (b)   (c)   .(d)

Das heißt, dass für die einzelnen Einträge auch negative Werte zugelassen sind. Die Masken für MI^{add} werden am besten direkt über die Differenz zwischen gegebenem und gesuchtem Grauwert gewählt. Ein Bereich wird in diesem Fall durch Addition von Grauwertdifferenz zwischen dem Bereich selbst und seiner Umgebung ausgeblendet oder durch Addition mit einem Wert im gesamten Gebiet gewichtet. Weiterhin ist eine Veränderung der externen Kräfte der Bildregistrierung durch additives Einfügen bestimmter Muster möglich. Diese Möglichkeit wird hier aufgrund ihrer Komplexität nicht näher betrachtet (mehr dazu in [6]).

4   Ergebnisse

Die oben vorgestellten Distanzmaße wurden mit 18 CT-Aufnahmen des Abdominalbereichs eines Patienten getestet. Eine Aufnahme wurde dazu als Referenz gesetzt, die restlichen als Template. Die Grauwerte der Bilder gehen dabei von 0 bis 3895. Alle 17 Registrierungen wurden jeweils mit SSD, MI, SSD^{mix} und MI^{add} als Distanzmaß berechnet und den elastischen Parametern $\mu = 10$ und $\lambda = 135$. Ein Beispiel mit den notwendigen zu gewichtenden Bildbereichen zeigt Abb. 1, wobei eine spezielle Farbdarstellung gewählt wurde, um die Gewebeübergänge zu verdeutlichen. Die zu registrierenden monomodalen Bilder sind dabei durch unterschiedliche Grauwerte im Darmbereich und geringe Grauwertdifferenzen zwischen einigen Bereichen problematisch für eine ungewichtete Registrierung. Aus Platzgründen gehen wir hier nur auf einen Bereich mit geringen Grauwertunterschieden ein, in dem eine ungenügende Transformation im Template deutlich ist (Abb. 3(a)). Das Ziel des Vergleichs ist es, ein optimales Distanzmaß für solche Problemfälle zu finden. Ein erster Versuch mit MI behebt dabei die Probleme nicht (Abb. 3(b)). Beide gewichteten Distanzmaße hingegen können durch eine Gewichtung, bei SSD^{mix} durch den Faktor 7 und bei MI^{add} durch den Wert 1000, eine deutlich bessere Übereinstimmung der Gewebebereiche bewirken (Abb. 3(c) und 3(d)). Dabei ist der Aufwand, in den sowohl der Berechnungsaufwand des Distanzmaßes als auch die Schwierigkeiten bei der Maskenaufstellung eingehen, für SSD^{mix} geringer als für MI^{add}.

Abb. 2. Ergebnisse des rechten unteren Bereichs aus Abb. 1 im Vergleich zur Referenz (e). Bei eine Registrierung mit SSD (a) und MI (b) stimmen die Gewebeübergänge nicht überein. Durch die Wahl von SSD^{mix} (c) oder MI^{add} (d) kann dies erreicht werden

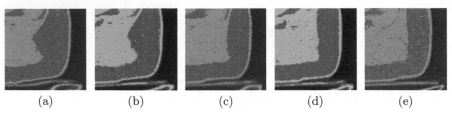

(a)   (b)   (c)   (d)   (e)

5 Diskussion

In manchen Fällen der monomodalen Bildregistrierung sind weder SSD noch MI als Distanzmaß ausreichend. Hier ist es notwendig, auf gewichtete Distanzmaße zurückzugreifen. Wir haben dazu zwei Distanzmaße, SSD^{mix} und MI^{add}, verglichen. Beide sind im Fall einer monomodalen Bildregistrierung gleich gut geeignet, die Registrierungsergebnisse zu verbessern, wobei zwei Punkte für die Anwendung von SSD^{mix} sprechen: Zum einen ist die Wahl der Masken für SSD^{mix} intuitiver als für MI^{add}, zum anderen ist der Rechenaufwand für SSD^{mix} vergleichbar zu SSD und damit geringer als für MI oder MI^{add}. Nächste Schritte sind weitere Untersuchungen zur Wahl der Masken, gerade für MI^{add}, um Strategien für einen effizienten Maskenaufbau zu entwickeln.

Literaturverzeichnis

1. Modersitzki J. Numerical Methods for Image Registration. Oxford University Press; 2003.
2. Hajnal JV, Hill DLG, Hawkes DJ. Medical Image Registration. CRC Press, Boca Raton; 2001.
3. Maintz JBA, Viergever MA. A survey of medical image registration. Medical Image Analysis 1998;2(1):1–36.
4. Viola PA, Wells III WM. Alignment by maximization of mutual information. In: Fifth International Conference on Computer Vision, IEEE; 1995. 16–23.
5. Schumacher H, Fischer B, Franz A. Weighted non-rigid image registration. submitted 2006.
6. Ens K, Schumacher H, Franz A, Fischer B. Improved elastic medical image registration using mutual information. Procs SPIE 2007.

Hybrid Spline-Based Elastic Image Registration Using Analytic Solutions of the Navier Equation

Stefan Wörz and Karl Rohr

University of Heidelberg, IPMB, and DKFZ Heidelberg,
Dept. Bioinformatics and Functional Genomics, Biomedical Computer Vision Group
Im Neuenheimer Feld 364, 69120 Heidelberg, Germany
Email: s.woerz@dkfz.de

Abstract. We introduce a new hybrid approach for spline-based elastic image registration using both point landmarks and intensity information. As underlying deformation model we use Gaussian elastic body splines (GEBS), which are solutions of the Navier equation of linear elasticity under Gaussian forces. We also incorporate landmark localization uncertainties represented by weight matrices to cope with anisotropic errors. The hybrid registration approach is formulated as an energy-minimizing functional that incorporates landmark and intensity information as well as a regularization based on GEBS. Since the approach is based on a physical deformation model, cross-effects in elastic deformations can be taken into account. We demonstrate the applicability of our scheme based on MR images of the brain. It turns out that the new scheme achieves more accurate results compared to a pure landmark-based as well as a pure intensity-based scheme.

1 Introduction

The registration of biomedical images is an important task, however, it is difficult and challenging. One reason is that in many applications it is still not quite clear which type of image information is optimal for matching. Another reason is that the spectrum of possible geometric differences is relatively large. Previous work on biomedical image registration can be characterized based on the nature of the transformation (e.g., rigid, nonrigid) as well as on the used image information (e.g., landmark-based, intensity-based). While rigid registration schemes are computationally efficient, they do not allow to cope with local differences between corresponding image data. Therefore, nonrigid (elastic) registration schemes are required (for a survey see [1]). Regarding the used image information, approaches are often based on either landmarks or intensity information. Main advantages of *landmark-based* approaches are computational efficiency, the fact that they can cope with large geometric differences, and the easy and intuitive incorporation of user-interaction. In contrast, main advantages of *intensity-based* approaches are that more image information is taken into account and that no segmentation is necessary (higher level of automation).

Elastic registration schemes are generally based on an energy functional or the related partial differential equation. One possibility is to numerically compute solutions using finite differences or the finite element method, which, however, is computationally expensive. For numeric schemes to improve the efficiency, see, for example, [2]. Alternatively, *spline-based* approaches can be used for elastic registration, which are often based on a nonuniform grid of control points (landmarks). Examples of such schemes are based on thin-plate splines (TPS, e.g., [3]), elastic body splines (EBS, [4]), and Gaussian EBS (GEBS, e.g., [5]-[8]). TPS are based on the bending energy of a thin plate, which represents a relatively coarse deformation model. In comparison, EBS and GEBS are derived from the Navier equation (partial differential equation), which describes the deformation of elastic tissues (bodies) under certain forces. GEBS in comparison to EBS have the advantage that more realistic image forces are used (Gaussian instead of polynomial forces).

Over the past few years, approaches that combine landmark-based and intensity-based methods have gained increased interest since advantages of both types of methods can be combined. However, so far only few *spline-based* registration approaches exist that use both landmarks and intensity information (e.g., [9, 10, 6, 7]). Typically, the intensity information is only used to determine optimal positions of the control points (e.g., [6, 7]) or to establish landmark correspondences, i.e. the landmarks and intensity information are not directly combined. In addition, often a physical deformation model is not used (e.g., [9, 10]). Furthermore, in landmark-based approaches generally an *interpolation* scheme is applied that forces corresponding landmarks to exactly match each other (e.g., [4, 5, 6]). The underlying assumption is that the landmark positions are known exactly. In real applications, however, landmark extraction is always prone to error. Therefore, to take these localization uncertainties into account, *approximation* schemes have been proposed, e.g., for TPS [3] and GEBS [8]. Note, however, that in these approaches only landmarks have been used but not intensity information.

In contrast to previous spline-based approaches, the central idea of our new approach is to directly combine the landmark and intensity information in a single energy functional as well as to include a regularization based on GEBS. In addition, we incorporate landmark localization uncertainties to cope with anisotropic errors. Since GEBS include a material parameter (Poisson ratio) that defines the ratio between transverse contraction and longitudinal dilation of an elastic material, cross-effects can be taken into account (which is not the case for, e.g., TPS). Moreover, since GEBS incorporate Gaussian forces we have a free parameter (the standard deviation) to control the locality of the transformation, and, therefore, GEBS are well suited for the registration of local differences.

2 Hybrid Gaussian Elastic Body Splines (GEBS)

We have developed a new hybrid approach for spline-based elastic image registration using both landmarks and intensity information. As underlying deformation

model we use Gaussian elastic body splines (GEBS), which are derived from the
Navier equation (for details see, e.g., [5, 8]). To compute the deformation field
$\mathbf{u}$ for registering the source image g_1 with the target image g_2 based on landmark and intensity information, we introduce an energy-minimizing functional
$J_{\text{Hybrid}}(\mathbf{u})$, which consists of four terms:

$$J_{\text{Hybrid}} = J_{\text{Data,I}}(g_1, g_2, \mathbf{u}^I) + \lambda_I \left\|\mathbf{u}^I - \mathbf{u}\right\|^2 + \lambda_L \left\|\mathbf{u}^L - \mathbf{u}\right\|^2 + \lambda_{El} J_{El}(\mathbf{u}) \quad (1)$$

Besides the searched deformation field $\mathbf{u}$, the functional comprises two deformation fields $\mathbf{u}^I$ and $\mathbf{u}^L$, which are computed based on the intensity and landmark
information, respectively (λ_I, λ_L, and λ_{El} are scalar weights).

Concerning the *intensity* information, the first term of (1) represents an intensity similarity measure between the deformed source image and the target
image. Here, we use the sum-of-squared intensity differences as similarity measure. The second term couples the intensity-based deformation field $\mathbf{u}^I$ with $\mathbf{u}$
using the Euclidean distance between both deformation fields.

Regarding the *landmark* information, the deformation field $\mathbf{u}^L$ is computed
based on the landmark correspondences using GEBS. To incorporate localization
uncertainties of landmarks, we employ the approximation scheme proposed in
[8]. With this scheme the landmarks are individually weighted according to their
localization uncertainties, which allows to control the influence of the landmarks
on the registration result. The localization uncertainties are characterized by
weight matrices, i.e. anisotropic landmark errors are taken into account. The
third term of (1) couples the landmark-based deformation field $\mathbf{u}^L$ with $\mathbf{u}$.

Finally, the fourth term represents the *regularization* of the deformation field
$\mathbf{u}$. In our case, J_{El} is based on the matrix-valued basis function of GEBS. By
minimizing the functional J_{Hybrid}, the resulting deformation field $\mathbf{u}$ is, on the one
hand, similar to the deformation field obtained from the landmark correspon-
dences, and, on the other hand, the intensities of the deformed source image are
similar to those of the target image. In addition, the regularization using GEBS
constraints the deformation field to physically plausible deformations.

An efficient way of minimizing J_{Hybrid} is to minimize it alternatingly w.r.t. $\mathbf{u}^I$
and $\mathbf{u}$. For the minimization w.r.t. $\mathbf{u}^I$, the following functional is relevant

$$J_{\text{Data,I}}(g_1, g_2, \mathbf{u}^I) + \lambda_I \left\|\mathbf{u}^I - \mathbf{u}\right\|^2 \quad (2)$$

This functional has the advantage that it can be stated independently for each
voxel, and that for each voxel only sums of squared differences are used. Therefore, (2) can be efficiently minimized using the method of Levenberg/Marquardt.
For the minimization w.r.t. $\mathbf{u}$, the following functional has to be considered

$$\lambda_I \left\|\mathbf{u}^I - \mathbf{u}\right\|^2 + \lambda_L \left\|\mathbf{u}^L - \mathbf{u}\right\|^2 + \lambda_{El} J_{El}(\mathbf{u}) \quad (3)$$

Interestingly, for minimizing (3) an explicit solution can be stated $\mathbf{u}(\mathbf{x}) = \mathbf{G}(\mathbf{x}) *$
$\left[\mathbf{u}^I(\mathbf{x}) - \mathbf{u}^L(\mathbf{x})\right] + \mathbf{u}^L(\mathbf{x})$, where "$*$" denotes the convolution of a matrix-valued
function with a vector field and $\mathbf{G}$ is the matrix-valued GEBS basis function.

Fig. 1. Registration of 2D MR brain images: Pre- (top left) and postsurgical image (bottom left) as well as the (inverse) deformation fields (top) and registered source images (bottom) using a pure landmark-based approach (middle left), a pure intensity-based approach (middle right), and using the new hybrid approach (right)

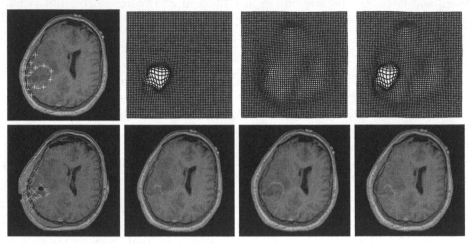

3   Experimental Results

We have applied the new hybrid registration approach to register 2D MR images of the human head. In this application the task is to register pre- and postsurgical MR images of the human brain. Fig. 1 shows 2D MR images of a patient before (source image, top left) and after (target image, bottom left) the resection of a tumor. 17 landmarks have been manually placed along the contours of the tumor and the resection area (indicated by crosses). Fig. 1 shows the (inverse) deformation fields (top) and registered source images (bottom) using a pure landmark-based approach (middle left), a pure intensity-based approach (middle right), and using the new hybrid approach based on GEBS (right). It turned out that using only *landmark* information (middle left) the vicinity of the tumor and resection area are well registered whereas regions without landmarks are not deformed. As a consequence, the mean intensity error improved by only 4.6% w.r.t. the unregistered case. In contrast, using only *intensity* information (middle right) yields deformations in different parts of the head with an improvement of the mean intensity error by 12.8%. However, the tumor has not been registered. Using the new *hybrid* approach the registration result is significantly improved in comparison to the previous two approaches since the tumor and resection area are well registered and, in addition, other parts of the head (see Fig. 1, right). Here, the mean intensity error for the whole image improved by 13.0%.

4   Conclusion

The presented hybrid elastic approach combines landmarks and intensity information as well as a regularization based on Gaussian elastic body splines (GEBS), which are analytic solutions of the Navier equation. In comparison to existing spline-based approaches, the new scheme combines a number of advantages. A main advantage is that the hybrid approach directly combines landmarks and intensity information, and hence exploits advantages from both landmark-based and intensity-based approaches. In contrast, existing spline-based approaches often use intensity information only to localize control points or to establish landmark correspondences. Moreover, the new registration approach takes into account anisotropic localization uncertainties of the landmark positions. We have demonstrated the applicability of our new registration approach based on MR brain images. From the experiments it turned out that the hybrid approach achieves more accurate registration results in comparison to a pure landmark-based approach and a pure intensity-based scheme.

Acknowledgment

This work has been funded by the Deutsche Forschungsgemeinschaft (DFG) within the project ELASTIR (RO 2471/2). The original images and the tumor outlines have kindly been provided by OA Dr. med. U. Spetzger and Prof. Dr. J.-M. Gilsbach, Neurosurgical Clinic, University Hospital Aachen of the RWTH.

References

1. Zitova B, Flusser J. Image registration methods: A survey. Image and Vision Computing 2003;24:977–1000.
2. Modersitzki J, Fischer B. Optimal image registration with a guaranteed one-to-one point match. Procs BVM 2003; 1–5.
3. Rohr K, Stiehl HS, Sprengel R, et al. Landmark-based elastic registration using approximating thin-plate splines. IEEE Trans Med Imaging 2001;20(6):526–534.
4. Davis MH, Khotanzad A, Flaming DP, et al. A physics-based coordinate transformation for 3D image matching. IEEE Trans Med Imaging 1997;16(3):317–328.
5. Kohlrausch J, Rohr K, Stiehl HS. A new class of elastic body splines for nonrigid registration of medical images. J Mathematical Imaging and Vision 2005;23(3):253–280.
6. Pekar V, Gladilin E, Rohr K. An adaptive irregular grid approach for 3-D deformable image registration. Phys Med Biol 2006;51:361–377.
7. Franz A, Carlson IC, Renisch S. An adaptive irregular grid approach using SIFT features for elastic medical image registration. Procs BVM 2006; 201–205.
8. Wörz S, Rohr K. Physics-based elastic image registration using splines and including landmark localization uncertainties. LNCS 2006;4191:678–685.
9. Cachier P, Mangin JF, Pennec X, et al. Multisubject non-rigid registration of brain MRI using intensity and geometric features. LNCS 2001;2208:734–742.
10. Rohr K, Cathier P, Wörz S. Elastic registration of electrophoresis images using intensity information and point landmarks. Pattern Recognition 2004;37(5):1035–1048.

An Efficient Registration Algorithm for Advanced Fusion of 2D/3D Angiographic Data

Martin Groher[1], Ralf-Thorsten Hoffmann[2], Christoph Zech[2],
Maximilian Reiser[2], Nassir Navab[1]

[1]Lehrstuhl für Informatikanwendungen in der Medizin, TU München
[2]Klinische Radiologie des Klinikums Grosshadern, LMU München
Email: groher@cs.tum.edu

Abstract. Computed tomography angiography (CTA) is often used for
pre-interventional diagnosis and planning, whereas nowadays, mostly 2D
angiograms are acquired for intra-interventional catheter guidance. Spatial information from pre-interventional scans is not transferred to the
intervention yet since existing 2D-3D registration methods either require
a good initial manual alignment or have rather long runtime and thus
lack clinical usefulness. We propose a fast and automatic method for
2D-3D registration and evaluate methods for intra-interventional visualization and navigation. Moreover, we introduce an easy clinical workflow for transferring a planned roadmap from pre-interventional 3D to
intra-interventional 2D using the registration. We demonstrate the good
quality of fit and the fast runtime of the algorithm on one phantom and
three patient data sets.

1 Introduction

Catheterizations are carried out on a daily basis in many hospitals. Very often, a
3D pre-interventional computed tomography angiography (CTA) is acquired for
pathology detection and procedure planning. During the treatment, only 2D projections (e.g. digitally subtracted angiography, DSA) are acquired for navigating
the catheter to the region of interest. A registration and proper visualization of
pre- and intra-interventional data during the procedure would help the physician
to navigate the catheter through the vessel system. We propose a registration
algorithm whose runtime is only depended on the number of junctions in the 3D
vasculature (mostly 20-30) and thus outperforms most other 2D-3D registration
algorithms based on non-linear optimization (see [1, 2, 3, 4] for the most recent
methods).

2 Method

Rigid 2D-3D registration aims at recovering the 6 degrees of freedom (DOF)
providing the viewing parameters of 2D image capture. The 6 DOFs are also
referred to as the extrinsic parameters $[R|t]$ of a perspective projection,

$$x = PX = K[R|t]X$$

$P \in \mathbb{R}^{3 \times 4}$ projects a homogeneous 3D point X onto a homogeneous 2D point x and can be decomposed into K (intrinsic parameters) and rotation R and translation $t = (t_x, t_y, t_z)^T$ (extrinsic parameters).

In order to produce feature coordinates to register, we segment the arterial vasculature in 3D from an angiographic phase of a CTA and in 2D from a DSA using region growing. We then extract centerline graphs with a thinning and wave propagation algorithm [5]. Only the bifurcations in the 3D and 2D data sets are used as features for registration. State-of-the-art angiographic C-arm devices store lots of information concerning imaging geometry. Each 2D angiogram is provided with the calibration matrix K, a source-to-object distance (STO[1]), and a source-to-detector distance (STD). Moreover, a primary and secondary rotation angle provide a rather decent estimate of the rotation matrix R.

We use all this information to produce initial image as well as object coordinates of the extracted vessel trees. For all node coordinates of the 2D centerline graph $\tilde{x}_i$ we undo the transformation specific to the imaging device

$$x_i = K^{-1}\tilde{x}_i$$

For all node coordinates of the 3D centerline graph $\tilde{X}_i$, we apply an initial transformation including primary/secondary angle in $\tilde{R}$ and an approximate z-translation $\tilde{t} = (0, 0, \text{STD} - \text{STO})^T$

$$X_i = \tilde{X}_i\tilde{R} + \tilde{t}$$

2.1 Registration of t_x and t_y

In order to find a value for x- and y-translation we assume rotation and z-translation given and try to establish correspondences between bifurcations using translation-invariant feature descriptors. From the different descriptors proposed in the literature, we have chosen the *shape context* descriptor of Belongie et al [6] since it describes features by their relative translation to all other features in the same shape and is independent of intensity neighborhoods. This inherent translational invariance is followed by a rotational invariance for small rotations which holds for our scenario. For each bifurcation of the 2D and projected 3D graph we create a histogram including all translation vectors to all other nodes of the graph (bifurcations and sampling nodes of vessel segments) binned over log-polar coordinates. To find a corresponding bifurcation to v_i in one graph, we determine the minimal "distance" $d_{\min}$ between histograms h_i, h_j[2] of all bifurcations v_j in the other graph

$$d_{\min} = \min_j \sum_k (h_i(k) - h_j(k))^2$$

---

[1] The *STO* is actually a source-to-table distance, but is called source-to-object distance in the DICOM header

[2] the histograms contain normalized polar coordinates

where k is the number of bins in each histogram. Here, we do not require a one-to-one correspondence solution (i.e. one feature might correspond to more than one feature in the other graph). We allow this inexact modelling of the correspondence problem because we just try to find one best correspondence and discard the others. This implementation speeds up the matching process compared to the original implementation using a bipartite graph matching algorithm.

Since there are many false matches due to segmentation errors, overlay, and deformation changes, we try to iteratively find one "best" correspondence between two bifurcations to receive x- and y-translations. For that, we iteratively translate the 3D graph in x- and y-direction parallel to the image plane such that a projected 3D bifurcation is laid over its corresponding 2D bifurcation. A cost function f_{topo}, described in [1], is evaluated and the (x, y)-translation yielding the lowest value is chosen.[3] This search algorithm for the best (x, y)-translation is linear in the number of bifurcations in the 3D graph (mostly between 20 and 50) and thus requires only a small and fixed number of cost function evaluations, which results in a speed-up compared to other registration algorithms based on non-linear optimization.

---

[3] f_{topo} uses geometric distances between bifurcations as well as topological information to rate the similarity between 3D and 2D graph

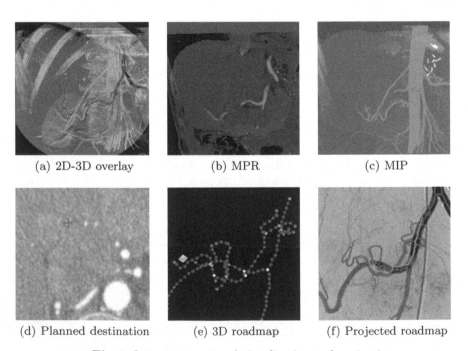

(a) 2D-3D overlay   (b) MPR   (c) MIP

(d) Planned destination   (e) 3D roadmap   (f) Projected roadmap

Fig. 1. Intra-interventional visualization and navigation

3 Experiments and Results

We have evaluated our approach on a rigid phantom for which a ground truth pose was created through intensity-based registration. Moreover, we asked physicians to register the patient data sets manually. In all cases, the pose could be recovered within 2-6 seconds. Deviations from the ground truth registration were in the range of 0.3mm for x- and y-translations, 10mm for z-translation, and $< 5°$ for rotations. We want to emphasize that a better accuracy could be reached (e.g. with a non-linear optimization taking this method as initialization step), but the goal of intra-interventional visualization and road- mapping only requires a rough alignment according to physicians. We therefore discarded the optimization for the sake of speed and thus intra-interventional usability.

3.1 Intra-interventional Visualization and Navigation

Once registered, the pre-interventionally acquired 3D CTA data can be transferred to the interventional room for improved orientation, navigation, and road-mapping. We have shown two different visualization techniques to physicians asking for their feedback. Moreover, a simple planning tool for the pre-interventional data was implemented that allowed physicians to create a 3D roadmap before the intervention. After the registration process this roadmap can be projected onto the current DSA highlighting the vessel path the catheter should take to reach the region of interest.

Direct volume rendering can be used to project the 3D data from the same viewpoint as the current DSA image. The resulting 2D image can be blended over the actual 2D DSA for 2D-3D overlay (fig. 1(a)). The fused images are shown on one monitor as an "In-place visualization" [7].

Multi-planar reconstruction (MPR) is a rendering technique to display a 2D slice of the volume with an arbitrary cutting plane. On a second monitor, we offer a cutting plane visualizing a slice perpendicular to the viewing direction in the middle of the volume. A slider translates the cutting plane along the viewing direction (fig. 1(b)). Since vessels have a much brighter intensity than surrounding tissue we allow maximum intensity projections (MIP) from partial volumes, too (fig. 1(c)). If the partial volume is properly defined, a manual browsing through slices can be avoided.

According to physicians the 2D-3D overlay on one view does not improve 3D perception in the interventional room. The 3D volume is projected and, since the registration information is to be kept, should not be transformed and seen from any other viewpoint. Thus, the overlay is only giving additional 2D, but not 3D perception. The MPR visualization was favored because it resembles the rendering of orthogonal slices radiologists are used to from diagnostic procedures. Moreover, if shown on a second monitor, it does not influence the 2D DSA and can be used as general orientation whereas fine-grained navigation is done on fluoroscopic/DSA images. By showing different slices and/or MIPs a 3D perception can be created. Although In-place visualization of registered data is preferred when fusing different 3D data sets [7], in the case of 2D-3D data fusion out-of-place visualization proves to be the better choice.

3.2 Roadmapping Tool

With the roadmapping tool, an interventionalist can plan a procedure pre-interventionally on the CTA data by simply clicking on the vessel branch to be embolized (fig. 1(d)). A shortest path is automatically calculated using the segmented vasculature's centerline. The path is followed to the main vessel by increasing vessel diameter. This roadmap can be visualized on the extracted 3D vasculature for orientation (fig. 1(e)) and projected with the registration parameters onto the current 2D image for improved catheter navigation (fig. 1(f)). This planning feature received very positive feedback from physicians since navigation through the vessel system can be significantly improved by roadmap projection.

4   Discussion

We introduced a fast 2D-3D registration algorithm working on junctions of vessel systems which is the only visible structure in catheter interventions. We are well aware that the resulting registration parameters are only near to an optimal solution. However, they are sufficient for the physician to be able to discern vessels and for the system to project a planned roadmap. Moreover, we evaluated different visualization techniques and proposed a clinical workflow for interventional planning in 3D and 2D roadmapping. We received a positive feedback from physicians and will now focus on a more extensive clinical study to further evaluate the method.

References

1. Groher M, Padoy N, Jakobs TF, Navab N. New CTA protocol and 2D-3D registration method for liver catheterization. LNCS 2006;4190:873–881.
2. Jomier J, Bullitt E, v Horn M, Pathak C, Aylward SR. 3D/2D model-to-image registration applied to TIPS surgery. LNCS 2006;4191:662–669.
3. Florin C, Williams J, Khamene A, Paragios N. Registration of 3D angiographic and x-ray images using sequential monte Carlo Sampling. LNCS 2005;3765:427–436.
4. Turgeon GA, Lehmann G, Guiraudon G, et al. 2D-3D registration of coronary angiograms for cardiac procedure planning and guidance. Med Phys 2005;32:3737–3749.
5. Zahlten C, Jürgens H, Peitgen HO. Reconstruction of branching blood vessels from CT-data. In: Eurographics Workshop of Visualization in Scientific Computing. Springer; 1994. 161–168.
6. Belongie S, Malik J, Puzicha J. Shape matching and object recognition using shape contexts. IEEE Trans PAMI 2002;24:509–522.
7. Tory M. Mental registration of 2D and 3D visualizations: An empirical study. In: Procs IEEE Visualization Conference. Seattle, Washington, USA; 2003. 49.

Registrierung von Aufnahmen des Augenhintergrundes zur Erstellung großflächiger Kompositionsaufnahmen

Daniel Baumgarten[1], Axel Doering[2], Michael Trost[2]

[1]Institut für Biomedizinische Technik und Informatik, Technische Universität Ilmenau
[2]R&D Software, Carl Zeiss Meditec AG, Jena
Email: daniel.baumgarten@tu-ilmenau.de

Zusammenfassung. Wir präsentieren einen automatischen Algorithmus zur Registrierung und Überlagerung von Fundusbildern zu großflächigen Kompositionsaufnahmen. Das Verfahren kombiniert flächenbasierte und punktbasierte Ansätze. Als Ähnlichkeitsmaß dient jeweils der normierte Korrelationskoeffizient, der sich im Vergleich zur Transinformation als robuster erwies und schneller zu berechnen ist. Den Transformationen der Bilder liegt ein quadratisches Modell zugrunde, das die annähernd sphärische Oberfläche der Retina berücksichtigt und anhand visueller Bewertung ausgewählt wurde. Bei der Validierung an realen klinischen Daten erwies sich der vorgestellte Algorithmus als robust und genau. Die Grenzen des Verfahrens bilden sehr unscharfe Bilder und solche, die nur sehr wenig relevante Strukturen enthalten.

1 Einleitung

Für die frühe Diagnose von Netzhauterkrankungen wie der Diabetischen Retinopathie empfiehlt sich eine ständige Beobachtung des Augenhintergrundes durch den Augenarzt oder im Rahmen von Screening-Untersuchungen. Dafür ist es erforderlich, die Fundusaufnahmen, die aufgrund des beschränkten Zugangs durch die Pupille jeweils nur einen kleinen Ausschnitt der Retina zeigen, zu großflächigen Kompositionsbildern zusammenzusetzen.

2 Stand der Forschung

Verschiedene Faktoren stellen hohe Ansprüche an die Verfahren zur Registrierung von Fundusaufnahmen. Die gekrümmte Fläche der Retina, unterschiedliche Beleuchtungsverhältnisse zwischen den Bildern, unterschiedliche Ausleuchtungen und strukturlose Bereiche innerhalb eines Bildes sowie nichtlineare Verzerrungen bilden hierbei die größten Probleme. In der Literatur lassen sich zwei Verfahren unterscheiden:

- *Flächenbasierte* (globale) Registrieralgorithmen [1, 2, 3] nutzen die Intensitätswerte der Bildpunkte. Die Registrierung erfolgt durch Maximierung eines Ähnlichkeitsmaßes des gesamten Überlappungsbereichs der Bilder.

- *Punktbasierte* (lokale) Registrieralgorithmen [4, 5] stützen sich dagegen auf ausgewählte, charakteristische Punkte. Es werden Punktkorrespondenzen zwischen den Bildern ermittelt, an die eine Transformation angepasst wird.

Ziel unserer Arbeiten ist die Entwicklung eines Algorithmus für den praktischen Einsatz in einer Funduskamera. Das Verfahren soll besonders zuverlässig und genau arbeiten und großflächige Kompositionsaufnahmen in einer für den Anwender akzeptablen Zeit berechnen. Um die Nachteile beider Ansätze zu umgehen, kombiniert das vorgestellte Verfahren ähnlich dem von Chanwimaluang et al. beschriebenen Algorithmus flächenbasierte und punktbasierte Ansätze [6]. Im Unterschied dazu werden die Punktkorrespondenzen durch ein Blockmatching-Verfahren bestimmt, dass die Verteilung und Validität der Passpunkte sicherstellt. Damit ist es möglich, auch in der Peripherie der Retina Passpunkte zuverlässig und in ausreichender Anzahl zu detektieren. Zudem wird der normierte Korrelationskoeffizient anstelle der Transinformation als Ähnlichkeitsmaß verwendet, der sich als robuster erwies und deutlich schneller zu berechnen ist.

3   Methoden

Im ersten Schritt des von uns entwickelten Algorithmus wird eine grobe Verschiebung für alle möglichen Bildpaare bestimmt. Dazu werden in den auf eine geringere Auflösung skalierten Bildern die Blutgefäße durch ein Template-Matching hervorgehoben, um globale Bildanteile zu unterdrücken und Beleuchtungsunterschiede zwischen den Bildern auszugleichen [7]. Als Vorlage dient dabei eine Gauss-Kurve, mit der sich der Querschnitt eines Gefäßes grob approximieren lässt, über einer festen Länge. Das Template wird in mehreren Richtungen angewendet. Im Frequenzbereich wird die Kreuzkorrelationsfunktion der Gefäßbilder berechnet, deren Maximum der gesuchten Verschiebung entspricht. Die Verschiebung wird als gültig bewertet, falls der Wert des Maximums über einer Schwelle σ_V liegt. Anhand der Anzahl der gültigen Verschiebungen und deren Mittelwert wird ein Ankerbild bestimmt, in dessen Koordinatensystem alle weiteren Bilder transformiert werden.

Für alle Bildpaare mit gültiger Vorpositionierung werden, ausgehend von der bestimmten Verschiebung, die Punktkorrespondenzen ermittelt. Dazu wird ein Blockmatching-Algorithmus angewendet, der in mehreren Auflösungsstufen zu einem ausgewählten Block des Ausgangsbildes den korrespondierenden Block im Zielbild bestimmt. In jeder Stufe wird zur Reduzierung der Anzahl der Ähnlichkeitsmaßberechnungen eine Diamant-Suchstrategie [8] eingesetzt. Um die Validität und eine gute Verteilung der Passpunkte über den Überlappungsbereich zu gewährleisten, wird dieser in Kacheln unterteilt. In jeder Kachel werden durch ein Doppelschwellwertkriterium maximal zwei Passpunktpaare ausgewählt. Die ersten beiden Passpunktpaare, deren Ähnlichkeitsmaß über einer Schwelle σ_1 liegt, werden akzeptiert und die Suche für diese Kachel abgebrochen. Wurden nach einer maximalen Anzahl untersuchter Blockpaare keine zwei gefunden, werden die besten übrigen Paare verwendet, sofern deren Ähnlichkeitsmaß über einer Schwelle σ_2 liegt.

Abb. 1. Verteilung des NKK (links) und der TI (rechts) für Verschiebungen zwischen zwei Fundusbildern

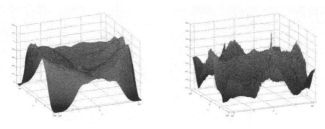

Aus den Korrespondenzen werden die Parameter der Transformation aller Bilder in das Koordinatensystem des Ankerbildes berechnet. Die Passpunktpaare eines Bildes mit dem Ankerbild und allen bereits registrierten Bildern ergeben mit dem gewählten Transformationsmodell ein überbestimmtes Gleichungssystem, aus dem die Parameter durch Ausgleichsrechnung nach der Methode der kleinsten Quadrate geschätzt werden. Nach einer initialen Berechnung wird iterativ das Paar mit dem größten Fehler entfernt und aus den verbliebenen eine neue Transformation berechnet, bis dieser unter einem Schwellwert liegt. Damit werden mögliche Ausreißer und Fehlregistrierungen entfernt, die die Transformation verfälschen können.

Nach der Berechnung der entsprechenden Parameter werden die Bilder transformiert. Vor der Überlagerung wird durch Segmentierung mit einem für jedes Bild individuell bestimmten Schwellwert eine Maske bestimmt. Aus dieser wird durch Tiefpassfilterung die Wichtung der Bildpunkte für die Überlagerung berechnet. Die Transparenz der Bilder nimmt so zum Rand hin zu, damit werden die Übergänge zwischen den Einzelbildern in der Bildmontage geglättet und die Regionen der Feldblende komplett ausgeblendet.

4 Ergebnisse

Für die Verwendung als Ähnlichkeitsmaß in der Vorpositionierung wurden der normierte Korrelationskoeffizient und die Transinformation untersucht. Lediglich die Verteilungen des NKK weisen einen deutlich erkennbaren und steilen Gipfel an der Position der gesuchten Verschiebung auf. Die dominierenden Anteile der Verteilungen der TI sind die zum Rand hin für große Verschiebungen stark ansteigenden Werte sowie ein Gipfel für die nicht gegeneinander verschobenen Bilder. Ursache ist jeweils die große Überlappung der homogenen Hintergrundbereiche [3]. Abb. 1 zeigt die Verteilung des NKK und der TI für ein Bildpaar.

Vier Transformationsmodelle wurden auf ihre Eignung für die Registrierung von Fundusbildern untersucht. Dazu wurden unter Nutzung dieser Modelle berechnete Bildmontagen visuell bewertet. Reichen die Freiheitsgrade eines Modells für die auftretenden Verzerrungen nicht aus, so sind Abweichungen sowie Sprünge an den Bildübergängen zu erkennen. 2 zeigt Ausschnitte von Bildmon-

Abb. 2. Ausschnitte einer Bildmontage für verschiedene Transformationsmodelle: Translation (a), affine (b), quadratische (c) und kubische Transformation (d)

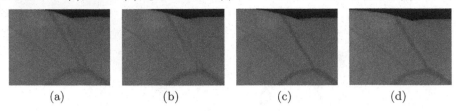

(a)   (b)   (c)   (d)

tagen, die aus denselben Bildern mit verschiedenen Transformationsmodellen berechnet wurden. Bei Translation und affiner Transformation sind deutliche Abweichungen erkennbar, für das quadratische und das kubische Transformationsmodell liegen die Gefäße exakt übereinander. Quantitative Untersuchungen bestätigen diese Beobachtungen.

Unser Verfahren wurde zur Validierung und Bewertung auf unterschiedliche Bildsätze angewendet. Dafür wurden bei 12 gesunden Probanden mit der Funduskamera VISUCAM© PRO NM unter Nutzung der 7-Felder-Methode, die an die ETDRS-Felddefinitionen angelehnt ist, jeweils sieben Bilder mit einem Bildwinkel von 30° oder 45° aufgenommen. Zudem wurden 14 Bildsätze von Tumorpatienten aus klinischen Untersuchungen verwendet. Pro Patient wurden ohne vorgegebenes Protokoll 25 bis 40 Bilder mit einem Bildwinkel von 45° aufgenommen.

Für die mit der VISUCAM© aufgenommenen Bildsätze konnten jeweils alle Bilder montiert werden, die Montagen weisen keine sichtbaren Fehlregistrierungen oder Schattengefäße auf. Bei der Berechnung von Kompositionsaufnahmen aus den Bildsätzen von Tumorpatienten konnten in einigen Fällen nicht alle Aufnahmen registriert werden. Die nicht hinzugefügten Bilder lagen meist in der Peripherie der Retina und enthielten damit kaum Strukturen. Zudem waren sie sehr unscharf. Auch diese Bildmontagen zeigen keine Fehlregistrierungen. Der mittlere Registrierungsfehler lag für alle Bildsätze unter zwei Bildpunkten. Die Übergänge zwischen den Einzelbildern sind in allen Fällen nicht mehr zu erkennen. 3 zeigt Beispiele für Bildmontagen aus den unterschiedlichen Testbildsätzen.

5 Diskussion

Diese Arbeit präsentiert einen automatischen Algorithmus zur Registrierung von Fundusbildern und deren Überlagerung zu Kompositionsaufnahmen. Als Ähnlichkeitsmaß für die flächenbasierte Vorpositionierung wird der normierte Korrelationskoeffizient gewählt. Unsere Untersuchungen zeigen, dass eine lineare Transformation (Translation, affine Transformation) als geometrisches Modell für die Verzerrung zwischen Fundusbildern nicht ausreicht. Gegenüber der quadratischen bringt die kubische Transformation keine erkennbare Verbesserung der Bildmontagen. Deshalb und aufgrund der höheren numerischen Instabilität

Abb. 3. Kompositionsbilder aus Aufnahmen der VISUCAM© (links) und Tumorpatienten (rechts)

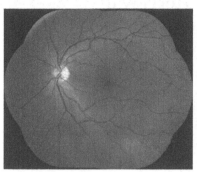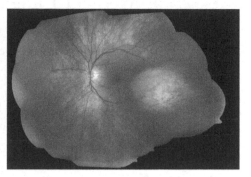

der kubischen Transformation wurde das quadratische Modell dem entwickelten Algorithmus zugrunde gelegt.

Mit dem vorgestellten Algorithmus lassen sich unter Nutzung dieser Erkenntnisse Fundusbilder unterschiedlicher Größe, Qualität und Beleuchtungsverhältnisse robust und exakt registrieren. Die berechneten Bildmontagen weisen keine sichtbaren Fehler auf. Weiterführende Arbeiten beschäftigen sich mit der weiteren Verbesserung der Zuverlässigkeit des Algorithmus, insbesondere gegen unscharfe Bilder und solche, die wenig Struktur enthalten. Darüber hinaus wurde der Algorithmus in einem Software-Modul implementiert und in die Gerätesoftware der Funduskamera VISUCAM® PRO NM der Carl Zeiss Meditec AG integriert. Damit ist es dem Anwender möglich, unmittelbar nach Aufnahme der Bilder eine Bildmontage zu erzeugen.

Literaturverzeichnis

1. Ritter N, Owens R, Cooper J, et al. Registration of stereo and temporal images of the retina. IEEE Trans Med Imaging 1999;18(5):404–418.
2. Voss K, Ortmann W, Süße H. Bildmatching und Bewegungskompensation bei Fundus-Bildern. In: Procs DAGM; 1998. 439–446.
3. Pluim JPW, Maintz JBA, Viergever MA. Mutual information based registration of medical images: A survey. IEEE Trans Med Imaging 2003;20(8):986–1004.
4. Can A, Stewart CV, Roysam B, Tanenbaum HL. A feature-based technique for joint, linear estimation of high-order image-to-mosaic transformations: Mosaicing the curved human retina. IEEE Trans PAMI 2002;24(3):412–419.
5. Laliberté F, Gagnon L, Sheng Y. Registration and fusion of retinal images: An evaluation study. IEEE Trans Med Imaging 2003;22(5):661–673.
6. Chanwimaluang T, Fan G, Fransen SR. Hybrid retinal image registration. IEEE Trans Inf Technol Biomed 2006;10(1):129–142.
7. Chaudhuri S, Chatterjee S, Katz N, Nelson M, Goldbaum M. Detection of blood vessels in retinal images using two-dimensional matched filters. IEEE Trans Med Imaging 1989;8(3):263–269.
8. Zhu S, Ma KK. A new diamond search algorithm for fast block matching motion estimation. IEEE Trans Image Process 2000;92(2):287–290.

Interfacing Global and Local CBIR Systems for Medical Image Retrieval

Sameer K. Antani[1], Thomas M. Deserno[1,2], L. Rodney Long[1],
Mark O. Güld[2], Leif Neve[1], George R. Thoma[1]

[1]National Library of Medicine, National Institutes of Health, Bethesda, MD, USA
[2]Dept. of Medical Informatics, Aachen University of Technology (RWTH), Germany
Email: santani@mail.nih.gov

Abstract. Contemporary picture archiving and communication systems are limited in managing large and varied image collections, because content-based image retrieval (CBIR) methods are unavailable. In this paper, an XML-based data and resource exchange framework is defined using open standards and software to enable specialized CBIR systems to act as geographically distributed toolkits. The approach enables communication and collaboration between two or more geographically separated complementary systems with possibly different architectures and developed on different platforms, and specialized for different image modalities and characteristics. The resulting synergy provides the user with a rich functionality operating within a familiar Web browser interface, making the combined system portable and independent of location and underlying user operating systems. We describe the coupling of the Image Retrieval in Medical Applications (IRMA) system and the Spine Pathology and Image Retrieval System (SPIRS) as proof of this concept.

1 Introduction

There has been an explosive growth in the acquisition and use of images in clinical medicine, medical research, and education [1]. In current picture archiving and communication systems (PACS), retrieval of image information is done using limited text keywords in special fields in the image header (e.g., patient identifier). Since these keywords do not capture the richness of features depicted in the image itself, content-based image retrieval (CBIR) has received significant attention in the literature as a promising technique to facilitate improved image management in PACS systems [2, 3]. With this approach, rather than limiting queries to textual keywords, users can also provide an example image or image feature (e.g., color, texture, or shape computed from a region of interest) to find similar images of the same modality, anatomical region, and disease along with the matching associated text records. In spite of this research interest, the challenging nature and variety of medical image data have contributed to the absence of CBIR in contemporary PACS. CBIR requires specialized methods specific to each image type and content detail. Some systems tend to focus on particular image types, while others that are less specific with respect to particular anatomy tend to concentrate more on image discrimination by overall appearance, and any pathological similarity is only in the gross overall view.

2   State of the Art and New Contribution

As proof of concept, we describe the collaboration between two leading, complementary geographically distributed CBIR systems:

- The Image Retrieval in Medical Applications (IRMA) Project[1] undertaken at the Aachen University of Technology (RWTH) [3, 4] aims to provide visually rich image management through CBIR techniques applied to medical images using intensity distribution and texture measures taken globally over the entire image. This approach permits queries on a heterogeneous image collection and helps identify images that are similar with respect to global features, e.g., all chest x-rays in the AP (anterior-posterior) view. The IRMA system lacks the ability for finding particular pathology that may be localized in particular regions within the image.
- The Spine Pathology and Image Retrieval System (SPIRS)[2] [5, 6, 7] at the U.S. National Library of Medicine provides localized vertebral shape-based CBIR methods for pathologically sensitive retrieval of digitized spine x-rays and associated person metadata that come from the Second U.S. National Health and Nutrition Examination Survey (NHANES II). In the SPIRS system, the images in the collection must be homogeneous, i.e., a single type imaging the same anatomy in the same view, e.g., vertebral pathology expressed in spine x-ray images in the sagittal plane.

Combining the strengths of these two complementary technologies of whole image and local feature-based retrieval is unique and valuable to find images that are not only similar in overall appearance but also with locally expressed pathology. This is accomplished through use of an XML-based service protocol to access particular internal methods in these systems.

3   System Background

3.1   Image Retrieval in Medical Applications

IRMA has developed and implemented high-level CBIR methods with application to medico-diagnostic tasks on radiological image archives. Current image data consists of radiographs, with future plans to include medical images from arbitrary modalities. IRMA is a system where methods are treated as black boxes with an input and an output connected as a directed graph [8]. Using this paradigm, new algorithms can be integrated into a Web-based query interface

---

[1] http://irma-project.org
[2] http://archive.nlm.nih.gov/spirs

with relative ease. IRMA caches intermediate results to improve efficiency and support its query logging capability. Distributed processing is also enabled by assigning the set of methods particular to a query or user interaction to one of the daemon services running on network-connected computers.

3.2 Spine Pathology and Image Retrieval System

SPIRS provides a Web-based interface, implemented as a Java applet, for performing image retrieval on a database of digitized spine x-rays using the morphological shape of the vertebral body. Its framework of shape indexing and retrieval algorithms communicate with external users through a Java servlet. SPIRS enables CBIR for the large databases of image and patient data using rich hybrid image and text query methods. A shape query editor enables sketching or selecting and/or modifying an existing shape in the database. It also supports advanced mechanisms like multiple partial shape queries. Additionally, text fields enable users to supplement visual queries with other relevant data. A customizable window displays the top matching vertebrae and related text data. SPIRS also offers a service of its core shape similarity algorithms and data with a predefined DTD. It is being extended and generalized to include color, texture, and spatial location in uterine cervix images from the National Cancer Institute [7].

4 Roadmap

The interfacing of the SPIRS and IRMA systems has been divided into the following phases, each phase adding enhancements and features to the combined system. This paper covers Phases 1 and 2 of this development:

1. *Whole shape matching*: The entire vertebral shapes are used in computing similarity. Additionally, the query shapes are selected from those within the database of pre-segmented vertebrae. Query shape modifications or user sketches are not supported.
2. *Similarity method selection*: SPIRS enables support for additional shape similarity algorithms. The user can select a shape similarity method at query time. A list of available methods and server status are provided by SPIRS.
3. *Partial shape matching*: The IRMA user will be able to specify multiple non-overlapping partial shapes and provide weights to indicate their relative importance.
4. *Shape matching by user-sketch*: The IRMA user will be allowed to alter pre-existing database shapes or sketch new shapes. Additionally, the user may specify a threshold for shape similarity scores to limit the number of results.
5. *Combined retrieval*: The IRMA user may securely upload his own spine x-ray image to find similar x-ray images using its global similarity algorithms. Shapes selected within a matching image may then be passed on to SPIRS for local similarity searches.

Fig. 1. Fragment of the SPIRS-IRMA DTD showing query and result elements

```
<!ELEMENT spirs_irma (querystatus|algorithms|query|queryresult)>

<!ELEMENT algorithmidlist (algorithmid+)>
<!ELEMENT algorithmid (#PCDATA)>
<!ELEMENT query (algorithmid,contour)>
<!ELEMENT algorithmid (#PCDATA)>
<!ELEMENT contour (pointlist)>
<!ELEMENT pointlist (point+)>
<!ELEMENT point (x,y)>
<!ELEMENT x (#PCDATA)>
<!ELEMENT y (#PCDATA)>

<!ELEMENT queryresult (neighborlist)>
<!ELEMENT neighborlist (neighbor*)>
<!ELEMENT neighbor (imagetag,vertebranum,similarityscore)>
<!ELEMENT imagetag (#PCDATA)>
<!ELEMENT vertebranum (#PCDATA)>
<!ELEMENT similarityscore (#PCDATA)>
```

5   Method

A loosely-coupled Internet-based distributed computing framework, such as the SPIRS-IRMA interface relies extensively on a robust communications protocol and an open standard data exchange format.

The elements in the XML file, styled to a predefined DTD, are designed toward particular events, e.g., the `<querystatus>` element is used to determine if a desired service is available and to obtain a list of currently available services, the `<query>` element is used by IRMA to make shape queries, and the `<queryresult>` element populated by SPIRS provides the results. A fragment of the DTD is shown in Figure 1. The XML data exchange is implemented on top of the standard hypertext transfer protocol (HTTP). This allows easy adoption into any Web server infrastructure without affecting the firewall settings. The SPIRS service is accessed through a pre-defined URL.

5.1   IRMA Methods for Interacting with SPIRS

As noted above, IRMA methods are treated as black boxes. This eases the addition of new SPIRS-IRMA coupling code to provide the communication interface with SPIRS and perform necessary conversion to and from the XML transport format. An additional required conversion is from the image-vertebra identifiers used in SPIRS to equivalent IRMA image IDs. The response to a query can be visualized using the existing Web-based IRMA interface.

5.2   SPIRS Service for External Queries

SPIRS implements the service gateway as a Java servlet which is the entry point for all service requests and acts as a mediator between client requests and server-side components. It manages multiple simultaneous connections as separate sessions and queues requests to the core SPIRS engine. It also translates query components that require information from the MySQL text database in SPIRS into SQL queries. Finally, the gateway is also responsible for formatting responses from server-side components and the MySQL database into the XML response format and sending them to the client.

5.3   Relevance Feedback for SPIRS-IRMA

IRMA supports relevance feedback by allowing the user to specify the degree of relevance on results from an initial CBIR query. The set of "relevance specified" images can form a new IRMA query which, however, cannot be directly applied to SPIRS since it uses only a single shape as query. In the modified method: (i) the contour vectors for all elements included in the feedback are collected; (ii) each of these vectors is then used to individually query SPIRS, which breaks down the feedback query into a series of single queries; (iii) the query refinement is performed thereafter as a post-processing step on the set of these single-query results.

6   Results and Conclusion

This paper describes the SPIRS-IRMA collaborative CBIR system, which enables users to pose shape queries local to a particular image region through the interface of a CBIR system that inherently supports only overall image similarity. The communication is done over HTTP using XML tags that conform to a predefined "SPIRS-IRMA interface" DTD. The development of this system is planned in several phases. The first two phases which allow vertebral whole shape queries, with user selection of similarity methods, is currently completed, and work on subsequent phases is in progress. A screen-capture of the SPIRS-IRMA system, which is accessible from the IRMA Website, is shown in Figure 2.

Acknowledgement

This research was supported by the Intramural Research Program of the U.S. National Institutes of Health (NIH), National Library of Medicine (NLM), and Lister Hill National Center for Biomedical Communications (LHNCBC).

References

1. Andriole KP, Morin RL. Transforming medical imaging: The first SCAR TRIP [TM] conference. A position paper from the SCAR TRIP[TM] subcommittee of the SCAR research and development committee. J Digital Imaging 2006;19(1):6–16.
2. Müller H, Michoux N, Bandon D, Geissbuhler A. A review of content-based image retrieval systems in medical applications: Clinical benefits and future directions. Int J Med Info 2004;73(1):1–23.

Fig. 2. The SPIRS-IRMA Web interface

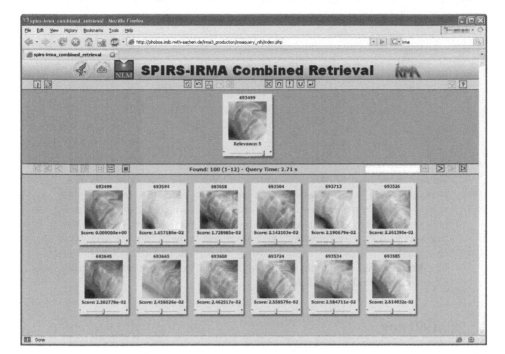

3. Lehmann TM, Güld MO, Thies C, et al. Content-based image retrieval in medical applications. Methods Info Med 2004;43(4):354–61.
4. Thies C, Güld MO, Fischer B, Lehmann TM. Content-based queries on the CasImage database within the IRMA framework. LNCS 2005;3491:781–92.
5. Antani S, Long LR, Thoma GR. Content-based image retrieval for large biomedical image archives. In: Proc 11th World Cong Medical Informatics; 2004. 829–33.
6. Long LR, Antani SK, Thoma GR. Image informatics at a national research center. Comp Med Imaging & Graphics 2005;29:171–93.
7. Thoma GR, Long LR, Antani SK. Biomedical imaging research and development: knowledge from images in the medical enterprise. Technical Report Lister Hill National Ctr for Biomedical Communications, US National Library of Medicine, NIH 2006;LHNCBC-TR-2006-002.
8. Güld MO, Thies C, Fischer B, Lehmann TM. A generic concept for the implementation of medical image retrieval systems. Int J Med Info 2006;In Press.

Anwendung der Random-Walker-Segmentierung für die Strahlentherapieplanung

Gerhard Lechsel, Tianguang Zhang und Rolf Bendl

Abteilung Medizinische Physik in der Strahlentherapie,
Deutsches Krebsforschungszentrum, 69120 Heidelberg
Email: g.lechsel@dkfz.de

Zusammenfassung. Die Anwendbarkeit der Random-Walker-Segmentierung (RWS) in der Strahlentherapieplanung wird untersucht. Hierzu wurde die RWS in ein Bestrahlungsplanungssystem integriert. Nach einem standardisierten Verfahren wurden die Ergebnisse der RWS mit der Segmentierung eines Strahlentherapeuten verglichen. Für die quantitative Analyse wurde die Segmentierung für die Blase durchgeführt. Das Ergebnis wird bezüglich des mittleren Abstandes der Konturen und eines Überdeckungsmaßes verglichen.

1 Einleitung

Die moderne Strahlentherapie hat das Ziel durch ionisierende Strahlung einen hohen Grad an Tumorkontrolle bei gleichzeitiger Schonung gesunden Gewebes zu erreichen. Hierzu müssen bei der Planung in den Bilddaten neben dem Zielvolumen umliegende Risikostrukturen (Organe die geschont werden sollen) segmentiert werden. Für die Planung wird in einem CT-Datensatz eine 3D-Segmentierung durchgeführt. Eine manuelle Segmentierung ist dabei sehr zeitaufwändig, weil mehrere Risikostrukturen in den einzelnen Schichten eingezeichnet werden müssen (für die Bestrahlung der Prostata sind dies beispielweise Rektum und Blase). Ziel der Bildverarbeitung ist es daher, dem Strahlentherapeuten geeignete Segmentierungswerkzeuge zur Verfügung zu stellen, um die 3D-Segmentierung der Risikoorgane zu beschleunigen.

2 Stand der Forschung und Fortschritt durch den Beitrag

Neben rein grauwertbasierten Segmentierungsverfahren (z.B. Region Growing) haben sich aufgrund des schwachen Kontrastes von Weichteilgewebe in CT-Bilddaten modellbasierte Verfahren, wie aktive Konturmodelle oder Point Distribution Modelle PDM, entwickelt. Ein neuerer Ansatz von Leo Grady [1] benutzt Graph-Cut-Verfahren, um eine Segmentierung zu realisieren. Hierzu wird der Bilddatensatz in einen Graphen mit Knoten und Kanten überführt. Mit Hilfe von als Label markierten Knoten wird der erstellte Graph in zwei oder mehr Teilgraphen zerlegt. Diese Zerlegung wird aufgrund der Grauwertinformation in den Bilddaten durchgeführt. Die Teilgraphen entsprechen schließlich einer Segmentierung des Bilddatensatzes.

Im Rahmen dieser Arbeit sollen die Segmentierungsergebnisse dieses Algorithmus für die Strahlentherapieplanung quantitativ untersucht werden. Hierzu wurde der Algorithmus implementiert und in das Bildverarbeitungsmodul eines Planungssystems [2] integriert. Da es sich beim Random-Walker-Algorithmus um ein interaktives Segmentierungsverfahren handelt, wurde eine Anleitung für die Segmentierung eines Organs entworfen und diese zur Segmentierung der Blase angewendet. Das Segmentierungsergebnis wurde dann mit der Segmentierung des Strahlentherapeuten für die Therapieplanung verglichen. Ziel ist es herauszufinden, ob die Segmentierung mit Hilfe des neuen Verfahrens effektiver (zeitlich schneller und mit vergleichbarer Genauigkeit) durchgeführt werden kann.

3 Methoden

Grundlage des implementierten Segmentierungsverfahrens ist der von Leo Grady [1] vorgeschlagene Random-Walker-Algorithmus. Dieser und seine Integration ins Planungssystem sind Voraussetzung für die quantitative Analyse.

3.1 Random-Walker-Algorithmus

Der Algorithmus gehört zur Klasse der Graph-Cut Methoden. Hierfür wird das Bild in einen Graphen $G = (V, E)$ überführt. Hierbei ist V die Menge der Knoten, die den Voxel eines Bildes entsprechen, und E eine Menge von Kanten, die jeweils benachbarte Voxel verbinden. Den einzelnen Kanten wird ein Gewicht zugeordnet. Dieses wird bei Leo Grady mit einer Gauß-Funktion ermittelt. Das Gewicht der Kante w_{ij}, das die Voxel i und j mit den Grauwerten g_i und g_j verbindet, wird berechnet aus $w_{ij} = \exp\left(-\beta(g_j - g_i)^2\right)$. Der Parameter β beschreibt den Einfluss der Bilddaten auf die Segmentierung (ein Standardwert von $\beta = 8$ hat sich bewährt).

Für die Zerlegung des Graphen in Teilgraphen, also der Segmentierung des zugrunde liegenden Bildes, werden einzelne Knoten des Graphen mit Label versehen. Dabei müssen mindestens zwei unterschiedliche Label benutzt werden. Die nicht als Label markierten Knoten werden bei der Zerlegung den verschieden Label zugeordnet. Für die Zuordnung wird die Random-Walker-Theorie verwendet. Ein Random-Walker der von einem bestimmten Knoten startet kann einen Nachbarknoten mit einer Wahrscheinlichkeit erreichen, die dem Gewicht der Kante w_{ij} entspricht. Liesse man den Random-Walker unendlich oft von diesem Voxel starten, könnte man für die unterschiedlichen Label die zugehörige Wahrscheinlichkeit bestimmen, mit der jedes Label erreicht wird. Für die Segmentierung wird das Voxel dem Label mit der größten Erreichungswahrscheinlichkeit zugeordnet.

3.2   Iteratives Lösungsverfahren

Dieses mathematische Problem der Bestimmung der Wahrscheinlichkeiten lässt sich analytisch lösen, aufgrund der Komplexität jedoch nicht in akzeptabler Zeit. Das Aufstellen des zugehörigen linearen Gleichungssystems wird ebenfalls von Grady [1] beschrieben.

Für die Lösung des linearen Gleichungssystems haben wir verschiedene Lösungsansätze (analytische und iterative Verfahren) bezüglich Genauigkeit und Schnelligkeit getestet. Das Gleichungssystem lässt sich durch eine symmetrische, dünn besetzte Matrix darstellen. Das Conjugate-Gradient-Verfahren erwies sich hierbei als effektivstes Lösungsverfahren. Dieses benötigt einen zusätzlichen Parameter ε, der die Rechengenauigkeit des Verfahrens angibt. Für die Berechnungen benutzen wir eine Genauigkeit von $\varepsilon = 0,001$, was sich als guter Kompromiss zwischen Schnelligkeit und Korrektheit der Lösung erwies.

3.3   Verwendete Vergleichsmaße

Zur Bewertung des Verfahrens wird der mittlere Abstand der Oberflächen der Segmentierungen vom Strahlentherapeuten und vom Algorithmus sowie der Dice-Koeffizient bestimmt [3]. Der mittlere Abstand $D(A, B)$ wird für den Vergleich der Ergebnisse berechnet aus der Formel

$$D(A, B) = \frac{\sum_{a \in A} \min_{b \in B} d(a, b)}{|A|} \tag{1}$$

wobei A die Menge der Punkte auf der mit dem Random-Walker-Algorithmus segmentierten Oberfläche sind B die vom Strahlentherapeuten segmentierte Oberfläche und $d(a, b)$ ein Abstandsmaß ist. Der Dice-Koeffizienten C_D ist bestimmt durch

$$C_D = \frac{2|A \cap B|}{|A| + |B|} \tag{2}$$

wobei A die Menge der Voxel der Segmentierung mit dem Random-Walker und B die Menge der Voxel der Segmentierung des Strahlentherapeuten entspricht.

4   Ergebnisse

Für die Auswertung wurde die Segmentierung der Blase von verschiedenen Bilddatensätzen standardisiert durchgeführt. Wir beschränken uns auf die Segmentierung nur eines Organs, obwohl der Algorithmus in der Lage ist, mehrere Organe gleichzeitig zu segmentieren und dadurch auch eine bessere Trennung von benachbarten Organen verspricht. Für eine Vergleichbarkeit von unterschiedlichen Patientendaten ist die Segmentierung nur eines Organs jedoch aussagekräftiger.

In jeweils drei orthogonalen Ansichten (transversal, frontal, sagittal) werden die Label für die Blase und den Hintergrund eingezeichnet (Abb. 1). Die Schicht schneidet dabei das Organ möglichst zentral. Die Label für die Blase

Abb. 1. Segmentierung mit dem Random-Walker: transversal, saggital und frontal

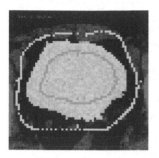 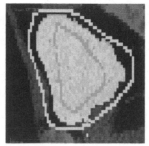 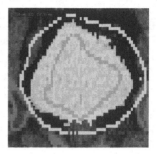

werden innerhalb des Organs in etwa 3-5 Voxel Abstand zum Rand von Hand eingezeichnet. Die Label für den Background entsprechend außerhalb.

Damit ist eine robuste Initialisierung des Random-Walker-Algorithmus gegeben. Das Segmentierungsergebnis ist unabhängig von einzelnen Label-Punkten. Die Blase muss in drei Ansichten insgesamt sechs Mal umfahren werden (drei Mal innerhalb und drei Mal außerhalb). Das Umfahren des Randes für das Einzeichnen der Label muss jedoch nicht mit der gleichen Sorgfalt durchgeführt werden, wie beim Einzeichnen einer Kontur für die Segmentierung der Blase.

Der Algorithmus wurde dahingehend erweitert, dass für die Aufstellung des Gleichungssystems nicht alle Voxel des Bilddatensatzes verwendet werden. Da in drei orthogonalen Schichten die Blase umfahren wird, werden für die Berechnung nur die Voxel innerhalb des kleinsten Rechtecks verwendet, das gerade alle Label enthält. Dadurch wird die Komplexität des Gleichungssystems verringert und die Rechenzeit erheblich reduziert.

Tab. 1 zeigt die Ergebnisse unserer Analyse. 10 verschiedene Datensätze wurden segmentiert. In der Tabelle sind diese nach der Größe des Volumens geordnet, für das die Berechnung durchgeführt wurde. Der Zeitbedarf für die Segmentierung hängt zum einen von dieser Größe ab, aber auch von der Konvergenz des iterativen Lösungsverfahren (für die Berechnung wurde $\varepsilon = 0,001$ gewählt). Für eine vollständige 3D-Segmentierung einer Blase ist mit einem Zeitbedarf von etwa 30 s zu rechnen (benutzt wurde ein PC mit 2,4 GHz, 1,0 GB RAM). Segmentierungen mit einem Dice-Koeffizienten größer als 80 % waren zufriedenstellend. Bei Patient Nr. 2 traten die größten Abweichungen auf. In der Nachbarschaft zur Prostata, also dem relevanten Bereich für die Therapieplanung traten hier erhebliche Abweichungen auf, da hier keine Kanten sichtbar waren. Korrekturen in diesem Bereich wären auch bei anderen Segmentierungen nötig gewesen.

5 Diskussion

Bei dem implementierten Segmentierungs-Algorithmus handelt es sich um ein einfach zu bedienendes, robustes und parallel anwendbares Verfahren. Einfach heißt für die Anwendung, dass die Initialisierung des Algorithmus durch das

Tabelle 1. Vergleich der Segmentierung der Blase durch einen Strahlentherapeut und mit Hilfe des Random-Walker-Algorithmus (in Voxel)

Patient (Nr.)	Volumen für Berechnung	Volumen der Blase	Mittlerer Abstand	Überdeckung (in Prozent)	Zeit (in Sekunden)
1	491 840	121 844	1,43 ± 0,06	89,4	40,29
2	452 790	76 142	3,53 ± 0,16	77,3	26,37
3	413 409	90 075	1,50 ± 0,06	90,0	38,57
4	412 020	102 053	1,42 ± 0,07	87,0	44,14
5	357 616	95 933	1,17 ± 0,07	91,0	32,60
6	283 954	43 224	1,84 ± 0,07	82,3	9,28
7	270 375	66 973	1,66 ± 0,07	89,9	17,32
8	252 370	39 643	0,99 ± 0,03	91,3	16,00
9	170 544	33 662	1,85 ± 0,09	86,6	9,48
10	139 320	36 615	1,36 ± 0,07	90,2	8,51

Einzeichnen der Label intuitiv ist. Darüber hinaus können durch das Verwenden mehrer Label mehrere Organe in einem Berechnungsschritt segmentiert werden.

Bei der Segmentierung der Blase kann es zum Auslaufen der Oberfläche im Grenzbereich zur Prostata kommen. Die Korrektur der Segmentierung erfolgt durch das Einzeichnen zusätzlicher Label für den Hintergrund in diesem Bereich. Für die Analyse wurde diese Korrektur nicht berücksichtigt, da sich dieser Schritt nicht standardisiert beschreiben lässt. Die erneute Berechnung des Gleichungssystems nach dem Hinzufügen von Labelpunkten erfordert jedoch weniger Zeit als die Neuberechnung des Gleichungssystems, da das iterative Verfahren von uns mit der vorhandenen Lösung initialisiert wird.

Eine verbesserte Segmentierung lässt sich dadurch erreichen, dass benachbarte Organe gleichzeitig segmentiert werden. Durch das hinzufügen von Label für die Prostata kann, z. B., die Grenze zur Blase besser identifiziert werden. Gerade die Segmentierung mehrerer Strukturen gleichzeitig ist ein wesentlicher Vorteil dieses Algorithmus.

Es hat sich gezeigt, dass der Algorithmus für eine interaktive Segmentierung geeignet ist. Er ist ausreichend schnell, um die Zeit für das Einzeichnen von Risikoorganen (nicht nur wie gezeigt der Blase) zu reduzieren.

Literaturverzeichnis

1. Grady L, Schwartz EL. Isoperimetric graph partitioning for image segmentation. IEEE Trans Pattern Anal Mach Intell 2006;28(3):469–475.
2. Bendl R, Pross J, Schlegel W. VIRTUOS: A program for virtual radiotherapy Simulation. CAR 1993; 822–823.
3. Heimann T, Thorn M, et al. Empirische Vergleichsmaße für die Evaluation von Segmentierungsergebnissen. Procs BVM 2004; 165–169.

Erstellung eines anatomischen Templates zur Zielvolumendefinition der Zervixregion für die Bestrahlungsplanung

Detlef Richter[1], Soulimane Abdellaoui[1,2], Faisel Bekkaoui[1,2]
Karsten Berthold[1,2] und Gerd Straßmann[2]

[1]Fachbereich Informatik, Fachhochschule Wiesbaden, D-65197 Wiesbaden
[2]Klinik für Strahlentherapie, Philipps-Universität Marburg, D-35043 Marburg
Email: richter@informatik.fh-wiesbaden.de

Zusammenfassung. Es wird ein Algorithmus zur halbautomatischen Erzeugung von Templates aus konturierten CT-Datensätzen der Zervix zur Bestrahlungsplanung vorgestellt. Die Anpassung des Templates an individuelle Datensätze erfolgt durch Verwendung anatomischer Landmarken. Diese bilden ein Landmarkenmodell, das für die Berechnung der Parameter für eine affine 3D Transformation des Templates verwendet wird.

1 Problemstellung

Die Bestrahlungsplanung beim Zervixkarzinom beinhaltet in der Regel die Konturierung der Tumorregion und der dazugehörigen ableitenden Lymphwege. In mehr als der Hälfte der Fälle wurde der Tumor bereits operativ entfernt. Die Automatisierung der postoperativen Zielvolumendefinition ist ein Problem mit zwei schwierig zu erfassenden Vorgaben. Erstens ist das Zielvolumen von der präoperativen irregulären Tumorform und der individuellen Patientenanatomie abhängig. Zweitens basiert die Zielvolumendefinition in großem Maße auf der individuellen Erfahrung des Arztes, der sich an anatomischen Landmarken und verschiedenen Organstrukturen orientiert. Diese Landmarken sind Lymphknotengruppen oder Gefäße, die einen festen Bezug zur anatomischen Struktur der Zervixregion beziehungsweise zu Knochenpunkten haben. Dementsprechend basiert die individuelle Zielvolumendefinition für eine 3D-konformale Bestrahlungsplanung trotz unterschiedlicher Anatomie der Individuen auf ähnlich geformten Zielvolumina. Es liegt daher nahe, ein Template aus mehreren CT-Datensätzen zu generieren. Für die Berechnung der notwendigen Transformationsparameter wird eine affine Transformation, die eine Translation, Rotation und eine in jeder Dimension unabhängige Skalierung einschließt, verwendet.

2 Stand der Forschung und Fortschritt durch den Beitrag

Aus den wenigen Arbeiten, die zu dem Thema der automatischen Zielvolumendefinition publiziert wurden, sind folgende Studien erwähnenswert. Ein Verfahren

[1] wurde zur Autosegmentierung von Leber, Lunge und Rückenmark entwickelt. Dieses Verfahren greift auf einen Atlas, in dem die komplette Organanatomie modelliert wurde, zurück. Das Organmodell wird dann schichtweise nach einer interaktiven Definition von sieben anatomischen Landmarken auf den individuellen CT-Datensatz übertragen und durch Snake-Algorithmen über eine Energiefunktion angepasst. Die Energiefunktionen verlangen kontrastreiche Strukturen zur Konturanpassung. In einem zweiten Verfahren [2] zur Definition von Risikostrukturen im Hirn werden zwei Datensätze, ein hoch aufgelöster, künstlich erzeugter und perfekt symmetrischer Datensatz und ein Atlas aus dem ersten Datensatz, verwendet. Um die Parameter für eine elastische 3D Transformation zu erhalten, wurde der künstlich erzeugte Datensatz in einem zweistufigen Verfahren mit einer rigiden und einer nicht rigiden Transformation an den Patientendatensatz angepasst und anschließend mit den so gewonnenen Parametern der Atlas mit einer elastischen Transformation auf die Patientendaten übertragen. Beide Verfahren nach [1] und [2] verwenden einen aufwendig manuell erstellten Atlas. Andere Methoden wie beispielsweise Statistical Shape Models mit nichtrigiden Transformationen sind auf gut separierbare Oberflächen der zu transformierenden Objekte angewiesen [3].

Durch das vorgestellte Verfahren können Templates von Zielvolumina, die nicht durch Gewebestrukturen definiert sind, einfach erstellt werden. Es sind keine aufwendig manuell vorbereiteten Atlanten wie bei [1] und [2] bzw. kontrastreiche Konturen wie bei [1] notwendig. Ebenso setzt das Verfahren keine definierten Organoberflächen zur Template-Erstellung wie bei [3] voraus. Eine 3D Anpassung des Templates an den individuellen Datensatz erfolgt durch Definition von einzelnen anatomischen Strukturen, die ein Landmarkenmodell definieren. Wie in [2] werden aus diesem Landmarkenmodell die Transformationsparameter berechnet. Das Verfahren kann zur Erstellung von Templates weiterer anatomischer Regionen angewendet werden. Speziell bei nicht durch Atlanten definierbaren Zielvolumina wird deren Definition durch dieses Verfahren objektiviert.

3   Methoden

Die Erstellung des Templates erfolgt in zwei Schritten. Zuerst wird ein Landmarkenmodell erstellt, aus dem die Parameter zur Transformation gewonnen werden. Im zweiten Schritt wird aus den konturierten Zielvolumina mithilfe der im ersten Schritt gewonnenen Parameter das Template erstellt. Für die Anwendung des Templates werden in dem individuellen Datensatz interaktiv die anatomischen Landmarken definiert und die Transformationsparameter berechnet. Mit diesen Parametern wird dann das Template auf den Datensatz übertragen.

3.1   Erstellung des Landmarkenmodells

Für die Erstellung des Landmarkenmodells [4, 5] wurden interaktiv fünf Lymphknoten und die Schwerpunkte der obersten und untersten Kontur definiert und

Abb. 1. Landmarkenmodell: Landmarken der CT-Datensätze (a), Kontur aus den interaktiv definierten Stützpunkten [6] (b), Zusammenfassung der Konturpunkte (c)

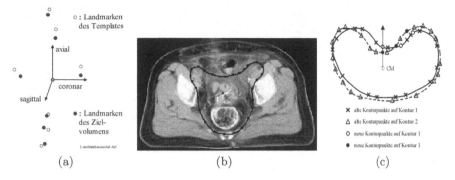

(a)   (b)   (c)

als anatomische Landmarken verwendet. Die Schwerpunkte der Landmarken eines jeden Datensatzes wurden berechnet und diese durch eine Translation zur Deckung gebracht. Anschließend wurden die Landmarken durch Rotation und Skalierung der einzelnen Datensätze so angepasst, dass die Summe der Fehlerquadrate der Euklidischen Abstände minimal ist. Die Transformationsmatrizen $A_n, n = 1 \ldots N$ der affinen Transformationen der N einzelnen Datensätze werden mit Hilfe von Tensorprodukten berechnet. Diese Tensorprodukte werden aus den Koordinaten der Landmarken gebildet. Die Matrizen A_n beinhalten nur die Rotation und konstante Skalierungen in jeder Dimension. Die aufeinander angepassten Landmarken werden nacheinander gewichtet zu einem Landmarkenmodell zusammengefasst (Abb. 1a). Zum Abschluß wird für jeden der N Datensätze eine 3D Transformationsmatrix B_n, bestehend aus einer Translation, einer Rotation und der Skalierung in jeder Dimension, bezogen auf das Landmarkenmodell, berechnet.

3.2 Erstellung des Templates

Für die Erstellung des Templates [4, 5] werden die Zielvolumina der einzelnen Datensätze durch Stützpunkte in einzelnen ausgewählten Schichten im Abstand von ca. 5 mm interaktiv definiert und diese durch geschlossene Hermite kubische Splines zu Konturen ergänzt (Abb. 1b) [6]. Auf die Konturstützpunkte wird dann die 3D Transformationsmatrix B_n angewendet. Dadurch können die ursprünglichen Stützpunkte aus einzelnen Schichten des Datensatzes in andere Schichten transformiert werden. Daher werden aus dem Drahtgittermodell der Konturen neue Stützpunkte in den neuen Schichten berechnet. Nachdem dieser Vorgang für alle N Datensätze durchgeführt wurde, werden auf den N einzelnen Konturen neue Stützpunkte in Bezug auf gleiche Anzahl pro Kontur, gleichen gegenseitigen Abstand und gleicher Phasenlage bezüglich einer vorgegebenen Richtung vom Schwerpunkt (CM) aus berechnet und die entstehenden singulären Punktwolken als Schwerpunkte zusammengefasst. In Abb. 1c wurden aus Gründen der Übersichtlichkeit nur drei neue Konturpunkte eingezeichnet.

Abb. 2. Definition der Volumina A, B und C zur Berechnung des Ähnlichkeitsindex

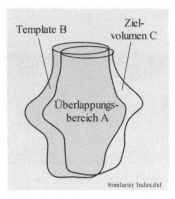

Diese so erhaltenen Punkte bilden als Konturmodell das Template. Es hat in Bezug auf das Landmarkenmodell eine konforme Lage.

3.3   Anwendung des Templates

Die Überlagerung des Templates auf einen individuellen CT-Datensatz basiert auf einem analogen Verfahren, mit dem das Template erstellt wurde. Zu Beginn werden die anatomischen Landmarken im individuellen Datensatz in der von der Software vorgegebenen Reihenfolge von dem Strahlentherapeuten definiert. Dadurch wird das Korrepondenzproblem der individuellen Landmarken zum Landmarkenmodell umgangen. Das Landmarkenmodell wird auf die Landmarken der Patientin mit dem bereits beschriebenen Verfahren approximiert. Man erhält somit eine Transformationsmatrix $(B_{N+1})^{-1}$ mit dem das Konturmodell auf alle Schichten des individuellen Datensatz übertragen wird.

4   Ergebnisse

Für die Erzeugung des Atlas standen für die vorliegende Arbeit 12 CT-Datensätze zur Verfügung. Die Evaluation der Ergebnisse wurde mit Hilfe eines Ähnlichkeitsindex AI (Abb. 2) durchgeführt: $AI = \frac{A}{B+C-A} \cdot 100$ in Prozent, wobei A das gemeinsame überlappende Volumen zwischen dem automatisch generierten und dem manuell konturierten Zielvolumen, B das automatisch erzeugte Template und C das manuell konturierte Zielvolumen ist. Von den N = 12 verfügbaren Datensätzen wurde durch Überlagerung eines aus N-1 = 11 Datensätzen erzeugten Templates auf den 12. Datensatz der Ähnlichkeitsindex AI berechnet. Die Ähnlichkeit zwischen dem manuell und dem automatisch definierten Zielvolumen beträgt im Durchschnitt 50 %, was als erste Näherung zur Zielvolumendefinition ausreichend ist. Weiterhin ergibt sich im Gegensatz zur konventionellen Zielvolumendefintion eine Zeitersparnis von ca. 40%.

Die entwickelte Software wurde auf einer Intel Pentium-4 CPU mit 2.6 GHz und 1024 MBytes getestet. Die Erstellung eines Templates aus den bereits konturierten Datensätzen dauert durchschnittlich 8 sec. Die Anpassung des Templates auf einen individuellen CT-Datensatz dauert nach der interaktiven Definition der anatomischen Landmarken ca. 200 ms.

5 Diskussion

Die durchgeführten Tests zeigen, dass die Anwendung einer affinen Transformation zur Erstellung eines Templates und dessen Anwendung zu befriedigenden Ergebnissen führt, sofern die anatomischen Regionen nicht allzu großen Formvariationen unterworfen sind. Die Erstellung der Templates erfolgt aus den konturierten Strukturen. Die automatische Zielvolumendefinition verkürzt beim Zervixkarzinom die Bestrahlungsplanungszeit. Ein nicht zu vernachlässigender Teil der aufgewendeten Zeit liegt in der Nachbearbeitung des automatisch definierten Zielvolumens. Es ist daher notwendig, die Nachbearbeitungszeit zu verringern. Allerdings sind von den in der vorliegenden Arbeit verwendeten anatomischen Strukturen fünf im Wesentlichen in der sagittalen Ebene und zwei in der axialen Ebene zu finden, weshalb die räumliche Anpassung, speziell am oberen und unteren Ende der Zervix noch nicht optimal ist. Eine andere Auswahl der anatomischen Landmarken, sofern diese definiert werden können, kann die Nachbearbeitungszeit weiter verringern.

Neben der Zeitersparnis bringt die Verwendung eines Templates speziell bei den nicht durch Gewebestrukturen begrenzten Zielvolumina den Vorteil einer Definition nach objektiven Kriterien. Für Strahlentherapeuten in der Ausbildung bietet die automatische Vorgabe eines Zielvolumens eine große Hilfestellung.

Literaturverzeichnis

1. Qatarneh S, et al. Evaluation of a segmentation procedure to delineate organs for use in construction of a radiation therapy planning atlas. Int J Medi Inform 2003;69:39–55.
2. Bondiau PY, et al. Atlas-based automatic segmentation of MR images: Validation study on the brainstem in radiotherapy context. Int J Radiation Oncology Biol Phys 2005;61:289–298.
3. Heitz G, et al. Shape model generation using nonrigid deformation of a template mesh. Procs SPIE 2005.
4. Abdellaoui S. Erstellung eines 3D Atlas ausgewählter Strukturen durch affine Transformation anatomischer Landmarken. Master's thesis. University of Applied Sciences of Darmstadt & University of Applied Sciences of Wiesbaden; 2006.
5. Richter D, Abdellaoui S, Straßmann G. Semiautomatic CT-based definition of target volumes using anatomical landmarks. Procs EURASIP Conference Biosignal 2006; 227–229.
6. Janecek J. Contouring and 3D Modelling of Organ Structures for Conformal Treatment Planning in Radiotherapy. Master's thesis. Brno University of Technology & University of Applied Sciences of Wiesbaden; 2005.

Präoperative Simulation von Rohrprothesen und Y-Stents zur endovaskulären Behandlung von Stenosen und Aneurysmen

Jan Egger[1,2], Stefan Großkopf[2], Bernd Freisleben[1]

[1]Philipps-Universität Marburg, FB Mathematik und Informatik, 35032 Marburg
[2]Siemens Computed Tomography, 91301 Forchheim
Email: jan.egger.ext@siemens.com

Zusammenfassung. Die endovaskuläre Behandlung von Gefäßerkrankungen erfordert zur Wahl eines passenden Stents die Kenntnis der individuellen Gefäßabmaße. Wir stellen eine Methode vor, mit der Rohrprothesen und Y-Stents zusammen mit den präoperativen CT-Daten visualisiert werden. Die verwendete physikalische Simulation ermöglicht darüber hinaus die Simulation des Verhaltens unterschiedlicher Stent-Bauarten beim Expandieren in der Arterie. So kann überprüft werden, ob ein ausgewählter Stent richtig bemessen ist. Zur Simulation des physikalischen Verhaltens wird das Verfahren der Aktiven Konturen (ACM) angewandt. Die Initialkontur entspricht dem zusammengefalteten Stent. Zum Generieren der Initialkontur werden zuerst die vaskulären Strukturen segmentiert. Danach wird die Gefäßmittellinie berechnet. Ausgehend davon wird ein Initialstent konstruiert, der unter Berücksichtigung von internen und externen Kräften expandiert. In diesem Beitrag werden Ergebnisse der Stent-Simulation für unterschiedliche Krankheitsbilder (BAA, TAA, Iliac Aneurysma, Karotis Stenose) präsentiert, um den Wert für die Stent-Planung zu demonstrieren.

1 Einleitung

Stenosen und Aneurysmen werden seit den frühen 1990er Jahren auch endovaskulär behandelt. Bei dieser Form der Behandlung wird – im Gegensatz zur offenen Operation – nur ein kleiner Schnitt unter lokaler Anästhesie zum Einführen der Prothese benötigt.

Der zusammengefaltete Stent wird im allgemeinen von der Beinarterie ausgehend bis zur Stenose oder dem Aneurysma vorgeschoben und dort expandiert. Diese Behandlungsform ist insbesondere für Risikopatienten – für die keine offene Operation in Frage kommt – geeignet. Klinische Studien [1, 2, 3, 4] haben gezeigt, dass die Ergebnisse eines endovaskulären Eingriffs vergleichbar sind mit der klassischen offenen Operation.

2 Stand der Forschung und Fortschritt durch den Beitrag

In [5] werden zwei Methoden zur Simulation und Visualisierung von Rohrprothesen vorgestellt: Zum einen ein geometrischer Ansatz und zum anderen ein

Ansatz, der das Verfahren der Aktiven Konturen anwendet. Beide Verfahren wurden aber nur für die Simulation von nicht verzweigten Stents in Aneurysmen entwickelt und getestet.

Ein Ansatz zur Simulation und Visualisierung von Rohrprothesen in Gefäßen wird in [6] beschrieben, der sich im Detail vom hier vorgestellten Verfahren unterscheidet: der Stent wird durch eine externe Kraft an eine virtuelle Gefäßmittellinie gebunden. Diese Kraft hat keinen Bezug zu den physikalischen Eigenschaften realer Stents, da die Mittellinie nur virtuell existiert.

In [7, 8] wird die Modellierung von verzweigten Stents durch ein geschlossenes ACM vorgestellt. Diese Modellierung unterstützt insbesondere die komplexe Planung von Bauchaortenaneurysma(BAA)-Stents.

Die hier vorgestellte Methode ist insbesondere in der Lage die Dilatation der Gefäßwände im Bereich einer Stenose zu Modellieren. Darüber hinaus wird der von uns vorgestellte Ansatz anhand einer Reihe realer Datensätze unterschiedlicher Krankheitsbilder demonstriert.

3 Methoden

Für die Simulation der Stents wurden die Methoden aus [7, 5, 8] erweitert. Sie erfordern eine vorherige Segmentierung der zu behandelnden Arterie. Dazu wird ein Saatpunkt-basiertes Regionen-Wachstumsverfahren verwendet, das die Voxel anhand ihrer Grauwerte der Arterie zuordnet.

Anschließend wird die Mittellinie der segmentierten Arterie zum Beispiel durch einen Skelettierungsalgorithmus ermittelt [9]. Für die Simulation der Stents wird ein Initialstent mit einem benutzerdefinierten Durchmesser konstruiert. Für die Konstruktion des Initialstents werden Strahlen radial von der Mittellinie der Arterie ausgesendet. Aus der Richtung und der vorgegebenen Länge der Strahlen ergeben sich dann die Oberflächenpunkte des Initialstents. Im Anschluss an diese geometrische Konstruktion wird der Stent durch ein ACM deformiert – ein rein geometrisches Verfahren hat sich in [5] als weniger realistisch herausgestellt.

Das ACM Verfahren realisiert externe und interne Kräfte und basiert auf der Technik von [10, 11]. Interne Kräfte in horizontaler, vertikaler und diagonaler Richtung simulieren das elastische Verhalten des Stents. Die externen Kräfte ziehen bzw. drücken den Stent in Richtung Arterienwand und werden durch die folgende Gleichung approximiert (Abb. 1)

$$F_{ext} = F_{Vessel} + F_{Balloon} + F_{Dilate} \qquad (1)$$

Eine externe Kraft mit expandierender Wirkung ist dabei die Ballonkraft $F_{Balloon}$, die das Anpressen des Stents an die Gefäßwand z.B. durch einen Ballonkatheter simuliert. Durch einen vorgegebenen maximalen Durchmesser weitet sich der virtuelle Stent im Bereich des Aneurysmas nur so weit, wie es der reale Stent aufgrund seiner Konstruktion zulässt.

Abb. 1. Zusammenspiel von F_{Vessel}, F_{Dilate} und F_{Balloon}: F_{Dilate} dilatiert das Gefäß um Δr

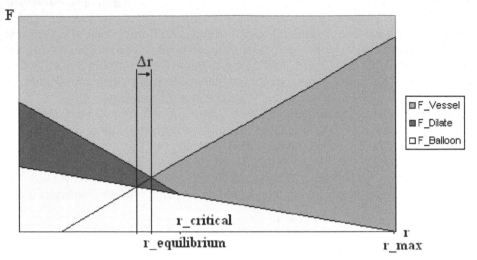

Die Kraft zur Dilatation des Gefäßes im Bereich einer Stenose wird durch die externe Kraft F_{Dilate} modelliert

$$F_{\text{Dilate}} = \begin{cases} c_d \left(r_{\text{critical}} - r\right) & r < r_{\text{critical}} \\ 0 & r \geqslant r_{\text{critical}} \end{cases} \tag{2}$$

Um die Verengung zu erweitern, übt F_{Dilate} im Bereich einer Stenose einen zusätzlichen Druck aus. Die Federkonstante c_d kann größer gewählt werden als die Federkonstante c_b zur Modellierung der Ballonkraft F_{Balloon}.

Der Betrag der externen Kraft $F_{\text{Vessel}} = \text{Vessel} \nabla D(x, y, z)$ wird aus der Distanzbild der segmentierten Arterie gewonnen und simuliert den Widerstand der Arteriewand.

4   Ergebnisse

Die Methoden wurden innerhalb der MeVisLab Plattform realisiert. Für die Evaluierung wurden sowohl Datensätze aus der klinischen Routine (BAA, TAA, Karotis Stenosen, Iliac Aneurysmen) als auch Phantomdatensätze verwendet. Die speziellen Material- und Ausdehnungseigenschaften der Stents konnten durch das ACM angemessen simuliert werden (Abb. 2).

Als rechenintensiv stellte sich die Aufstellung und Berechnung der Steifigkeitsmatrix für das ACM heraus. Die Anzahl der Oberflächenpunkte des Stents gibt die Größe der Steifigkeitsmatrix vor. Zur Simulation einer Y-Prothese müssen im allgemeinen mehr Oberflächenpunkte verwendet werden als bei einer Rohrprothese. Die Rechenzeiten für die Lösung des Gleichungssystems reichen dementsprechend von ca. 60 bis 90 Sekunden auf einer Intel Xeon CPU, 3 GHz,

Abb. 2. Simulationsergebnisse: Rohrprothese Iliac Aneurysma (a), Rohrprothese TAA (b), Rohrprothese BAA (c), Y-Prothese BAA (d), Initialstent Karotis Stenose (e), Rohrprothese Karotis Stenose (f)

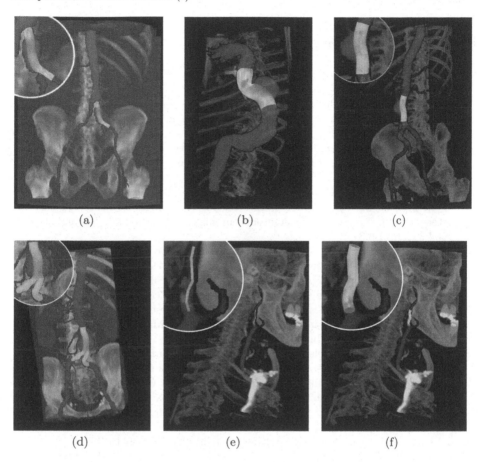

(a)   (b)   (c)

(d)   (e)   (f)

3 GB RAM, Windows XP Professional 2002. Ein Iterationsschritt des ACM benötigt weniger als eine Sekunde und ist somit nicht zeitkritisch.

5 Diskussion

Wir stellen einen umfassenden Ansatz zur Simulation von Stents vor, der in der Lage ist, Stents in Aneurysmen und Stenosen zu simulieren und zu visualisieren. Dazu wurde eine Methode, die auf dem numerischen Verfahren der Aktiven Konturen basiert, entwickelt und verifiziert. Bei allen Varianten kann ein behandelnder Arzt somit vor dem Eingriff bei der Auswahl des Stents durch die Simulation unterstützt werden.

Unser Verfahren ist ein Beitrag zur Unterstützung der komplexen Planung von Stenting in BAAs, aber auch in anderen Aneurysmen und Stenosen. Langfristig gesehen könnte eine exaktere Planung des Eingriffs auf der Grundlage der Simulation dazu beitragen, die mit dem endovaskulären Eingriff verbundene Mortalitätsrate zu senken.

Literaturverzeichnis

1. Blankensteijn JD. Impact of the EVAR-1 and DREAM trials. Endovascular Today 2005;3:33–37.
2. Blankensteijn JD, de Jong SE, Prinssen M, et al. Two-year outcomes after conventional or endovascular repair of abdominal aortic aneurysms. N Engl J Med 2005;352(23):2398–2405.
3. Hacke W. Stent-protected percutaneous angioplasty of the carotid artery vs. endarterectomy (SPACE). Presented at the European Stroke Conference, Brussels; 2006.
4. Yadav JS, Wholey MH, Kuntz RE, et al. Stenting and angioplasty with protection in patients at high risk for endarterectomy investigators: Protected carotid-artery stenting versus endarterectomy in high risk patients. N Engl J Med 2004;351(15):1493–1501.
5. Egger J, Großkopf S, Freisleben B. Comparison of two methods for preoperative visualization of stent grafts in CT-data. In: CURAC; 2006. 140–141.
6. Florez-Valencia L, Montagnat J, Orkisz M. 3D graphical models for vascular-stent pose simulation. Machine Graphics & Vision 2004;13(3):235–248.
7. Egger J. Selektion und Visualisierung von Endoprothesen (Stent Grafts) zur Therapieplanung von Bauchaortenaneurysmen (BAA). Master's thesis. Hochschule Darmstadt, Fachbereich Informatik; 2006.
8. Egger J, Großkopf S, Freisleben B. Simulation of bifurcated stent grafts to treat abdominal aortic aneurysms (AAA). Procs SPIE Medical Imaging 2007.
9. Boskamp T, Rinck D, Link F, Kuemmerlen B, Stamm G, Mildenberger P. A new vessel analysis tool for morphometric quantification and visualization of vessels in CT and MR imaging data sets. Radiographics 2004;24(1):287–297.
10. Kass M, Witkin A, Terzopoulos D. Constraints on deformable models: Recovering 3D shape and nongrid motion. Artificial Intelligence 1988;36(1):91–123.
11. Kass M, Witkin A, Terzopoulos D. Snakes: Active contour models. International Journal of Computer Vision 1987;1(4):321–331.

Bayesian Vessel Extraction for Planning of Radiofrequency-Ablation

Stephan Zidowitz[1], Johann Drexl[1], Tim Kröger[2], Tobias Preusser[2],
Felix Ritter[1], Andreas Weihusen[1], Heinz-Otto Peitgen[1]

[1]MeVis Research GmbH, Universitätsallee 29, 28359 Bremen
[2]CeVis - Center for Complex Systems and Visualization, Department of Mathematics
and Computer Science, University of Bremen, Universitätsallee 29, 28359 Bremen
Email: zidowitz@mevis.de

Abstract. The software-assisted planning of radiofrequency-ablation of
liver tumors calls for robust and fast methods to segment the tumor and
surrounding vascular structures from clinical data to allow a numerical
estimation, whether a complete thermal destruction of the tumor is feasible taking the cooling effect of the vessels into account. As the clinical
workflow in radiofrequency-ablation does not allow for time consuming
planning procedures, the implementation of robust and fast segmentation algorithms is critical in building a streamlined software application
tailored to the clinical needs. To suppress typical artifacts in clinical CT
or MRT data - like inhomogeneous background density due to the imaging procedure - a Bayesian background compensation is developed, which
subsequently allows a robust segmentation of the vessels by fast threshold based algorithms. The presented Bayesian background compensation
has proven to handle a wide range of image perturbances in MRT and CT
data and leads to a fast and reliable identification of vascular structures
in clinical data.

1 Introduction

To assist the complete thermal destruction of the tumor in radiofrequency-
therapy a software-assisted image based planning of the ablation must consider
the extension of the tumor as well as the vascular structures in the vicinity of
the tumor, to incorporate the cooling effect of the vessels. Hence the software-
assisted planning of radiofrequency-ablation of liver tumors calls for robust and
fast methods to segment the tumor and the surrounding vascular structures from
clinical data. However, the use of fast threshold based algorithms is prevented by
inhomogeneous image intensities present in clinical CT and MRT data. A reliable
reduction of this image perturbances subsequently speeds up the segmentation
procedures and leads to a fast and robust one-click segmentation of relevant
anatomical structures. As the clinical workflow in radiofrequency-ablation does
not allow for time consuming planning procedures, the implementation of robust
and fast segmentation algorithms is critical in building a streamlined software
application tailored to the clinical needs.

2   State of the Art and New Contribution

The problem of removing intensity nonuniformity from MRT images has been extensively addressed by many researchers [1]. Beside homomorphic unsharp masking and other filtering techniques [2] the problem of nonuniformity is addressed using an approach becoming known under the name nonparametric nonuniform intensity normalization [3]. In this a gain field is estimated to sharpen the histogramm of the MRT data. Other researchers look uppon the intensity correction as intrinsic part of the enclosing classification and segmentation problem [4]. Commonly these algorithms for the inhomogeneity correction in MRT data rely on the estimation of multiplicative correction factors, whereas the method presented here is based on an additive two-component model. Comparable methods are used for background compensation in astrophysics [5, 6]. The proposed method has proven suitable to handle a wide range of image perturbances in MRT and CT data likewise. While we exploit the local intensity only, the statistical model provides in addition an easy to use framework to incorporate more sophisticated image measures if needed.

3   Methods

The widespread problem of separating vascular structures from parenchymal background in inhomogeneous clinical CT or MRT images is solved with Bayesian probability theory. To capture the defining characteristics of the images - namely that the parenchymal regions are smoother than the vascular structures - a two-component mixture model is used. Given the MRT image intensity $\{y_i\}$ at each voxel i, our complemetary hypotheses for the measurement process are

$(\mathcal{B})$ y_i is purly background: $y_i = b_i + \epsilon_i$
$(\mathcal{S})$ y_i contains signal contribution: $y_i = b_i + s_i + \epsilon_i$

While the first hypothesis specifies that the image intensity consists only of background b_i spoiled with noise ϵ_i, the complementary hypothesis specifies the case where additional signal intensity s_i contributes to the image. An additional assumption is that the background is smoother than the signal. This is enforced by approximating the data by a linear combination of smooth basis functions, namely by modelling the background using B-spline approximation of the data. Spline approximation incorporating smoothness constraints is superior to filtering techniques in dealing with given situation of data inhomogenities with a wide range of spacial scales [7]. As the spline approximation are used as filter for this application, the smoothing parameters of the B-splines - primarily the distance between basis functions - are not derived from the data but choosen a priory.

The image noise $\{\epsilon_i\}$ is approximated with Gaussian or Poisson statistic

$$\text{Gaussian:}\quad p(y_i|\xi_i) = (2\pi\sigma^2)\exp\left[-\frac{(\xi_i - y_i)^2}{2\sigma^2}\right]$$

$$\text{Poisson:}\quad p(y_i|\xi_i) = \frac{y_i^{\xi_i}}{\xi_i!}\exp\left(-y_i\right)$$

where the expected value ξ_i is given by the background $\xi_i = b_i$ for $\mathcal{B}$ or by the background with additional signal contribution $\xi_i = b_i + s_i$ for hypothesis $\mathcal{S}$ respectively.

The signal contribution is descripted probablistically in terms of its prior distribution. Assuming, we know only the average value λ of the signal intensity, the prior distribution is given by an exponential function (for positive signal intensities)

$$p(y_i|\lambda) = \frac{\exp\left[-\frac{y_i}{\lambda}\right]}{\lambda}$$

Using this prior, the likelihood for the hypothesis "*(S) y_i contains signal contribution*" is obtained by marginalizing the noise probability over the signal. For positive signal intensities this leads to

Gaussian: $\quad p_{(\mathcal{S})}(y_i|b_i,\lambda) = \frac{1}{2\lambda}\left\{1 + \text{erf}\left[\frac{\lambda(y_i-b_i)-\sigma^2}{\lambda\sqrt{2\sigma^2}}\right]\right\}\exp\left[\frac{-2\lambda(y_i-b_i)+\sigma^2}{2\lambda^2}\right]$

Poisson: $\quad p_{(\mathcal{S})}(y_i|b_i,\lambda) = \frac{\exp\left[\frac{b_i}{\lambda}\right]}{\lambda(1+\lambda^{-1})^{y_i+1}}\frac{\Gamma\left[(y_i+1),b_i(1+\lambda^{-1})\right]}{\Gamma[y_i+1]}$

where $\Gamma[a,x]$ is the incomplete Gamma-function and $\Gamma[a] = \Gamma[a,0]$. The extension to negative signale intensities is straightforward.

For the mixture model the prior probability for the two complementary hypotheses is chosen to be independent of the localization: $p_{(\mathcal{B})} = \beta$ and $p_{(\mathcal{S})} = 1 - \beta$.

While the background intensities $\{b_i\}$ are calculated using spline approximation of the data, the probility parameters σ, λ, and β are estimated by histogram analysis of the remaining image intensities. Subsequently for each voxel the probability of not being background is calculated. Afterwards, a fast threshold based region growing algorithm is used on this probability map to segment the vascular structures.

4   Results

Combining a threshold based region growing algorithm with a Bayesian background compensation, we were able to implement a robust one-click segmentation of vascular structures for clinical CT and MRT data of the liver. The background compensation is based on two successive steps: First the background intensity variations are approximated as illustrated in figure 1. Taking the induced shift of the intensities into account, the probility parameters σ, λ, and β are extracted by fitting the modelized intensity distribution to the histogram of the remaining image intensities. Figure 2 exemplifies the gain for the archivable segmentation result. The presented combination of the developed statistical data analysis with a simple threshold based region growing ensures a robust and fast vascular segmentation with results comparable to data segmentations with more sophisticated, time consuming algorithms.

Fig. 1. Left: Slice of clinical MRT-data of the liver with typical data inhomogeneties; Right: Corresponding slice of the smoothed background intensity calculated by spline approximation (MRI is courtesy of Prof. Broelsch, University Hospital Essen)

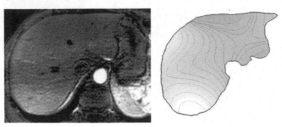

Fig. 2. Vascular structure segmented by region growing algorithm with optimized global threshold: Segmentation based on original MRT-data (left); Corresponding object segmented from probability map resulting from the bayesian data analysis (right)

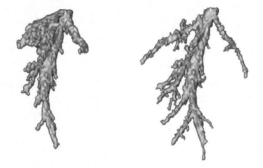

5   Discussion

The presented Bayesian background compensation has proven to handle a wide range of image perturbances in MRT and CT data and leads to a fast and reliable identification of vascular structure in clinical data. The presented background compensation is robust, fully automatic, and requires litte image specific knowledge. Hence it is attractive as a preprocessing step for further data analysis. Moreover, the statistical model provides an easy to use framework to incorporate more sophisticated image measures if needed. The incorporation of this algorithm improves the robustness and speed of the segmentation algorithms. This robust segmentation is a mandatory part of the carefully tailored workflow for the software-assisted patient individual planning of radiofrequency-ablation of liver tumors.

Bundling the presented vascular segmentation with a robust tumor segmentation [8], an interactive positioning of a virtual applicator-model and a numerical estimation of the region destroyed by the induced thermal energy, a clinical applicable software-assistant for the patient individual planning of radiofrequency-ablation is developed [9]. Extracting anatomical information about the tumor and the close by vascular structures from clinical data, the implemented software-assistant allows to approximate the effect of the radiofrequency-ablation taking the cooling effect of local vessels into account [10]. Tailored to the clinical needs, this application makes a patient individual planning of the radiofrequency-ablation available in a clinical feasible workflow. Thereby the developed software-assisted patient individual planning reduces uncertainty in the planned applicator positioning and supports the evaluation of the achievable thermal destruction. This enhances the confidence in achieving a complete thermal destruction of the tumor.

6 Acknowledgement

The research leading to this publication has been supported by the German Federal Ministry of Education and Research under grant number 01EZ0010 and 01BE03C as part of the cooperation projects VICORA and FUSION.

References

1. Arnold JB, Liow JS, Schaper KA, et al. Qualitative and quantitative evaluation of six algorithms for correcting intensity nonuniformity effects. Neuroimage 2001;13:931–943.
2. Brinkmann BH, Manduca A, Robb RA. Optimized homomorphic unsharp masking for MR grayscale inhomogeneity correction. IEEE Trans Med Imaging 1998;17:161–171.
3. Sled JG, Zijdenbos AP, Evans AC. A nonparametric method for automatic correction of intensity nonuniformity in MRI data. IEEE Trans Med Imaging 1998;17:87–97.
4. Shattuck DW, Sandor-Leahy SR, Schaper KA, et al. Magnetic resonance image tissue classification using a partial volume model. Neuroimage 2001;13:856–876.
5. Fischer R, Hanson KM, V Dose V, von Der LindenW. Background estimation in experimental spectra. Phys Rev E Stat Phys Plasmas Fluids Relat Interdiscip Topics 2000 Feb ;61 (2):1152 -60 2000;61:1152–1160.
6. Guglielmetti F, Fischer R, Dose V. Mixture modeling for background and sources separation in x-ray astronomical images. American Institut of Physics; 2004. 111–118.
7. Schumaker LL, Utreras FI. On generalized cross validation for tensor smoothing splines. SIAM J Sci Stat Comput 1990;11(4):713–731.
8. Bornemann L, Kuhnigk JM, Dicken V, et al. OncoTREAT - A software assistant for oncological therapy monitoring. Procs CARS 2005; 429–434.
9. Weihusen A, Ritter F, Pereira P, et al. Towards a workflow-oriented software assistance for the radiofrequency ablation. Lecture Notes in Informatics 2006;93:507–513.
10. Kröger T, Altrogge I, Preusser T, et al. Numerical simulation of radio frequency ablation with state dependent material parameters in three space dimensions. LNCS 2006;4191:380–388.

Computergestützte 3D-Operationsplanung zur präoperativen Repositionierung von Knochenfragmenten bei komplizierten Knochenbrüchen

Kai Bestmann[1], Jan Ehrhardt[2], Daniel Briem[3], Johannes Rüger[3], Stefan Müller[1], Heinz Handels[2]

[1]Institut für Computervisualistik, Universität Koblenz, 56070 Koblenz
[2]Institut für Medizinische Informatik
[3]Klinik für Unfall-, Hand- und Wiederherstellungschirurgie
[2,3]Universitätsklinikum Hamburg-Eppendorf, 20246 Hamburg
Email: j.ehrhardt@uke.uni-hamburg.de

Zusammenfassung. In diesem Beitrag wird das Softwaresystem PRO-FRAPS zur virtuellen Repositionierung von Knochenfragmenten bei komplexen Frakturen vorgestellt. Mittels verschiedener Visualisierungstechniken, wie z.B. Farb- und Transparenzdarstellungen, wird die räumliche Zusammensetzung der Fraktur dem Anwender verdeutlicht. Die detailierte Analyse eng beieinander liegender und verdeckter Fragmente wird dabei durch eine Explosionsdarstellung ermöglicht. Die Einzelschritte der vollständigen Repositionierung werden in einer Transformationshistorie dokumentiert und für die spätere intraoperative Umsetzung ausgegeben. Eine integrierte Kollisionserkennung gewährleistet stets gültige Fragmentpositionen. PROFRAPS wurde an zwei Trümmerfrakturen getestet. Eine quantitative Evaluation der Laufzeit ergab, dass die Kollisionserkennung auch für sehr komplexe Frakturen in Echtzeit erfolgt. Die vorgestellte Anwendung ermöglicht damit die detaillierte Planung der Fragmentrepositionierung für eine Operation, indem komplizierte Knochenbrüche präoperativ umfassend analysiert und virtuell repositioniert werden.

1 Einleitung

In zahlreichen medizinischen Anwendungen haben sich computergestützte Techniken für die Operationsplanung, –simulation und –durchführung in der chirurgischen Praxis etabliert [1, 2, 3]. Auch im Bereich der Unfallchirurgie existieren (teils kommerzielle) computergestützte Systeme, deren Einsatzgebiete jedoch häufig auf Standardeingriffe, wie z.B. einfache Schaft– oder Gelenkfrakturen, beschränkt sind [1, 4, 5, 6, 7]. Sie werden oftmals zur Unterstützung der intraoperativen Repositionierung und Fixierung unter Verwendung fluoroskopischer Bildgebung eingesetzt. Für die Planung komplizierter Knochenfrakturen, wie z.B. bei Trümmerbrüchen im Gelenkbereich, sind diese Anwendungen nur eingeschränkt einsetzbar.

Im klinischen Alltag der Unfallchirurgie werden bei Trümmerfrakturen zumeist Volumendaten mit Hilfe der Computertomographie erzeugt. Die Fraktur wird anschließend anhand der Schichtansichten des vorliegenden Volumens analysiert und die anstehende Operation geplant. Eine 3D–Visualisierung der Fraktur unterstützt einen Chirurgen bei diesen Aufgaben. Sie gibt dem Betrachter einen erweiterten Eindruck der räumlichen Zusammenhänge zwischen den einzelnen Frakturelementen. Aber auch diese Darstellungsform weist Schwächen auf. Es existieren Frakturen, bei denen Knochenteile vollständig eingeschlossen und daher nicht sichtbar sind. Zudem gibt eine statische 3D-Ansicht zusammen mit Schichtbildern oftmals unzureichenden Aufschluss über die Komplexität der Positions- und Orientierungsabweichung von der natürlichen Position und Ausrichtung wieder. Um ein umfassendes Verständnis der Fraktursituation bei komplexen Trümmerbrüchen zu ermöglichen, sind daher eine erweiterte 3D–Visualisierung und eine interaktive Manipulation der Knochenteile bezüglich Darstellung und Positionierung sinnvoll.

In der hier vorgestellten Arbeit wurde das Softwaresytem PROFRAPS zur präoperativen Planung von Gelenkfrakturen entwickelt. Mittels verschiedener Visualisierungstechniken wie z.B. der Transparenz– und Explosionsdarstellung wird die räumliche Konstellation und Beschaffenheit der Knochenfragmente verdeutlicht. Die Knochenfragmente können interaktiv repositioniert werden. Dabei werden die Repositionierungsschritte der Frakturteile vollständig dokumentiert und nach Abschluss der Planung in einer für den Arzt geeigneten Form ausgegeben. Durch die Verwendung von Kollisionserkennungsverfahren wird die Repositionierung in der virtuellen Szene erleichtert und die Gültigkeit der Fragmentpositionen sichergestellt.

2   Methoden

In einem Vorverarbeitungsschritt werden aus den CT–Datensätzen Oberflächenmodelle der einzelnen Knochenteile konstruiert. Diese werden zusammen mit den CT–Daten in die Anwendung (Abb. 1) eingeladen. Mittels verschiedener Visualisierungstechniken, wie z.B. Farb– und Transparenzdarstellungen, wird die räumliche Zusammensetzung der Fraktur dem Anwender verdeutlicht. Zusätzlich ermöglicht eine Explosionsdarstellung der gesamten Knochenfraktur die Übersicht über die vorhandenen Frakturelemente und lässt zudem die Analyse eng beieinander liegender und verdeckter Fragmente zu (Abb. 2). Es besteht die Option, die orthogonalen Schichtansichten mit den Konturen der Knochenteile aus der veränderbaren 3D-Szene zu überlagern, wodurch eine Beziehung zwischen der für den Arzt gewohnten 2D– und der 3D–Darstellung hergestellt wird.

Die Repositionierung der Frakturteile erfolgt durch rigide Transformationen, wobei Rotationen um frei definierbare Punkte oder Achsen erlaubt werden. Rotationspunkte oder –achsen werden entweder in der 3D-Ansicht auf den Objektoberflächen oder in einer der orthogonalen Schichtansichten definiert. Die durchgeführten Transformationen einzelner oder gruppierter Objekte werden in

Abb. 1. Benutzeroberfläche von PROFRAPS: Links oben ist die 3D–Darstellung der gesamten Fraktur zu finden. Darunter befinden sich die drei verschiedenen Schichtenansichten, wobei die Konturen der Knochenfragmente jeweils überlagert dargestellt sind

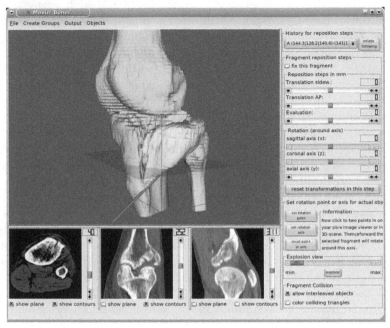

einer Transformationshistorie hinterlegt. Dies ermöglicht die Bewegungsabläufe der Repositionierung nachträglich zu betrachten.

Wahlweise kann während der Transformation von Knochenfragmenten eine Kollisionserkennung zwischen den einzelnen Objekten durchgeführt werden. Dazu wurde die Softwarebibliothek V-Collide [8] mit VTK verknüpft. V-Collide wurde nach dem Vergleich mit anderen Kollisionsbibliotheken ausgewählt, da es mit triangulierten, beliebig komplexen *polygon–soups* umgehen kann und zugleich eine ausreichend schnelle Verarbeitung bietet. Die Kollisionserkennung gewährleistet eine gültige Fragmentposition während der Korrektur. Alternativ ist die Möglichkeit gegeben, Überschneidungen und Berührungspunkte von Fragmenten farblich hervorzuheben (Abb. 3).

Der Repositionierungsprozess einer Fraktur kann im XML–Format dokumentiert und gespeichert werden. Dabei werden alle Teiltransformationen und Darstellungseigenschaften der Knochenfragmente gesichert. Die Modell– und Volumendaten bleiben unverändert. Es besteht zudem die Möglichkeit pro Fragment die Teiltransformationen oder eine einzige durch Faktorisierung ermittelte Gesamttransformation der Repositionierung im HTML–Format auszugeben. In diese druckbare Ausgabe können beliebig viele, interaktiv wählbare 3D–Szenendarstellungen eingefügt werden. Ein Ausdruck dieses Reports kann während der Operation als Hilfestellung genutzt werden, ohne dass zusätzliche

Gerätschaften im Operationssaal notwendig sind. Er dient der Betrachtung der einzelnen Repositionierungsschritte und dem Verstehen der räumlichen Zusammenhänge.

3 Ergebnisse

PROFRAPS wurde anhand zweier Trümmerfrakturen getestet. Eine Fraktur des Knies bestand dabei aus fünf Fragmenten. Bei der zweiten Fraktur handelte es sich um eine Fraktur der Hüfte, bestehend aus acht Fragmenten. Die Anzahl der Dreiecke, aus denen die verwendeten 3D-Objekte bestanden, lag zwischen 6384 und 225516. Bei den Tests wurden verschieden große und komplexe Knochenmodelle willkürlich durch die Szene bewegt. Der Repositionierungsprozess der Knochenfragmente konnte auch bei aktiver Kollisionserkennung in Echtzeit erfolgen. Hierbei wurden Berechnungsszeiten von weniger als 0.001 Sekunden benötigt, wodurch eine Anbindung von haptischen Ein- und Ausgabegeräten möglich wird. Die optionale farbliche Markierung kollidierender Objektdreiecke bei Transformationen verursachte jedoch eine Frequenz von weit weniger als 25 Hz, da alle von der Kollision betroffenen Modelldreiecke ermittelt und neu dargestellt werden müssen.

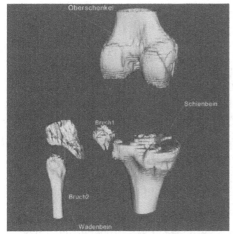

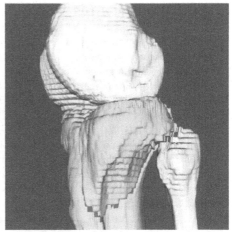

Abb. 2. Das Bild illustriert die Explosionsdarstellung einer Kniefraktur, in der die Fragmente auseinandergezogen und beschriftet werden. Zudem sind die Bewegungspfade der Fragmente, ausgehend von Szenenmittelpunkt, eingezeichnet.

Abb. 3. Das linke Bild zeigt eine Szene, bei der kollidierende Dreiecke am Tibiaschaft mit der Farbe rot hervorgehoben werden.

4   Diskussion

PROFRAPS ermöglicht die Planung der einzelnen Schritte der Fragmentrepositionierung für eine Operation, indem komplizierte Knochenbrüche präoperativ analysiert und virtuell korrigiert werden. Dazu werden die Fragmente unterschiedlich dargestellt. Die Explosionsdarstellung findet bei den Medizinern großen Zuspruch, um eine Übersicht über die vorhandenen Fragmente zu gewinnen. Die Kollisionserkennung arbeitet in Echtzeit und erleichtert die Ermittlung von reproduzierbaren und gültigen Planungsergebnissen.

Der Zeitaufwand für die Segmentierung der Frakturelemente und die 3D-Modellerstellung ist derzeit noch zu hoch, um die Anwendung im medizinischen Alltag anwenden zu können. Deshalb ist für diesen Prozess eine Optimierung geplant. Zudem gilt es die Qualität der 3D–Modelle zu verbessern, ohne dabei notwendige Informationen zu verlieren. Für die Lehre von Studierenden der Medizin außerhalb des Klinikalltags ist eine Nutzung bereits jetzt schon möglich.

In zukünftigen Arbeiten soll PROFRAPS um weitere Komponenten erweitert werden: die Anbindung haptischer Ein- und Ausgabegeräte [9], Verfahren zur automatischen Repositionierung und die Integration von Fixationsobjekten sowie Methoden, um den Interaktionsaufwand bei der Segmentierung der Fraktursegmente zu reduzieren.

Literaturverzeichnis

1. Schep NWL, Broeders IAMJ, van der Werken C. Computer assisted orthopaedic and trauma surgery: State of the art and future perspectives. Injury 2003;34(4):299–306.
2. Börner M, Lahmer A, Bauer A, Stier U. Experiences with the ROBODOC system in more than 1000 cases. Procs CARS 1998; 689–693.
3. Viceconti M, Lattanzi R, Antonietti B, et al. CT-based surgical planning software improves the accuracy of THR preoperative planning. Med Eng Phys 2003;25(5):371–377.
4. Gosling T, Westphal R, Hufner T, et al. Robot-assisted fracture reduction: A preliminary study in the femur shaft. Med Biol Eng Comput 2005;43(1):115–120.
5. Marschollek M, Teistler M, Bott OJ, et al. Pre-operative dynamic interactive exploration of complex articular fractures using a novel 3D navigation tool. Methods Inf Med 2006;45(4):384–388.
6. Joskowicz L, Milgrom C, Simkin A, et al. FRACAS: A system for computer-aided image-guided long bone fracture surgery. Comput Aided Surg 1998;3(6):271–288.
7. BrainLab AG. Kapellenstr. 12, Feldkirchen, Germany. VectorVision - Trauma; 2006.
8. Hudson TC, Lin MC, Cohen J, et al. V-COLLIDE: accelerated collision detection for VRML. In: Procs VRML. New York: ACM Press; 1997. 117–121.
9. Färber M, Drescher F, Ehrhardt J, et al. Integration von haptischen Ein-/Ausgabegeräten zur intuitiven Interaktion mit virtuellen Körpern in OP-Planungssysteme. In: Procs GMDS. Leipzig; 2006. 71–72.

MITK als telekonferenzfähiges PlugIn in der CHILI-Workstation

Michael Hasselberg, Ivo Wolf, Marco Nolden, Mathias Seitel, H.P. Meinzer,
Uwe Engelmann

Abteilung für Medizinische und Biologische Informatik,
Deutsches Krebsforschungszentrum, 69120 Heidelberg
Email: mbi@dkfz-heidelberg.de

Zusammenfassung. Die Arbeit beschreibt eine Lösung zur Realisierung von telekonferenz-fähigen Zusatzmodulen (PlugIns) mit dem Toolkit MITK innerhalb der CHILI-Workstation (CHILI GmbH, Heidelberg). Das CHILI-System bietet die Möglichkeit der Erweiterung durch PlugIns und stellt ein API für Telekonferenzen zur Verfügung. Um ein Zusatzmodul telekonferenz-fähig zu machen, mussten bisher eine Vielzahl spezifischer Anpassungen vorgenommen werden. Die hier vorgestellte Lösung kapselt die meisten der erforderlichen Anpassungen innerhalb des Toolkits MITK, sodass der Entwickler nur wenige zusätzliche Regeln bei der Erstellung eines telekonferenzfähigen PlugIns beachten muss.

1 Einleitung

Digitale Diagnose-, Labor- und Bilddaten von Patienten sind grundlegende Entscheidungsfaktoren von Ärzten. Die Aufbereitung der digitalen Informationen übernehmen zunehmend spezielle, auf klinische Anforderungen zugeschnittene Softwarelösungen. Im modernen Klinikalltag werden digitalen Bilddaten durch ein Picture Archiving and Communication System (PACS) verteilt, befundet und archiviert. Die Workstation des CHILI-PACS (CHILI GmbH, Heidelberg) besitzt die Eigenschaft der Erweiterbarkeit durch PlugIns und bietet darüber hinaus Telekonferenzfunktionen, die auch von PlugIns genutzt werden können [1, 2]. Sowohl von CHILI selbst, als auch von anderen Entwicklern werden CHILI-PlugIns realisiert, die sich nahtlos in die Umgebung der Workstation einbetten und Spezialfunktionen z.B. für Volumenvisualisierung [3] oder die virtuelle Chirurgie bereitstellen [4].

Am Deutschen Krebsforschungszentrum (DKFZ) in Heidelberg wird das Medical Imaging Interaction Toolkit (MITK) entwickelt, das als Plattform für die Erstellung von fortgeschrittenen Bildverarbeitungsanwendungen dient [5]. Auch MITK-Anwendungen laufen als PlugIn in der CHILI-Umgebung. Abbildung 1 zeigt ein Beispiel für eine MITK-Anwendung innerhalb der CHILI-Workstation.

Ziel dieser Arbeit war es, die Telekonferenzfähigkeit der CHILI-Workstation auch für MITK-PlugIns so nutzbar zu machen, dass zukünftige MITK-Entwickler diese Funktionalität mit möglichst geringem Zusatzaufwand nutzen können.

Abb. 1. MITK als PlugIn in CHILI. Im Folgenden werden die Basiselemente von CHI-LI (A-C) und MITK (1-3) benannt: Datenbankschnittstelle (A), digitaler Lichtkasten (B), CHILI-Kontrollbereich (C), Kontrollbereich der Menübar (1), dreidimensionaler Arbeitsbereich (2), Kontrollbereich der PlugIn-Funktionalitäten (3)

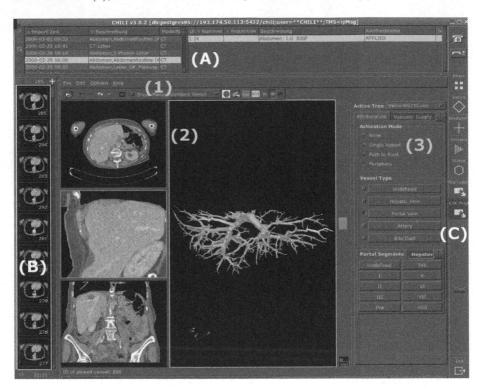

2   Stand der Forschung und Fortschritt durch den Beitrag

Telekonferenzsysteme können in drei verschiedene grundsätzliche Systemfamilien unterteilt werden:

1. Videokonferenzsysteme (Übertragung von Bild und Ton und ggf. mit einem „Whiteboard" für gemeinsame Notizen),
2. Application-Sharing-Systeme (gemeinsames Arbeiten an einem System, dessen Ein- und Ausgaben auf mehrere, räumlich entfernte Displays verteilt werden) und
3. Systeme für das computerunterstützte kooperative Arbeiten (computer supported cooperative work, CSCW).

Die letztgenannten Systeme sind sich ihrer Konferenzfunktionalität bewusst und explizit für das kooperative Arbeiten konzipiert. Dieser Ansatz ist der aufwändigste von den drei genannten, aber für die Bearbeitung großer Datensätze, wie das in der medizinischen Bildverarbeitung in der Regel der Fall ist, besser geeignet, als die anderen o.g. Systeme. Der wesentliche Vorteil ist, dass bei Interaktionen nicht gesamte Bildschirminhalte zu den anderen Konferenzteilnehmern übertragen werden müssen, sondern nur Synchronisationsbefehle ausgetauscht werden und sich die Systeme auf diese Weise gegenseitig „fernsteuern". Benutzerinteraktionen in der graphischen Benutzungsschnittstelle (Events) eines Systems werden an die anderen Konferenzpartner übertragen und dort synchron ausgeführt, als wären die Eingaben dort lokal ausgeführt worden.

In MITK werden die Bilddaten durch Interaktion mit dem Kontroll- und Arbeitsbereich aufbereitet. Somit ist jede Aktion im Kontrollbereich und Arbeitsbereich ein wichtiger neuer Ausgangspunkt für den folgenden Schritt. Das Versenden von Bildvolumen nach jedem Verarbeitungsschritt ist wegen des hohen Datenaufkommens inakzeptabel. Diese Arbeit wurde deshalb auf den Austausch von Ereignissen, die zur Änderung führen, also den CSCW-Konzepten folgend aufgebaut. Die Ereignisse lösen bei den Konferenzpartnern dieselben Operationen aus und führen so zu identischen Resultaten. Mit diesem Ansatz setzt man voraus, dass nicht jeder Teilnehmer willkürlich Aktionen auf den Arbeits- oder Kontrollbereich ausführen darf. Alle Aktionen müssen vollständig und abgeschlossen sein. Das bedeutet z.B., dass beim Zeichnen eines Polygons kein anderer Teilnehmer das Datenobjekt bearbeiten oder verschieben darf, bis die Transaktion abgeschlossen ist. Im MITK gibt es ein Interaktionskonzept, das gemäß der Automatentheorie nach Mealy umgesetzt wurde [6]. Es ermöglicht nicht nur die sichere Überführung eines Zustandes in einen neuen, sondern auch die Möglichkeit sie später rückgängig zu machen (Undo).

3 Methoden

Die Telekonferenz baut auf der ipMsg-Bibliothek der CHILI-Workstation auf. Die Bibliothek stellt grundlegende Kommunikationsbausteine zur Verfügung [1]. MITK nutzt Methoden der ipMsg-Bibliothek, um CHILI-Partnerapplikationen untereinander zu synchronisieren.

Der Ereignismechanismus von MITK verarbeitet Positionen in 3D Weltkoordinaten. Das Graphical User Interface (GUI) von Qt in Version 3 kann darüber hinaus alle Ereignisse für den Kontrollbereich wie z.B. Dialogfelder und Buttonklicks, die für die Werkzeug- und Filterauswahl wichtig sind, identifizieren und versenden. Die Verwendung von Qt-Koordinaten ist nicht ausreichend, weil bei den Konferenzteilnehmern unterschiedliche Bildschirmauflösungen zu unterschiedlichen Darstellungen führen würden. Für eine stabile Telekonferenz müssen Ereignisse aus Qt und MITK berücksichtigt werden.

Um eine Konferenz durchzuführen, muss gewährleistet sein, dass Teilnehmer Aktionen wie das Zeichnen eines Polygons störungsfrei zum Abschluss bringen können. Dazu wurde ein Token eingeführt, welches in einer Konferenz mit beliebig vielen Teilnehmern genau einmal vorkommt. Für alle Interaktionen mit dem MITK-PlugIn muss das Token vorliegen, gegebenenfalls wird es automatisch beantragt.

Die Anzeige des Mauszeigers ist in einer Telekonferenz ein nützliches Instrument, bspw. zum Hinweis auf anatomische Besonderheiten. Bewegungen des Mauszeigers werden auch ohne vorliegendes Token angezeigt. Da das Layout bei verschiedenen Bildschirmauflösungen variieren kann, ist eine korrekte Darstellung des Mauszeigers im Bereich der Qt-GUI-Elemente i.A. nicht möglich. Im Arbeitsbereich dank der Weltkoordinaten kann jedoch die 2D-Position des Mauszeigers exakt rekonstruiert werden. Um nicht die gesamte Szene neu rendern zu müssen, wird der OpenGL-Buffer nach dem Rendern der Szene zwischengespeichert und mit einem Mauszeiger an der jeweils aktuellen Position überlagert dargestellt.

4   Ergebnisse

In der vorliegenden Arbeit wurde MITK als PlugIn für die CHILI-Workstation durch die vorgenommenen Erweiterungen in der Ereignisbehandlung telekonferenzfähig gemacht. Experten verschiedenster Disziplinen können z.b. miteinander eine computergestützte Operationsplanung beraten. Für den Anwender ist nur wenig Lernaufwand notwendig, um in einer Telekonferenz zu arbeiten. Der MITK-Softwareentwickler hat in der Regel nur den zusätzlichen Aufwand die Kontrollelemente eindeutig zu benennen. Zudem muss darauf geachtet werden, dass keine Displaykoordinaten sondern ausschließlich 3D-Weltkoordinaten verwendet werden.

4.1   Laufzeitverhalten

Das Laufzeitverhalten im gewählten Ansatz ist nicht abhängig von den Datengrößen der Bildobjekte und der Darstellungsqualität. Eine Verzögerung im Reaktionsverhalten der Anwendung ist durch die reine Ereignisbehandlung kaum wahrnehmbar.

Das implementierte Token-Prinzip setzt geringe Latenzzeiten im Netzwerk voraus. Hohe Latenzzeiten würden zu einem verzögerten Arbeiten führen.

4.2   Arbeits- und Kontrollbereich

Die Fenster des Arbeitsbereiches müssen hier für 2D und 3D getrennt betrachtet werden. Im Standardfall visualisieren drei Fenster das Bildobjekt in 2D, typischerweise werden die orthogonalen Schnitte dargestellt. Das vierte Fenster stellt die Szene dreidimensional dar, während die Darstellung des Bildobjekts in 2D während einer Telekonferenz immer synchronisiert ist, konnten in MITK in 3D bis jetzt nicht bei allen Interaktionen in einen synchronisierten Zustand gebracht werden. Der Ereignismechanismus in 3D wird an dieser Stelle derzeit noch nicht immer mit dem Mechanismus von MITK gesteuert, sondern direkt durch das Visualization Toolkit (VTK). Das Resultat kann in diesem Fall eine veränderte Lage des Bildobjekts sein.

Die Darstellung des Mauszeigers wurde für die 2D-Ansichten durch die Nutzung des OpenGL-Speichers leistungsoptimiert umgesetzt. Die Position des Zeigers wird exakt auf dem Bildobjekt gezeichnet. Im 3D-Arbeitsbereich konnte die Ansicht des Mauszeigers bisher noch nicht zufriedenstellend umgesetzt werden.

Der Kontrollbereich konnte für die meisten Anwendungen telekonferenzfähig gemacht werden.

5 Diskussion

Die Telekonferenz für MITK ist ein neuer Schritt, um MITK-Funktionalitäten besser in den radiologischen Arbeitsplatz zu integrieren. Die Qualität der Telekonferenz kann auf Grundlage dieser Arbeit als stabil bezeichnet werden. Verschiedenste Erweiterungen für die MITK-Applikation sind ohne Anpassungen telekonferenzfähig. Eine Schwachstelle ist die Ereignisbehandlung für den Kontrollbereich über Qt, weil bei den Konferenzteilnehmern nicht alle Objekte eindeutig zugeordnet werden können. Dieses Problem wird mit dem Upgrade auf die Version 4 von Qt behoben und schrittweise umgesetzt.

Auf der Grundlage dieser Arbeit können räumlich entfernte Experten komplexe Fragestellungen gemeinsam in interaktiven Telekonferenzen bearbeiten, was Diagnose und Therapie qualitativ verbessert und vor allem zeitlich beschleunigt.

Literaturverzeichnis

1. Engelmann U, Schröter A, Baur U, Schwab M, et al. Openness in (tele-) radiology workstations: The CHILI plugin concept. Procs CARS 1998;(2-3):437–442.
2. Engelmann U, Schröter A, Münch H, Meinzer HP. Die plattformunabhängige Befundungs-Workstation CHILI/Qt mit PlugIns für die Segmentierung und Visualisierung von 3- und 4-dimensionalen Datensiätzen. Fortsch Röntenstr 2004;176:274.
3. Evers H, Mayer A, Engelmann U, Schröter A, et al. Extending a teleradiology system by tools for visualization and volumetric analysis through a plug-in mechanism. Int J Med Inform 1999;53(2-3):265–275.
4. Glombitza G, Evers H, Hassfeld S, Engelmann U, Meinzer HP. Virtual surgery in a (tele-) radiology framework. IEEE Trans ITB 1999;(3):186–196.
5. Wolf I, Vetter M, Wegner I, Bottger T, et al. The Medical Imaging Interaction Toolkit. Medical Image Analysis 2005;9:594–604.
6. Wegner I, Vetter M, Wolf I, Meinzer HP. Ein generisches Interaktionskonzept mit Undo für die medizinische Bildverarbeitung. Procs BVM 2004; 150–154.

Subject-Based Regional Anaesthesia Simulator Combining Image Processing and Virtual Reality

Sebastian Ullrich[1], Benedikt Fischer[2], Alexandre Ntouba[3], Jakob T. Valvoda[1], Andreas Prescher[4], Torsten Kuhlen[1], Thomas M. Deserno[2], Rolf Rossaint[3]

[1]Virtual Reality Group, RWTH Aachen University
[2]Institute of Medical Informatics, University Hospital Aachen
[3]Clinic of Anaesthesia, University Hospital Aachen
[4]Institute for Neuroanatomy, University Hospital Aachen
Email: s.ullrich@rz.rwth-aachen.de

Abstract. In this paper, a novel virtual reality-based simulator for regional anaesthesia is presented. Individual datasets of patients with nerve cords are created from medical scans with the help of advanced segmentation and registration algorithms. Techniques for interaction and immersive visualization are utilized by the simulator to improve training of medical residents.

1 Introduction

Regional anaesthesia encompasses several techniques for blocking the nerve supply to specific parts of the human body. Common techniques for upper and lower extremities are the axillary brachial plexus block and the femoral nerve block, respectively. After positioning the patient, the needle insertion site is determined with the help of surface and anatomic landmarks. An electric nerve stimulator is connected to the needle used for the procedure in order to locate nerve cords with muscular response (e.g., twitches in the hand or knee). After successful localization, local anesthetic is injected to block the desired nerve.

One essential requirement for simulation is a precise, anatomic plausible model of the nerve cords. In addition, representations of bones, blood vessels, musculature and skin tissue are needed to frame the peripheral nerve system. Current technology of medical image acquisition does not capture nerve tissue sufficiently. Therefore, advanced segmentation algorithms must be researched. The simulation itself should allow to train all steps of a typical procedure as described above. Currently, there is no extendable, software-based simulator for regional anaesthesia. Even though specialized haptics solutions are used by the applications described in the following section, clinical acceptance is very low. Reasons are restrictions to single datasets, rigid virtual patients that can not be repositioned, no proper training of needle insertion site localization and lack of simulators with support for peripheral block. On this account, training is still done on living patients. However, because errors in anaesthesiology can be lethal, there is an urgent necessity to find alternatives for training in medical education.

Fig. 1. Overview of the system

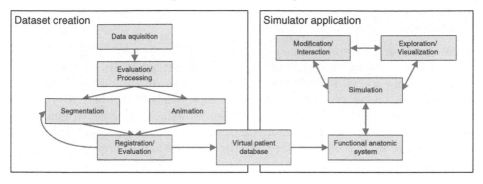

2   State of the Art and Motivation

The related work comprises segmentation and registration for dataset creation and simulation approaches.

The creation of appropriate datasets requires segmentation and registration of volumetric data from medical diagnostic imaging. Segmentation approaches for volumetric data can be divided into voxel-, surface-, and region-based as well as hybrid variants [1]. Standard registration approaches include point-to-point correspondence [2], extensions of the iterative closest point method for elastic registration [3], thin plate splines [4], boundary mapping [5], computational fluid dynamics [6], as well as daemon-based registration [7], which have been used already for mappings between an atlas and patient data [8].

A comprehensive overview of medical simulators is given in [9]. We have focused our research on topics related to regional anaesthesia. There are many needle simulators for different areas of applications, e.g., acupuncture [10], lumbar puncture [11, 12] and intravenous procedures [13]. Even though there are examples for epidural blocking procedures [14, 15], these approaches are based on static datasets (i.e., due to a rigid vertebral column the virtual patient can not bend forward) and are not adaptable to peripheral blocks of limbs.

3   Methods

The entire data flow is visualized in Figure 1. The two major parts, dataset creation and simulator application are linked via a virtual patient database.

3.1   Dataset Creation and Processing

Data acquisition and processing. The primary goal of data acquisition is to collect suitable/feasible data for segmentation of peripheral nerve cords. Therefore, initial efforts are focused on experimenting with parameters and time constants involved in relaxation processes of the tissue nuclei to improve contrast of magnet resonance imaging (MRI). In order to create a representative database, medical imaging is being conducted on different constitutional types.

Segmentation. A hybrid segmentation approach is applied. While structures such as skin, bones and musculature are clearly separated in the MRI scans, the nerve cords are not visualized with sufficient contrast to support an automatic segmentation. Therefore, a knowledge-based approach is used, where the relative position of the nerve cords and the arteries is defined in order to guide the segmentation process. In particular, the structural prototypes that have been defined in [16] are extended to the three-dimensional data source.

Registration. The registration has to match atlas-based information to the contents of the patient-specific images. At the current state, a daemon-based approach is favored, which has been successfully applied for similar purposes [8].

Animation. Typical muscular responses of the limbs induced by electric nerve stimulation are captured with optical tracking of markers attached to sections of the extremities. Additionally, the movement of single digits is captured with a data glove. The raw data of both approaches is used to compute the joint movements and store it as an animation sequence. With retargeting approaches, the data can be applied to all constitutional types and must be recorded only once.

3.2   Simulator Application

The simulator application is being developed for virtual environments and consists of several modules (Fig. 1). The work is based on an extensible architecture that combines data, simulation, visualization and interaction [17].

Functional anatomy system. Data separation is a fundamental aspect of the proposed architecture. We conceived a structured approach that resembles the human organism as defined by the systematic and functional anatomy. To share common data and to create interlinks between algorithms, abstract control entities are designed that emulate the basic setup of physiological systems. The model-view-controller pattern is utilized to establish a separation of algorithms and data.

Simulation. The simulation algorithms operate on the data provided by the functional anatomy system. An interactively induced change of the pose of a virtual patient (for a procedure) is resolved by kinematic solutions and moves anatomical structures that are attached to each other accordingly. For nerve impulse transmission, a tree structure of nerve cords is implemented. This network is also used for visualization, collision detection and animation. Finite element-based deformation algorithms are being adapted for needle penetration.

Fig. 2. MRI slice with N. femoralis (a), prototype of the simulator on a Desktop-VR system (b) and interactive changes in posture of a virtual patient (c)

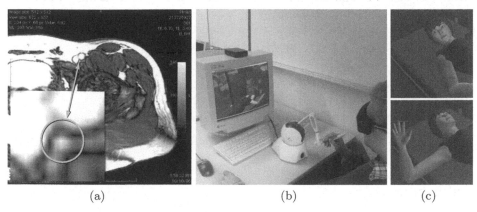

(a)   (b)   (c)

Visualization. Visualization is needed to enable an explorative analysis and to interactively render realistic geometric representations of the virtual patient and the instruments. We use vertex blending techniques to render the deformable skin surface. For evaluation purposes, the skin can be turned transparent to reveal anatomic visualizations of virtual bones, musculature, vessels and nerves.

Interaction. Besides anatomic realism, one of the most important requirements is an intuitive interaction interface. Therefore, the interaction algorithms support different input devices and allow to record a session during training for later evaluation. Customized haptic input devices are used for palpation to localize the needle insertion site realistically and are also used for needle operation.

4 Results

Several series of medical imaging scans have been evaluated. In comparison, MRI scans have yielded the best results (Fig. 2a), which can be explained by the anatomical soft tissue properties of nerve filaments. Segmentation algorithms are being adapted.

The architecture for the simulation of a virtual patient has been implemented. Virtual musculature and nerve cords are already simulated and can also be visualized. The application can be used in various virtual environments, varying from Desktop-VR to large projection environments (Fig. 2b). Several algorithms for interaction techniques are being adapted (Fig. 2c).

5 Discussion and Conclusion

Datasets containing nerve cords are created with the help of hybrid segmentation algorithms that are in addition knowledge-based guided. The system renders an anatomical patient specific model in virtual environments that can be explored, intuitively controlled and manipulated. Additionally, evaluations are conducted by medical experts on a regular base to insure authentic data sets and plausible simulation. The final goal is to use the developed software as a new educational device for training of regional anaesthesia procedures.

Acknowledgments

This work was funded by the START-Programm (UK Aachen) and also supported by a grant from the German Research Foundation (DFG, KU 1132, LE 1108, RO 2000).

References

1. Lehmann TM, Hiltner J, Handels H. Handbuch der Medizinischen Informatik. 2nd ed. Carl Hanser Verlag; 2005. 361–424.
2. Moshfeghi M. Elastic matching of multimodality medical images. CVGIP: Graphical Models and Image Processing 1991; 271–282.
3. Rangarajan A, Chui H, Mjolsness E, et al. A robust point matching algorithm for autoradiograph alignment. Medical Image Analysis 1997;4(1):379–398.
4. Barret HH, Gmitro AF, editors. Information Processing in Medical Imaging. Springer; 1991. 326–342.
5. Davatzikos CA, Prince JL, Bryan RN. Image registration based on boundary mapping. IEEE Trans Med Imaging 1996;15(1):112–115.
6. Christensen GE. Deformable shape models for anatomy. Ph.D. thesis. Sever Institute of Technology, Washington University, St. Louis, MO, USA; 1994.
7. Thirion JP. Image matching as a diffusion process: An analogy with Maxwell's demons. Medical Image Analysis 1998;2(3):243–260.
8. Handels H, Horsch A, Lehmann TM, Meinzer HP. Bildverarbeitung für die Medizin. Springer; 2001.
9. Liu A, Tendick F, Cleary K, Kaufmann C. A survey of surgical simulation: Applications, technology, and education. Presence 2003;12(6):599–614.
10. Leung KM, Heng PA, Sun H, Wong TT. A haptic needle manipulation simulator for chinese acupuncture. In: Procs MMVR; 2003. 187–189.
11. Gorman P, Krummel T, Webster R, Smith M, Hutchens D. A prototype haptic lumbar puncture simulator. In: Procs MMVR; 2000. 106–109.
12. Färber M, Heller J, Handels H. Virtual reality simulator for the training of lumbar punctures. In: Procs CURAC; 2006. 126–127.
13. Rawn CL, Reznek MA, et al. Validation of an IV insertion simulator: Establishing a standard simulator evaluation protocol. In: Procs MMVR; 2002.
14. Blezek DJ, Robb RA, Martin DP. Virtual reality simulation of regional anaesthesia for training of residents. In: HICSS; 2000. 5022–5029.
15. Glassenberg R. Virtual epidural. In: Procs IMMS; 2004.
16. Fischer B, Winkler B, Thies C, Güld MO, Lehmann TM. Strukturprototypen zur Modellierung medizinischer Bildinhalte. Procs BVM 2006; 71–75.
17. Valvoda JT, Kuhlen T, Bischof CH. Interactive virtual humanoids for virtual environments. In: Eurographics Symposium on Virtual Environments; 2006. 9–12.

Visualisierung von Gefäßsystemen mit MPU Implicits

Christian Schumann[1,2], Steffen Oeltze[1], Ragnar Bade[1], Bernhard Preim[1]

[1]Institut für Simulation und Graphik, Uni Magdeburg, 39106 Magdeburg
[2]MeVis Research - Center for Medical Image Computing, Uni Bremen, 28359 Bremen
Email: schumann@mevis.de

Zusammenfassung. Wir präsentieren eine Methode zur Visualisierung von Gefäßstrukturen basierend auf dem Segmentierungsergebnis aus kontrastmittelverstärkten Bilddaten. Im Gegensatz zu modellbasierten Verfahren wird die Morphologie der darzustellenden Gefäße exakt wiedergegeben. Dies ermöglicht neben einer Anwendung in der Therapieplanung und der medizinischen Ausbildung auch einen Einsatz in der Gefäßdiagnostik. Basierend auf dem Segmentierungsergebnis wird zunächst eine Punktwolke generiert. Diese wird mit Hilfe von Multi-level Partition of Unity Implicits (MPU Implicits) in eine Oberfläche überführt und automatisch parametriert. Somit kann effizient eine glatte, artefaktfreie Oberfläche erzeugt werden.

1 Einleitung

Eine qualitativ hochwertige Darstellung von Gefäßstrukturen ist von hohem Interesse für Diagnostik und Therapieplanung. Während bei der Therapieplanung vor allem die Topologie eines Gefäßbaumes im Vordergrund steht, erfordert die Diagnostik eine genaue Wiedergabe der Gefäßmorphologie, um auch pathologische Veränderungen korrekt repräsentieren zu können. Für beide Anwendungsgebiete ist die Erzeugung einer glatten Gefäßoberfläche ohne störende treppenartige Artefakte wünschenswert. Eine weitere Anforderung stellt die korrekte Rekonstruktion von Verzweigungen und dünnen Strukturen dar. In dieser Arbeit werden implizite Oberflächen genutzt, um einen Kompromiss zwischen der geforderten Genauigkeit und der gewünschten qualitativ hochwertigen Darstellung zu erzielen, wobei keine Modellannahmen zugrunde gelegt werden.

Methoden zur Gefäßvisualisierung lassen sich in modellbasierte und modellfreie Verfahren unterteilen. Modellbasierte Verfahren rekonstruieren die Gefäßoberfläche auf Grundlage des Gefäßskeletts sowie assoziierter Querschnittsinformationen. Zumeist wird hierbei die vereinfachende Annahme von kreisrunden Gefäßquerschnitten zu Grunde gelegt, welche für nicht-pathologische Gefäße oft zutrifft. Implizite Oberflächen wurden bereits eingesetzt, um auf Basis eines solchen Modells eine qualitativ hochwertige Rekonstruktion zu erzeugen [1]. Während modellbasierte Verfahren die Topologie des Gefäßbaumes veranschaulichen und somit für die Therapieplanung geeignet sind, ist eine Gefäßdiagnose durch die Annahme kreisrunder Gefäßquerschnitte nicht möglich. Modellfreie

Verfahren stellen daher die Gefäße entweder direkt dar (z.B. Maximum Intensity Projection) oder rekonstruieren die Gefäßoberfläche basierend auf dem Segmentierungsergebnis aus kontrastmittelverstärkten Bilddaten. Beispielhaft hierfür ist der Marching-Cubes-Algorithmus. Die so erzeugten Oberflächen leiden jedoch unter starken treppenartigen Artefakten. Die Nutzung eines Low-Pass-Filters [2] sowie ähnlicher Glättungsverfahren reduziert diese zwar, führt jedoch besonders bei dünnen Gefäßen zu einem starken Volumenverlust [3]. Constrained Elastic Surface Nets [4] beschränken diesen Verlust durch eine Restriktion der Variabilität des Netzes; können das Schrumpfen besonders dünner Gefäße jedoch nicht verhindern [5]. In [6] werden MPU Implicits [7] genutzt, um aus einer auf den Bilddaten basierenden Punktwolke anatomische Strukturen zu rekonstruieren. Das Verfahren scheitert an dünnen verzweigten Strukturen, da diese durch zu wenig Punkte beschrieben werden.

2   Methoden

MPU Implicits approximieren eine über Punkte und assoziierte Normalenvektoren definierte Punktwolke durch eine implizite Oberfläche. Durch den Parameter ϵ_0 kann hierbei bestimmt werden, wie genau die Oberfläche die Punkte annähert. Die Punktwolke wird auf Basis eines Octree's unterteilt. Die Punkte innerhalb einer Zelle werden lokal durch eine quadratische Funktion approximiert. Ist die Abweichung dieser Fläche von den Punkten in der Zelle größer als ϵ_0, so wird die Zelle rekursiv weiter unterteilt, bis für jede Blattzelle des Octree's eine genügend genaue lokale Approximation ermittelt wurde. Anschließend werden die lokalen Approximationen durch Wichtungsfunktionen zu einer globalen Approximation zusammengefasst. Eine polygonale Repräsentation der Oberfläche wird mit Hilfe von Bloomenthal's Implicit Polygonizer generiert [8]. Bei Nutzung eines hohen Wertes für ϵ_0 kann das Verfahren eine treppenartige Anordnung der Punkte der Punktwolke ausgleichen. Um eine hohe Genauigkeit garantieren zu können, ist jedoch ein geringes ϵ_0 nötig. Es gilt also, eine treppenartige Anordnung der Punkte zu vermeiden. MPU Implicits können Daten mit variierender Dichte verarbeiten. Das Verfahren erzeugt jedoch kugelförmige Artefakte, wenn Details durch zu wenig Punkte beschrieben werden. Die Dichte der Punktwolke muss also hoch genug sein, um auch dünne Zweige adäquat darstellen zu können.

2.1   Punktwolkengenerierung

In [6] werden die Punkte der Punktwolke im Zentrum der Randvoxel des Segmentierungsergebnisses platziert. Ein Zweig, der nur ein Voxel stark ist, würde so nur durch eine Linie statt eine Oberfläche repräsentiert werden. Statt dessen schlagen wir eine fallbasierte Platzierung der Punkte innerhalb des Volumens der äußeren Randvoxel vor. Dies sind jene Hintergrundvoxel, die zu Objektvoxeln benachbart sind. Es wird je nach Anordnung von Objektvoxeln in der Nachbarschaft eines äußeren Randvoxels entschieden, ob ein Punkt im Zentrum des Voxels oder auf einer der Grenzflächen erzeugt wird (siehe Abb. 1, links).

Abb. 1. Fallbasierte Platzierung der Punkte (links). Überabtastung an dünnen Strukturen (Mitte). Verringerung treppenartiger Artefakte durch Hinzufügen weiterer Subvoxel (rechts)

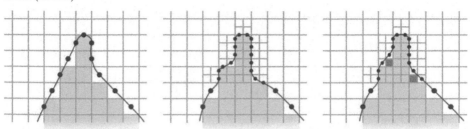

Auf diese Weise wird eine treppenartige Anordnung der Punkte verhindert. Die Platzierung der Punkte auf Basis des Voxelgitters führt jedoch dazu, dass dünne Strukturen durch zu wenig Punkte beschrieben werden. Daher führen wir eine Überabtastung des Voxelgitters durch. Damit diese nicht in einer zu großen Menge an Punkten resultiert, wird die Überabtastung auf die äußeren Randvoxel an dünnen Strukturen beschränkt (Abb. 1, Mitte). Zur Erkennung dünner Strukturen nutzen wir ein morphologisches Opening mit einem $3 \times 3 \times 3$ - Strukturelement. Jedes äußere Randvoxel, das zu einer dünnen Struktur benachbart ist, wird in acht Subvoxel unterteilt. Die Extraktion der Punkte auf Basis dieser Subvoxel erfolgt auf die selbe Weise, wie zuvor für Voxel beschrieben. Um eine treppenartige Anordnung der Punkte bei Nutzung des überabgetasteten Voxelgitters zu verhindern, werden vor der Punktextraktion zusätzliche Subvoxel als Objektsubvoxel markiert (Abb. 1, rechts; siehe [5] für Details). Die mit den Punkten assoziierten Normalenvektoren werden mit Hilfe des Grauwertgradienten berechnet. Bevor die Punktwolke zur Erzeugung der MPU Implicits genutzt wird, wird sie in Weltkoordinaten überführt. Die erzeugte Oberfläche liegt somit ebenfalls in Weltkoordinaten vor.

2.2 Parameterbestimmung

Die Generierung und Polygonalisierung der MPU Implicits kann durch eine Vielzahl von Parametern beeinflusst werden. Eine manuelle Ermittlung geeigneter Werte für diese Parameter ist sehr zeitaufwändig und würde einen praktischen Einsatz der vorgestellten Methode erschweren. Deswegen erweitern wir unser Verfahren um eine automatische Parameterbestimmung. Für einige Parameter können heuristisch bestimmte Werte als Standard genutzt werden. So legen wir zum Beispiel die Anzahl der für die lokalen Approximationen benötigten Punkte auf 200 fest, um eine möglichst glatte Rekonstruktion zu erreichen. Die Werte anderer Parameter (z.B. ϵ_0) werden individuell für jeden Datensatz abhängig von der Ausdehnung der Punktwolke sowie der Größe der Voxel festgelegt. Eine ausführliche Erläuterung der Parameterbestimmung ist in [5] zu finden.

Abb. 2. Rekonstruktion eines Bronchialbaumes mit MPU Implicits (links). Rekonstruktion eines Aneurysmas mit Marching Cubes (rechts oben), Convolution Surfaces (rechts Mitte) und MPU Implicits (rechts unten). Höhere Genauigkeit gegenüber Convolution Surfaces und Reduktion von Artefakten gegenüber Marching Cubes sind die wesentlichen Vorteile der MPU Implicits

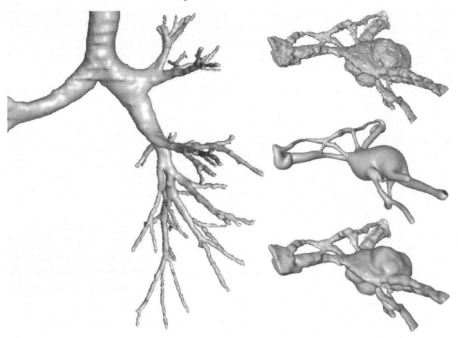

3   Ergebnisse

Das Verfahren wurde für verschiedene Gefäßsysteme (Lebergefäßbaum, Bronchialbaum, zerebrale Gefäße, Aneurysma) getestet. Für jeden der Datensätze konnten unter Nutzung der berechneten Parameterwerte artefaktfreie, glatt wirkende Oberflächen erzeugt werden (siehe Abb. 2). Dünne Zweige, Verzweigungen und pathologische Veränderungen werden korrekt rekonstruiert. Die Berechnungszeiten für den Bronchialbaum ($343 \times 193 \times 259$ Voxel) und das Aneurysma ($129 \times 107 \times 45$ Voxel) betragen 38 bzw. 5 Sekunden, wobei ca. 30% der Zeit für die Punktwolkengenerierung benötigt werden. Die Berechnungsdauer hängt hierbei sowohl von der Auflösung der Ausgangsdaten als auch von der Komplexität der beschriebenen Struktur ab.

Um die Abweichung vom Segmentierungsergebnis zu messen, wurden die Oberflächen von vier Datensätzen mit den entsprechenden Marching-Cubes-Ergebnissen verglichen. Die Abweichung beträgt im Mittel 0,188 Voxeldiagonalen, das Maximum liegt bei 1,5 Voxeldiagonalen und ist somit äußerst gering. Bei Convolution Surfaces ist die Abweichung mit durchschnittlich 0,5 Voxeldiagonalen weitaus höher (maximale Abweichung: ca. 5 Voxeldiagonalen). Die Glattheit der erzeugten Oberflächen wurde durch eine Analyse der Verteilung von

Krümmungswerten auf der Oberfläche mit Hilfe von AMIRA untersucht. Bei einer Marching Cubes-Rekonstruktion sind hohe und niedrige Krümmungswerte gleichmäßig auf der Oberfläche verteilt. Dies resultiert aus den treppenartigen Artefakten der Rekonstruktion. Bei der MPU Implicits-basierten Rekonstruktion korrespondiert die Verteilung der Krümmungswerte hingegen mit der Verteilung der Gefäßradien. Dicke Äste weisen nur geringe Krümmungswerte auf, während dünne Äste durch hohe Krümmungswerte gekennzeichnet sind. Treppenartige Artefakte sind somit nicht vorhanden.

4 Diskussion

Das vorgestellte Verfahren ist in der Lage, auf Basis des Segmentierungsergebnisses eine genaue und glatt wirkende Oberfläche eines Gefäßbaumes zu rekonstruieren. Es ist für eine Anwendung im Bereich der Therapieplanung *und* der Diagnostik geeignet. Für einen Einsatz in der Therapieplanung ist jedoch die Verbindung der Oberfläche mit einem Gefäßmodell wünschenswert, um eine einfache Exploration des Gefäßbaumes zu ermöglichen. Durch die vorgeschlagene automatische Parameterberechnung entfällt die zeitaufwändige manuelle Anpassung der Parameterwerte für die Erzeugung und Polygonalisierung der MPU Implicits für verschiedene Datensätze. Die benötigte Berechnungsdauer liegt im Bereich von Sekunden. Ein Einsatz des Verfahrens im klinischen Alltag scheint daher möglich. Eine weitere Erhöhung der Effizienz wäre dennoch wünschenswert. Dies wäre zum Beispiel durch Nutzung eines adaptiven Polygonalisierungsverfahrens möglich. Die Genauigkeit des Verfahrens kann weiter erhöht werden, indem für kleine Vertiefungen eine ähnliche adaptive Überabtastung angewendet wird, wie sie für dünne Zweige vorgeschlagen wurde.

Literaturverzeichnis

1. Oeltze S, Preim B. Visualization of Vascular Structures: Method, Validation and Evaluation. IEEE Transactions on Medical Imaging 2005;24(4):1–9.
2. Taubin Gabriel. A Signal Processing Approach to Fair Surface Design. In: Proc. of SIGGRAPH; 1995. 351–358.
3. Bade R, Haase J, Preim B. Comparison of Fundamental Mesh Smoothing Algorithms for Medical Surface Models. In: SimVis; 2006. 289–304.
4. Gibson SFF. Constrained Elastic Surface Nets: Generating Smooth Surfaces from Binary Segmented Data. In: Proc. of MICCAI '98; 1998. 888–898.
5. Schumann Christian. Visualisierung baumartiger anatomischer Strukturen mit MPU Implicits. Master's thesis. Universität Magdeburg, Fakultät für Informatik; 2006.
6. Braude I. Smooth 3D Surface Reconstruction from Contours of Biological Data with MPU Implicits. Master's thesis. Drexel University; 2005.
7. Ohtake Y, Belyaev A, Alexa M, et al. Multi-level Partition of Unity Implicits. ACM Transactions on Graphics 2003;22(3):463–470.
8. Bloomenthal J. An Implicit Surface Polygonizer. Graphics Gems IV 1994; 324–349.

Integrierte Visualisierung kardialer MR-Daten zur Beurteilung von Funktion, Perfusion und Vitalität des Myokards

Lydia Paasche[1], Steffen Oeltze[1], Frank Grothues[2], Anja Hennemuth[3],
Caroline Kühnel[3] und Bernhard Preim[1]

[1]Institut für Simulation und Graphik, Otto-von-Guericke-Universität Magdeburg
[2]Klinik für Kardiologie, Angiologie and Pneumologie,
Otto-von-Guericke-Universität Magdeburg
[3]MeVis Research, 28359 Bremen
Email: stoeltze@isg.cs.uni-magdeburg.de

Zusammenfassung. Wir präsentieren die integrierte Visualisierung von linksventrikulären Funktionsparametern, First-Pass (FP) Perfusions- und Late Enhancement (LE) Daten für die Diagnostik der Koronaren Herzkrankheit (KHK). Die Visualisierung basiert auf einem 3d-Modell des linken Ventrikels und einfachen geometrischen Primitiven (Glyphen), deren Farbe und Größe in Abhängigkeit von den Datenwerten variieren. Die kombinierte Darstellung von Funktionsparametern und LE-Daten kann die Abgrenzung von temporär inaktivem, aber vitalem Myokard und Narbengewebe unterstützen. Eine Integration von FP-Perfusions-Daten ermöglicht zudem die Differenzierung von *hibernating* (chronisch minderdurchblutet) und *stunned* (verzögerte Erholung) Myokard.

1 Einleitung

Der Zustand des Myokards (Herzmuskel) ist bei der KHK-Diagnostik von elementarer Bedeutung. Die KHK ist gekennzeichnet durch Verengungen (Stenosen) oder Verschlüsse der Koronararterien und stellt weltweit eine der führenden Todesursachen in den Industrieländern dar. Eine Koronarstenose führt abhängig von ihrem Schweregrad zu einer Minderdurchblutung (Ischämie) des Myokards. Ein kompletter Verschluss resultiert bei fehlender kompensatorischer Blutversorung aus anderen Koronararterien (Kollateralgefäße) in einem Myokardinfarkt. Die kardiale MR-Diagnostik erlaubt die qualitative und semiquantitative Untersuchung der Durchblutung (FP-Perfusion), die Beurteilung der Myokardfunktion sowie die Differenzierung zwischen Narbengewebe und noch vitalem Myokard (LE). Bei der Funktionsdiagnostik des Myokards werden die Parameter regionale Wanddicke, Wanddickenzunahme und Wandbewegung sowie die globale Funktion des linken Ventrikels beurteilt. In FP-Perfusionsuntersuchungen (4d) ist der Verlauf der Signalintensitätszunahme des Myokards nach intravenöser Kontrastmittelgabe (KM) Grundlage der Differenzierung zwischen ischämischem (durchblutungsgestörtem) und nicht-ischämischem (normal perfundiertem) Myokard.

Hierauf basierend können z.B. eventuell vorhandene Koronarstenosen detektiert bzw. auf ihre hämodynamische Relevanz hin beurteilt werden. Die LE-Daten werden häufig zusätzlich zur FP-Perfusionsuntersuchung ca. 5-20 Minuten nach der KM-Applikation akquiriert. Narbenareale stellen sich bei dieser Aufnahmetechnik mit einem hyperintensen Signal dar.

Wir präsentieren eine integrierte Visualisierung der obigen Daten basierend auf Glyphen und einem 3d-Modell des linken Ventrikels aus den LE-Daten. Eine Kombination von LE-Daten und Funktionsparametern unterstützt die Abgrenzung von Narbengewebe und temporär inaktivem, aber vitalem Myokard. Letzteres kann durch die Integration von FP-Perfusions-Daten in *hibernating* (Perfusionsdefizit) und *stunned* (normale Perfusion) Myokard unterschieden werden.

2   Stand der Forschung und Fortschritt durch den Beitrag

Bisherige Verfahren widmen sich der integrierten Visualisierung mehrerer Parameter des KM-Verlaufs aus FP-Perfusionsdaten [1], [2] und der Kombination von LE- und FP-Perfusionsdaten [3] bzw. von LE-Daten und Funktionsparametern [4], [5]. In [1] werden Multiparametervisualisierungen zur Exploration verschiedener Parameter des KM-Verlaufs vorgestellt. In dem Softwareassistenten MeVisCardioPerfusion [2] ist eine erweiterte Version des Bull's Eye Plots (BEP) integriert, welche die Gegenüberstellung korrespondierender Parameter der Ruhe-/Stress-Perfusion gestattet. Zur Unterscheidung zwischen ischämischem und infarziertem Gewebe, schlagen [3] die Kombination von LE- und FP-Perfusionsdaten vor. Hierzu wird die Infarktnarbe segmentiert und im BEP den Ergebnissen der Perfusionsanalyse überlagert. Die automatische Identifikation von *hibernating* Myokard wird in [4] vorgestellt. Dazu werden Wanddickenzunahme und Transmuralität der Infarktnarbe (Anteil vernarbten Gewebes an der Wanddicke) bestimmt, miteinander gewichtet und auf der aus den LE-Daten extrahierten Ventrikeloberfläche farbkodiert. Dies erlaubt die visuelle Detektion von Gebieten mit einem Funktionsausfall aber ohne hyperintenses Signal in den LE-Daten. In [5] wird der Softwareassistent HeAT zur Analyse der Myokardfunktion nach einem Infarkt vorgestellt. Hierzu werden die Ergebnisse der Funktionsanalyse auf die LE-Daten registriert. Die schichtweise Überlagerung der Daten ermöglicht dann eine statistische Auswertung der Funktion im Infarktgebiet.

Existierende Arbeiten konzentrieren sich auf die Kombination von max. 2 unterschiedlichen Datentypen. Wir präsentieren die integrierte Visualisierung von Funktionsparametern, FP-Perfusions- und LE-Daten. Die Verwendung von Glyphen ist inspiriert durch [6], welche die auf einem Modell basierende Myokardkontraktion visualisieren. Bei der integrierten Darstellung steht die Adaptivität der Visualisierung im Vordergrund. Der Nutzer kann sowohl die zu kombinierenden Daten abhängig von der klinischen Fragestellung wählen, als auch Darstellungsattribute interaktiv beeinflussen. Standardeinstellungen beschleunigen eine initiale Beurteilung.

3   Material und Methoden

Zur Erprobung der Algorithmen wurden MR-Daten einer Infarktpatientenstudie mit 15 Probanden genutzt. Die Bilder der Perfusions- und Funktionsmessungen (4d Cine MR) und die Bilder der Vitalitätsmessung (3d LE-MR) sind in Kurzachsenschnitten aufgenommen. Die Bildaufnahme erfolgte mit einem 3T System (TRIO, Siemens): FP-Perfusion (Matrix = 192×115, Schichtanzahl = 4, Zeitpunkte = 40, Schichtdicke = 6mm), Funktion ($256 \times 146 \times 10 \times 30$, 6mm), LE ($256 \times 139 \times 10 \times 1$, 8mm).

3.1   Vorverarbeitungsschritte

Zur Bewegungskorrektur sowie zum Matching der Phasen der FP-Perfusionsdaten wird eine Kombination von starrer und elastischer Registrierung, mit Mutual Information als Ähnlichkeitsmaß, genutzt. Das Myokard wird in allen Bilddaten mit Hilfe eines LiveWire-Verfahrens [7] segmentiert. Für eine integrierte Visualisierung werden die Daten der Endsystole (ES) und Enddiastole (ED) aus den Funktionsmessungen und die FP-Perfusiondaten auf die LE-Daten registriert. Die Registrierung erfolgt manuell durch ein rigides Verfahren. Aus den FP-Perfusionsdaten werden Parameter [8] berechnet, welche die Kontrastmittelanreicherung charakterisieren, und in Parametervolumina $\{P\}$ abgespeichert. Die Infarktnarbe wird in den LE-Daten mittels eines Schwellwertverfahrens segmentiert [3]. Basierend auf der Segmentierung des Myokards zur ES und ED in den Bildern der Funktionsmessung werden Isooberflächen von Endokard und Epikard mit Hilfe des *Marching Cubes* Algorithmus generiert. Die Wanddickenzunahme wird aus der zur ES und ED mittels euklidischer Distanzmaße berechneten Wanddicke ermittelt und in den Knoten des Epikardmodells zur ED (Epi_{ED}) gespeichert. Die ED wird gewählt, da auch die LE-Daten zu diesem Zeitpunkt aufgenommen wurden.

3.2   Integration von Funktion, FP-Perfusion und Late Enhancement

Problematisch bei der Integration von Funktion, FP-Perfusion und LE sind die unterschiedlichen Aufnahmezeitpunkte sowie die verschiedene Schichtdicke und Schichtanzahl. Im Folgenden wird exemplarisch anhand der beiden erstgenannten Datentypen eine Lösung dieses Problems beschrieben. Zur gemeinsamen Darstellung von Wanddickenzunahme und FP-Perfusionsparametern wird Epi_{ED} in den Voxelraum des FP-Perfusionsdatensatzes transformiert. Die Transformationsmatrix basiert auf der Inversen der für die FP-Perfusionsdaten bekannten Transformation von Voxel- in Weltkoordinaten. Für jeden Knoten des Modells kann nun bestimmt werden, in welchem Voxel V_i des FP-Perfusionsdatensatzes er sich befindet. Basierend auf den Knoten, die einem Voxel zugewiesen werden können, wird ein Datensatz mit den Dimensionen des FP-Perfusionsdatensatzes angelegt. Die mittlere Wanddickenzunahme wird für jedes neue Voxel $V_{i_{new}}$ aus allen Knoten bestimmt, die in V_i liegen. Damit ist eine Korrespondenz zwischen Funktion und FP-Perfusion erzeugt worden.

Abb. 1. Silhouette des linken Ventrikels mit Narbe als opakes Oberflächenmodell und Lage des Septums: Glyphen repräsentieren die Wanddickenzunahme und das Maximum der Kontrastmittelanreicherung (Peak Enhancement) der FP-Perfusion (links) bzw. Peak Enhancement und Anstieg der Kontrastmittelanreicherung (Up-Slope) (rechts)

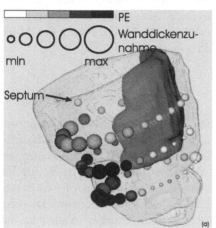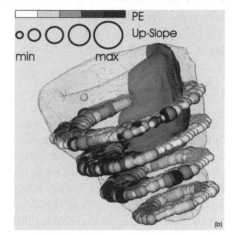

Die Repräsentation der Daten basiert auf einfachen geometrischen Primitiven, so genannten Glyphen, auf deren Attribute die Datenwerte abgebildet werden. Sollen z.B. die Wanddickenzunahme und ein Parameter aus $\{P\}$ zusammen dargestellt werden, wird das Myokard in den zugehörigen Datensätzen in eine beliebige Anzahl an Segmenten oder AHA-konform in 17 Segmente [9] unterteilt. Die Datenwerte in den Segmenten werden gemittelt und beeinflussen die Größe und Farbe der Glyphen. Über Farbskalen und Skalierungsstufen, welche durch den jeweiligen Maximal- und Minimalwert des Parameters begrenzt sind, wird das entsprechende Attribut der Glyphen gesetzt. Die Korrelation zwischen den dargestellten Parametern der kardialen MRT-Untersuchung und den Attributen des Glyphen kann vom Nutzer interaktiv beeinflusst werden. Zu Testzwecken wurde eine einfache Kugelform des Glyphen gewählt.

Die Platzierung der Glyphen ist der segmentweisen Unterteilung des Myokards angepasst. Für die Positionierung wird dabei der Schwerpunkt des Segments bestimmt, wobei nur Voxel betrachtet werden, die innerhalb des Myokards liegen. Mit einer einfachen Matrixmultiplikation können die so ermittelten Positionen im Voxelraum in das Weltkoordinatensystem transformiert und zusammen mit dem Modell des linken Ventrikels angezeigt werden (Abb. 1, links). Eine voxelweise Platzierung der Glyphen ist ebenfalls möglich und erleichtert z.B. die Analyse mehrerer Parameter der FP-Perfusion (Abb. 1, rechts).

4   Ergebnisse

In den Testdaten sind lokale Korrelationen von minderdurchblutetem und kontraktionsarmem Gewebe zu erkennen (Abb. 1, links). Die nutzerdefinierte Segmenteinteilung des Myokards erlaubt eine genauere Untersuchung von krankhaftem und gesundem Muskelgewebe als die Standardsegmentierung der AHA. Zur Abgrenzung von Narbengewebe und temporär inaktivem, aber vitalem Myokard kann die Infarktnarbe eingeblendet und die Wanddickenzunahme auf die Glyphengröße abgebildet werden. Eine anschließende Differenzierung zwischen *hibernating* und *stunned* Myokard, wird durch die Abbildung eines Parameters der FP-Perfusion auf die Glyphenfarbe unterstützt. Der Nutzer kann die Abbildungen und die Wahl der Parameter interaktiv beeinflussen.

5   Diskussion

Das vorgestellte Verfahren ermöglicht die integrierte und adaptive Visualisierung von linksventrikulären Funktionsparametern, FP-Perfusions- und LE-Daten. Erste Anwendungen haben gezeigt, dass eine Lokalisation und Differenzierung verschiedener krankhafter Veränderungen des Myokards unterstützt wird. Zur Validierung dieser Aussagen müssten Datensätze einer Verlaufskontrolle vorliegen. Techniken zur Formänderung der Glyphen, z.B. für die Kodierung eines weiteren Parameters, sind zu entwickeln und hinsichtlich der menschlichen Wahrnehmung zu diskutieren.

Literaturverzeichnis

1. Oeltze S, Grothues F, Hennemuth A, et al. Integrated visualization of morphologic and perfusion data for the analysis of coronary artery disease. Procs Eurographics 2006; 131–138.
2. Kuehnel C, Hennemuth A, Boskamp T, et al. New software assistants for cardiovascular diagnosis. Procs Informatik für den Menschen 2006;Band 1:491 – 498.
3. Breeuwer M, Paetsch I, Nagel E, et al. The detection of normal, ischemic and infarcted myocardial tissue using MRI. Procs CARS 2003;1256:1153–1158.
4. Noble NMI. Information Alignment and Extraction from Cardiac Magnetic Resonance Images. Ph.D. thesis. King's College London; 2004.
5. Säring D, Stork A, Juchheim S, et al. HeAT: A software assistant for the analysis of LV remodeling after myocardial infarction in 4D-MR follow-up studies. Procs Informatik für Menschen 2006;Band 1:537–543.
6. Wü BC, Lobb R, Young AA. The visualization of myocardial strain for the improved analysis of cardiac mechanics. Procs GRAPHITE 2004; 90–99.
7. Schenk A, Prause G, Peitgen HO. Local cost computation for efficient segmentation of 3D objects with live wire. Procs SPIE 2001;4322:1357–1367.
8. Al-Saadi N, Gross M, Bornstedt A, et al. Comparison of various parameters for determining an index of myocardial perfusion reserve in detecting coronary stenosis with cardiovascular MRT. Z Kardiol 2001;90:824–34.
9. Cerqueira MD, Weissman NJ, Dilsizian V, et al. Standardized myocardial segmentation and nomenclature for tomographic imaging of the heart. Int J Cardiovasc Imaging 2002; 539–542.

Improving Depth Perception in Medical AR
A Virtual Vision Panel to the Inside of the Patient

Christoph Bichlmeier[1], Tobias Sielhorst[1], Sandro M. Heining[2], Nassir Navab[1]

[1]Chair for Computer Aided Medical Procedures (CAMP), I-16,
Technische Universität München, Boltzmannstraße 3, 85748 Garching, Germany
[2]Trauma Surgery Department, Klinikum Innenstadt,
LMU München, Nußbaumstraße 20, 80336 München, Germany
Email: bichlmei@cs.tum.edu

Abstract. We present the in-situ visualization of medical data taken from CT or MRI scans in real-time using a video see-through head mounted display (HMD). One of the challenges to improve acceptance of augmented reality (AR) for medical purpose is to overcome the misleading depth perception. This problem is caused by a restriction of such systems. Virtual entities of the AR scene can only be presented superimposed onto real imagery. Occlusion is the most effective depth cue [1] and let e.g. a correctly positioned visualization of the spinal column appear in front of the real skin. We present a technique to handle this problem and introduce a *Virtual Window* superimposed onto the real skin of the patient to create the feeling of getting a view on the inside of the patient. Due to motion of the observer the frame of the window covers and uncovers fragments of the visualized bones and tissue and enables the depth cues motion parallax and occlusion, which correct the perceptive misinformation. An earlier experiment has shown the perceptive advantage of the window. Therefore seven different visualization modes of the spinal column were evaluated regarding depth perception. This paper introduces the technical realization of the window.

1 Introduction

Real-time in-situ visualization of medical data is getting increasing attention and has been a subject of intensive research and development during the last decade [2], [3], [4]. Watching a stack of radiography is time and space consuming within the firm work flow in an operating room (OR). Physicians have to associate the imagery of anatomical regions with their proper position on the patient. Medical augmented reality allows for the examination of medical imagery like radiography right on the patient. Three dimensional visualizations can be observed by moving with a head mounted display around the AR scene. Several systems [5, 2, 6] that are custom made for medical procedures tend to meet the requirements for accuracy and to integrate their display devices seamlessly into the operational work flow.

Fig. 1. Opaque surface model occludes real thorax. Therefore it is perceived in front of the body although the vertebrae is positioned correctly. Even if the visualization is semi-transparent like the direct volume rendered vertebrae we do not perceive the bones at their proper position. Right figure shows some components of our AR setup including a plastic phantom and the HMD

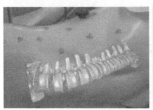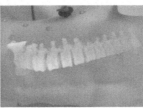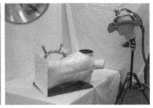

2   State of the Art and New Contribution

Depth perception has become a major issue of current research in medical AR. Virtual data is superimposed on real imagery and visual depth perception is disturbed (Fig. 1). The problem has been identified as early as 14 years ago in the first publication about medical augmented reality [7]. This group tasked the problem by rendering a "synthetic hole" ... "around ultrasound images in an attempt to avoid conflicting visual cues." In an earlier paper Tobias Sielhorst et al. described an experiment that evaluated seven different visualization modes for the spinal column regarding depth perception [8]. This paper describes the technical realization of one of the winners of the evaluation. This is a virtual window that can be overlaid onto the skin and provides a bordered view onto the spinal column inside the patient. Due to the virtual window depth perception of the visualized medical data can be corrected.

3   Method

Medical data taken from a CT or MRI scan is presented using a stereoscopic video see-through HMD. The whole tracking system that allows for tracking the observer wearing the HMD, the patient and several surgical instruments is described at [8]. We use direct volume rendering and presegmented surface models to visualize the data.

3.1   Position the Window

Placing the window to get the desired view into the patient can be performed without touching or moving the patient. While positioning the window, the observer wearing the HMD views a frame (Fig. 2) and guides it to the area of interest by moving his or her head. When the frame is at the desired position, the window can be set by key press. The size is adjustable by mouse interaction, which can be performed by an assistant on an external monitor that shows a copy of the imagery presented by the displays of the HMD. The window adopts the shape of the skin. Therefore we add an augmentation of the skin presented as a surface model. The frame of the window defines the borders of a structured 2D grid consisting of a certain number of grid points. For every grid point a so-called picking algorithm examines the depth buffer at its corresponding pixel and recalculates three dimensional information of the nearest virtual object, which is in our case the surface model of the skin. After determination of their position in 3D space, the grid points are connected to compose a transparent surface. When the window surface is defined, it is used to mask the part of the scene, which is inside the thorax. Therefore we employ the so-called stencil buffer. The stencil buffer is an additional buffer besides the color buffer and depth buffer found on modern computer graphics hardware and can be used to limit the area of rendering. In our application the area is limited to the window when the visualized tissue or bones are drawn. Finally the window surface itself is rendered.

3.2   Window Design & Perceptive Advantage

The window was equipped with some design features to intensify the depth cues. Certain material parameters let the window appear like glass. Highlight effects due to the virtual light conditions support depth perception. Highlights on the window change the color of objects behind the window or even partially occlude these objects. The window plane is mapped with a simply structured texture, which enhances the depth cue motion parallax. Due to motion of the observer the texture on the window seams to move relatively faster than objects behind the window. The background of the virtual objects seen through the window can be set to transparent or opaque.

Cutting et al. summarized the most important binocular and monocular depth cues [1]. Our AR scene is perceived binocularly with the two color cameras mounted on the HMD. Stereopsis is realized by the slightly different perspectives of the two cameras. Convergence is predefined by the orientation of the cameras. The window enhances perceptive information about depth because it partially occludes the vertebrae. The frame of the window covers and uncovers parts of the spinal column while the observer is moving. The latter depth cue motion parallax is after occlusion and stereopsis the third most effective source of information about depth [1].

4   Results

The virtual window helps to overcome the misleading depth perception caused by the superimposed virtual spinal column onto the real thorax. Regarding depth perception an earlier experiment [8] compared seven different visualization modes of the spinal column including the virtual window. The virtual window was evaluated as one of the best methods. The method of posing the window interactively into the scene has the advantage that the surgeon or personnel of the OR do not have to touch the patient or use a further instrument that has to be kept sterile and wasts space. The observer wearing the HMD can easily position and

Fig. 2. Volume rendered spinal column and setup of the window. Frame can be guided by head movement to the required area

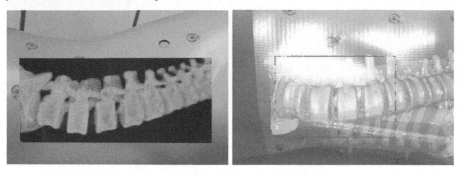

Fig. 3. Sequence shows the window from different perspectives with a surface model of the spinal column

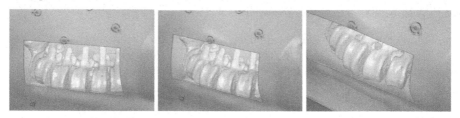

reposition the window by moving his or her head. Figures 3 show a sequence while the observer is moving the HMD respective the thorax with the attached window.

5   Discussion

We presented the virtual window regarding spine surgery to provide a intuitive view on the visualization of the vertebrae. However, the window can be used for further medical application, which will be part of our future work. Future work will also concern the optimization of setting up the window to avoid wasting precious time in the medical work flow, variation and evaluation of different designs, i.e. shape of the window and structure of the texture mapped on the window plane, to achieve the best depth perception and integration of augmented surgical instruments.

6   Acknowledgment

Special thanks to Frank Sauer, Ali Khamene, and Sebastian Vogt from Siemens Corporate Research (SCR) for the design, setup, and implementation of the in-situ visualization system RAMP they provided us. Thanks to A.R.T. GmbH for providing cameras and software for the outside-in tracking system. We also want to express our gratitude to the radiologists and surgeons of the Klinikum Innenstadt München for their precious contribution in obtaining medical data and evaluating our systems. Thanks also to Joerg Traub, Marco Feuerstein, Stefan Wiesner and Philipp Stefan of the NARVIS group for their support. This work was granted by the BFS within the NARVIS project (www.narvis.org).

References

1. Cutting JE, Vishton PM. Perceiving layout and knowing distances: The integration, relative potency, and contextual use of different information about depth. In: Epstein W, Rogers S, editors. Perception of Space and Motion; 1995. 69–117.
2. Birkfellner W, Figl M, Huber K, et al. A head-mounted operating binocular for augmented reality visualization in medicine: Design and initial evaluation. IEEE Trans Med Imaging 2002;21(8):991–997.
3. King AP, Edwards PJ, Maurer CR Jr, det al. Stereo augmented reality in the surgical microscope 2000;9(4):360–368.
4. Sauer F, Khamene A, Bascle B, Vogt S, Rubinob GJ. Augmented reality visualization in iMRI operating room: System description and pre-clinical testing. Procs SPIE 2002;4681:446–454.
5. Sauer F, Khamene A, Vogt S. An augmented reality navigation system with a single-camera tracker: System design and needle biopsy phantom trial. LNCS 2002;2489:116–124.
6. King AP, Edwards PJ, Maurer CR Jr, et al. Design and evaluation of a system for microscope-assisted guided interventions. IEEE Trans Med Imaging 2000;19(11):1082–1093.
7. Bajura M, Fuchs H, Ohbuchi R. Merging virtual objects with the real world: Seeing ultrasound imagery within the patient. In: Procs Computer Graphics and Interactive Techniques. ACM Press; 1992. 203–210.
8. Sielhorst T, Bichlmeier C, Heining SM, Navab N. Depth perception a major issue in medical AR: Evaluation study by twenty surgeons. In: Procs MICCAI; 2006.

Cardiac C-Arm CT

SNR Enhancement by Combining Multiple Retrospectively Motion Corrected FDK-like Reconstructions

M. Prümmer[1], L. Wigström[2,3], R. Fahrig[2], G. Lauritsch[4], J. Hornegger[1]

[1]Institute of Pattern Recognition, FA University Erlangen-Nuremberg, Germany
[2]Department of Radiology, Stanford University, USA
[3]Center for Medical Image Science and Visualization, Linköping University, Sweden
[4]Siemens AG, Medical Solutions, Forchheim, Germany
Email: pruemmer@informatik.uni-erlangen.de

Abstract. Cardiac C-arm CT is a promising technique that enables 3D cardiac image acquisition and real-time fluoroscopy on the same system. Retrospective ECG gating techniques have already been adapted from clinical cardiac CT that allow 3D reconstruction using retrospectively gated projection images of a multi-sweep C-arm CT scan according to the desired cardiac phase. However, it is known that retrospective gating of projection data does not provide an optimal signal-to-noise-ratio (SNR) since the measured projection data is only partially considered during the reconstruction. In this work we introduce a new reconstruction technique for cardiac C-arm CT that provides increased SNR by including additional corrected and resampled filtered back-projections (FBP) from temporal windows outside of the targeted reconstruction phase. We take advantage of several motion corrected FDK-like reconstructions of the subject to increase SNR. In the presented results, using in vivo data from an animal model, the SNR could be increased by approximately 30 percent.

1 Introduction

The combination of real-time projection imaging with 3D imaging modalities in the interventional suite is becoming more important as procedures increase in complexity. One such combination, x-ray fluoroscopy with cardiac C-arm CT, is under development. Retrospectively ECG gated FDK [1] reconstructions (RG-FDK) provide promising image quality for cardiac C-arm CT as shown by Lauritsch et al. [2]. Image presentation during a procedure often requires new imaging algorithms for segmentation and image registration, and such algorithms have stringent need for high image quality including signal-to-noise ratio (SNR) and contrast-to-noise ratio (CNR). In cardiac C-arm CT, the retrospective selection of projection images whose ECG time is closest to the cardiac phase that is desired for reconstruction considers only $\frac{1}{N_s}$ of the measured projection data of an e.g. $N_s \times 4s$ multi-sweep scan, which does not maximize the potential SNR of the 3D reconstructions. In this work we introduce a technique that allows use of all projection images from a multi-sweep scan and therefore can provide enhanced SNR in the reconstructed volume. A similar approach for respiratory motion correction and SNR enhancement was introduced by Li et al. [3]. The approach we introduce is a trade-off between the spatial resolution provided by a retrospectively ECG gated FDK reconstruction using only a selected subset of all acquired projection images and a reconstruction that uses all measured projection data (and therefore has good SNR) but may exhibit reduced spatial resolution due to approximations applied during the temporally dependent spatial motion correction.

2 Methods

Let P be the set that contains all acquired projection images of a multi-sweep scan, then P^t is a subset of P that provides the retrospectively selected projection images of cardiac phase t (defined in percent between subsequent R-peaks); for each projection angle one projection image is selected that is closest to the cardiac phase t. P^t_β denotes the β-th projection image where the index β is ordered according to an increasing projection angle of a short-scan projection data set P^t. The cardiac phase of a projection image is denoted by $\tau(P^t_\beta)$. The *effective cardiac phase* (ECP) of a reconstruction using the set of images P^t is

$$\tau_E(t) = \frac{1}{|P^t|} \sum_{\beta=1}^{|P^t|} \tau(P^t_\beta) \tag{1}$$

As mentioned above we have a trade-off between spatial resolution and SNR enhancement due to an approximate motion correction scheme. A RG-FDK volume of the desired cardiac phase t_r is reconstructed to provide a baseline of spatial resolution where the projection images are retrospectively selected such that the observed ECP $\tau_E(t)$ is closest to t_r. This volume is denoted by $f^{RG}_{t_r}(\boldsymbol{x})$ and $\boldsymbol{x}$ is a 3D grid of the reconstructed volume intensities. It can be seen as a first sample from multiple volume reconstructions that are later combined to enhance SNR. However, during the reconstruction of $f^{RG}_{t_r}(\boldsymbol{x})$ only $\frac{1}{N_s}$ of the projection data is used. To make use of the remaining unused projection data, we apply retrospective motion correction.

2.1 Retrospective Motion Correction

As shown by Prümmer et al. [4] increased temporal resolution can be achieved by computing a 4D motion vector field $\boldsymbol{U}(t)$ (MVF) of the subjects' individual heart motion using image registration as introduced by Modersitzki [5]. The 3D MVF $\boldsymbol{u}_t := \boldsymbol{U}_{t_r}(t)$ describes the relative 3D deformation of each voxel between a selected *reference cardiac phase* t_r (RCP) that is desired for a reconstruction with enhanced SNR, and cardiac phase t. The MVF is combined with an FDK-like algorithm [4] that allows a temporally dependent spatial warping of the filtered-backprojections $\tilde{P}^t_{\beta_i}(\boldsymbol{x})$. Since we apply a voxel-driven back-projection the FBPs are defined on the 3D grid $\boldsymbol{x}$. The integral in the FDK-like algorithm [1], that we call FDK-4D, over all discrete β_i can be written as the sum

$$\tilde{f}_{t_r}(\boldsymbol{x}) = \sum_{i=1}^{|P^{tr}|} \tilde{P}^t_{\beta_i}(\boldsymbol{x} - \boldsymbol{u}_{\tau(P^t_{\beta_i})}) \qquad (2)$$

of the temporally dependent spatially warped FBPs according to the MVF. This allows the use of additional projection images during the reconstruction that would, due to their cardiac phase, otherwise introduce motion artifacts.

2.2   Multiple Volume Reconstruction

Since we correct for motion we can create several e.g. N_m arbitrary subsets P^l of projection images for a short-scan, that are not retrospectively gated. For each of the N_m subsets a motion corrected volume $\tilde{f}^l_{t_r}(\boldsymbol{x})$ according to (2) is reconstructed using FDK-4D. The selection strategy of the projection data implies that each measured projection image of a multi-sweep scan is contained in at least one of the subsets P^l. The multiple volume reconstructions are then voxel-wise combined using a 1D Gaussian window $G^{\mu\boldsymbol{x}}_\sigma(i)$ where the mean $\mu_{\boldsymbol{x}} := f^{RG}_{t_r}(\boldsymbol{x})$ is defined by the voxel intensity of the RG-FDK reconstruction f^{RG}, i is the intensity and standard deviation σ. The SNR enhanced reconstruction f^{SNR} using the proposed algorithm, that we call Multiple-Volume-FDK (MV-FDK), is then given by

$$f^{SNR}_{t_r}(\boldsymbol{x}) = \frac{1}{1 + \sum\limits_{l=1}^{N_m} G^{\mu\boldsymbol{x}}_\sigma(\tilde{f}^l_{t_r}(\boldsymbol{x}))} \left(\sum_{l=1}^{N_m} G^{\mu\boldsymbol{x}}_\sigma(\tilde{f}^l_{t_r}(\boldsymbol{x}))\tilde{f}^l_{t_r}(\boldsymbol{x}) + f^{RG}_{t_r}(\boldsymbol{x}) \right) \qquad (3)$$

3   Results

To investigate improvement of image quality using the MV-FDK algorithm, a series of ten RG-FDK reconstructions (using 191 retrospective selected projections for the reconstruction) was performed. These initial reconstructions were used to compute the MVF relative to the cardiac phase $t_r = 80$. Using the FDK-4D algorithm six motion corrected volumes, each of which using a partially distinct set of projection images, were reconstructed such that all 1146 acquired and (according to their phase distance to $t_r = 80$) spatially warped projection images were considered during MV-FDK reconstruction. Different standard deviations σ for the Gaussian weighting between the multiple reconstructions where investigated as shown in Figure 1. The MV-FDK reconstructions are compared against the RG-FDK reconstruction. The between the arrows measured SNR (defined as the ratio of the mean intensity value to the standard deviation) is $(\sigma, SNR) = (15, 66.07), (30, 73.58), (60, 74.45), (90, 74.14), (120, 73.94), (150, 73.73), (200, 73.73), (RG - FDK, 57.7)$ (see Fig. 1). An example of representative image quality of a RG-FDK reconstruction in comparison with an MV-FDK reconstruction is shown in Figure 2.

Fig. 1. Intensity profile plot along a line as shown in the top left image. The image shows a slice of an MV-FDK reconstruction (6 × 4s multi-sweep scan, using 1146 projection images during reconstruction). The intensity profile of the complete line is shown in the top right panel. A magnification of the intensity profile measured between both arrows is shown in the bottom panel. Each MV-FDK reconstruction is a combination of six reconstructions, that are reconstructed using several partially distinct subsets of the acquired projection data. Inside the left ventricle the intensity profile of the MV-FDK reconstruction is more homogeneous compared to the RG-FDK reconstruction

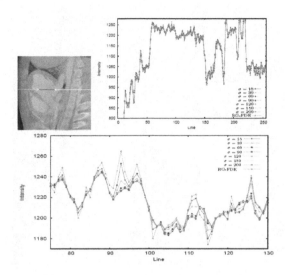

4 Conclusion and Discussion

We could show that using the MV-FDK algorithm the SNR can be improved by approximately 30 percent compared to a standard RG-FDK reconstruction. The measured intensity profile inside the ventricle shows a higher SNR. Intensity variations inside high density regions like the contrast filled ventricle are decreased and the location of edges remain while only a very slight blurring is noticed such that improved segmentation results for clinical applications can be expected. In conclusion we can say that improvement of SNR by including additional corrected and resampled projections from cardiac phases outside the temporal window of the targeted reconstruction phase during reconstruction can be achieved.

5 Acknowledgments

This work was supported by Siemens AG, Medical Solutions, Forchheim, Germany, NIH grant R01 EB 003524 and by the Lucas Foundation, HipGraphics, Towson, Maryland, USA, BaCaTec and by Deutsche Forschungsgemeinschaft (DFG), SFB 603, TP C10.

226 M. Prümmer et al.

Fig. 2. Column (a) shows three orthogonal multi-planar reconstructions (MPRs) of the heart from an animal model using RG-FDK where 191 retrospectively selected projection images were used ($t_r = 80$). Column (b) shows a multiple-volume FDK reconstruction considering 1146 acquired projection images from a $6 \times 4s$ scan. The standard deviation of the Gaussian kernel used for the MV-FDK reconstruction (b) was $\sigma = 60$. The MV-FDK reconstruction (b) is less noisy compared to the RG-FDK reconstruction (a) while edges in principle remain as provided by the RG-FDK approach

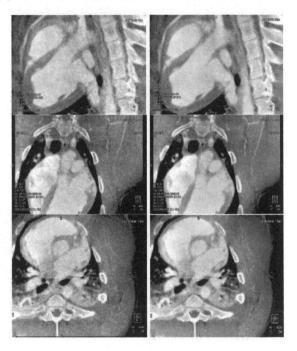

References

1. Feldkamp LA, Davies LC, Kress JW. Practical cone-beam algorithm. J Opt Soc Am A1 1984:612–619.
2. Lauritsch G, Boese J, Wigström L, Kemeth H, Fahrig R. Towards Cardiac C-arm Computed Tomography. IEEE Trans Med Imaging 2006;25:922–934.
3. Li T, Schreibmann E, Thorndyke B, Tillman G, Boyer A, Koong A, et al. Radiation dose reduction in four-dimensional computed tomography. Med Phys 2005;32(12):3650–3660.
4. Prümmer M, Wigström L, Hornegger J, Boese J, Lauritsch G, Strobel N, et al. Cardiac C-Arm CT: Efficient motion correction for 4D-FBP. Procs IEEE Medical Imaging Conference, San Diego, 2006, accepted for publication.
5. Modersitzki J. Numerical Methods for Image Registration. Oxford University Press, 2004.

Photon Attenuation Correction in Misregistered Cardiac PET/CT

A. Martinez-Möller[1,2], N. Navab[2], M. Schwaiger[1], S.G. Nekolla[1]

[1]Nuklearmedizinische Klinik der TU München
[2]Computer Assisted Medical Procedures and Augmented Reality, TU München
Email: a.martinez-moller@lrz.tu-muenchen.de

Abstract. PET-CT misalignment has been reported as a source of arte-facts in cardiac PET/CT due to a biased photon attenuation correction. Using the data from 28 cardiac PET/CT rest/stress examinations, PET-CT misalignment was corrected using three different methods: manual registration, automatic mutual information based image registration and an emission-driven correction algorithm. The clinical effects of the re-alignment were quantitatively assessed, and significant changes were ob-served in 6 out of 28 examinations (21.4%), in 5 of these studies resulting in the disappearance of large apparent perfusion defects. These results in-dicate that the excellent specificity of PET for the detection of perfusion defects could be compromised when CT-based attenuation correction is done without correction of PET-CT misalignment.

1 Introduction

Positron emission tomography (PET) is a functional imaging technique which provides volumetric images of the distribution of a radiotracer in the body. This is achieved through the detection of 511 keV photons produced by the anni-hilation of positrons emitted by the radiotracer. However, only a fraction of the photons is being detected, as a significant part is being *attenuated* (either scattered or absorbed) through interactions within the body, according to the following formula:

$$A = A_0 \exp^{-\oint \mu(x)dx} \qquad (1)$$

where A_0 is the flow of initial photons, A the flow of photons which go through the trajectory without suffering attenuation, and μ the coefficient of attenua-tion for each of the body regions within each photon's trajectory. Therefore, a correction for photon attenuation is necessary for accurate quantification of PET images. This is done through the obtention of attenuation maps containing the coefficient μ for each part of the body [1]. Since the introduction of com-bined PET/CT scanners, the attenuation map is usually computed by a bilinear scaling of X-ray tissue radiodensity as measured using CT [2].

One fundamental assumption of the attenuation correction is the accurate spatial registration of the PET emission data and the attenuation maps. How-ever, even when using combined PET/CT scanners, a potential misregistration

Fig. 1. On the top row, fused PET/CT examination without attenuation correction showing a clear misregistration. On the bottom, the same examination after attenuation correction. A notable decrease of activity is observed in the misregistered areas of the myocardium due to a biased attenuation correction

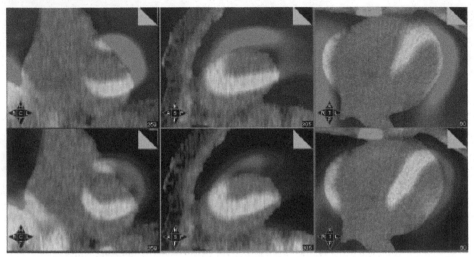

can be found between both modalities as a result of non simultaneous acquisition and differences in temporal resolution between PET and CT. Such a misregistration can lead to artefacts in the attenuation corrected PET image, as can be seen in Fig. 1.

2   State of the Art and New Contribution

To our knowledge, no studies have reported on the effects of the misregistration for cardiac PET/CT yet. In contrast, the problem of emission-transmission misalignment in cardiac imaging -due to pharmacological stress, patient breathing or other patient motion- has been previously investigated using PET with rotating sources [3, 4], SPECT [5] and SPECT/CT [6].

This work provides new information regarding frequency and extent of cardiac PET-CT misregistration, evaluates the clinical impact of such a misregistration due to artefacts caused by biased photon attenuation correction, and proposes potential solutions to minimize these artefacts.

3   Methods

28 consecutive patients (20 men and 8 women, age 63±12y) with suspected coronary artery disease (CAD) were enrolled in this study. All patients had been referred for a cardiac PET/CT rest/stress perfusion study to evaluate the functional impact of CAD. Imaging was performed on a Siemens Biograph 16 PET/CT (Siemens Medical Solutions, Erlangen, Germany).

Transmission data for the thorax were acquired with a low-dose CT scan (120 kV, 26 mA) performed in shallow breathing. After that, patients received a 300 to 500 MBq injection of ^{13}N-labelled NH_3 and the PET image was acquired for 10 minutes. Image data from 5 min p.i. to 10 min p.i. was summed and used for further analysis.

3.1   PET-CT Registration

In order to investigate the clinical effects of PET-CT misalignment we sought to remove the misregistration by realigning the CT to the PET and repeating the PET reconstruction with the aligned CT-based attenuation map. For this purpose, a registration program was developed using IDL (Interactive Data Language, RSI Inc. Boulder, CO, USA), allowing three different possibilities to realign the PET and CT examinations: manual registration (only translational motion allowed), automatic mutual information based registration (exhaustive search within the translational space), and an "emission driven" correction method to modify the heart outline based on the PET data.

The emission driven correction is an in-house developed method based on the following assumption: if there is tracer uptake corresponding to the left ventricle (LV) in the PET image, the corresponding voxel in the CT should contain cardiac tissue. However, in case there is an inconsistency and the voxel contains lung tissue and therefore nearly no attenuation, the value of the voxel is modified to match that of cardiac tissue. As this operation was only to be applied in the LV. a fully automatic segmentation of the LV from the PET scan was required, and performed by means of a spatially localized thresholding, as the LV has always high NH_3 uptake. The segmentation and modification of the attenuation map required less than one second runtime using a standard personal computer.

For each PET examination, all three realignment techniques mentioned above were separately applied, and the PET raw data was reconstructed again hsing each of the realigned CT. The tracer uptake was quantified before and after realignment by spatially sampling the left ventricle and projecting the measured activity on a polar map basis. The polar map was then divided in 17 segments according to the AHA17 model [7] and compared to a normal NH_3 perfusion map. Segments where the uptake differed by more than 2.5 standard deviations were considered as perfusion defects.

4   Results

The average misalignment between the PET and CT datasets assessed by manual registration was 6.1±6.3 mm. The spatial distribution of the motion was as follows: left-right 1.3±2.2 mm (range: 0 - 5.1 mm), anterior-posterior 1.6±2.9 mm (range: 0 - 15.4 mm), head-feet 4.7±6.1 mm (range: 0 - 23.6 mm). Head-feet motion represented the major component of the misalignment, in agreement with the main direction of the breathing motion. The maximum value of the misalignment for an examination was 29 mm.

The defect size as quantified by comparison to a normal database changed by more than 10 %LV in 6 out of 28 patients (21.4%), all of them following a manual realignment greater than 10 mm. In 5 of the 6 patients, the perfusion defect - which ranged between 15 and 46 %LV- was fully artifactual and disappeared after reconstruction with the realigned CT-based attenuation map.

Automatic mutual information based image registration was not successful for the registration of PET and CT cardiac images. The effects of a misaligned heart in the were largely compensated by a reasonably well aligned thorax, so that the registration indicated that the original pose was always the best alignment. Subsequently, we tested a more regional approach by applying the registration to a manually defined volume of interest around the heart. Unfortunately, this technique did not produce better results, as the low correlation between the functional information provided by PET and the anatomical detail provided by CT made mutual information fail, being incapable of properly assessing the agreement between both poses when limited to the cardiac region only.

The emission-driven method had results equivalent to those obtained by manual registration. The correlation between the variation of measured uptake produced by both methods was high ($R^2 = 0.74$, $p < 0.001$) and good agreement was seen for large misregistration-induced defects.

5 Discussion

The results in this study indicate that PET-CT misregistration occurs frequently in cardiac perfusion studies and can have important clinical consequences. Changes of the defect size larger than 10% of the myocardium were observed in 6 out of 28 patients (21.4%), fact which which could compromise the otherwise excellent specificity of PET for the detection of perfusion defects.

Realignment of CT to PET and repetition of the PET reconstruction minimizes the artefacts induced by a biased photon attenuation correction. Although automatic registration would be the optimal approach, we obtained disappointing results for the cardiac region, indicating that manual registration is the only solid option. Alternatively to manual registration, the proposed emission-driven correction yielded equivalent results, having the advantages of being fast and fully automatic.

References

1. Zaidi H, Hasegawa BH. Determination of the attenuation map in emission tomography. J Nucl Med 2003;44:291–315.
2. Kinahan P, Hasegawa BH, Beyer T. X-ray-based attenuation correction for positron emission tomography/computed tomography scanners. Sem Nucl Med 2003;33(3):166–179.
3. Loghin C, Sdringola S, Gould KL. Common artifacts in PET myocardial perfusion images due to attenuation-emission misregistration: Clinical significance, causes and solutions. J Nucl Med 2004;45:1029–1039.

4. McCord ME, Bacharach SL, Bonow RO, et al. Misalignment between PET transmission and emission scans: Its effect on myocardial imaging. J Nucl Med 1992;33:1209–1213.
5. Matsunari I, Boning G, Ziegler SI. Effects of misalignment between transmission and emission scans on attenuation-corrected cardiac SPECT. J Nucl Med 1998;39:411–416.
6. Fricke H, Fricke E, Weise R, et al. A method to remove artifacts in attenuation-corrected myocardial perfusion SPECT introduced by misalignment between emission scan and CT-derived attenuation maps. J Nucl Med 2004;45:1619–1625.
7. Cerqueira MD, Weissman NJ, Dilsizian V. Standardized myocardial segmentation and nomenclature for tomographic imaging of the heart: A statement for healthcare professionals from the cardiac imaging committee of the council on clinical cardiology of the American Heart Association. Circulation 2002;105:539–542.

Separate CT-Reconstruction for Orientation and Position Adaptive Wavelet Denoising

Anja Borsdorf[1,2], Rainer Raupach[2], Joachim Hornegger[1]

[1]Chair for Pattern Recognition, Friedrich-Alexander-University Erlangen-Nuremberg
[2]Siemens Medical Solutions, Forchheim
Email: anja.borsdorf@informatik.uni-erlangen.de

Abstract. The projection data measured in computed tomography (CT) and, consequently, the slices reconstructed from these data are noisy. For a reliable diagnosis and subsequent image processing, like segmentation, the ratio between relevant tissue contrasts and the noise amplitude must be sufficiently large. By separate reconstruction from even and odd numbered projections, two images can be computed, which only differ with respect to noise. We show that these images allow an orientation and position adaptive noise estimation for level-dependent threshold determination in the wavelet domain.

1 Introduction

In computed tomography (CT), the projections acquired at the detector are noisy, predominantly caused by quantum statistics. This noise propagates through the reconstruction algorithm to the reconstructed slices. Pixel noise in the images can be reduced by increasing the radiation dose or by choosing a smoothing reconstruction [1]. However, with respect to patient care, the least possible radiation dose is required and a smoothing reconstruction lowers image resolution. This shows that pixel noise in the images cannot be reduced arbitrarily.

Nevertheless, an increased signal-to-noise ratio is beneficial for a reliable diagnosis and subsequent image processing, like registration or segmentation. This paper presents a new wavelet based method for edge-preserving noise reduction in CT-images.

2 State of the Art and New Contribution

A very important requirement for any noise reduction in medical images is that all clinically relevant image content must be preserved. A common approach for edge-preserving noise reduction is wavelet thresholding, based on the work of Donoho and Johnstone [2]. The input image is decomposed into wavelet coefficients. Insignificant detail coefficients below a defined threshold are erased, but those with larger values are preserved. The noise suppressed image is obtained

Fig. 1. Block diagram of the noise reduction method

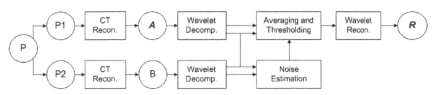

by an inverse wavelet transformation from the modified coefficients. The difficulty is to find a suitable threshold, especially for noise with spatially varying power and directed noise, which is commonly present in CT-images. Choosing the threshold too high may lead to visible loss of image structures, but the effect of noise suppression may be insufficient, if the threshold was chosen too low. Therefore, a reliable estimation of noise for threshold determination is one of the main issues.

We show that the local and orientation dependent noise power in CT can be estimated from two separately reconstructed images, which only differ with respect to image noise. Therefore, the noise reduction method adapts itself to the noise power and allows for the reduction of spatially varying and oriented noise.

3   Methods

3.1   Overview

An overview of the noise reduction method is shown in Fig. 1. First, two images A and B are generated, which only differ with respect to image noise. In CT, this can be achieved by separate reconstruction from disjoint subsets of projections $P1 \subset P$ and $P2 \subset P$, with $P1 \cap P2 = \emptyset$. More precisely, one image is reconstructed from the even and the other from the odd numbered projections. The two resulting images include the same information but different noise. Both images are decomposed by a two dimensional stationary wavelet transformation (SWT) [3]. After this transformation, at each decomposition level, four two-dimensional blocks of coefficients are available for both images: the lowpass filtered approximation image C and three detail images W^H, W^V and W^D including high frequency structures in horizontal (H), vertical (V) and diagonal (D) direction, together with noise in the respective frequency bands. The computation of the differences between the detail coefficients of the two input images shows just the noise in the respective frequency band and orientation. These noise images can then be used for the estimation of the spatial and orientation dependent standard deviation of noise in A and B. From this estimation, a thresholding mask is computed and applied to the averaged detail coefficients of the input images. The computation of the inverse wavelet transformation from the modified coefficients results in a noise-suppressed image. This again corresponds to the reconstruction from the complete set of projections but with improved signal-to-noise ratio.

3.2   Threshold Determination

The two images A and B only differ with respect to image noise, but include the same information

$$A = S + N_A, \quad B = S + N_B \tag{1}$$

where S represents information and $N_A \neq N_B$ noise included in image A and B, respectively. The standard deviations of noise in the two separately reconstructed images can be assumed to be equivalent ($\sigma_A \approx \sigma_B$), because the number of contributing quanta for both images is approximately the same. However, the noise level in A and B is increased by a factor of $\sqrt{2}$ in comparison to the reconstruction from the complete set of projections or the average of the two input images $M = 0.5(A + B)$. It can be assumed that we have zero-mean noise in both images. By the computation of the difference image

$$D = A - B = N_A - N_B \tag{2}$$

we get a noise-image free of structures. The standard deviations σ_A and σ_B of noise can be approximated from the standard deviation in the difference image σ_D by

$$\sigma_A = \sigma_B = \frac{\sigma_D}{\sqrt{2}} \tag{3}$$

Thus, the standard deviation of noise in the average image M results in:

$$\sigma_M = \frac{\sigma_A}{\sqrt{2}} = \frac{\sigma_D}{2} \tag{4}$$

In order to compute a level and orientation dependent threshold for denoising in the wavelet domain, noise in the different frequency bands and orientations should be estimated in separation. The discrete wavelet transformation is a linear transformation. Therefore, the differences between the detail coefficients can also be directly used for noise estimation. At each decomposition level l the difference images

$$D_l^H = W_{Al}^H - W_{Bl}^H, \quad D_l^V = W_{Al}^V - W_{Bl}^V, \quad D_l^D = W_{Al}^D - W_{Bl}^D \tag{5}$$

between the detail coefficients are computed, where the subscripts A and B correspond to the two images. These difference images are then used for the estimation of noise in the respective frequency band and orientation. In CT-images, the noise power is spatially varying. Therefore, noise should be estimated position dependent. In order to achieve this, a region of $m \times m$ pixels is chosen around each position in the difference image and the standard deviations of the pixel values are locally computed within these regions. Thus, we obtain three images σ_l^H, σ_l^V and σ_l^D with the local standard deviations of noise in the difference images in the horizontal, vertical and diagonal directions. Together with Eq. (4), orientation, position and level dependent thresholds are computed

$$\tau_l^H = k\frac{\sigma_l^H}{2}, \quad \tau_l^V = k\frac{\sigma_l^V}{2}, \quad \tau_l^D = k\frac{\sigma_l^D}{2} \tag{6}$$

Fig. 2. Example of orientation and position dependent threshold at the first decomposition level for thoracic image with strongly directed noise

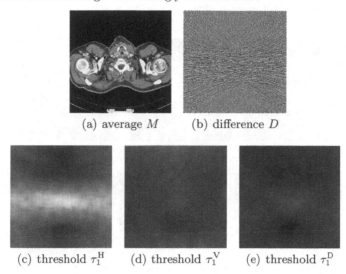

(a) average M (b) difference D

(c) threshold τ_1^H (d) threshold τ_1^V (e) threshold τ_1^D

The constant k controls the amount of noise suppression. With increasing k more noise is removed. In Fig. 3(c)- 3(e) the thresholds computed with $m = 32$ for the first decomposition level in the horizontal, vertical and diagonal directions are shown for a thorax-slice (see average of input images in Fig. 3(a)) with strongly directed noise (see difference of input images in Fig. 3(b)).

3.3   Averaging and Thresholding

The computed thresholds from Eq. (6) are then applied to the averaged wavelet coefficients of the input images. We perform a *hard* thresholding, meaning that all coefficients with an absolute value below the threshold are set to zero and values above are kept unchanged. The final noise suppressed image is computed by an inverse wavelet transformation from the averaged and weighted wavelet coefficients of the input images.

4   Results

In Fig. 4(d) and 4(f), zoomed-in noise suppressed results from the proposed method applied to a thoracic image (see Fig. 3(a)) are shown for two different settings of k. Further, the difference images (Fig. 4(e), 4(g)) between the denoised and average of input images (Fig. 4(a)) are displayed. The images are compared to the denoising result achieved with the *SWT De-noising 2D* tool from the Matlab wavelet toolbox [4] (see Fig. 4(b) and 4(c)). All computations were performed using a Haar wavelet decomposition up to the fourth decomposition level. For denoising in Matlab, we used a *Balance Sparsity-Norm* hard thresholding method with a non-white-noise model.

Fig. 3. Denoising result of the proposed method in pixel region taken from thorax-slice with strongly directed noise. Center and window settings used for displaying CT-images: $c = 50$, $w = 400$. Center and window settings used for displaying difference images: $c = 0$, $w = 30$

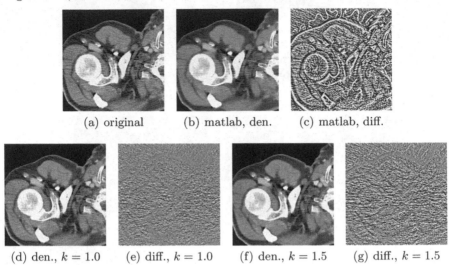

(a) original   (b) matlab, den.   (c) matlab, diff.

(d) den., $k = 1.0$ (e) diff., $k = 1.0$ (f) den., $k = 1.5$ (g) diff., $k = 1.5$

5   Discussion

The difference image in Fig. 4(c) shows that standard wavelet denoising methods reduce noise in the images but also blurr edges. The reason for this is that no reliable noise estimation is possible if just one CT-image is available. In contrast, the proposed method adapts itself to the spatially varying noise power in the different frequency bands and orientations and, therefore, performs much better especially in images with directed noise.

References

1. Kalender WA. Computed Tomography. Munich: Publics MCD Werbeagentur GmbH; 2000.
2. Donoho DL, Johnstone IM. Ideal spatial adaptation by wavelet shrinkage. Biometrika 1994;81(3):425–455.
3. Coifman RR, Donoho DL. Translation invariant denoising. Lecture Notes in Statistics: Wavelets and Statistics 1995;103:125–150.
4. Mathworks Inc. Wavelet Toolbox; 2006. http://www.mathworks.com/products/wavelet/.

Assessment of Renal Function from 3D Dynamic Contrast Enhanced MR Images Using Independent Component Analysis

Frank G. Zöllner[1,2], Marek Kocinski[3], Arvid Lundervold[2], Jarle Rørvik[1]

[1]Department for Radiology, University of Bergen, 5021 Bergen, Norway,
[2]Department of Biomedicine, University of Bergen, 5009 Bergen, Norway,
[3]Institute of Electronics, Technical University of Lodz, 90-924 Lodz, Poland
Email: frank.zoellner@biomed.uib.no

Abstract. In this paper we present an automated, unsupervised, data-driven approach to assess renal function from 3D DCE-MR images. Applying independent component analysis to four different data sets acquired at different field strengths and with different measurement techniques, we show that functional regions in the human kidney can be recovered by a subset of independent components. Time intensity curves, reflecting perfusion in the kidney can be extracted from the processed data. The procedure may allow non-invasive, local assessment of renal function (e.g. glomerular filtration rate, GFR) from the image time series in future.

1 Introduction

Diagnosis of renal dysfunction is today based on blood test and urine sampling (e.g. plasma creatinine, creatinine clearance). These indirect measures are rather imperfect, since e.g. a significant change in creatinine level is only detectable until a 60% function loss has occurred. Furthermore, these measures do not give a split function between left and right kidney.

To overcome these limitations dynamic imaging of the kidneys is an emerging technique for a more accurate assessment of the local renal function [1, 2]. By using dynamic contrast enhanced magnetic resonance imaging (DCE-MRI), the passage of the contrast agent through the organ is reflected by intensity changes over time in the images. From the extracted regional time intensity curves, parameters such as blood flow and time of arrival of contrast agent can be estimated. Thus, a very precise assessment of renal function in the different compartments of the kidney is possible. However, this approach assumes proper motion correction (image registration) has been performed previous to the time course analysis, since the kidneys are non-rigid moving organs where complex voxel-displacements during data collection are caused by respiration and pulsations.

The emerging clinical interest in this kind of imaging studies stems partly from the fact that renovascular disease are rapidly increasing in the population, and can often progress to end stage renal disease (ESRD) requiring dialysis or kidney transplantation. Another diagnostic problem with relevance to the present study is early graft failure detection, where perfusion defects in the kidney transplant can occur at an early stage.

In this work we introduce an unsupervised, data-driven time course analysis method for regional assessment of renal function. By applying independent component analysis (ICA) to motion-corrected DCE MRI data we can automatically segment the 3D+time image into separate regions representing functional compartments of the kidney, e.g. the renal cortex, medulla, and pelvis. From each of these compartments we can obtain time intensity curves that provide valuable information about tissue perfusion and glomerular filtration, and thus renal function.

2   State of the Art and New Contribution

Assessment of renal function using DCE-MRI is typically based on manual or semi-automated delineation of regions of interest (ROIs) in the recorded images (e.g. [3]). This procedure is time consuming, expensive and error prone [4], and subject to intra- and inter-observer variations. Computational approaches can help overcome these limitations and provide more objective and reproducible results.

ICA of dynamic MR image acquisitions was first introduced by McKeown et al. [5], studying BOLD fMRI of brain. Since then, several different ICA algorithms and techniques have been proposed for the analysis of brain imaging data, including analysis of the 'default network' at resting state fMRI, and in group studies (cf. [6, 7]). To our knowledge, this is the first report using ICA in the study of human kidney DCE-MRI recordings obtained at 1.5 and 3T scanners with different pulse sequences and temporal and spatial resolutions (cf. [8]). The motivation for using ICA on images from moving kidneys was twofold (i) manual segmentation of functional compartments of the kidneys are time consuming and difficult since information is distributed in both time and space, (ii) renal physiology is relatively simple (compared to the brain), where we expect at least three sources contributing to the observed time courses, i.e. an early contrast enhancing cortical compartment, a late enhancing pelvic compartment, and an intermediate medullary compartment.

3   Methods

Briefly, ICA is a method for separating a multivariate signal $\mathbf{x} = (x_1, \ldots, x_p)$, into statistically independent components (or sources) $\mathbf{s} = (s_1, \ldots, s_q)$, $q \leq p$. This can be formulated as $\mathbf{x} = \mathbf{A}\mathbf{s}$ where $\mathbf{A}$ is the mixing matrix, and $\mathbf{A}$ and $\mathbf{s}$ are unknown. By inverting to $\hat{\mathbf{s}} = \mathbf{W}\mathbf{x}$, we can identify $\mathbf{W}$ as the unmixing matrix we wish to estimate, such that the statistical independence of the estimated sources $\hat{\mathbf{s}}$ is maximised, i.e. estimating maximum nongaussianity [9].

Table 1. Study data: A = 1.5 T Siemens Symphony, B = 3.0 T Signa Excite GE

ID	Scanner	Sequence	Resolution [mm]	Size	Timing
1	A	FLASH	1.48x1.48x3.00	256x256x20x20	not equidistant
2	A	VIBE	1.48x1.48x3.00	256x256x20x118	1 volume per 2.5s
3	B	LAVA	0.86x0.86x1.20	512x512x44x60	1 volume per 3.0s
4	B	LAVA	1.72x1.71x2.40	256x256x22x60	1 volume per 3.7s

In our case we consider time courses $\mathbf{x}^i$ of the DCE-MRI data set for each voxel i in a subregion containing the kidneys, where p is the number of time frames. The task solved by the ICA algorithm is estimation of $\mathbf{s}^i$ (consisting of q components) that might contribute to the functional relevant subregions of the kidney, or represent the surrounding tissue. Initially, the 4D data is preprocessed. First step is motion correction, applying a non-rigid registration procedure [10]. Thereafter, to discriminate between left and right kidney function, we used a k-means clustering procedure, as in [11], to automatically separate the two kidneys.

For ICA analysis we used the fastICA algorithm to our preprocessed data. Prior to the calculation we reduced the dimension of the time series using principle component analysis (PCA) and whitening as suggested in [9]. A suitable number of PCs and ICs was eroded by applying the ICASSO method [12] which provides two measures on the stability of the ICA estimates (using clustering). The I_q coefficient measures the compactness of the clusters, the R-index (I_R) the similarity between the found ICs.

Furthermore, we projected the transformed data back into image space for assessing the location and spatial extension of the ICs, and for calculation of time intensity curves to identify functional parts of the kidney and verify the results qualitatively.

4 Results

We tested our approach on four data sets acquired from healthy volunteers. We used different field strength, pulse sequences, and spatial and temporal resolutions (cf. Tab. 1). A Gadolinium based contrast agent (Omniscan, GE Healthcare) were used in all experiments. The experiments were approved by the regional ethical committee.

For data analysis, the ICASSO and fastICA were applied to the 3D voxel time courses. By exploratory analysis of possible dimension reductions I_R showed a local minimum at 5 indicating a possible good solution [12]. In addition I_q showed high compactness values (≥ 0.8) for all five independent components. As non-linearity $g(u)$ used in the fixed point algorithm we select $g(u) = u^3$.

The resulting ICA signal was projected back into image space to visually inspect regions represented by the independent components. Figure 1 depicts the computed functional regions of the left kidney of data set 3. For the renal cortex, medulla, and pelvis region the corresponding time intensity curves are plotted. The other two independent components (data omitted due to limited

Fig. 1. Anatomically and functionally distinct regions and their corresponding time intensity curves resulting from ICA analysis of the left kidney of data set 3. The renal compartments are superimposed on the original slice images from frame 10. The corresponding mean time intensity curves (bold) and the standard deviations (error bars) are plotted to the right. Top to bottom: cortex, medulla, and pelvis.

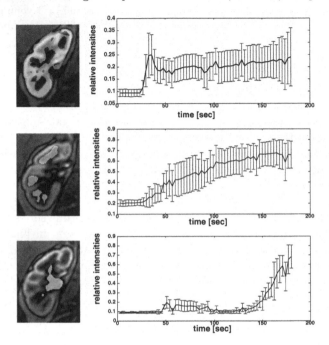

space) depict background voxels and voxels of partial volume effects. Similar results were obtained for the other data sets being analysed.

5   Discussion

We have presented an automated, unsupervised, data-driven ICA approach to assess renal function from 3D DCE-MR images of the human kidneys. Our results demonstrate that ICA is a powerful tool for segmenting time course information and functional 3D regions in the kidney. Using the ICASSO explorative visualisation method with bootstrapping, we found high statistical reliability and stability of the estimated independent components. Moreover, the regional mean time intensity curves in our healthy volunteers was close to those reported in [3]. A prerequisite for ICA analysis is proper volume-by-volume image registration since uncorrected large voxel displacements will introduce erroneous time courses and unreliable results [8]. However, the independent component analysis was also effective in detection of gross movements (e.g. when the breath-holding period ended), enabling assessment of registration performance, as the time courses belonging to these ICs had distinct spikes at times where misregistration occurred.

Thus, it seems that periodic or stochastic voxel displacements is a source of information that can be captured by independent components much in the same way as background voxels or voxels subject to partial volume effects can be. Whether this information will be detected or not, will also depend on the number of independent components that are specified or being estimated.

Ongoing research is directed toward comparison of the independent component regions obtained by ICA analysis, and the segmentation results obtained by conventional k-means clustering of the time courses [11]. Using data-driven volume segmentation of the DCE-MR image recordings and transformation of time-intensity curves into time-concentration curves, we will explore local glomerular filtration rate (GFR) quantification using pharmacokinetic modelling (e.g. [13]).

References

1. Michaely H, Herrmann K, Nael K, et al. Functional renal imaging: Nonvascular renal disease. Abdominal Imaging 2006.
2. Prasad PV. Functional MRI of the kidney: tools for translational studies of pathophysiology of renal disease. Am J Physiol Renal Physiol 2006;290(5):F958–F974.
3. Huang AJ, Lee VS, Rusinek H. Functional renal MR imaging. Magn Reson Imaging Clin N Am 2004;12(3):469–86, vi.
4. de Priester JA, den Boer JA, Giele EL, et al. MR renography: an algorithm for calculation and correction of cortical volume averaging in medullary renographs. J Magn Reson Imaging 2000;12(3):453–459.
5. McKeown MJ, Makeig S, Brown GB, et al. Analysis of fMRI data by blind separation into independent spatial components. Human Brain Mapping 1998;6:160–188.
6. Calhoun VD, Adali T, Hansen LK, et al. ICA of Functional MRI Data: An Overview. In: Proc. 4th International Symposium on Independent Component Analysis and Blind Signal Separation (ICA2003); 2003. 281–287.
7. Calhoun VD, Adali T. Unmixing fMRI with independent component analysis. IEEE Eng Med Biol Mag 2006;25(2):79–90.
8. Zöllner FG, Kocinski M, Lundervold A. Assessment of kidney function from motion-corrected DCE-MRI voxel time-courses using independent component analysis. In: Int. Workshop on Mining Brain Dynamics. Bergen, Norway; 2006.
9. Hyvärinen A, Karhunen J, Oja E. Independent Component Analysis. Wiley Interscience; 2001.
10. Sance R, Rogelj P, Ledesma-Carbayo MJ, et al. Motion correction in dynamic DCE-MRI studies for the evaluation of the renal function. MAGMA 2006;19(Supplement 7):106–107.
11. Zöllner FG, Sance R, Anderlik A, et al. Towards quantification of kidney function by clustering volumetric MRI perfusion time series. MAGMA 2006;19(Supplement 7):103–104.
12. Himberg J, Hyvärinen A. Icasso: software for investigating the reliability of ICA estimates by clustering and visualization. In: Proc. 2003 IEEE Workshop on Neural Networks for Signal Processing (NNSP2003); 2003. 259–268.
13. Michoux N, Vallee JP, Pechere-Bertschi A, et al. Analysis of contrast-enhanced MR images to assess renal function. Magn Reson Mater Phy 2006;19:167–179.

Determination of Mitotic Delays in 3D Fluorescence Microscopy Images of Human Cells Using an Error-Correcting Finite State Machine

Nathalie Harder[1], Felipe Mora-Bermúdez[2], William J. Godinez[1],
Jan Ellenberg[2], Roland Eils[1] and Karl Rohr[1]

[1]University of Heidelberg, IPMB, and DKFZ Heidelberg, Dept. Bioinformatics and
Functional Genomics, Im Neuenheimer Feld 364, D-69120 Heidelberg,
[2]European Molecular Biology Laboratory (EMBL), Gene Expression and Cell
Biology/Biophysics Programmes, Meyerhofstrasse 1, D-69117 Heidelberg
Email: n.harder@dkfz-heidelberg.de

Abstract. In high-throughput cell phenotype screens large amounts of image data are acquired. The evaluation of these microscopy images requires automated image analysis methods. Here we introduce a computational scheme to process 3D multi-cell image sequences as they are produced in large-scale RNAi experiments. We describe an approach to automatically segment, track, and classify cell nuclei into seven different mitotic phases. In particular, we present an algorithm based on a finite state machine to check the consistency of the resulting sequence of mitotic phases and to correct classification errors. Our approach enables automated determination of the duration of the single phases and thus the identification of cell cultures with delayed mitotic progression.

1 Introduction

RNA interference (RNAi) is an effective tool for identifying the biological function of genes. With this method genes are systematically silenced and the resulting morphological changes are analyzed. However, such large-scale screens provide large amounts of data which require tools for automated image analysis.

Our work is carried out within the project MitoCheck, which has the goal to explore the processes of cell division (mitosis) in human cells at a molecular level. In this project RNAi secondary screens are performed and fluorescence microscopy image sequences of the treated cell cultures are acquired to study the effects of the silenced genes on mitosis. This contribution is concerned with the automated evaluation of an assay for studying delays in mitotic phases, which are caused by gene silencing. Thus, the duration of the different phases of cell division has to be measured for the treated cells and compared with the normal cells from control experiments. Therefore, cells have to be observed throughout their life cycle and for each time point the respective phase has to be determined.

Automated analysis of high-throughput cell phenotype screens plays an increasingly important role. Approaches to analyse single-frame multi-cell 2D images from large-scale experiments have been described, e.g., in [1]. Recently,

Fig. 1. Image analysis workflow: (1) Maximum intensity projection of multi-cell 3D images, (2) Segmentation and tracking in 2D, (3) Extraction of 3D ROIs that include single cells,(4) Selection of most informative slices, (5) Feature extraction, (6) Classification, (7) Consistency check, error correction, and determination of phase durations

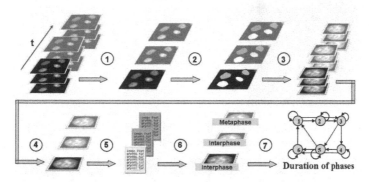

work has been done on automatically processing multi-cell 2D image sequences for cell cycle analysis. With these approaches, cells are segmented, tracked, and classified given phase-contrast [2] or fluorescence [3] microscopy images. In [2, 3] cells or cell nuclei are classified into a maximum of four phases. In [4] 3D image sequences are processed and cell nuclei are classified into seven cell cycle phases but no consistency check of the resulting phase sequences has been performed.

Our approach allows to analyze 3D multi-cell image sequences from a confocal fluorescence microscope. We classify cell nuclei into seven mitotic phases. To this end, we have developed a workflow that comprises segmentation, tracking of splitting nuclei, extraction of static and dynamic features, and classification. In particular, we present a scheme to check the consistency of the resulting sequences of mitotic phases of cells based on biological constraints. This scheme is based on a finite state machine which enables to automatically resolve errors using the confusion probabilities of the classifier. As a result, we can determine the lengths of the seven mitotic phases of cell nuclei automatically.

2   Methods

Image analysis workflow To analyze the mitotic phases high-resolution confocal fluorescence microscopy 3D images of the DNA are acquired which consist of three confocal planes (slices). Because of technical reasons in the image acquisition process the number of slices is restricted to three. During mitosis the cell changes its shape (gets more rounded) and therefore in different phases the DNA is visible in different slices. Using multi-cell images that contain cells in different mitotic phases, it is impossible to define one slice per time step that well represents the DNA of all cells. Therefore, we have developed the workflow shown in Fig. 1. First, we apply a maximum intensity projection (MIP) for each time step, resulting in 2D images (Fig. 2 (left)). Based on these MIP images we

Fig. 2. (left) Original 3D image (Maximum intensity projection), (right) 1-4: Example for the tracking of a mitotic nucleus in four consecutive time-steps, 4a: Result without mitosis detection, 4b: Result after mitosis detection and track merging

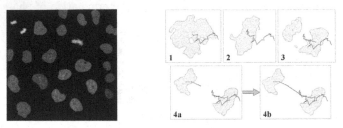

Fig. 3. Example images for the seven different mitotic phases (from left to right): inter-, pro-, prometa-, meta-, ana- 1, ana- 2, and telophase

perform segmentation and tracking to determine the correspondences in subsequent frames. We now go back to the 3D images and define 3D ROIs for each cell based on the segmentation and tracking result. For each 3D ROI we choose the most informative slice and extract static and dynamic features. Then we apply a classifier which results in a sequence of mitotic phases for each cell trajectory. Finally, the resulting phase sequences are parsed with a finite state machine to check their consistency, resolve inconsistencies, and determine the phase lengths.

Segmentation and tracking of mitotic cell nuclei For segmentation we apply region-adaptive thresholding which proved to be fast and robust in our application. This scheme computes local intensity thresholds in overlapping image regions using histogram-based threshold selection. To analyze the mitotic behavior of single cells, a tracking scheme is required that determines the temporal connections for splitting objects. We have developed the following two-step scheme: First, initial, non-splitting trajectories are established, and second, mitotic events are detected and the related trajectories are merged resulting in tree-structured trajectories (Fig. 2 (right)). For more details see [4].

Feature extraction and classification To compute image features we select for each cell nucleus its individual most informative slice. Our experiments showed that the maximum total intensity performs very well as selection criterion. Within the most informative slice we compute static and dynamic image features. The static features comprise object- and edge-related features, texture features, grey scale invariants, and Zernike moments. As dynamic features we compute the difference of object size, intensity mean and standard deviation, and circularity for each nucleus to its predecessor and successor. We apply a support vector machine (SVM) classifier with a radial basis function (RBF) ker-

Fig. 4. Finite state machine to check the consistency of the computed phase sequences

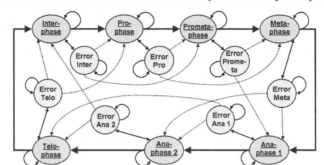

nel to classify the nuclei into the classes interphase, prophase, prometaphase, metaphase, anaphase 1, anaphase 2, and Telophase (Fig. 3).

Consistency check and error correction In order to determine the phase lengths automatically it is necessary that the computed phase sequences are consistent (which is not always the case due to classification errors). Therefore, we have developed a finite state machine (FSM) that accepts only biologically possible phase sequences. Each phase is represented by one state of the FSM. The possible phase transitions are represented by the state relations. Fig. 4 shows a sketch of the FSM; for clarity only the most important relations are displayed. The FSM contains error states to resolve inconsistencies. An error state is quit if the following phase is a valid phase. Then the most likely phase for the error state is determined based on the confusion probabilities of the classifier that have been established using cross-validation on the training set. In one run of the FSM inconsistencies of length 1 are completely corrected. Errors of length larger than 1 can be successively resolved in multiple runs of the FSM. In addition, the FSM determines the phase durations.

3   Results

Our experiments are based on four multi-cell 3D image sequences each consisting of 124 time steps. 29 cell nuclei have been segmented and tracked over 124 time steps resulting in 4225 single cell 3D image stacks (note that the cells proliferate). Some few trajectories have been manually corrected since our tracking scheme currently detects 80% of the occurring mitoses. We have performed a kind of two-fold cross-validation on the 29 available trajectories where in each loop 18 tracks have been used for training and 11 tracks for testing. In each cross-validation loop first the confusion probabilities were determined using a five-fold cross-validation on the training set. Then, the classifier was trained with the whole training set and tested with the test set. We obtain an overall classification

Table 1. Sample numbers and classification accuracies for each class (22 tracks tested)

	Inter	Pro	Prometa	Meta	Ana1	Ana2	Telo
No. of samples	2986	51	36	76	14	50	152
Class. accuracy	99.0%	84.3%	94.4%	79.0%	57.1%	86.0%	69.7%

accuracy of 96.6% (the sample numbers and accuracies per class for both cross-validation loops are given in Tab. 1). The resulting phase sequences for the 22 classified trajectories were processed with the finite state machine using the confusion matrices determined on the training sets to resolve consistency errors. Finally, the corrected phase sequences have been compared with the manually assigned correct phases (ground truth). It turned out that all inconsistencies of length 1 have been resolved in the first run of the FSM. Applying the FSM a second time on the corrected sequences resolved also all inconsistencies of length 2. Longer inconsistencies have partly been resolved. Note that this correction step is essential for determining the phase lengths automatically.

4 Discussion

We have presented an approach for automated analysis of the duration of mitotic phases in 3D confocal microscopy image sequences. Our approach segments and tracks splitting nuclei and thus determines cell pedigrees. By using static and dynamic features our scheme classifies the cells into seven mitotic phases. The consistency of the computed phase sequences is checked and inconsistencies are resolved using a priori knowledge. Finally, the phase durations are determined.

In future work, we plan to improve the performance of the tracking and classification schemes by including additional image features. We will also apply our approach to a larger number of image sequences and evaluate its performance.

Acknowledgment

This work has been supported by the EU project MitoCheck.

References

1. Perlman ZE, Slack MD, Feng Y, et al. Multidimensional drug profiling by automated microscopy. Science 2004;306:1194–1198.
2. Yang F, Mackey MA, Ianzini F, et al. Cell segmentation, tracking, and mitosis detection using temporal context. LNCS 2005;3749:302–309.
3. Padfield DR, Rittscher J, Sebastian T, et al. Spatio-temporal cell cycle analysis using 3D level set segmentation of unstained nuclei in line scan confocal fluorescence images. Procs ISBI 2006; 1036–1039.
4. Harder N, Bermúdez F, Godinez WJ, et al. Automated analysis of the mitotic phases of human cells in 3D fluorescence microscopy image sequences. LNCS 2006;4190:840–848.

Network Snakes for the Segmentation of Adjacent Cells in Confocal Images

Matthias Butenuth[1] and Fritz Jetzek[2]

[1]Institut für Photogrammetrie und GeoInformation,
Leibniz Universität Hannover, 30167 Hannover
[2]Evotec Technologies GmbH, 22525 Hamburg
Email: butenuth@ipi.uni-hannover.de

Abstract. Network snakes constitute one of the latest advances in the research of image segmentation techniques: they integrate topology into active contour models. This concept is applied to the problem of delineating biological cells in confocal images and is compared to results obtained with a current state-of-the-art segmentation method. Lacking a representative gold standard for this task, we adjust the well-established measure of segmentation quality developed by Pratt to our requirements and discuss the matching result of network snakes on one hand and conventional algorithms on the other. The work concludes with a discussion of some characteristic features and flaws of the approach.

1 Introduction

The advent of high content screening facilities by means of image acquisition from confocal laser scanning microscopes has significantly changed the conditions of pharmaceutical target research in recent years. One of the needs that arose is the task of automatically segmenting cell culture images. Information relevant to biological research includes cell properties like shape, size, and intensity distribution, which use the exact boundaries of cells.

The general problem of image segmentation still remains largely unsolved with respect to the sophisticated demands of medical applications. With the availability of multi-channel fluorescence labelings, image segmentation can often be split into smaller problems, for example, by detecting cell nuclei in one channel first, and subsequently using the prior information for the segmentation of cells in the second channel. However, machine-dependent artifacts like noise and object-typical characteristics like homogeneous areas in the intensity distribution at cell boundaries still provide major difficulties.

Enhancing well-known active contour models, which are only defined for closed object boundaries, a new methodology called *network snakes* [1] was introduced having the possibility to delineate objects, which form a network and thus interact during the optimization process. Cells are often adjacent with only one visible boundary in between. Therefore, network snakes can be used to detect the cell boundaries without intersection or overlap of the individual cells.

The next section contains some thoughts about the segmentation and modeling of cells. In addition, network snakes are shortly summarized to provide a base for introducing topology to the traditional concept. In section 3 the methodology to delineate cells using network snakes is described. In order to evaluate the proposed method, a conventional method is used to derive a reference. Subsequently, both methods are validated with the measure of segmentation quality introduced by Pratt [2]. Finally, some concluding remarks are given.

2   State of the Art and New Contribution

Image analysis for cell segmentation still follows paradigms that have been developed years ago, the most prominent ones being global and local thresholding techniques and the watershed transform [3]. A lot of research has been performed on the topic, but the aspect of modeling the natural properties of the objects of interest is largely neglected, even though it is obvious that this would improve the segmentation process [4]. In contrary, the presented network snakes approach follows a modeling scheme in that it does not restrict the detection of boundaries to a mere analysis of local intensity distributions, but takes energy minimization considerations into account that correspond more closely to cytoplasmic membrane morphology of adjacent cells.

The total energy of a traditional snake, to be minimized, is defined as [5]

$$E_{snake}^* = \int\limits_0^1 E_{snake}(v(s))ds = \int\limits_0^1 \left(E_{img}(v(s)) + E_{int}(v(s)) \right) ds \qquad (1)$$

where $E_{img}(v(s))$ represents the image energy and $E_{int}(v(s))$ the internal energy. A minimum of the total energy E_{snake}^* can be derived by solving the respective Euler equations [5]. The derivatives are approximated with finite differences since they can not be computed analytically. The Euler equations read

$$\alpha_i(v_i - v_{i-1}) - \alpha_{i+1}(v_{i+1} - v_i) \qquad (2)$$
$$+ \beta_{i-1}(v_{i-2} - 2v_{i-1} + v_i) - 2\beta_i(v_{i-1} - 2v_i + v_{i+1} + \beta_{i+1}(v_i - 2v_{i+1} + v_{i+2})$$
$$+ f_v(v) = 0$$

and can be rewritten in matrix form as

$$Av + f_v(v) = 0 \qquad (3)$$

Equation 3 can be solved iteratively by introducing a step size γ. Finally, a solution can be derived by matrix inversion

$$v_t = (A + \gamma I)^{-1}(\gamma v_{t-1} - \kappa f_v(v_{t-1})) \qquad (4)$$

where I is the identity matrix and κ is an additional parameter in order to control the weight between internal and image energy.

The minimization of the internal energy during the optimization process is only defined for closed object boundaries, i.e. $v_0 = v_n$ [5]. A new methodology was presented to overcome this limitation, called network snakes [1]. Integrating the topology into the energy minimization process causes a problem when solving equations 2 and 3: the derivatives approximated by finite differences are not defined for nodes with a degree $\rho(v) \neq 2$, because the required neighboring nodes are either not available or exist multiple times. A new definition of the total energy is proposed, which enables control at the common nodal point v_n, in that case with a degree $\rho(v) = 3$ with $v_n = v_{a_n} = v_{b_n} = v_{c_n}$ [1]

$$\beta(v_{a_n} - v_{a_{n-1}}) - \beta(v_{a_{n-1}} - v_{a_{n-2}}) + f_{v_a}(v_a) = 0$$
$$\beta(v_{b_n} - v_{b_{n-1}}) - \beta(v_{b_{n-1}} - v_{b_{n-2}}) + f_{v_b}(v_b) = 0 \qquad (5)$$
$$\beta(v_{c_n} - v_{c_{n-1}}) - \beta(v_{c_{n-1}} - v_{c_{n-2}}) + f_{v_c}(v_c) = 0$$

v_a, v_b and v_c represent three contours, each ending in a common nodal point v_n. The energy definition of equation 5 allows for a minimization process to control the shape of each contour segment separately even though they end in one common point. The new definition is straightforward for nodes with a degree $\rho(v) = 1$ and $\rho(v) > 3$, which are not used in this work. Of course, the proposed method requires a given topology, which is assumed to be correct.

3   Methods

Two different segmentation methods are compared for delineating biological cells in confocal images. A method using network snakes is proposed on one hand and a conventional method is presented on the other. The strategy of both methods is divided into two parts: at first, the image representing the cell nuclei is used to derive a coarse initialization. In a second step, both techniques are applied to the cytoplasm image to obtain the cell boundaries.

Concerning the use of network snakes, the required initialization is accomplished by means of a segmentation of the relative homogeneous background in the cell nuclei image utilizing a region growing algorithm. Subsequently, a skeleton is computed to yield a coarse initial network representing the boundaries between adjacent cells. Since each cell nucleus is located within the associated cell membrane, the skeleton can be used to derive the topology of the network. At that time a somewhat inaccurate geometrical position is tolerated. In the second step of the strategy the initial boundaries between the cells are used to initialize the network snakes approach and to optimize the preliminary boundaries deriving the final results.

For reasons of comparison, we also apply a conventional segmentation algorithm[1] to the same data as follows [6]: The nuclei image is transformed into a binary image using a sliding window to compute local thresholds for the intensity distribution. The resulting binary image is assumed to contain all nuclei

---

[1] Acapella data analysis software, Evotec Technologies GmbH

Fig. 1. Validation of the segmentation: (a) cell boundaries as calculated with network snakes, (b) corresponding result with conventional segmentation method, (c) Pratt values for all pairs of cell boundaries from both results

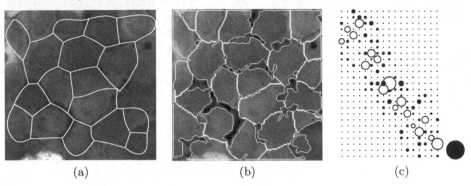

(a)　　　　　　　　　(b)　　　　　　　　　(c)

to be detected. A connected-component-labeling of this data yields a stencil of separate objects. Objects with low contrast are eliminated in order to remove artifacts erroneously detected as nuclei. The final step is carried out on the cytoplasm image exploiting the nuclei locations as seed objects for a watershed transform that delivers the final borders of the cytoplasm.

For the validation of the results a measure introduced by Pratt [2, pp. 497] is utilized, originally intended to evaluate the automatic detection of lines. The measure

$$R = \frac{1}{I_N} \sum_{i=1}^{I_A} \frac{1}{1 + \delta\left(x_i, I\right)} \tag{6}$$

compares the distances $\delta\left(x_i, I\right)$ of claimed boundary pixels $x_i \in A$ to assumed ideal boundary pixels I with $I_N = max\left(I_I, I_A\right)$. Equation 6 yields a range of $]0..1]$ where values close to 0 correspond to high discrepancies and a value of 1 corresponds to an ideal matching of a pair of boundaries.

4　Results

Results of the proposed method using network snakes and using the conventional method are presented in figure 1. 17 cells are detected applying the network snakes approach (Fig. 1a), and 25 cells are segmented with the conventional watershed-based algorithm (Fig. 1b). Figure 1c illustrates the Pratt values for all pairs of cell boundaries from the two segmentation techniques. The 25 rows and 17 columns of the table correspond to the objects from the conventional and from the network snake approach, respectively. The Pratt values are given in circles, where larger circles correspond to a better match of the pair. To enhance the result, circle radii have been computed as $(1 + R)^2 - 1$. In order to provide a scale, the black circle at the bottom right is given, which represents an ideal match $R = 1$. Those circles that actually denote pairs of objects that belong to an identical cell are depicted with a white filling.

Three important observations can be made from the analysis. First, those circles that denote correct correspondences are by far the largest; this means segmentation with network snakes performs well enough to identify cells. Of course, the underlying assumption is based on correct reference data contributed by the conventional method. Second, the matching scores are smaller than the ideal value of 1. This distortion is due to the nature of both techniques: While conventional treatment of local intensities is bound to have a frayed border, the modeled shape behavior of snakes let boundaries appear smoother. However, it is this difference in the borders that decreases the interpretability of the Pratt value. Third, the proposed method using network snakes does not consider incomplete cells at the image boundary and, thus, less cells are segmented. Independently of image border effects any cells have been extracted successfully.

5 Discussion

This contribution compares a new segmentation technique of delineating adjacent cells in confocal images – the analysis with network snakes – to a typical conventional algorithm. It is known that the construction of a gold standard for segmentation evaluation is problematic. The used Pratt method is meaningful, even though it can not cover an overall set of assessment criteria. The comparison cannot conclude whether the candidate algorithm performs better than the standard but it can give an impression of its quality *in terms of* the state-of-the-art. Considering the vast differences that human testers produce in manually segmented images, we claim that the proposed method is justifiable. An important conclusion relates to the shape behavior of the cell boundaries: within the network snakes approach the modeled shape is represented in a smoother and more natural way compared to the watershed-based conventional approach, which could not be reflected in the evaluation in a positive manner.

References

1. Butenuth M. Segmentation of Imagery Using Network Snakes. International Archives of Photogrammetry, Remote Sensing and Spatial Information Sciences 2006;36(3):1-6.
2. Pratt WK. Digital Image Processing. Wiley-Interscience, New York; 1978.
3. Roerdink JBTM, Meijster A. The watershed transform: Definitions, algorithms and parallelization strategies. Fundamenta Informaticae 2001;41:187–228.
4. Jetzek F, Rahn CD, Dreschler-Fischer L. Ein geometrisches Modell für die Zellsegmentierung. Procs BVM 2006; 121–125.
5. Kass M, Witkin A, Terzopoulos D. Snakes: Active contour models. Int J Comp Vis 1988;1(4):321–331.
6. Wählby C, Lindblad J, Vondrus M, Bengtsson E, Björkesten L. Algorithms for cytoplasm segmentation of fluorescence labelled cells. Analytical Cellular Pathology 2002;24(2–3):101–111.

Berandungsgenaue Segmentierung von Plasma und Nucleus bei Leukozyten

Thomas Rehn[1,2], Thorsten Zerfaß[1], Thomas Wittenberg[1]

[1]Fraunhofer-Institut für Integrierte Schaltungen IIS, Erlangen
[2]Universität Magdeburg
Email: thorsten.zerfass@iis.fraunhofer.de

Zusammenfassung. Die exakte Segmentierung von Zellkern und Zellplasma weißer Blutzellen bildet die Grundlage für die Erstellung eines automatischen, bildbasierten Differentialblutbildes. In diesem Beitrag wird ein Verfahren zur entsprechenden Segmentierung von Leukozyten vorgestellt. Nach einer Vorverarbeitung durch einen Kuwahara-Filter wird ein Fast-Marching-Verfahren zur Bestimmung der groben Zellumrisse bestimmt. Um die Zellfläche zu erhalten, wird anschließend ein Kürzester-Pfad-Algorithmus angewandt. Die Markierung des Zellkerns erfolgt durch eine Schwellenwertoperation. Eine Evaluierung des Verfahrens wurde auf einer repräsentativen Stichprobe von 80 Bildern durchgeführt und mit einer Handsegmentierung auf der Basis des Dice-Koeffizient und sowie der Hausdorff-Distanz verglichen.

1 Einleitung

Die sichere Erkennung und exakte Segmentierung von weißen Blutzellen (Leukozyten) in gefärbten Ausstrichen des peripheren Blutes bildet die Grundlage für eine automatische, bildbasierte Erstellung eines sog. Differenzialblutbildes im Kontext der medizinischen Labordiagnostik (sog. Computer Assistierte Mikroskopie – CAM). Die Vielfältigkeit der in einem Blutausstrich auftretenden weißen Blutzellen, verbunden mit ihrer jeweils charakteristischen Farbverteilung und Texturierung, erhöhen die Schwierigkeit bei der Klassifikation im Rahmen einer vollständigen Automatisierung. Während die automatische Detektion und Segmentierung weisser Blutzellen in digitalen Bildern mittlerweiler zum Stand der Technik gehört, ist die anschließende berandungsgenaue Segmentierung von Zellkern und speziell des Zellplasmas im Hinblick einer nachfolgenden Klassifikation noch nicht zufiedenstellend gelöst.

2 Stand der Forschung und Fortschritt durch den Beitrag

Bekannte Ansätze zur Segmentierung von Zellplasma *und* Zellkern weißer Blutzellen greifen oftmals auf Schwellwertverfahren zurück [1, 2]. Ein in [3] vorgeschlagenes Verfahren führt zusätzlich wahrscheinlichkeitstheoretische Elemente ein, um eine Unterscheidung in Hintergrund, rote Blutkörperchen, sowie Kern und Plasma der Leukozyten zu treffen. Ein Active Contour-Verfahren zur Zellumrissbestimmung kommt in [4] zum Einsatz. Der in [5] vorgestellte Ansatz setzt auf Scale-Space-Filtering zur Bestimmung des Zellkerns und 3D-Watershed-Clustering des ins HSV-Modell transformierten Bildes.

Im Gegensatz zu den genannten Ansätzen wird in diesem Beitrag ein neuartiger Ansatz vorgestellt werden, der Level-Set- und Fast-Marching-Methoden mit einem Kürzester-Pfad-Algorithmus kombiniert, um eine vollständige und berandungsgenaue Segmentierung von Zellkern und Zellplasma zu erreichen.

3   Methoden

Als Ausgangsmaterial wurden Lichtmikroskopaufnahmen von Blutabstrichen verwendet, die mit einer MGG-Färbung behandelt wurden. Entsprechende farbliche Charakteristika finden ihren Niederschlag in der Wahl der Parametrisierung des folgenden Verfahrens. Um die Segmentierung automatisch durchführen zu können wurde ein dreistufiger Algorithmus entwickelt, der sich grob in Bildvorverarbeitung, Auffinden von Kern und Plasma und Nachbearbeitung und Feinkorrektur unterteilen lässt.

3.1   Vorverarbeitung

Da einige Bildelemente wie rote Blutkörperchen (bläulicher Rand durch die Färbung und Optik) und Granulozyten (Textur mit relativ hochfrequente farblicher Varianz) lokal mit atypischen oder den Hauptalgorithmus störenden Eigenschaften versehen sind, werden die Bilder mit einem kantenerhaltenden und rauschunterdrückenden Kuwahara-Filter vorverarbeitet [6].

3.2   Finden von Kern und Plasma

Um die Empfindlichkeit gegenüber Schwankungen der Farbkomponenten weiter zu reduzieren, findet die weitere Verarbeitung nach einer Transformation des RGB-Eingangsbildes im HSV-Modell statt. Als erstes werden mittels eines Schwellenwertverfahrens (Thresholding) Kandidaten für den relativ einfach grob zu lokalisierenden Zellkern (dunkle Blaufärbung) bestimmt. Diese dienen zunächst weniger zur Markierung als viel mehr zur Mittelpunktsbestimmung der Zelle. Innerhalb dieser Kandidatenmenge N werden zufällig n Punkte $S \subset N$ ausgewählt und derjenige, der $\min_{x \in S} \sum_{y \in S} d(x, y)$ erfüllt, also den geringsten Abstand zu allen anderen Punkten aus S hat, zum vorläufigen Mittelpunkt m_{seed} erklärt. Als nächstes folgt die Bestimmung von Punkten knapp außerhalb des Zellplasmas beziehungsweise eine Markierung des letzteren, um die Kontur der Zelle erfassen zu können. Hierbei kommt ein Fast-Marching-Algorithmus zum Einsatz [7], der eine diskrete Variante der Eikonal-Gleichung $\|\nabla u(x)\| F(x) = 1$ in u löst, welche die Ausbreitung einer Welle, ausgehend von m_{seed} in Abhängigkeit der den Pixeln zu Grunde liegenden Farbeigenschaften F, simuliert. Im Optimalfall ist durch $\{u < F(m_{seed}) + \varepsilon\}$ mit geeigneter Funktion

F und ε bereits die Zelle beschrieben. Dass dies in der Realität fast nie gegeben ist, liegt zumeist in der unscharfen Trennung der weißen und roten Zellen begründet; das Resultat ist aber zumeist sehr gut geeignet um mit einem anderen Verfahren eine vollständige Trennung herbeizuführen. Als brauchbar für die Segmentierung von Leukozyten hat sich die Funktion F von der folgenden Struktur herausgestellt:

$$F(x) = \begin{cases} \beta & \text{falls } c(x) \geq \alpha_1 \vee (c(x) \geq \alpha_2 \wedge v(x) \leq \gamma) \\ 0 & \text{sonst} \end{cases} \tag{1}$$

Hierbei ist mit $c(x)$ die Summe der drei Farbkomponenten im RGB-Raum und mit $v(x)$ die Value-Komponente im HSV-Modell im Punkte x bezeichnet. Die Parameter sind so zu wählen, dass mittels α_1 der Bild-Hintergrund und α_2 bzw. γ alles außerhalb von Hintergrund, Zellkern ($c(x) < \alpha_2$) und Zellplasma ($v(x) > \gamma$) erfasst wird. Um nicht von einer speziellen Farbsituation abhängig zu sein, wurde eine iterative Anpassung des wichtigen Parameters γ implementiert, α_1 und α_2 können für Bilderserien unter gleichen Aufnahmebedingungen unverändert bleiben. Der Wert von γ wird von einem niedrigen Niveau ausgehend schrittweise erhöht, bis bei Lauf in Nord-, Süd-, West- und Ostrichtung von Punkten nahe von m_{seed} jeweils Punkte p_N, p_S, p_W, p_O aus $\{u > F(m_{\text{seed}}) + \varepsilon\}$ gefunden werden, die nach Wahl der Parameter den Bereich außerhalb der Zelle markieren sollen. Anschließend kann mittels eines Wegfindungsalgorithmus ein Pfad entlang der Kontur der Zelle bestimmt werden. So führt eine Dijkstra-Variante unter Verwendung einer farbabhängigen Kostenfunktion $c(x,y)$ für die (gerichtete) Kante zwischen benachbarten Punkte x und y (8er Nachbarschaft) mit

$$c(x,y) = \|x - y\|_2 \cdot \left(1 + \alpha \mathbf{1}_{\{u < F(m_{\text{seed}}) + \varepsilon\}}(y)\right) +$$
$$\beta \|m_{\text{seed}} - y\|_2 + \gamma \mathbf{1}_{H_{blue}}(h(y)) \tag{2}$$

zur gewünschten Trennung der Zelle von ihrer Umgebung, wobei $h(x)$ den Hue-Wert im HSV-Modell im Punkt x und H_{blue} eine Untermenge des blauen Hue-Wertebereichs, sowie $\mathbf{1}_A(x)$ die Indikatorfunktion der Menge A bezeichnet. Die Parameter α und γ sorgen dafür, dass der Pfad möglichst nicht über die bläulich gefärbte Zelle verläuft, während β den Weg auch nicht allzu weit von der Zelle wegführen lässt.

Auf solche Weise bestimmte Pfade, die die vier Punkte p_N, p_S, p_W, p_O durch vier Teilpfade verbinden, markieren oftmals den Zellenumriss schon recht genau. Das oben beschriebene Schwellwertverfahren zur Bestimmung des Zellkerns ist zwar geeignet einen guten Ausgangspunkt m_{seed} innerhalb der zu segmentierenden Zelle zu finden, hat sich jedoch als ungeeignet erwiesen den vollen für das menschliche Auge als solchen wahrnehmbaren Zellkern zu erfassen. Für diese Aufgabe wurde ein anderes Schwellwertverfahren, das beim Verhältnis zwischen Blau- und Grün-Kanal des RGB-Eingangsbildes ansetzt, verwendet.

Abb. 1. Von links nach rechts: Ausgangsbild, $u(x)$ mittels Fast-Marching-Algorithmus, Ergebnis vor und nach der Nachbearbeitung

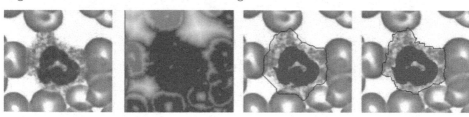

3.3   Nachverarbeitung

Da es sich gezeigt hat, dass mit Hilfe des oben beschriebenen Verfahrens bestimmte Pfade Konkavitäten des Zellplasmas nicht gerecht werden, ist eine Nachbearbeitung des Pfades notwendig. Dabei genügt es den Pfad punktweise in Richtung m_{seed} zu verschieben, solange sich die Punkte auf dem durch die Farbe klar zu erkennenden Hintergrund oder auf auch roten Blutkörperchen befinden. Die so erhaltene Punktemenge, jeweils durch Kanten verbunden und geglättet, stellt das Ergebnis des gesamten Verfahrens das Zellplasma betreffend dar.

Auch der Zellkern bedarf eines Nachverarbeitungschrittes, der mittels eines morphologischen Open-Close-Filters störende, isoliert liegende Punkte entfernt.

4   Ergebnisse

Die Leistungsfähigkeit des vorgestellten Algorithmus wurde anhand einer Sammlung von 80 Proben überprüft, die die verschiedensten Typen von Leukozyten enthält. Dabei wurde mit Hilfe verschiedener Kenngrößen die Qualität der automatischen Segmentierung mit einer zuvor per Hand durchgeführten Segmentierung verglichen. Bei der Evaluation zum Einsatz kamen zum einen der Dice-Koeffizient

$$C_D(A, B) = \frac{2|A \cap B|}{|A| + |B|} \tag{3}$$

sowie eine normierte Hausdorff-Metrik

$$H(A, B) = \frac{\max_{x \in A} \min_{y \in B} \|x - y\| + \max_{y \in B} \min_{x \in A} \|x - y\|}{2 \max\{\operatorname{diam} A, \operatorname{diam} B\}} \tag{4}$$

Die Ergebnisse sind für Zellkern und -plasma getrennt in Tabelle 1 aufgeführt. Die optischen Eindrücke der Segmentierungsergebnisse, die in Abb. 2 zu sehen sind, bestätigen die guten Resultate der Evaluierung durch Kennzahlen.

5   Diskussion

In diesem Beitrag wird ein Verfahren zur Segmentierung von Leukozyten in Kern und Plasma in Bildern von Blutausstrichen vorgestellt. Nach einer Vorverarbeitung durch einen Kuwahara-Filter wird ein Fast-Marching-Verfahren zur

Abb. 2. Beispiele für Segmentierungsergebnisse von Zellkern und Zellplasma

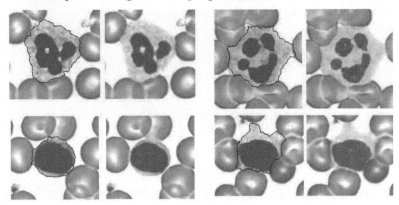

Tabelle 1. Ergebnisse der Evaluation für eine Serie von **80** Bildern

	C_D	H
Zellplasma	0.94 ± 0.02	0.91 ± 0.03
Zellkern	0.94 ± 0.02	0.90 ± 0.04

Bestimmung der groben Zellumrisse bestimmt und dann ein Kürzester-Pfad-Algorithmus, der zum großen Teil auf den bestimmten Level Sets operiert angewandt, um die Zellfläche zu erhalten. Die Markierung des Zellkerns kann im Wesentlichen durch reine Schwellwertoperationen erfolgen. Die damit erzielten Ergebnisse erreichen bei einer Evaluierung sowohl auf visueller Basis als auch mittels Standard-Maßzahlen wie Dice-Koeffizient und Hausdorff-Distanz gute Ergebnisse.

Literaturverzeichnis

1. Cseke I. A fast segmentation scheme for white blood cell images. In: 11th IAPR Int. Conf. on Pattern Recognition Vol.III: Image, Speech & Signal Analysis; 1992. 530–533.
2. Liao Q, Deng Y. An accurate segmentation method for white blood cell images. In: IEEE Intl. Sym. on Biomedical Imaging; 2002. 245–248.
3. Ramoser H, Laurain V, Bischof H, et al. Leukocyte segmentation and classification in blood-smear images. IEEE Engineering in Medicine and Biology Society 2005; 3371–3374.
4. Ongun G, Halici U, Leblebicioglu K, et al. An automated differential blood count system. IEEE Eng in Med and Biology 2001;3:2583–2586.
5. Jiang K, Liao QM, Xiong Y. A novel white blood cell segmentation scheme based on feature space clustering. Soft Comput 2006;10(1):12–19.
6. Chen S, Shih TY. On the evaluation of edge preserving smoothing filter. In: Proceedings of Geoinformatics; 2002. paper C43.
7. Sethian JA. Levelset methods and fast marching methods. Cambridge University Press; 1999.

Chromatinmuster-basierte Zellklassifizierung für die DNS-Bildzytometrie an Mundschleimhaut-Abstrichen

Timna Schneider[1], André Bell[1], Gerlind Herberich[1], Dietrich Meyer-Ebrecht,[1] Alfred Böcking[2], Til Aach[1]

[1]Lehrstuhl für Bildverarbeitung, RWTH Aachen, 52064 Aachen
[2]Institut für Cythopathologie, Heinrich-Heine-Universität, 40225 Düsseldorf
Email: timna.schneider@lfb.rwth-aachen.de

Zusammenfassung. Mit zytopathologischen Methoden kann Krebs sehr früh schon anhand geringfügiger Normabweichungen in einzelnen Zellen erkannt werden. Nachteil ist oft der derzeit benötigte Zeitaufwand eines Zytopathologen, der insbesondere einen Einsatz als Screening-Verfahren ausschliesst. Eine wichtige zytologische Diagnosemethode ist die DNS-Bildzytometrie. Um deren Zeitaufwand zu reduzieren, müssen für die Messung relevante Zellen automatisch detektiert werden. Für Epithelien der Mundschleimhaut vergleichen wir daher verschiedene Varianten des k-Nächste-Nachbarn-Klassifikators (kNN), um zwischen sicher gesunden und krebsverdächtigen Zellbildern zu unterscheiden. Geeignete Merkmalskombinationen wurden durch das Floating-Search-Verfahren ausgewählt.

1 Einleitung

Die DNS-Bildzytometrie ordnet jeder Zelle als objektive Messgröße ihren DNS-Gehalt zu. Nach dem stöchiometrischen Färben einer Probe nach Feulgen werden dazu die integralen optischen Dichten der Kerne berechnet. Um aus diesen den DNS-Gehalt zu bestimmen, werden zunächst Referenzzellen gesucht. In Abstrichen der Mundschleimhaut sind das gesunde Epithelzellen mit doppeltem Chromosomensatz (2c) als DNS-Gehalt. Der DNS-Gehalt der diagnostisch relevanten Analysezellen, also von auffällig veränderten und damit krebsverdächtigen Epithelien, läßt sich dann aus dem Verhältnis ihrer optischen Dichten zu der Dichte der Referenzzellen berechnen. Basierend auf einem Histogramm des DNS-Gehaltes der ausgewählten Analysezellen wird schliesslich die Diagnose gestellt.

Die manuelle Selektion von Referenz- und Analysezellen ist zeitaufwändig und sollte durch eine automatische Vorauswahl messrelevanter Zellen unterstützt werden. Dies wird bei Mundschleimhaut-Präparaten dadurch erschwert, dass Referenz- und krebsverdächtige Analysezellen nicht aus verschiedenen Zelltypen gewählt werden können, sondern an demselben Zelltyp unterschieden werden müssen. Neben morphologischen Auffälligkeiten ist dabei das Chromatinmuster, d.h. die Textur innerhalb des Zellkerns, von entscheidender Bedeutung.

2   Stand der Forschung

Für die standardisierte DNS-Bildzytometrie [1] werden durch den Zytopathologen interaktiv neben ca. 30 normalen Referenzzellen ca. 300 auffällige, zu messende Analysezellen ausgewählt. Eine andere Vorgehensweise besteht im automatischen Messen des DNS-Gehalts *aller* auf dem Objektträger vorhandenen Exemplare des Analysezelltyps. Dies ermöglicht zwar einen Einsatz als Screening-Verfahren und ist auch bei fehlendem Fachpersonal einsetzbar, wenn die Anzahl von Krebszellen in einem Präparat aber im Verhältnis zur Anzahl gesunder Zellen eher gering ist, kann es zu falsch-negativen Diagnosen kommen. Die DNS-Verteilung einer Krebszellpopulation wird dann im Histogramm von derjenigen der gesunden Population überlagert und somit nicht wahrnehmbar. Eine Tumorzell-positive Diagnose kann daher nur bei Detektion von unter Umständen selten vorkommenden Zellen mit abnormal hohem DNS-Gehalt gestellt werden. Für die Automatisierung wollen wir aber die Sensitivität der manuell durchgeführten DNS-Bildzytometrie erreichen. Dies soll durch eine automatische Auswahl auffällig veränderter Zellen erfolgen, anhand deren DNS-Verteilung letztlich entschieden wird, ob die Veränderung tatsächlich Krebs entspricht.

Existierende Ansätze für diagnostische Systeme arbeiten basierend auf morphologischer und textureller Analyse von meist morphologisch gefärbten Zellen [2, 3, 4]. Neben reinen Formmerkmalen finden häufig moment- oder histogrammbasierte Texturmerkmale Anwendung [5]. Spezielle weitere Merkmale für die Chromatinmusteranalyse finden sich in [5, 6].

3   Methoden

Unsere Basis-Merkmalsmenge besteht aus morphologischen Merkmalen wie Fläche, Umfang, Formfaktor, sowie aus Fourier-Deskriptor-basierten Merkmalen. Weiterhin verwenden wir affin invariante momentbasierte Merkmale [7], sowie zusätzlich unabhängige momentbasierte Merkmale [8]. Diese sind berechnet für die Kernmaske als Erweiterung der morphologischen Merkmale, sowie für Extinction- [5] und Flat-Texture-Bild [5] als Texturmerkmale. Extinction- und Flat-Texture-Bild basieren beide auf dem Grünkanal des Originalbildes. Hinzu kommen histogrammbasierte Merkmale über das topologische Gradientenbild [5] und Merkmale wie Klumpigkeit, Homogenität, Verdichtung des Chromatinmusters zum Kernrand nach [6]. Unsere Merkmalsmenge umfasst derzeit insgesamt 203 Merkmale zur Beschreibung von Zellkernmorphologie und -textur.

Für die Ermittlung geeigneter Merkmalskombinationen (ohne alle möglichen Kombinationen zu testen) verwenden wir als parameterloses Suchverfahren Sequential Forward Floating Search (SFFS) [9]. Die Bewertung verschiedener Merkmalskombinationen erfolgt dabei durch die Bhattacharyya-Distanz [10], das Scatter-Matrix-Kriterium [11] sowie Mutual-Information [12] als Gütefunktionen.

Anforderungen an den Klassifikator sind die Nachvollziehbarkeit des Klassifikationsalgorithmus und der Fehlklassifikationen durch den medizinischen Partner, wie auch ein Konfidenzmass für die erfolgte Klassenzuordnung. Dieses ermöglicht darüberhinaus eine Sortierung der Zellen nach Auffälligkeit. Ohne eine

Tabelle 1. Ergebnis der Merkmalsauswahl. Aufgelistet sind pro Merkmalsgruppe die Klassifikationsraten (A;R;G) von (A)nalyse- und (R)eferenzzellen, sowie gemittelter (G)esamtrate in Prozent, das Gütekriterium ((M)utual-Information, (S)catter-Matrix-Kriterium, (B)hattacharyya-Distanz), die Anzahl der Merkmale, sowie Anzahl nächster Nachbarn des kNN für die beste Gesamtrate der Trainingsmenge. Die beiden gefundenen Merkmalskombinationen für Chromatin+Momente und Gesamtmerkmale sind identisch.

Merkmalsgruppe	Klassifikationsrate (A;R;G)	Güte-kriterium	Anzahl Merkmale	Anzahl Nachbarn des kNN
Morphologie	75, 5; 92, 3; 85, 2	B	14	3
Grünkanal-Chromatin	92, 5; 95, 2; 94, 1	B	14	1
Extinction-Chromatin	90, 2; 96, 5; 93, 8	B	19	3
Chromatin+Momente	90, 7; 98, 3; 95, 1	M	2	4
Gesamtmerkmale	90, 7; 98, 3; 95, 1	M	2	4

sinnvolle Annahme über ein parametrisches Verteilungsmodell treffen zu können, verwenden wir deshalb kNN und Fuzzy-kNN (F-kNN) zur Unterscheidung von Analyse- und Referenzzellen. Der F-kNN [13] wurde einmal mit der vom Zytopathologen klassifizierten {0, 1}-Klassenzugehörigkeit der Trainingsdaten trainiert (F-kNN-a) und zum anderen mit einer zu den Klassenmittelpunkten abstandsgewichteten Klassenzugehörigkeit (F-kNN-b). Letzterer berücksichtigt insbesondere im Übergangsbereich zwischen Referenz- und Analysezellen, wie repräsentativ eine Zelle für eine Klasse ist. Als kNN trainierten wir eine Variante, die solange sucht, bis k Nachbarn der gleichen Klasse gefunden sind.

4   Experimente und Ergebnisse

Unsere Datenbasis besteht aus Feulgen-gefärbten, segmentierten Epithelzellkernen der Mundschleimhaut. Von einem Zytopathologen wurden 950 Referenzzellen aus 10 krebszellnegativen und 748 Analysezellen aus 5 krebszellpositiven Abstrich-Präparaten klassifiziert. Davon wurden 1300 Zellen als Trainingsmenge und 200 Referenz- sowie 198 Analysezellen als Validierungsmenge verwendet. Die Zellbilder wurden mit einem 63-fach Öl-Immersionsobjektiv und einer 3-Chip CCD-Kamera aufgenommen mit einer resultierenden Auflösung von $\approx 0.1\mu m$ Pixelkantenlänge.

Die Merkmale wurden auf den Bereich [0, 1] normalisiert und zu fünf verschiedenen Merkmalsgruppen zusammengefasst: Morphologie, Grünkanal-Chromatin, Extinction-Chromatin, Chromatin+Momente (Kombination beider Chroma-tin-Gruppen inkl. momentbasierter Merkmale auf Extinction- und Flat-Texture-Bild) und alle Merkmale zusammengefasst in Gesamtmerkmale. Für jede dieser Merkmalsgruppen wurden für alle drei Gütekriterien geeignete Merkmalskombinationen berechnet und durch Leave-one-out Cross-validation auf der Trainingsmenge mittels kNN-Klassifikator für k von 1, .., 10 bewertet (Tab. 1). Mit den besten Merkmalskombinationen pro Merkmalsgruppe wurden durch Klassifikation mit kNN und Fuzzy-kNN die Gesamt- und Einzelklassifikationsraten für

Tabelle 2. Validierung der Merkmalskombinationen und Klassifikatoren aus Tabelle 1 an der Validierungsmenge. Aufgelistet sind pro Merkmalsgruppe die Klassifikationsraten (A;R;G) von (A)nalyse- und (R)eferenzzellen, sowie die gemittelten (G)esamtraten der verschiedenen Klassifikatoren kNN, F-kNN-a, sowie F-kNN-b

Merkmalsgruppe	kNN (A;R;G)	F-kNN-a (A;R;G)	F-kNN-b (A;R;G)
Morphologie	$75, 3; 92, 5; 85, 4$	$77, 7; 88, 5; 83, 2$	$57, 6; 98, 5; 78, 1$
Grünkanal-Chromatin	$91, 9; 97, 5; 94, 7$	$91, 9; 97, 5; 94, 7$	$80, 3; 93, 0; 86, 7$
Extinction-Chromatin	$93, 9; 95, 5; 94, 7$	$91, 9; 94, 5; 93, 2$	$73, 7; 93, 0; 83, 4$
Chromatin+Momente/ Gesamtmerkmale	$92, 4; 98, 5; 95, 5$	$93, 9; 97, 5; 95, 7$	$65, 7; 85, 5; 75, 6$

die Validierungsmenge berechnet (Tab. 2). Die beiden Merkmale, die in Kombination die beste Trennrate erzielten, sind das Moment 0-ter Ordnung berechnet im Extinction-Bild (IMTOTE in [5]) als eine Schätzung der optischen Dichte, sowie der Median des Histogramms des topologischen Gradientenbildes (RG in [5]) des Grünkanals als ein Maß für die Inhomogenität der Chromatinverteilung.

5 Diskussion

Auffällig ist die durchgängig unterschiedliche Klassifikationsleistung zwischen beiden Zellklassen. Ein wesentlicher Grund liegt in der unterschiedlichen Anzahl von Trainingsdaten beider Klassen, so dass die Klasse der Analysezellen zukünftig um weitere Musterzellen erweitert, oder ein anderes Klassifikationsverfahren angewendet werden muss. Das vergleichsweise schwache Abschneiden des F-kNN-b zeigt, dass die Voraussetzung gleicher Varianz zwischen beiden Klassen nicht erfüllt ist. Eine Analyse der Klassifikationsergebnisse ergab, dass für 7 der 12 falsch klassifizierten Analysezellen der DNS-Gehalt im Bereich des c-Wertes von Referenzzellen (zwischen 1.8c und 2.21c) lag. Relevant für die DNS-Bildzytometrie ist die optische Dichte der Referenzzellen und damit ihr c-Wert, nicht jedoch eine mögliche Chromatinmuster-Aberration. Diese Fehlklassifikationen haben somit nur einen geringfügigen Einfluss auf das diagnostisch relevante DNS-Histogramm. Unter den Fehlklassifikationen befanden sich darüberhinaus meist ausschliesslich Zellen der Gegenklasse unter den nächsten Nachbarn (Abb. 1). Ein Einsatz des Verfahrens in der Routine, d.h. die Klassifikation von segmentierten Objekten auf verschiedenen Objektträgern, sowie eine Untersuchung des Einflusses von Färbevariabilitäten, können nun getestet werden. Die gefundene Merkmalskombination korreliert mit dem Vorgehen der Zytologen und läßt damit eine Nachvollziehbarkeit der Entscheidung des Klassifikators zu. Zukünftig ist zu untersuchen, ob eine Feulgenfarbspektrum angepasste Filterung zu einer weiteren Verbesserung der Klassifikationsraten führt.

Danksagung

Das Projekt wird vom Viktor-und-Mirka-Pollak-Fonds unterstützt.

Abb. 1. Falschklassifikationen aus F-kNN-a: Spalte a) enthält zwei klassifizierte Zellen der Validierungsmenge. In Zeile 1 ist eine fälschlich als Referenzzelle klassifizierte Analysezelle, in Zeile 2 eine als Analysezelle klassifizierte Referenzzelle dargestellt. die Spalten b) bis e) enthalten die 4 nächsten Nachbarn der Gegenklasse

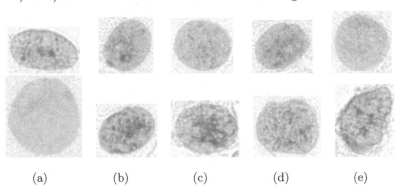

(a)   (b)   (c)   (d)   (e)

Literaturverzeichnis

1. Böcking A, et al. Consensus report of the ESACP task force on standardization of diagnostic DNA image cytometry. Anal Cell Pathol 1995;8(1):67–74.
2. Wittenberg T, Neubauer K, Küblbeck C, et al. Automatische Tumorerkennung bei unterschiedlichen Organen mittels Berechnung und Klassifikation von Texturmerkmalen. Procs BVM 2001; 377–381.
3. Fischer B, Palm C, Lehmann TM, et al. Selektion von Farbtexturmerkmalen zur Tumorklassifikation dermatoskopischer Fotografien. Procs BVM 2002; 338–341.
4. Zhou ZH, Jiang Y, Yang YB, et al. Lung cancer cell identification based on artificial neural network ensembles. Artif Intell Med 2002;24(1):25–36.
5. Rodenacker K, Bengtsson E. A feature set for cytometry on digitized microscopic images. Anal Cell Pathol 2003;25(1):1–36.
6. Young IT, Verbeek PW, Mayall BH. Characterization of chromatin distribution in cell nuclei. Cytometry 1986;7(5):467–474.
7. Reiss TH. Recognizing Planar Objecs Using Invariant Image Features. Springer; 1991.
8. Suk T, Flusser J. Graph Method for Generating Affine Moment Invariants. In: Procs ICPR. vol. 2; 2004. 192–195.
9. Pudil P, Novovičová J, Kittler J. Floating search methods in feature selection. Pattern Recognition Letters 1994;15(11):1119–1125.
10. Fukunaga K. Statistical Pattern Recognition. Academic Press; 1990.
11. Duda RO, et al. Pattern Classification. John Wiley & Sons; 2001.
12. Pluim JPW, Maintz JBA, Viergever MA. Mutual information based registration of medical images: a survey. IEEE Trans Med Imaging 2003;22(8):986–1004.
13. Keller JM, Gray MR, Givens JA. A Fuzzy K-Nearest Neighbor Algorithm. IEEE Trans Syst Man Cybern 1985;SMC-15(4):580–585.

Visual Computing zur Analyse von zerebralen arteriovenösen Malformationen in 3D- und 4D-MR Bilddaten

Dennis Säring[1], Jens Fiehler[2], Nils Forkert[1], Milena Piening[2], Heinz Handels[1]

[1]Institut für Medizinische Informatik
[2]Klinik und Poliklinik für Neuroradiologische Diagnostik und Intervention
Universitätsklinikum Hamburg-Eppendorf, 20246 Hamburg
Email: d.saering@uke.uni-hamburg.de

Zusammenfassung. Im Beitrag werden Verfahren zur Visualisierung und Analyse von zerebralen arteriovenösen Malformationen (AVM) präsentiert. Als Eingabe dienen hochaufgelöste 3D- sowie zeitlich-räumliche 4D-MRT-Daten. Ein Ziel dieser Arbeit ist die Kombination von räumlichen und zeitlichen Informationen. Bei der vorgestellten Methode wird zunächst in den 3D-MRT-Daten das Gefäßsystem segmentiert und daraus ein Oberflächenmodell erzeugt. In einem weiteren Schritt werden in den 4D-MRT-Daten für jedes Voxel der Signalverlauf über die Zeit analysiert und die berechneten Einströmzeitpunkte in einem 3D-Parameterbild gespeichert. Ein affines Registrierungsverfahren ermöglicht die farbcodierte Darstellung der zeitlichen Parameter in den räumlich hochaufgelösten Schichten und den Oberflächenmodellen. Diese kombinierte Visualisierung der komplizierten Struktur und der Hämodynamik unterstützt den Mediziner bei der räumlichen Beurteilung von AVM.

1 Einleitung

Die zerebrale arteriovenöse Malformation (AVM) ist eine Fehlbildung des Gefäßsystems im Gehirn. Durch eine AVM wird das sauerstoffreiche Blut von den arteriellen Gefäßen zum großen Teil direkt ohne Kapillarbett in die venösen Gefäße geleitet und es kann zu einer Sauerstoffunterversorgung des Gehirns kommen. Diese Kurzschlussverbindung erhöht durch den anormal hohen Blutdruck in den Venen das Risiko einer schweren intrazerebralen Blutung. Für die Behandlung von AVM stehen u.a. endovaskuläre Embolisation, neurochirurgische Operation und stereotaktische Radiochirurgie sowie deren Kombination zur Verfügung [1]. Hierbei sind Lokalisation und Quantifizierung der AVM, Detektion von zuführenden (Feeder) und abfließenden Gefäßen (draining veins) sowie Beurteilung des zeitlichen Einströmverlaufes des Blutes von besonderem Interesse. In der Klinik werden dazu neben der zeitlich hochaufgelösten digitalen 2D-Subtraktionsangiographie (DSA) auch neue 3D- und 4D-MRT-Aufnahmetechniken verwendet. Hierbei stellt die DSA als invasive Prozedur mit einer Komplikationsrate von bis zu 0,5% für Therapieverlaufskontrollen ein erhöhtes Risiko dar.

Das Softwaresystem AnToNIa[1] wurde zur kombinierten Visualisierung und Analyse von räumlichen und räumlich-zeitlichen MRT-Datensätzen entwickelt. Mit seiner Hilfe sollen nicht-invasive 3D- und 4D-MRT-Bildsequenzen kombiniert, qualitativ und quantitativ unter Verwendung neuer Visualsierungstechniken für AVM und Feeder analysiert und visuell mit der DSA verglichen werden. Der Grundgedanke ist hierbei, die zeitaufgelöste Information im dreidimensionalen Raum darzustellen und so eine Betrachtung aus beliebigen Betrachtungswinkeln und Schnittebenen zu ermöglichen. Die Informationen über die individuelle Struktur der AVM sollen die Therapieplanung und Verlaufskontrolle unterstützen.

2 Stand der Forschung und wesentlicher Fortschritt

Für die Diagnostik der AVM werden unterschiedliche bildgebende Verfahren eingesetzt. MRT-Daten ermöglichen u.a. die Differenzierung von kleinen AVM und die Erkennung von großen zuführenden und abführenden Gefäßen [2]. Die DSA erlaubt insbesondere eine präzise hämodynamische Diagnose und ist derzeit unerlässlich für die Prognoseeinschätzung und Therapieplanung. MRT-Datensätze mit annähernd ähnlicher zeitlicher Auflösung (0,5ms) sind erst durch die Entwicklung von 3T Hochfeldgeräten mit parallelen Bildgebungstechniken möglich geworden. Mit der Unterstützung durch AnToNIa soll untersucht werden, inwieweit die 4D-MRT-Datensätze eine Alternative zur DSA darstellen.

Die Anzahl der Veröffentlichungen, welche sich mit der Segmentierung, computergestützten Analyse und Visualisierung von Gefäßsystemen des Gehirns beschäftigen, ist hoch. Jedoch ist ein Segmentierungs- oder Analysetool speziell für die Problematik einer komplizierten arteriovenösen Malformation den Autoren nicht bekannt. In Bullitt [3] wird die AVM mit Volume-Rendering Technik in Kombination mit den Oberflächenmodellen der Gefäße dargestellt und so eine Visualisierung der komplizierten Struktur ermöglicht. Eine zusätzliche Kombination mit 4D-MRT-Bilddaten wird dort nicht beschrieben.

AnToNIa unterstützt durch semi-automatische Segmentierung und integrierte 3D-Visualisierungstechniken die Beurteilung der komplizierten räumlichen Strukturen der AVM. Durch die Registrierung von 3D- und 4D-MRT-Bilddaten wird das Einblenden zeitlicher Information über die Hämodynamik ermöglicht.

3 Methoden

Mit Hilfe von neuen parallelen Bildgebungstechniken, wie beispielsweise GRAPPA (generalized autocalibrating partially parallel acquisition), können zeitaufgelöste kontrastmittelgestützte 4D-TREAT-Sequenzen (time-resolved echo-shared MR-angiography) erzeugt werden, welche die Grundlage für die zeitliche

---

[1] Abkürzung für Analysis Tool for Neuro Imaging Data

Abb. 1. TOF MRT (a) und 3 TREAT Schichten (b-d) mit zeitlichem Abstand 6 ms

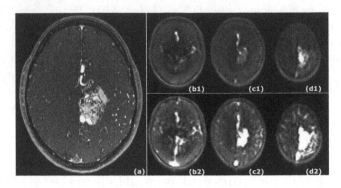

Analyse der Hämodynamik bilden. Die visuelle Bildqualität ist bei den 4D-TREAT-Bilddaten mit einer zeitlichen Auflösung von ca. 0,5 s und einer Voxelgröße von $1,875 \times 1,875 \times 5,0mm^3$ eher gering (Abb. 1 b-d). Daher werden zusätzlich nach Kontrastmittelgabe räumlich hochauflösende 3D TOF-MRA (time-of-flight) aufgenommen (Abb. 1a), welche durch einen verbesserten Blut-zu-Hintergrund-Kontrast und einer geringen Voxelgröße von $0,469 \times 0,469 \times 0,5mm^3$ eine detaillierte Segmentierung des Gefäßsystems und eine Quantifizierung von Größe und Lage [4] der AVM ermöglichen. AnToNIa wurde unter Verwendung der Toolkits ITK & VTK entwickelt. Klassen wurden problemorientiert angepasst und eigene Klassen in C++ implementiert.

3.1 Kombination von TREAT und TOF

Um die zeitliche Information der Dynamik des Blutes aus den TREAT-Bilddaten und die räumliche Auflösung der TOF-Bilddaten zu kombinieren, wird zunächst für jedes Voxel der Intensitätsverlauf über die Zeit analysiert (Abb. 2a-c). Darüber hinaus werden aus den zeitlichen Signalverläufen Parameter zur Charakterisierung der Hämodynamik extrahiert. Hierbei wird der Zeitpunkt, zu dem die Ableitung der Signalkurve maximal ist, als Einströmzeitpunkt definiert. Basierend auf dieser Definition werden voxelweise die Einströmzeitpunkte des Blutes berechnet, wodurch das zeitlich-räumliche Datenvolumen auf einen 3D-Datensatz reduziert wird.

In AnToNIa wird eine 3D-Maximum Intensity Projection (MIP) über alle Zeitpunkte aus den 4D-TREAT-Daten berechnet. Die 3D-MIP ermöglicht eine verbesserte Darstellung von charakteristischen Gefäßverläufen (Abb. 2e), die daraus entstandenen zusätzlichen Bildinformationen sind hilfreich für den Registrierungsprozess. Für das hier verwendete affine 3D-3D Registrierungsverfahren wird zunächst mittels Resampling die Auflösung der 3D-MIP an die der TOF-MRT-Bildsequenz angepasst und anschließend der hochskalierte MIP- mit dem TOF-MRT-Datensatz registriert. Die daraus berechnete Transformation ermöglicht eine direkte Übertragung der Einströmzeitpunkte auf die räumlich hochaufgelösten TOF-MRT-Daten. In Abb. 2 ist das Ergebnis der Registrierung im Schachbrett-View der MIP aus TOF (Abb. 2d) und TREAT-MIP dargestellt.

Abb. 2. Zeitlichen Intensitätsverlauf (b) und diskret approximierte Ableitungen für zwei Voxel aus den 4D TREAT (a). Ergebnis der 3D-3D Registrierung im Schachbrett-View (f) der MIP von beiden Datensätzen (d+e)

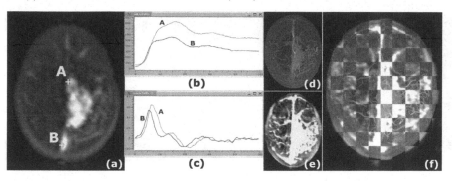

3.2   Analyse des Gefäßsystems

In dem 3D-TOF-Datensatz wird das individuelle Gefäßsystem mittels Region-Growing und manueller Korrektur in orthogonalen Sichten segmentiert. Aus der Segmentierung wird anschließend unter Verwendung des Marching-Cube-Algorithmus [5] ein 3D-Oberflächenmodell des Gefäßbaumes generiert. In An-ToNIa kann durch den Arzt im dreidimensionalen Raum mittels interaktiver Positionierung der orthogonalen Begrenzungsebenen ein Quader definiert werden, der als erste Approximation des Kerns der AVM verwendet wird.

Der Verlauf von Gefäßen in einer definierten Region außerhalb und innerhalb des Kernbereiches der AVM wird analysiert und farblich dargestellt. Die Klassifizierung in zufließende Arterien (Feeder) und abfließende Venen (draining veins) wird durch den Mediziner unter Verwendung einblendbaren Parameterinformationen über die Einströmzeitpunkte interaktiv vorgenommen (Abb. 3c).

4   Ergebnisse

Bei der Entwicklung der Analyse und Visualisierungstechniken von AnToNIa standen 12 Datensätze von Patienten mit AVM zur Verfügung. Zur Evaluation erster Ergebnisse wurde in den TOF-MRT-Bilddaten aller Patienten das Gefäßsystem segmentiert und ein Oberflächenmodell erzeugt. Anschließend wurden in 4D-TREAT-Datensätzen Einströmzeitpunkte berechnet und nach 3D-3D Registrierung farbcodiert in den 2D-TOF-Schichtbildern und auf dem 3D-Oberflächenmodell dargestellt (Abb. 3a+b). Die Darstellungen wurden von Experten als hilfreich für die Diagnose und Therapieplanung eingestuft. Die interaktive Navigation im 3D-Raum, Rotation und Zooming, sowie das optionale Ein- und Ausblenden der Zeitinformation von Gefäßstrukturen wurde als Vorteil gegenüber der DSA gesehen.

Abb. 3. Farbcodierte Darstellung der Einströmzeitpunkte auf TOF-MRT (a)und im 3D-Oberflächenmodell (b) sowie die farbliche Darstellung von zu- und abfließenden Gefäßen (c)

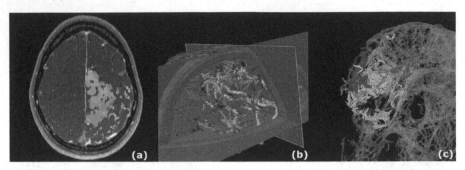

5   Diskussion

Es wurden neue Verfahren zur Visualisierung und Analyse von AVM präsentiert. Hierbei wurden aus zeitlich-räumlichen 4D-TREAT-Datensätzen Parameter für die Hämodynamik extrahiert und nach affiner Registrierung mit räumlich hochaufgelösten 3D-TOF-Bilddaten kombiniert visualisiert. Dabei können die extrahierten Parameter optional als starre Farbüberlagerung in den TOF-Schichten und im 3D-Gefäßmodell dargestellt werden. Für die nähere Zukunft ist geplant, das Analysis Tool for Neuro Imaging Data im Bereich der Segmentierung des Gefäßbaumes zu erweitern, um den Zeitaufwand des Segmentierungsprozesses zu reduzieren. Zusätzlich könnten Struktur- und Verlaufsanalysen des Gefäßbaumes, wie sie z.B. bei der Leberoperationsplanung eingesetzt werden, in Kombination mit der Hämodynamik eine automatische Detektion von zu- und abfließenden Gefäßen ermöglichen. Im Bereich der Visualisierung müssen weitere Techniken zur Real-Time-Visualisierung des Blutflusses entwickelt werden, um die starre Darstellung durch eine dynamische zu ersetzen.

Literaturverzeichnis

1. Grzyska U. Treatment of cerebral arteriovenous malformations. Hamburg Concept Clinical Neuroradiology 2004;14(1):41–47.
2. S Fasulakis, S Andronikou. Comparison of MR angiography and conventional angiography in the investigation of intracranial arteriovenous malformations and aneurysms in children. Pediatr Radiol 2003;33:378–384.
3. Bullitt E, et al. Computer-assisted visualization of arteriovenous malformations on the home personal computer. Neurosurgery 2001;48(3).
4. Spetzler RF, Martin NA. A proposed grading system for arteriovenous malformations. J Neurosurg 1986;65:467–483.
5. Lorenson WE, Cline HE. Marching cubes. Computer Graphics 1987;21(4):163–169.

Automatic Extraction of Symmetry Plane from Falx Cerebri Areas in CT Slices

Darius Grigaitis[1] and Mecislovas Meilunas[2]

[1]Department of Electronics Systems
[2]Department of Mathematical Modelling
Vilnius Gediminas Technical University, Naugarduko 41, LT-03227, Vilnius, Lithuania
Email: darius.grigaitis@el.vtu.lt

Abstract. We present the simple and fast symmetry plain detection algorithm, that recognizes Falx cerebri curve on each human brain computed thomogrpahy slice. Symmetry curves appear approximately on 30% images and using such images as reference it is possible to determine symmetry plane. We propose an algorithm based on hybrid methods, that allows detect symmetry plane with deviation angle until 25^0. The method is based on fuzzy logic that selects region of interest and symmetry curves. Direct pixels selection with evaluation of symmetry curve properties are used to calculate symmetry plane with high speed.

1 Introduction

Determination of symmetry plane (SP) on human brain images is a crucial task for further automatic analysis. Division of brain region into symmetric areas provides more accuracy in detection of brain structures and recognition of non-healthy regions of the brain like stroke, aneurism, tumor, etc. There are many methods to compute mid-sagitall symmetry plain of brain. Some of them measure cross correlation [1, 2, 3, 4] or Hough transform [5] or other features [6, 7, 8]. Disadvantage of such algorithms are time-consuming calculations, especially in the case of cross correlation method. Therefore high speed algorithms are required. One of possible ways is to use distributed computing or optimize existing algorithms. In our task the specific fast hybrid principle was used that extracts Falx cerebri feature (Fig. 1). The designed method uses direct point search method in order to increase noise resistance and avoid Hough transform floating point of angle calculations. Because our proposed algorithm works with only integer numbers, the time of calculation is less then 1 second to calculate symmetry plane using 50 images by 512×512 resolution with Pentium 4, 2.6GHz computer.

2 Method

Algorithm consists of four stages. First stage is image preprocessing, definition of the region of interest (ROI). The scope of future analysis is elimination of unnecessary image information for axis determination. The smaller brain view

Fig. 1. An example of symmetry curve in CT images of this same person: higher slice (left); lower slice (right)

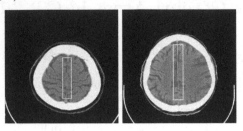

area helps to reach better filter response on symmetry curve (SC). In the second stage filtering is implemented in order to select narrow light curves (Fig. 1) called Falx Cerebri. Almost 30% CT images contain this information in human vertex area. Third stage is detection of symmetry axis. In this stage SC are converted into the lines in order to calculate SP. Conversion is implemented by simple separation of pixels by lines with some angle [9]. The last stage is related to SP calculation using symmetry lines coordinates detected in previous stage. For correct SP detection minimum two lines must be detected.

2.1   Definition of the Region of Interest

The proposed algorithm requires clean areas to detect SC. However, there are critical areas in CT images that possess properties similar to SC. This is left and right human brain areas, that after processing with SC filter appears as vertical curves. By this reason, left and right areas are removed and speed of SP detection increase, because the area of brain can be reduced more than in 40%. The algorithm executes from the calculation of the center point of brain view and diagonal lines (Fig. 2) that show corresponding areas of brain view in each slice.

The brain region in image is defined as gray valued pixels

$$S = \{(x,y), g(x,y) > 0\} \tag{1}$$

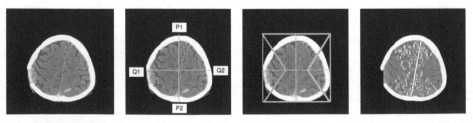

Fig. 2. Region of interest selection: initial image (left); center of object detection (middle left); diagonal lines for area separation (middle right); ROI after filtering (right)

Here, x, y - coordinates of pixels, $g(x, y)$ - human brain image with bone areas. In the beginning of ROI selection the boundaries of brain view are denoted as follows

$$Q_1(\underline{x}, y_l), \quad Q_2(\overline{x}, y_r)$$
$$P_1(x_b, \underline{y}), \quad P_2(x_t, \overline{y}) \tag{2}$$

Here, y_l, y_r - left and right pixels of objects in y coordinate, x_t, x_b - top and bottom pixels of objects in x coordinate , $\overline{x}$, $\underline{x}$, $\overline{y}$, $\underline{y}$ is left, right and top, bottom grey level view pixels positions

$$\underline{x} = \min_i \{x_i | (x_i, y_j)\} \in S, \quad \underline{y} = \min_i \{y_j | (x_i, y_j)\} \in S$$
$$\overline{x} = \max_i \{x_i | (x_i, y_j)\} \in S, \quad \overline{y} = \max_i \{y_j | (x_i, y_j)\} \in S \tag{3}$$

Using such information any line shown in Fig. 2 can be calculated. The gap between diagonal lines is ROI and SC can easily fit with 25 degrees angle or more. The shape of ROI is not significant, it was only important to remove left and right areas (Fig. 2) that filters recognize as parts of SC.

2.2   Detection of Symmetry Curve

Several types of filters that are related to symmetry curve properties was analyzed. In Fig. 3 is shown filters shapes that are used for analyzing its behavior on symmetry curve (SC). The maximum size of sliding window of filter was 10×10 pixels because symmetry curve can easily fit in it. The main property of symmetry curve is brighter pixels than other gray matter pixels entire image. Thus, the simple fuzzy filters for brightness comparison were constructed. These filters are suitable to recognize vertical light curves. Construction of tested filters Fig. 3 is shown. The main property of filters is that center pixels (black squares) are compared with surrounding pixels (white squares) by rule

$$I_b(x, y) = \begin{cases} 1, & g_{left}(x, y) \& g_{right}(x, y) > g_c(x, y) \\ 0, & \text{otherwise} \end{cases} \tag{4}$$

Here, $I_b(x, y)$ - center pixels of sliding window of binary images; $g_c(x, y)$ - center pixels of sliding window of gray scale images; $g_{left}(x, y)$, $g_{right}(x, y)$ - left and right pixels of sliding window of gray scale image.

For testing of filters we used 1462 images of 91 patients. 60% of slices where eliminated automatically because they have not SC property. As testing parameter the length of SC was used, that was calculated with fourth step of designed algorithm. The experiment showed that histograms of SC length of given filters differ slightly and shape of filter is not essential. Moreover, if the sliding window of filter becomes more simple than Fig. 4, then SC can not be detected, when SC appears very unclear. There is eventually strong relation between number of comparison in filter, brightness and length of SC pixels (Fig. 2).

Fig. 3. An example of used filters shapes for SC detection

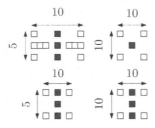

2.3   The Estimation of Symmetry Axis

In symmetry curve detection stage, sectors of filtered images are collected into lines $B = \{(x_i, y_i), g(x_i, y_i) > 0\}$. Here the Hough transform can be used, that can draw the line through the concentrated pixels [10, 5]. According noisy CT images we used direct point selection by lines with appropriate angle. In Fig. 4 is shown an example of lines positioning. First, two horizontal and parallel lines are used. Second, from the q_1 the lines are drawn by formula of standard line between two points. All straights positions are stored and used to produce all possible lines between horizontal lines. The number of possible lines is $M = q_n \cdot r_m$, which has set of pixels l_{ij} where $1 \leq i \leq m, 1 \leq j \leq m$ are set of filtered pixels (Fig. 2). Here m, n - lengths of horizontal lines. In estimation of symmetry line is important intersection of filtered pixels and produced lines $k_{ij} = \sum l_{ij} \cap B$. One of lines can represent symmetry axis in case when meets the requirements of $(i_0, j_0) = \arg\max(k_{ij} + \delta)$. The parameter $\delta = \sum_{s=1}^{k_{ij}} \sum_{p=1}^{P} \sum_{r=1}^{R} \sum_{l=1}^{L} (g_{ps}(x, y) - g_{lr}^{ps}(x, y))$ evaluates SC brightness of pixels by their neighbours. This simple addition dramatically increases k_{ij} value and symmetry axis can be detected even SC is represented with low number pixels. In this case the filtered image (Fig. 2 d) can contain more noise pixels than SC. Finally symmetry plane equation is derived using $N = 2K$ number of points in 30% slices. Here K is number of CT slices of single patient.

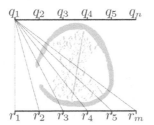

Fig. 4. An example of symmetry curve detection by lines, the bone area was placed to show proper image position

3   Results

Experiments with CT images showed that shape of filter is not essential and simplest filter shape can be used. The critical parameter that affect speed is forming of straights (Fig. 4). If only odd values of m, n are used to draw straights then time of calculation decreases more than 35%, but precision of SP detection decreases. To speed up an algorithm the straights are calculated once and copied to determine all possible angles between horizontal lines. For experiments we used 1462 CT images of 91 person. The SP were detected successfully for 89 persons. Visually all 89 images collections showed correct position of SC in $-25^0.. + 25^0$ angle interval. Because the symmetry curves appear only in human head vertex area, then symmetry axis are projected in to all slices. This algorithm can be used for magnetic nuclear resonance images also. For precision evaluation of formed SP the future analysis of comparison must be prepared.

References

1. Prima S, Ourselin S, Ayache N. Computation of the mid-sagittal plane in 3D brain images. IEEE Trans Med Imaging 2002; 122–138.
2. Tuzikov AV, Colliot O, Bloch I. Brain symmetry plane computation in MR images using inertia axes and optimization. Institute of Engineering Cybernetics Academy of Sciences of Republic Belarus: IEEE; 2002. 1051–4651.
3. Ardekani BA, Kershaw J, Braun M, Kanuo I. Automatic detection of the mid-sagittal plane in 3D brain images. IEEE Trans Med Imaging 1997;16:947–952.
4. Liu Y, Collins RT, Rothfus WE. Robust midsagittal plane extraction from normal and pathological 3D neuroradiology images. IEEE Trans Med Imaging 2001;20:175–192.
5. Brummer ME. Hough transform detection of the longitudinal fissure in tomographic head images. IEEE Trans Med Imaging 1991;10:74 – 81.
6. Anbazhagan P, Carass A, Bazin P, Prince JL. Automatic estimation of midsagittal plane and AC-PC alignment based on nonrigid registration. Procs IEEE Symp Biomed Imaging 2006; 828 – 831.
7. Prima S, Ourselin S, Ayache N. Computation of the mid-sagittal plane in 3D brain images. IEEE Trans Med Imaging 2002;21:122–138.
8. Smith S, Jenkinson M. Accurate robust symmetry estimation. Procs MICCAI 1999; 308–317.
9. Grigaitis D, Zitkevicius E, Usinskas A. Determination of symmetry axis on human brain CT image. Procs Bienlial Baltic Electronics Conf 2004; 165–168.
10. Gonzalez RC, E WoodsR. Digital Image Processing. Prentice-Hall, Inc.- Second Edition; 2002.

Automatic Quantification of DTI Parameters Along Fiber Bundles

Jan Klein, Simon Hermann, Olaf Konrad, Horst K. Hahn,
Heinz-Otto Peitgen

MeVis Research, 28359 Bremen
Email: klein@mevis.de

Abstract. We introduce a novel technique that allows for an automatic quantification of MR DTI parameters along arbitrarily oriented fiber bundles. Most previous methods require either a manual placement of ROIs, are limited to single fiber tracts, or are limited to bundles which are perpendicular to one of the three image planes. Thus, the quantification process is made much more time-efficient and robust by our new approach. We compare our technique with a manual quantification of an expert and show the similarity of the results. Furthermore, we demonstrate how to visualize the parameters at a certain position of the fiber bundle so that areas of interest can easily be examined.

1 Introduction

Over the last few years, diffusion tensor imaging (DTI) received increasing attention in the neurosurgical and neurological community with the motivation to identify white matter tracts afflicted by an individual pathology or tracts at risk for a given surgical approach [1]. An explicit geometrical reconstruction of white matter tracts has become available by fiber tracking based on DTI data [2].

Color-coded maps of fractional anisotropy (FA) computed from DTI data were successfully employed in several studies where it has been shown that modified parameters like FA, relative anisotropy or diffusion strength are an indicator of diseases affecting white matter tissue [3, 4, 5].

A pointwise assessment of those parameters was proposed along a single streamline combined with a visualization of uncertainties in [6]. Other quantification algorithms [4, 3, 5] use a manual definition of one or more ROIs which cover a certain fiber bundle at some slices of the image data. Within such ROIs, more robust parameters can be computed from several single parameters. In a previous work, we extended standard ROI-based techniques by considering partial volume effects so that fibrous and non-fibrous tissue can be classified [7]. Recently, it has been shown how to define fiber bundles implicitly and how to compute their parameters as integrals [8].

However, it is often desirable to determine the parameters along a whole fiber bundle as precisely as possible so that several ROIs have to be drawn manually via a multi-planar reconstruction. As this process is very time-consuming and error-prone, [9] proposed a semi-automatic algorithm where ROIs are placed on axial, sagittal, or coronal slices between two predefined ROIs automatically. As a consequence, reliable results can only be achieved if the fiber tracts are perpendicular to one of the three image planes. Moreover, curved fiber bundles cannot be handled by their approach and had to be divided into several parts.

1.1 Novel Contributions

In this paper, we propose a method that overcomes the problems mentioned above and that allows for an efficient and automatic quantification of MR DTI data along arbitrarily oriented fiber tracts. A parameter map, defined by a Delaunay triangulation, visualizes the distribution of all single data points contributing to one single parameter. In contrast to the method proposed by Fillard [10], we do not compute an average parameter by several single values that all have the same geodesic distance from a user-defined origin (ROI). Instead, we compute a reference plane depending on the local curvature of the fiber bundle, which is used afterwards to determine the nearest fiber points with corresponding parameters. Thus, more reasonable results may be achieved by our new approach when dealing with geometrically complex fiber bundles.

2   Methods

For a tumor patient suffering from a right hemispheric glioma (F, 73 y), echo-planar DTI data were acquired on a 1.5 T Siemens Sonata (image resolution 1.875 x 1.875 x 1.9 mm^3, 60 slices, 6 gradient directions). Using a deflection-based algorithm [11], we compute the fiber bundle which has to be quantified. During fiber tracking, the parameters of interest (e.g., the FA) are computed and stored at each fiber point. We developed a simple filtering tool, where fibers can be excluded from the bundle or can be cropped at their endings afterwards.

2.1   Quantification

For quantification, two steps have to be done. First, each fiber is resampled so that all fibers consist of the same number of equidistantly distributed fiber points as proposed in [12]. Using the resampled fibers, an average center line of all fibers is computed where its j-th point p_j is calculated by averaging all j-th points of all fibers: $p_j = \frac{\sum_{i=1}^{n} f_i(j)}{n}$. This center line yields to n reference planes $h_j : (\overrightarrow{x} - \overrightarrow{p_j}) \cdot (\overrightarrow{p_j} - \overrightarrow{p_{j+1}}) = 0$ which are used for the quantification.

In a second step, for each point of the center line, a corresponding quantification parameter v_j can be determined by $v_j = g(v(f_1(j)), ..., v(f_n(j)))$. There, $v(f_i(j))$ denotes a single parameter corresponding to fiber point $f_i(j)$, and g denotes an arbitrary function with n input parameters, e.g., it computes the average of the n values. However, there may be some outliers $f_i(j)$ which are far away from the plane h_j (Fig. 2). In this case, v_j would also be determined depending on unwanted outliers $v(f_i(j))$. Thus, we propose to replace them by $v(f_i(k))$ where $f_i(k)$ is the point with minimum distance to the plane h_j.

Fig. 1. We compared our new automatic quantification technique with our manual quantification [7]. (i): the reference plane (visualized as orange circle) is automatically determined by our new technique, FA=0.421. (ii): a ROI has to be drawn manually within our manual quantification tool, FA=0.464

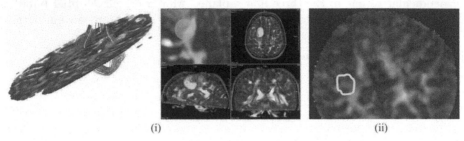

(i)   (ii)

2.2 Visualization

For visualizing all parameters contributing to v_j, we perform a Delaunay triangulation of the corresponding fiber points. The resulting triangles are shaded depending on the parameters $v(f_i(j))$. Simultaneously, the reference plane h_j and the fiber bundle are displayed in 3D. The user can interactively slide through the fiber bundle so that the parameter map and the plane are updated (Fig. 3).

3 Results

A fiber bundle, which is part of the corpus callosum and consists of $n = 50$ single fibers, was tracked and cropped at it endings (Fig. 3). The maximum number of fiber points along a fiber is 1183 so that we determined 1183 average, minimum, and maximum FA values, each of them computed by about 50 single parameter values. The results can be found in Fig. 3 (right). The whole computation including the center line and all FA values took much less than a second (AMD Athlon 64 X2 Dual, 3800+). Fig. 2 shows the distribution of all 50 parameters contributing to v_j (the plane h_j was chosen as displayed at the bottom of Fig. 3).

We also compared our technique with our manual quantification tool [7] which considers partial volume effects and which performs a classification of fibrous as well as non-fibrous tissue before the quantification. For several regions, we measured the average FA values by both methods, an example is shown in Fig. 1. The difference was always smaller than 0.05.

4 Discussion

Compared to a manual quantification, which takes at least 30 minutes for a reasonably detailed measurement of a fiber bundle (> 50 measured parameters), our new approach drastically reduces the time to a few milliseconds. For a fair comparison we have to mention that for a manual quantification the fiber tracking as well as the cropping and filtering (which takes us about one minute) have not to be done explicitly, but only implicitly by defining the ROIs.

Fig. 2. Left: there may be some outliers $f_i(j)$ which are far away from the plane h_j used for computing the quantification parameter v_j. In this case, we substitute $v(f_i(j))$ by $v(f_i(k))$ where $f_i(k)$ has the minimum distance to h_j. Right: Delaunay triangulation indicating the distribution of the single parameters (yellow) used for computing v_j (blue: low FA, red: high FA)

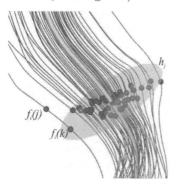
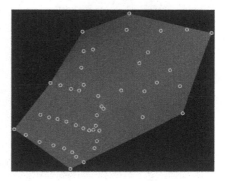

Initial experiments have shown that the differences between the manual and our new automatic quantification are at most 0.05. They may be explained by the manual determination of the plane, which is used for placing the ROI, as well as by the different algorithmic computation of the parameter values: the manual quantification needs a more complex function for computing the average FA value within an ROI, because it has to differentiate between FA values belonging to fibrous and to non-fibrous tissue. In contrast, this has not to be done by our novel approach because the preceding fiber tracking solves the problem so that only a simple function g depending on n input parameters can be used for the computation (see Section 2). In the future, we would like to use the idea of moving least squares for computing the center line. Furthermore, a more rigorous comparison between manual and automatic quantification has to be done depending on different data sets.

References

1. Yamada K, Kizu O, Mori S, et al. Brain fiber tracking with clinically feasible diffusion-tensor MR imaging: initial experience. Radiology 2003;227(1):295–301.
2. Mori S, Crain BJ, Chacko VP, et al. Three-dimensional tracking of axonal projections in the brain by magnetic resonance imaging. Ann Neurol 1999;45(2):265–269.
3. Tievsky AL, Ptak T, Farkas J. Investigation of apparent diffusion coefficient and diffusion tensor anisotropy in acute and chronic multiple sclerosis lesions. Am J Neuroradiol 1999;20(8):1491–1499.
4. Stahl R, Dietrich O, Teipel S, et al. Assessment of axonal degeneration on alzheimer's disease with diffusion tensor MRI. Radiologe 2003;43(7):566–575.
5. Tropine A, Vucurevic G, Delani P, et al. Contribution of diffusion tensor imaging to delineation of gliomas and glioblastomas. J Magn Reson Imaging 2004;20(6):905–912.
6. Jones DK, Travis AR, Eden G, et al. PASTA: Pointwise assessment of streamline tractography attributes. Magn Reson Med 2005;53:1462–1467.

276   J. Klein et al.

Fig. 3. Left: fiber bundle that we use for quantification. The center line is shown in yellow. Right: plot which shows maximum, minimum and average FA values along the fiber bundle. The vertical line corresponds to the orange plane h_j shown on the left

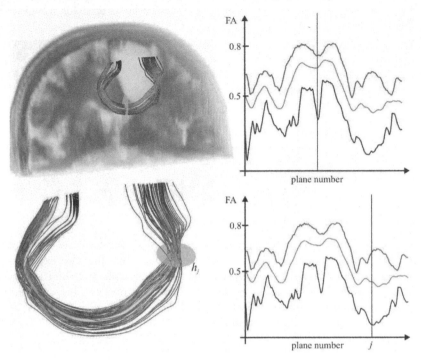

7. Schlüter M, Stieltjes B, Hahn HK, et al. Detection of tumour infiltration in axonal fibre bundles using diffusion tensor imaging. Int J Medical Robotics and Computer Assisted Surgery 2005;1:80–86.
8. Niethammer M, Bouix S, Westin CF, et al. Fiber bundle estimation and parametrization. In: Procs MICCAI'06; 2006. 252–259.
9. Aoki S, Iwata NK, Masutani Y, et al. Quantitative evaluation of the pyramidal tract segmented by diffusion tensor tractography: feasibility study in patients with amyotrophic lateral sclerosis. Radiation Medicine 2005;23(3):195–199.
10. Fillard P, Gilmore J, Lin W, et al. Quantitative analysis of white matter fiber properties along geodesic paths. In: Procs MICCAI'03; 2003. 16–23.
11. Schlüter M, Konrad O, Hahn HK, et al. White matter lesion phantom for diffusion tensor data and its application to the assessment of fiber tracking. Procs SPIE 2005;5746:835–844.
12. Enders F, Sauber N, Merhof D, et al. Visualization of white matter tracts with wrapped streamlines. In: Provs IEEE Visualization; 2005. 51–58.

Evaluierung von Erscheinungsmodellen für die Segmentierung mit statistischen Formmodellen

Sascha Münzing, Tobias Heimann, Ivo Wolf und Hans-Peter Meinzer

Abteilung für Medizinische und Biologische Informatik, DKFZ Heidelberg
Email: s.muenzing@dkfz-heidelberg.de

Zusammenfassung. Zur Segmentierung mit Formmodellen werden Erscheinungsmodelle benötigt, die eine exakte Anpassung an die Bilddaten ermöglichen. Wir haben Standardverfahren und nichtlineare Modellierungsmethoden für die 3D-Segmentierung erweitert und auf klinischen Leberdaten evaluiert. Mit nichtlinearen Erscheinungsmodellen wurden insgesamt deutlich bessere Ergebnisse erzielt. Dabei erbrachte die Erweiterung um einen generischen Ansatz zur Erhöhung der Datendichte eine zusätzliche signifikante Verbesserung.

1 Einleitung

Die Segmentierung ist ein wichtiger Schritt in vielen Bereichen der medizinischen Bildverarbeitung, wie z.B. in der Operationsplanung, Bestrahlungsplanung oder bildbasierter Diagnostik. Da medizinische Bilder häufig durch Rauschen und andere Artefakte gestört sind, ist zur automatische Erkennung und Extraktion von relevanten Gewebsstrukturen (z.B. der Leber oder dem Herz) oftmals Vorwissen nötig, d.h. ein internes Modell der erwarteten Form und/oder Intensitäten.

Bei Statistischen Formmodellen, auch als Active Shape Models [1] bekannt, wird Vorwissen aus Trainingsbildern gelernt. Dabei wird jedes Trainingsbild durch eine Menge von Punkten auf der Objektoberfläche repräsentiert, so genannten Landmarken. Aus den korrespondierenden Positionsdaten aller Trainingsbilder wird eine mittlere Form berechnet und anhand einer Hauptkomponentenanalyse die zugehörigen Varianzen ermittelt. Jedes Trainingsbild kann somit aus der mittleren Form zuzüglich einer Linearkombination von Verschiebungsvektoren beschrieben werden.

Um das generierte Formmodell zur Segmentierung verwenden zu können, müssen sich die Landmarken des Formmodells an die Bilddaten anpassen. Es wird, vergleichbar zum Formmodell, Vorwissen über die Landmarken benötigt, um das Aussehen an einer bestimmten Position, mit dem erwartenden Aussehen für einen gegebenen Landmarkenpunkt zu vergleichen. Hierzu werden so genannte Erscheinungsmodelle erstellt, die die Grauwertumgebung einer Landmarke anhand bestimmter Eigenschaften abbilden. Man spricht auch von lokalen Erscheinungsmodellen, da nicht die globale Erscheinung des ganzen Formmodells, sondern jeweils der lokale Bereich um eine Landmarke abgebildet wird.

2   Stand der Forschung und Fortschritt durch den Beitrag

In der ersten Version der Active Shape Models wurden die Landmarken mit einem simplen Gradientenprofil gesucht. Später folgten Statistische Modelle [2], bei denen das Aussehen einer Landmarke durch ein mittleres Profil aus allen Trainingsbildern, sowie die zugehörigen Kovarianzen modelliert wird. Normalverteilte Grauwerte werden damit korrekt abgebildet, um aber beliebige Verteilungen modellieren zu können, werden in neuerer Zeit nichtlineare Modelle verwendet. In [3] wird ein kNN-Klassifikator mit Grauwertprofilen verwendet, um sowohl die Objektgrenze, als auch Bereiche in der Landmarkenumgebung zu modellieren. In [4] wird ein Multiskalenklassifikator zur 2D-Segmentierung eingesetzt, bei dem anhand des Multi Local Jet Verfahrens differenzierte Bildmerkmale aus sogenannten locally orderless images berechnet werden. Diese Verfahren wurden für die 3D-Segmentierung erweitert und auf klinischen Daten der Leber evaluiert. Durch die einheitliche Datenbasis ist ein direkter Vergleich der Methoden gegeben.

3   Methoden

Die evaluierten Erscheinungsmodelle wurden zur Verwendung innerhalb eines Multiresolution-Frameworks entwickelt. Dabei wird für jedes CT Volumen eine Bildpyramide aus fünf verschiedenen Auflösungen R_0 bis R_4 erstellt. Auf der Originalauflösung R_0 beträgt die Schrittweite 1mm und auf den nachfolgenden Stufen wird diese jeweils verdoppelt. Für jede Auflösungsstufe werden separate Erscheinungsmodelle erstellt.

3.1   Standardverfahren

Bei der einfachsten Methode werden Landmarken anhand der stärksten Kante gesucht. Entlang der Oberflächennormalen wird ein normalisiertes Gradientenprofil der Länge $k = 2n + 1$ berechnet, mit jeweils n Punkten zu jeder Seite der Oberfläche. Hierbei besteht das Vorwissen lediglich aus der Annahme, dass der Grauwertgradient an der Position der Objektkante maximal sei.

Bei den Statistischen Modellen werden Grauwerte durch Profile der Länge k - analog zum obigen Modell - für jede Landmarke und aus allen Trainingsbildern extrahiert. Aus den gesammelten Profilen $\mathbf{g}_i = (g_1, g_2, \ldots, g_k)^{\mathrm{T}}$ wird zu jeder Landmarke ein mittleres Profil $\bar{\mathbf{g}}$ und eine Kovarianzmatrix $\mathbf{S}_g$ berechnet. Zur Anpassung einer Landmarke wird ein neues Profil $\mathbf{g}_s$ mit den Profilen aus der Verteilung verglichen, indem die quadrierte Mahalanobisdistanz $f(\mathbf{g}_s)$ berechnet wird

$$f(\mathbf{g}_s) = (\mathbf{g}_s - \bar{\mathbf{g}})^{\mathrm{T}} \mathbf{S}_g^{-1} (\mathbf{g}_s - \bar{\mathbf{g}}) \qquad (1)$$

Wenn das Profil $\mathbf{g}_s$ auf der optimalen Position liegt, ist die Mahalanobisdistanz minimal. Das Verfahren wurde mit einfachen Grauwertprofilen und normalisierten Gradientenprofilen evaluiert, da diese in [2] die besten Ergebnisse erzielten.

3.2 Nichtlineares Grauwertmodell

Beim nichtlinearen Grauwertmodell wird das Aussehen einer Landmarke anhand eines kNN-Klassifikators verteilungsfrei modelliert. Es werden Grauwertprofile der Länge $k = 2n + 1$ entlang der Oberflächennormalen abgetastet, aber im Gegensatz zum Statistischen Modell werden nicht nur Profile direkt auf der Objektgrenze (Kantenprofile) verwendet, sondern zusätzlich $2n$ Profile aus der Landmarkenumgebung (Umgebungsprofile), jeweils n Profile nach außen und n in Richtung zum Objektinneren. Die Menge der Trainingsprofile besteht also aus zwei Klassen. Die Wahrscheinlichkeit, dass ein Profil g_s aus einem neuen Bild auf dem Objektrand liegt, ist durch die Posteriori Wahrscheinlichkeit des kNN-Klassifikators gegeben

$$P(\text{Kantenpunkt}|g_s) = \frac{n_{\text{true}}}{k_{\text{nn}}} \tag{2}$$

wobei n_{true} die Anzahl der Kantenprofile aus den k_{nn} nächsten Nachbarn ist. Bei der NN-Suche werden die Trainingsprofile in einem KD-Tree gespeichert, wobei die Grauwerte eines Profils die Koordinaten eines k-dimensionalen Punktes darstellen. Gewöhnlich ist die resultierende Datendichte gering, deshalb wurde wie in [5] ein K-Means-Clustering durchgeführt. Durch dieses Verfahren kann man die Leber in ca. 20 Cluster einteilen und somit Daten aus durchschnittlich 128 Landmarken in einem Erscheinungsmodell zusammenfassen.

3.3 MultiLocalJet-Merkmale

Bei diesem nichtlinearen Erscheinungsmodell werden Landmarken nicht durch Grauwertprofile sondern durch differenzierte Merkmale aus Bildpunkten des Objekts und der angrenzenden Umgebung modelliert. Für ein Bild werden einzelne Voxel anhand des Localjet-Verfahrens als ein Taylorpolynom interpretiert. Die benötigten Taylorkoeffizienten sind die Ableitungen an einem Bildpunkt bis zum entsprechenden Grad des Polynoms. Auf den Skalenraum des Bildes angewendet, resultiert eine große Anzahl an Merkmalskombinationen. Wählt man fünf Auflösungsstufen und alle Ableitungen bis zum zweiten Grad (auch gemischte), erhält man für den 3D-Fall insgesamt 45 Merkmale. Um aus dieser Menge die besten Merkmale zu selektieren, wird zunächst eine klassifikatorabhängige Sequential Feature Forward Selection durchgeführt, wobei zu jeder Landmarke maximal 10 Merkmale ausgewählt werden. Zusammen mit einem kNN-Klassifikator ($k_{\text{nn}}=10$, $e^{-\text{Distanz}}$) ergibt sich ein Multiskalenklassifikator aus den besten Merkmalen für eine entsprechende Anwendung und einen bestimmten Bildbereich. Um in einem neuen Bild eine Landmarke zu lokalisieren, werden zunächst $k = 2n + 1$ Bildpunkte entlang der Oberflächennormalen klassifiziert

$$f(g) = \sum_{i=-n}^{-1} g_i + \sum_{i=0}^{+n} (1 - g_i) \tag{3}$$

Anhand der Kostenfunktion $f(g)$ wird die optimale Landmarkenposition als die Stelle definiert, an der die Wahrscheinlichkeit am größten ist, dass die Profilpunkte g_i innerhalb der Kontur $i = 0 \ldots + n$ tatsächlich zum Objekt gehören und die Punkte außerhalb $i = -n \ldots - 1$ zur Umgebung.

3.4   Evaluationsverfahren

Die Güte eines Erscheinungsmodells wird unabhängig von einem Suchverfahren für alle Trainingsbilder bestimmt, indem die Anpassung der Modelle an der Originallandmarkenposition und an drei Positionen auf jeder Seite der Oberfläche untersucht wird. Um die Bedingungen während einer Bildsuche zu simulieren, erfolgt eine Randomisierung der Landmarkenposition mit einer Varianz von 1 mm in der Originalauflösung entlang der Oberfläche (in den nachfolgenden Auflösungen jeweils verdoppelt). Gleichzeitig wird die Richtung des Normalenvektors mit einer Varianz von ungefähr zehn Grad randomisiert. Auf diese Art werden in jedem Trainingsbild zu jeder Landmarke 20 Stichproben entnommen. Der Index der Stelle mit der besten Anpassung (ein Bereich zwischen -3 und 3) wird gespeichert und zur Erzeugung eines Histogramms verwendet. Aus den Häufigkeiten der auftretenden Verschiebungen kann als Gütemaß der mittlere Quadratfehler berechnet werden [6].

4   Ergebnisse

Das Bildmaterial bestand aus 32 CT-Aufnahmen des Abdomens, mit einer Auflösung von 512x512 Voxeln in der Ebene und einer variierenden Anzahl von 60 bis 130 Schichten. Der Voxelabstand variiert in der Ebene zwischen 0,55mm und 0,8mm und der Schichtabstand beträgt meistens 3mm, in einigen Fällen 5mm.

Zu jedem Erscheinungsmodell sind in Abbildung 1 die mittleren quadratischen Fehler und in Abbildung 2 die entsprechenden Histogramme für alle fünf Auflösungsstufen dargestellt.

5   Diskussion

Das erreichbare Maximum wird durch die anisotropen Auflösungen der verwendeten Trainingsbilder und insbesondere in der Originalauflösung durch die Un-

Aufl. stufe	ohne Training	Statistische Modelle		Nichtlineare Modelle		
	Gradient	Intensität	Gradient	ungeclustert	geclustert	LocalJet
R0	2,97	2,92	1,85	1,67	1,63	1,22
R1	2,10	2,38	0,99	0,95	0,77	0,94
R2	2,36	2,22	0,99	0,86	0,57	1,27
R3	3,38	2,09	1,59	1,06	0,75	1,60
R4	3,56	1,84	1,48	1,26	1,02	1,84

Abb. 1. Tabelle der mittleren quadratischen Fehler der Erscheinungsmodelle

Abb. 2. Standardverfahren (oben): Stärkste Kante, Statistische Modelle mit Intensitätsprofil und normalisierten Gradientenprofil; Nichtlineare Modelle (unten): ungeclusterte und geclusterte Grauwertprofile, LocalJet-Merkmale

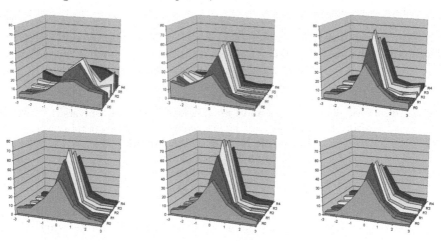

genauigkeiten bei den manuellen Segmentierungen (klinischer Goldstandard) begrenzt. Diese haben ab der zweiten Stufe R_1 durch die geringere Auflösung und größere Schrittweite immer weniger Einfluss. Die schlechteren Ergebnisse ab R_3 resultieren vermutlich aus den ab dieser Stufe relativ großen Profilen und der damit einhergehenden großen Bildvariationen, teilweise ragen die Profile sogar über den Bildrand hinaus.

Mit den besten nichtlinearen Modellen werden Landmarken im Vergleich zum besten Standardverfahren um durchschnittlich 30% besser abgebildet. Besonders das geclusterte Modell liefert insgesamt bessere Ergebnisse, darum soll in Zukunft auch das LocalJet-Modell um diesen Ansatz erweitert werden.

Literaturverzeichnis

1. Cootes TF, Taylor CJ, Cooper DH, Graham J. Active shape models: Their training and application. Comput Vis Image Underst 1995;61(1):38–59.
2. Cootes T, Taylor C. Active shape model search using local grey-level models: A quantitative evaluation. In: Procs BMVC. BMVA Press; 1993. 639–648.
3. de Bruijne M, van Ginneken B, Niessen WJ, et al. Active shape model segmentation using a non-linear appearance model: Application to 3D AAA segmentation. Inst. of Inform. and Comp. Sciences, Utrecht University; 2003.
4. van Ginneken B, Frangi AF, Staal JJ, et al. Active shape model segmentation with optimal features. IEEE Trans Med Imaging 2002;21(8):924–933.
5. Bacher MG, Pekar V, Kaus MR. Model-based segmentation of anatomical structures in MR images of the head and neck area. Procs BVM 2005.
6. Heimann T, Wolf I, Meinzer HP. Active shape models for a fully automated 3D segmentation of the liver: An evaluation on clinical data. Procs MICCAI 2006; 41–48.

Cognition Network Technology for Automated Holistic Analysis in Mammography

Günter Schmidt[1], Alexander Horsch[2], Rüdiger Schulz-Wendtland[3],
Sukhbansbir Kaur[1], Matthias Elter[5], Harald Sittek[4], Thomas Wittenberg[5],
Maria Athelogou[1], Gerd Binnig[1]

[1]Definiens AG, Munich
[2]Institute for Medical Statistics and Epidemiology, Technical University Munich
[3]Institute for Radiology of the University Erlangen-Nuremberg
[4]Diagnostic Mammacenter, Munich
[5]Fraunhofer-IIS, Erlangen
Email: gschmidt@definiens.com

Abstract. Digital mammography and comprehensive breast cancer screening approaches have led to the generation of a vast amount of image data. Since the visual inspection of a large set of images is expensive and to some extend also subjective, new methods for fully automated mammography image analysis are needed. The Definiens Cognition Network Technology (CNT) solves the image analysis problem by simulating human cognition processes using knowledge based and context dependent processing. It represents processed image data, image processing methods, and image objects and their definitions in a unified model which incorporates elements from semantic networks, description logics and functional programming. We present first steps towards a successful application of this technology on automated detection of masses and calcifications according to the ACR BI-RADS^{TM} standard.

1 Introduction

The Definiens Cognition Network Technology (CNT) has revolutionized automated image analysis for complex scenes. Since its invention in 1996 it has been applied with great success to a variety of image analysis tasks based on data from very different kind of sensors ranging from satellites equipped with radar or optical sensors, over electron or optical microscopes to three-dimensional computer tomographs [1, 2, 3].

CNT generates automatically a semantic object network from unstructured data such as images and database tables. This object network represents explicitly all user-relevant information about real world objects (e.g. breasts, nipples, and lesions) which was initially hidden in the input data. CNT is based on three pillars:

First, the automatic analysis of the data can be formulated in a knowledge-driven fashion. Knowledge about real world objects is explicitly specified in a semantic network of class objects. Each class object contains a fuzzy or a nearest neighbour classifier which is able to calculate the class membership of a data object. The fuzzy classifier may use any logical combination of object properties to calculate the membership according to user-defined fuzzy sets.

Second, based on the semantic network of class objects, a hierarchical object network is generated by iteratively segmenting and classifying the image and segments of it. In CNT data understanding in general and image understanding in particular is an iterative local and context depended process which uses the class network to generate in several steps a network of objects of interest on the basis of the input data. The resulting object network is a semantic network which consists of classified nodes and links carrying high-level properties. The classification connects the object network with the class network and provides the objects with a meaning. The object's properties characterize an object by calculating statistical properties from the underlying input data or by aggregating properties of connected objects. Frequently used image object properties represent spectral, texture, shape and relational information.

Third, the object network generation and processing is defined by process objects which are embedded in a processing hierarchy. Process objects modify the elements of the object network according to an algorithm and a process domain. The process domain specifies which subset of the object network will be used for algorithm execution or for further downstream processing. The domain specification uses the classification, the properties and the link information of objects. Through the links a meaningful navigation from those objects that are already identified as relevant to objects or regions that have to be processed in the next step becomes possible. The three most basic process algorithms in CNT are context-dependent classification, segmentation and information bundling. Each segmentation step creates a new data object from a set of objects and links this new object with each object in the set using a given link type. This enables the system to build dynamically image object hierarchies to analyze an image simultaneously on several scales to generate context for further processing. The information bundling updates automatically object properties such as pixel statistics if there are any changes in the semantic object network. This ensures the consistency of structure and information content at each time step. As the result of the CNT processing, all relevant image objects and their mutual relations are available for further analysis.

We applied this technology in the context of mammography to the holistic processing of complete patient records, including four mammogram images (cranio-caudal and medio lateral views of both breasts) and including patient metadata such as weight, age, medication, number of children and family history. The knowledge base comprise in depth anatomical and diagnosis-related information as provided by mammography experts and as specified in the ACR BI-RADS standard [4].

2   State of the Art and New Contribution

Since 1972 there are numerous approaches to automate mammography image analysis. These approaches can be categorized in the specific task and the methods used. Common tasks are the detection of breasts and nipples, the registration of views, the detection of masses and the detections of calcifications [5, 6]. There are pixel- and region-based methods used for detection of abnormal regions (masses, calcifications). In pixel-based approaches, several filters such as edge detection, Law's texture, Gaussian smoothing, adaptive thresholding and others generate a feature vector per pixel. This feature vector is then classified into "normal" and "abnormal" using nearest neighbour, fuzzy, neural network or Bayesian classifiers. Region-based methods generate simply connected regions using a segmentation of the pixel filter responses. For those regions features are calculated which form the bases for classification.

Our approach extends and unifies pixel- and region-based methods. The image analysis task is modelled by an iterative segmentation and classification. All knowledge about the objects (regions) to detect is stored in an explicit semantic class network. The filtering, segmentation and classification processes are context-dependent and utilise the information gained in previous analysis steps. The generated object network enables us to analyse all four images simultaneously so that findings in one image may be supported by findings in other views.

3   Methods

We obtain 200 complete patient data sets from the Diagnostic Mammazentrum Munich and the Institute for Diagnostic Radiology of the University Erlangen. Each data set consists of a cranio-caudal (cc) and a medio-lateral (ml) mammogram of one or two breasts. The data sets are manually annotated using a BI-RADS compatible software tool developed at the Fraunhofer-Institute for Integrated Circuits IIS. For data sets with BI-RADS category 4 and 5 a breast biopsy is performed to validate the findings.

To automate mammography image analysis, we develop a Cognition Network Language (CNL) script using the Definiens Developer software. CNL is a concrete implementation of the Cognition Network Technology featuring rapid script prototyping and a graphical user-interface for visual script development. The mammography CNL script comprises a class network which describes the breast anatomy and BI-RADS related categories for findings (Fig 1). To describe the anatomy, classes for breast, nipple, skin, pectoral muscle, duct, mass and calcification are defined. Each class includes several attributes to allow its more specific classification. For example, the breast is described by a relative gray value range within the image histogram and by a given minimal size. The nipple is described as a local object boundary feature in breast shape (protruding part of specific size) or a texture feature when segmenting breast tissue in a stripe near skin. The calcifications are classified using a combination of edge filter response, contrast and area. The CNL script uses these class descriptions to segment and identify the objects simultaneously in all available images of one patient data set. The implemented strategy is to find first breasts, then skin and nipples, pectoral muscle, calcifications and finally masses. For the final classification of objects we utilise object linking. This generic concept enables CNL processes to establish and retrieve semantic (named) links between objects in a set of images. To link objects between the two views of one breast, the position of the nipple provides a reference coordinate. Since two two-dimensional views are registered, we further use the fact that one object dimension must be the same in both views. This registration enables the system to identify corresponding, similar objects (masses and calcifications) in both views (cc/ml). If an object was found in both views, we increase its detection probability. Furthermore, the intra-view linking of calcifications enables their classification according to group properties such as *linear*, *branched*, *segmented* and *pleomorphic*. We intend to use linking between objects found in the left and right breast to enhance the detection accuracy of masses. All findings are classified according to BI-RADS standard. Each patient record is automatically classified in BI-RADS category 1 to 5. To evaluate the quality of the automated analysis, we compare the detection results with the manual annotations provided by the medical experts. To calculate the number of true positive findings, we determine for each visual annotation its relative pixel overlap with each automatically found segment bearing the same classification. If the relative pixel overlap and the segment's classification probability are greater than predefined thresholds, then the annotation is counted as true positive (hit). The number of false negatives (misses) is determined by subtracting the number of hits from the number of annotations. The number of false positives (false alarms) is determined by counting all segments bearing a finding and having a relative overlap to a visual annotation of the same class less than a predefined threshold.

4   Results

In a first experiment we developed a CNL script which is able to extract breast, nipples nd calcifications reliably in a data set from 11 patients (see Figure 1). The script automatically detects the view orientation and classifies the extracted breast object according to that view e.g. right breast cranio-caudal. The nipples were found in all images at the correct location, although the exact position is sometimes difficult to determine even for a human expert. Individual calcifications were detected and grouped using the links to create a basis for benign/malign classification. The found malign calcifications in 11 patient cases indicate a true positive rate of 100% (no masses detected yet). We are therefore very confident to implement a prototype system in the next months which will deliver a true positive rate of greater than 99% on the full dataset of 200 patients while keeping false alarms and misses less than 1%.

Fig. 1. Screenshot of Definiens Developer software with a preliminary CNL script. The left-top window shows the raw data of one patient, the manual annotated regions (blue) and one selected, automatically found, potentially malign group of calcifications (red). The right-top window shows the segmentation results for breasts (orange), nipples (red), calcifications (blue) and malign/benign calcification markers (red/green). The bottom window shows a detail of two found groups of calcifications, one malign (red) and one benign (green). The small frames at right shows sections of the class and process hierarchies

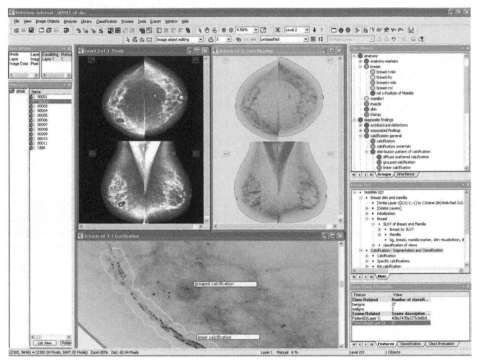

5   Summary

Already the first preliminary results of the knowledge driven approach for automated image analysis of mammograms described in this paper demonstrate the potential for the development of an analysis system with a very high degree of robustness and flexibility. The explicitly specified anatomical knowledge in the class network enables continuous improvement by medical experts and a transparency of decisions which are not achievable with other solutions such as neural networks. Based on Definiens platform technology "classical" concepts such as using various pixel image filters were embraces while the depth of analysis was extended by using a semantic (classified) object network. Moreover, the CNT implementation comprises an interactive scripting language, so that rapid solution development is possible. This enabled the detection of breasts, nipples and calcifications with high accuracy.

Acknowledgement

This work is part of the project Mammo-iCAD, thankfully funded by the Bavarian Research Foundation.

References

1. Athelogou M. Amobi 2 Abschlussbericht. Bayerische Forschungsstiftung; 2004.
2. Schaepe A, Urbani M, Leiderer R, Athelogou M. Fraktal hierarchische, prozess- und objektbasierte Bildanalyse. Procs BVM 2003.
3. Schoenmayer R, Athelogou M, et al. Automatisierte Segmentierung der Seitenventrikel des menschlichen Gehirns aus kernspintomographischen Datensaetzen. Procs BVM 2003; 83–87.
4. ACR BI-RADS Mammography. Deutsche Roentgengesellschaft, Thieme; 2006.
5. Sampat M, Markey M, Bovik A. Handbook of Image and Video Processing. Academic Press; 2005. 1195–1217.
6. Thangavel K, Karnan M, et al. Automatic detection of microcalcification in mammograms: A review. ICGST GVIP 2005;(5).

Pattern Recognition and Classification in High-Resolution Magnetic Resonance Spectra

Markus T. Wenzel, Bernd Merkel, Matthias Althaus, Heinz-Otto Peitgen

MeVis Research GmbH, Bremen, Germany
Email: wenzel|merkel|althaus|peitgen@mevis.de

Abstract. We show the impacts of various signal preprocessing techniques – dimensionality reduction and transformations – for high-resolution NMR spectra on the classification accuracy of different breast cancer tissue. Our results show that some preprocessing algorithms that are widely used nowadays will not reduce the data dimensionality in an information-preserving way: the classification accuracy drops. Besides showing the most successful preprocessing steps, we can report excellent results on a challenging classification problem.

1 Introduction

Despite growing research efforts on the identification of good prognostic factors for breast cancer, only few of them are proving clinically useful for identifying patients at minimal risk of relapse, patients with a worse prognosis, or patients likely to benefit from specific treatments. Traditional prognostic factors as lymph node status and tumor size are insufficiently accurate. Better or supplementary predictors of high-risk and treatment response are needed. Today, a number of new experimental methods are being explored to improve diagnostic and prognostic information on the genetic, protein or metabolite level, such as gene expression arrays, protein arrays and magnetic resonance spectroscopy (MRS), respectively. The MRS method gives a comprehensive window into tissue biochemistry and interrogates cancer tissue for diagnostic and prognostic markers. MRS of tissue specimens is an ex vivo technique with very high spectral resolution and signal-to-noise ratio. To explore the complex nature of such spectra with high reproducibility, automated classification schemes have to be implemented. There are many ways of processing [1, 2] and classifying [3, 4] NMR spectroscopic datasets. Our effort is to aid physicians in the everyday clinical routine of cancer diagnosis by automated high-resolution MR spectra classification.

2 State of the Art and New Contribution

In previous work carried out by DERR [5] various simple approaches for dimensionality reduction on high-resolution MRS spectra are compared. It is suggested to firstly refine the alignment of the spectra iteratively before performing piecewise integration such that neighbouring integration intervals overlap with a ratio that is selected to account for natural chemical shifts of metabolites. In a paper by BAUMGARTNER and co-workers [6] a method reducing spectral data with approximately 1500 dimensions is presented by employing a genetic algorithm that is constrained to deliver a maximum of 30 regions. This promising approach is to be explored for its ability to scale well with the dimensions of the data, which is work-in-progress.

Although a pathologist's expertise can determine the tumor grading of tissue biopsates with high accuracy, there are several disadvantages which the MRS diagnosis of tissue can overcome: the need for rather voluminous biopsates, the time-consuming procedure as such and therefore the elongated period of unwanted remaining in uncertainty for the patient. Additionally, not only the state can be determined from the spectra, but also a quantitative assessment of cancer indicating metabolites is possible. Moreover, the results of the basic research conducted here have the potential to be transferred to examinations of tissue by in-vivo MRS-Imaging methods, thus limiting the need for biopsy to cases where automatic classification results are ambiguous.

From the computer assisted diagnosis perspective, the first step is to identify methods to deal with the high dimensionality of the data in question. Therefore the impacts of various preprocessing steps on the final classification results are shown and compared. We believe this to be a major contribution to the systematic analysis of processing methods for high dimensionality data in general and for the assessment of spectral information based on MRS in particular.

3   Methods

Breast tissue biopsates have been WHO graded by pathology and measured by MRS. The complete dataset consists of 91 high resolution NMR spectra acquired on a Bruker Avance 600 spectrometer with a spectral width of 9kHz (see [7] for details). Of this dataset, 41 were rated to be of grading 0, two of grading 1, 26 of grading 2, 21 of grading 3 and one of grading 4. All classification results reported within this paper improve considerably (about 3%) when omitting the 3 samples of grading 1 and 4. Within an experimental pipeline approach consisting of three steps, we systematically modify the processing.

3.1   Alignment of Data

Upon acquisition of spectral data, reference points are manually set in the data. Therefore, instances are not correctly aligned with each other in general. This is a common problem in all research done where NMR spectral data is to be handled automatically. To overcome this unfavorable situation, we implemented an algorithm to estimate and correct this data misalignment. Regions present in all training spectra instances are identified manually. These regions are cut out and convolved with a a slightly broader region in all other examples. The peak of the convolution shows the respective "best fit" positions of the region in the test instance.

It is acknowledged, that all alignment performed by a rigid shift according to the displacement of only one section will only produce displacements in other regions. Still we achieved systematically increased classification rates after alignment, which may be due to fact that more important regions were now aligned with each other.

Advanced shifting algorithms – dynamic time warping (DTW) and correlation optimized warping (COW) – were also employed recently [8, 9]. Both were introduced for real-time processing of speech data, but were found to be useful in chemometrics as well. Our results with COW are more promising than those with DTW, but both require further research as to assess the side-effects, introduced with respect to the robustness of the overall system.

3.2   Transformations and Data Reduction

We performed data reduction with the following transformations on aligned and unaligned data, plus unchanged as control, ending up with four output datasets per input.

In subsampling every 5th and also every 6th data point with different starting points was kept.

For threshold-guided cutting we reduced the data to regions with signals above a threshold τ and longer than a threshold ρ. Only one configuration with $\tau = 800$ and $\rho = 0.034$ ppm was further considered, because the information loss seemed to worsen disproportionate to increasing τ and ρ, whereas the desired dimensionality reduction effect deteriorates disproportionate to decreasing thresholds. For the thresholds given above, the dimensionality approximately halves.

Additionally, we decomposed the data with predominantly biorthogonal wavelets, which were chosen based on prior experiences on mass spectrometric data. For further processing we used both detail and approximation coefficients from level 3 to 6, but also other wavelets like symlets and Daubechies were used.

Exhaustively searching all possible attribute combinations – although guaranteed to find the optimal solution – is clearly not feasible computationally on datasets of tens of thousands of attributes. A very common alternative is a feature selection, based on correlation, although it is doubted in [10]. The "Best First" forward selection (FS) method adds single best attributes iteratively unless some optimality criterion stops improving. FS is guaranteed to converge, but not necessarily to the optimal solution, because it will not combine individually inferior attributes, which may however perform better if combined. For our experiments, we used the WEKA implementation of this algorithm [11]. Also, we employed a Genetic Algorithm (GA) guided selection from the same toolbox, using its default parameters.

3.3   Evaluation by Classification

To evaluate the performance of the data alignment, data transformation, and dimensionality reduction techniques on our data, we chose the classification accu-

Table 1. Best classification results with forward selection

Method	# Attributes / Accuracy			
	Unaligned		Aligned	
Subsampling (5th)	42	74.7%	30	80.2%
Threshold+Subsampling	29	70.3%	35	71.4%
Bior3.7-Approx.3	24	70.3%	33	74.7%
Bior3.7-Det.3	37	76.9%	34	73.6%
Only FS	72	79.1%	66	81.3%
Only FS w/o grad.I+IV	78	83.0%	68	84.1%

racy as the performance measure. The input of this pipeline step are the datasets produced from the above preprocessing.

We compare the results of all feature reduction algorithms by applying a Random Forest classification algorithm to the reduced data [12]. Random Forests are collections of Random Trees built from randomly selected subsets of all training subjects, where the split at each node is performed based on a random selection of attributes. The parametrization of the number of random attributes used for each split in the trees was chosen based on suggestions of BREIMAN [12]. The number of random trees to build was determined by our experiments and finally fixed at 100 trees.

4 Results

In our experiments we found that subsampling worsens the classification accuracy while not substantially reducing the feature number. If, however, FS is applied on the subsampled data, 80.2% on the aligned data resulted.

Threshold-guided cutting in combination with subsampling the spectra performed worse, although the classification accuracy increases with FS. Doing a classification only on the wavelet-transformed spectra was not successful, but here with FS better accuracies were achieved.

Table 1 summarizes our results from the main set of experiments where the pipeline steps were varied. We give only the best accuracies together with the according configuration. As the GA guided selection performed worse on almost every approach, no results are in here.

Reducing the problem to a two-class-problem (benign vs. malignant), we achieved 92.0% sensitivity and 95.1% specificity on the aligned data by applying only FS without any previous transformation or data reduction.

5 Discussion

Our comparison of feature selection algorithms showed the unexpected superiority of Forward Selection over all competing approaches. The results generally improved after a coarse alignment of the instance vectors motivating further research in this area. A wavelet transformation did not improve classification results as expected. Nevertheless, since the accuracy did not drop significantly and since wavelet decomposition is a fast and widely used approach to dimensionality reduction, we will also explore these topics in the future.

Since we only examined the spectra from the lipid phase of the breast tissue we expect an improved classification result when the water soluble phase is also taken into account. In general, the classification on lipid-spectra is more challenging due to the high demand on the measurement accuracy [7], suggesting the possibility to generalize our approach on this data.

We wish to cross-check our results with other classifications schemes. In our ongoing research we implement projective classification schemes which promise to provide dimensionality reduction by projection and classification in a joint approach [9]. Besides, we are currently evaluating established methods of spectral analysis to be able to compare our findings better with widely acknowledged "ground truth" methods.

References

1. Vanhamme L, Sundin T, van Hecke P, van Huffel S. MR spectroscopic quantitation: A review of time-domain methods. NMR Biomed 2001;14:233–246.
2. Mierisová S, Ala-Korpela M. MR spectroscopy quantitation: a review of frequency domain methods. NMR Biomed 2001;14:247–259.
3. Hagberg G. From magnetic resonance spectroscopy to classification of tumors: A review of pattern recognition methods. NMR Biomed 1998;11:148–156.
4. Menze BH, Lichy MP, Bachert P, Kelm BM, Schlemmer HP, Hamprecht FA. Optimal classification of long echo time in vivo magnetic resonance spectra in the detection of recurrent brain tumors. NMR Biomed 2006;19:599–609.
5. Derr T. Medizinisch-diagnostische Anwendung neuronaler Netzwerke zur Analyse NMR-spektroskopischer Daten von Körperflüssigkeiten. Ph.D. thesis. Universität Bremen; 1997.
6. Baumgartner R, Ho TK, Somorjai R, Himmelreich U, Sorrell T. Complexity of magnetic resonance spectrum classification. Data Complexity in Pattern Recognition 2005.
7. Beckonert O, Monnerjahn J, Bonk U, Leibfritz D. Visualizing metabolic changes in breast-cancer tissue using 1H-NMR spectroscopy and self-organizing maps. NMR Biomed 2003;16:1–11.
8. Tomasi G, van den Berg F, Andersson C. Correlation optimized warping and dynamic time warping as preprocessing methods for chromatographic data. J Chemometrics 2004;18:231–241.
9. Wenzel MT, Merkel B, Althaus M, Peitgen HO. PCNSA for NMR spectroscopy breast tissue classification. In: ISMRM DP Spect WS; 2006.
10. Nikulin AE, Dolenko B, Bezabeh T, Somorjai RL. Near-optimal region selection for feature space reduction: Novel preprocessing methods for classifying MR spectra. NMR in Biomedicine 1998;11:209–216.
11. Witten IH, Frank E. Data Mining: Practical Machine Learning Tools and Techniques. 2nd ed. San Francisco: Morgan Kaufmann; 2005.
12. Breiman L. Random Forests. Machine Learning 2001;45:5–32.

Fully-Automatic Correction of the Erroneous Border Areas of an Aneurysm

J. Bruijns, F.J. Peters, R.P.M. Berretty, B. Barenbrug

Philips Research Eindhoven, The Netherlands
Email: Jan.Bruijns@philips.com

Abstract. Volume representations of blood vessels acquired by 3D rotational angiography are very suitable for diagnosing an aneurysm. We presented a fully-automatic aneurysm labelling method in a previous paper. In some cases, a portion of a "normal" vessel part connected to the aneurysm is incorrectly labelled as aneurysm. We developed a method to detect and correct these erroneous border areas. Application of this method gives better estimates for the aneurysm volumes.

1 Problem

Volume representations of blood vessels acquired by 3D rotational angiography show a clear distinction in gray values between tissue and vessel voxels [1]. These volume representations are very suitable for diagnosing an aneurysm. Physicians may treat an aneurysm by filling it with coils. Therefore, they need to know the volume of the aneurysm.

We developed a method for fully-automatic labelling of the aneurysm voxels after which the volume is computed by counting these voxels [2]. We use local distance thresholds to define a tight bounding surface around the aneurysm. This tight bounding surface should be located just outside the aneurysm where it borders to tissue. Elsewhere, it should intersect the "normal" vessel parts as close to the aneurysm as possible. The local distance thresholds are derived from border vessel voxels (i.e. vessel voxels connected to a tissue voxel). Since border vessel voxels are missing at an aneurysm neck, the tight bounding surface may bulge out into a "normal" vessel part. In such a case a portion of this vessel part is incorrectly labelled as aneurysm (Fig. 2.1, Fig. 2.3).

A possible solution to correct these erroneous labelled border areas of the aneurysm consists of first interactively creating a connection tube through such a border area, and next computing the neck outline. After the neck outline is computed, the aneurysm voxels in this border area are changed to "normal" vessel voxels [3]. The problem with this solution is that correcting all erroneous labelled border areas interactively may take a lot of time.

2 Related Work

Bruijne et al. [4] use model-based interactive segmentation of abdominal aortic aneurysms from CTA data and multi-spectral MR images. After manual delineation of the aneurysm sac in the first slice, the method automatically detects the contour in subsequent slices.

Bescos et al. [5] described a method for the measurement of intracranial aneurysms from 3D rotational angiography using gradient edge detection. Using 13 aneurysm phantoms, they showed that their method gives more accurate volume measurements than gray value thresholds selected by a human operator. But, they use manual segmentation to separate the aneurysm from the "normal" vessels.

Wong et al. [6] described a method for the detection of vascular abnormalities given a topologically and morphologically correct vascular segmentation (i.e., with no holes and cavities). They first create a model of the "normal" vessels. The abnormal vascular structures are then determined as the complement of the approximated "normal" vessels. But, to create the initial tubes per vessel section a human operator has to select two centerline endpoints in 3D space for each section between two branch points. These centerline endpoints should be located outside the abnormal vascular structures.

3   What Is New

To eliminate the time-consuming interaction, we have developed a method to automatically create as many of the required connection tubes as possible. For each created connection tube the neck outline is computed so that the erroneous aneurysm voxels in this border area are changed to "normal" vessel voxels.

We use the shape information extracted from the "normal" vessel parts to control this process. In our system, shape information extracted from a "normal" vessel part is stored in a *tube object* (tube for short). A tube consists of a series of consecutive probes [7]. A *probe* is a combination of a sphere, a plane through the center of the sphere and a number of shape parameters. After a tube is created by fully-automatic vessel tracing [8], the sphere centers are close to the central axis of the vessel, the planes are almost orthogonal to the vessel and each probe contains an ellipse representing the local cross-section of the probe's plane with the vessel surface. Note that the fully-automatic branch labelling method is extended to also create a node for each aneurysm neck.

4   Method

An erroneous labelled border area of the aneurysm is normally bounded by two necks. But not every neck pair defines an erroneously labelled border area. After all, there may exist neck pairs for which the connection tube travels through the inner area of the aneurysm (note that for faithful representation of the local vessel shape a connection tube does not connect the two necks but two remote cross-sections of the two "normal" vessel parts connected to these necks [3]). To prevent the inner area of the aneurysm from being changed, the necks of a border area neck pair must fulfill certain conditions. The most important ones are:

Fig. 1. A checkpoint on a peripheral connection tube

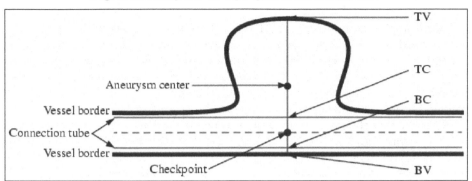

1. The vessel radii at the two neck nodes are about equal.
   A neck pair is rejected if one radius is less than or equal to the half of the other radius. It is very unlikely that two such vessel parts represent an "normal" continuous vessel part.
2. The connection tube travels through the periphery of the aneurysm.
   We check the location of the connection tube at five checkpoints on the central curve between the two neck centers. A checkpoint is OK if one of the following two conditions is fulfilled along the line through this checkpoint and the center of the aneurysm (Fig. 1):
   (a) The top of the aneurysm along this line TV is located above the top of the connection tube TC and the bottom of the connection tube BC is located below the bottom of the vessel BV (this case is not shown in Fig. 1).
   (b) The distance below the connection tube (BC located above BV as shown in Fig. 1) is less than the average neck radius r and the distance above the connection tube is much greater than the distance below the connection tube: $\| BC - BV \| < r \wedge \| TV - TC \| > \| BC - BV \| + r$
   The location of the vessel tube is OK if and only if all five checkpoints are OK.

Remarks:

1. If the aneurysm bulge does not block the "normal" vessel part completely, the erroneous labelled border area is defined by a single neck. So, not only all neck pairs but also each single neck is checked, applying similar conditions as used for each neck pair.
2. To detect as many erroneous labelled border areas as possible, the necks should be located as close to the aneurysm as possible (see [9]). Therefore, the necks have first been shifted as close to the real aneurysm as possible.

5   Results and Discussion

We have applied our method to 51 clinical volume datasets with a single aneurysm (16 of them with a resolution of 256x256x256, the rest 128x128x128 voxels), acquired with the 3D Integris system [10]. In 39 of these cases erroneous border areas were corrected. The total number of erroneous border areas corrected was 92 (an aneurysm can have more than one erroneous border area). No connection tube was generated through the inner area of an aneurysm.

The effect of the correction of the erroneous border areas can be perceived by comparing Fig. 2.1 with Fig. 2.2 and Fig. 2.3 with Fig. 2.4. These last two pictures reveal that our method is able to correct multiple connected erroneous border areas. Since the original vessel cross-sections are represented by the ellipses of the connection tube, tiny local bulges on the vessel surface result in a bumpy border between the aneurysm and the "normal" vessel section.

The mean number of aneurysm voxels changed is 12.5% of the number of aneurysm voxels, the maximum number of aneurysm voxels changed is 45.6% (a large relative correction may arise when the size of the real aneurysm is about the same as the size of the "normal" vessel part). Although some "normal" vessel voxels may be missed and some aneurysm voxels may be incorrectly changed, correction of the erroneous border areas gives better estimates for our clinical aneurysm volumes but a clinical validation of the accuracy of our aneurysm labelling method has yet to be done.

The average elapsed time for first shifting of the aneurysm necks as close to the real aneurysm as possible followed by fully-automatic correction of the erroneous border areas of an 128x128x128 volume is 15.5 seconds on an SGI Octane (300MHz MIPS R12000 + MIPS R12010 FPU) and 2.4 seconds on a Linux PC (2.8GHz Pentium 4). The average elapsed time for an 256x256x256 volume is 131.2 seconds on the SGI Octane and 16.6 seconds on the Linux PC. So, the elapsed time scales almost linearly with the number of voxels of the volume.

References

1. Kemkers R, de Beek JOp, Aerts H, et al. 3D-rotational angiography: First clinical application with use of a standard Philips C-arm system. In: Proc. CAR 98. Tokyo, Japan; 1998. 182–187.
2. Bruijns J. Local distance thresholds for enhanced aneurysm labelling. Procs BVM 2005; 148–152.
3. Bruijns J, Peters FJ, Berretty RPM, et al. Computer-aided treatment planning of an aneurysm: The connection tube and the neck outline. In: Proc. VMV. Erlangen, Germany; 2005. 265–272.
4. de Bruijne M, van Ginneken B, Viergever MA, et al. Interactive segmentation of abdominal aortic aneurysms in CTA images. Med Image Anal 2004;8(2):127–138.
5. Bescos JO, Slob MJ, Slump CH, et al. Volume measurement of intracranial aneurysms from 3D rotational angiography: Improvement of accuracy by gradient edge detection. AJNR Am J Neuroradiol 2005;26(10):2569–2572.

6. Wong WCK, Chung ACS. Augmented vessels for quantitative analysis of vascular abnormalities and endovascular treatment planning. IEEE Trans Med Imaging 2006;25(6):655–684.
7. Bruijns J. Semi-automatic shape extraction from tube-like geometry. In: Proc. VMV. Saarbruecken, Germany; 2000. 347–355.
8. Bruijns J. Fully-automatic branch labelling of voxel vessel structures. In: Proc. VMV. Stuttgart, Germany; 2001. 341–350.
9. Bruijns J, Peters FJ, Berretty RPM, et al. Shifting of the aneurysm necks for enhanced aneurysm labelling. Procs BVM 2006; 141–145.
10. Philips-Medical-Systems-Nederland. INTEGRIS 3D-RA. Instructions for use. Release 2.2. Philips Medical Systems Nederland. Best, The Netherlands; 2001.

Pictures

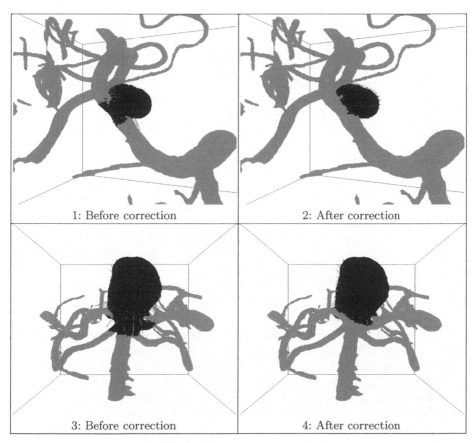

1: Before correction   2: After correction

3: Before correction   4: After correction

Fig. 2. Two aneurysm cases

Real-Time Image Mosaic for Endoscopic Video Sequences

Wolfgang Konen[1], Beate Breiderhoff[1], Martin Scholz[2]

[1]Institut für Informatik, Fachhochschule Köln, 51643 Gummersbach
[2]Neurochirurgische Universitätsklinik, Ruhr-Universität Bochum, 44892 Bochum
Email: wolfgang.konen@gm.fh-koeln.de

Abstract. We present an algorithm capable of making in real time image mosaics with enlarged field-of-view from the endoscopic video data stream. The algorithm is based on the method of Kourogi et al. (1999) which we extend to the case of endoscopic masks. The algorithm automatically finds the optimal affine transform between video frames and builds the enlarged field-of-view as an intervention-free side task. We apply our algorithm to endoscopic video sequences and compare it to the well-known image-mosaicing algorithm of Szeliski (1994). Our method turns out to be more robust, more than 3 times faster, having at the same time a 4 times smaller average motion estimation error: 0.19 pixel instead of 0.72 pixel between successive frames.

1 Introduction

In endoscopic interventions the surgeon has often to deal with a rather limited field of view which can cause navigational difficulties. It would be therefore desirable to have a tool which combines automatically many endoscopic video frames to a larger, metrically accurate field-of-view ('panoramic overview'). To our knowledge such an endeavour has not been undertaken so far, with the exception of a very recent (Oct'06) paper [1] which was brought to our attention after submitting this paper. They show interesting results obtained independently on endoscopic retinal images. Our approach is similar, using and evaluating a new method based on optical flow.

Many algorithms on image mosaicing are known, however only relatively few of them can work fully automatic, e.g. [2, 3, 1, 4] and under real-time conditions [2, 1, 4]. Except for [1] they have not yet been applied to endoscopic video. On the other hand, interesting work on combining and improving endoscopic images exist: Wald et al. [5] combine two endoscopic frames using manual control points and show how the image quality can be improved by using a smoothing cross dissolve technique. Vogt et al. [6] show how to reduce colour errors and mark specular lights in endoscopic images. This is an important prerequisite for image mosaics.

Fig. 1. The main idea of Kourogi's algorithm shown for the 1D-case

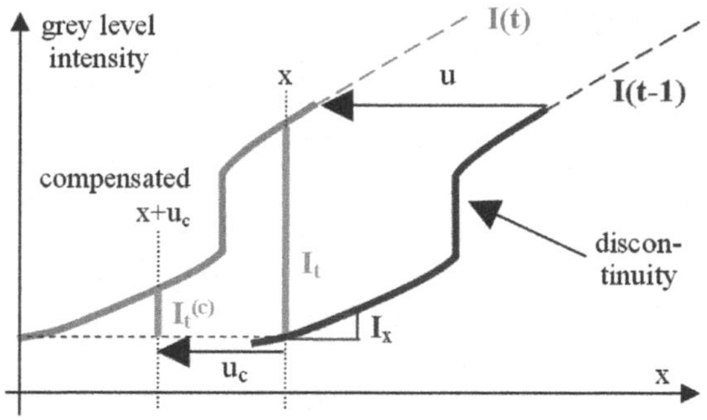

2   Methods

The goal of Kourogi's algorithm [2] is to estimate the motion field between successive frames $I(t-1)$ and $I(t)$ of a video sequence. This is done with an improved optical flow algorithm which calculates at each pixel (x, y) the so-called pseudo motion

$$\begin{pmatrix} u_p \\ v_p \end{pmatrix} = \begin{pmatrix} -I_t^{(c)}/I_x \\ -I_t^{(c)}/I_y \end{pmatrix} + \begin{pmatrix} u_c \\ v_c \end{pmatrix} \text{ with } I_t^{(c)} = I(x + u_c, y + v_c, t) - I(x, y, t-1)$$

where I_x and I_y denote the spatial gradient and (u_c, v_c) is the so-called compensated motion at this pixel location. If we set $(u_c, v_c) = 0$ then $I_t^{(c)}$ becomes the time derivative I_t and we have the usual pseudo motion equation, which is however known to be non-robust and bound to fail at discontinuities or non-linearities in grey level distribution (Fig. 1). Due to the shown discontinuity the estimate $-I_t/I_x$ will be larger than the true motion u. If, on the other hand, u_c is an estimate for the true motion, it is likely that we avoid the discontinuity and get with $-I_t^{(c)}/I_x + u_c$ a good estimate for u. Note that $I_t^{(c)}$ has to be calculated with subpixel accuracy.

Our algorithm proceeds now as follows: First the compensated motion is initialized either with zero or with an estimate from the previous frame. Then the following steps are carried out in a loop:

1. Calculate the pseudo motion for each pixel of the endoscopic mask.
2. Accept only those pixel which fulfil the following criteria:
   (a) I_x and I_y are not 0,
   (b) $(x + u_p, y + v_p)$ is inside the endoscopic mask, and
   (c) $|I(x + u_p, y + v_p, t - I(x, y, t-1)| < T$. Here, T is a suitable grey level threshold, e.g. $T = 5$.

3. Find the affine parameters $\mathbf{a} = \{a_1, \ldots, a_6\}$ for a global motion field best-fitting the pseudo motion at all accepted pixel locations i, i.e. solve the overdetermined system of equations

$$a_1 x_i + a_2 y_i + a_3 = u_{p,i} \quad \text{and} \quad a_4 x_i + a_5 y_i + a_6 = v_{p,i} \qquad (1)$$

in a least-square sense. Use the motion field given by $\mathbf{a}$ as a new estimate for (u_c, v_c) and continue with step (1.).

The loop is terminated either after a fixed number of iterations or when the change in the global motion field drops below a certain threshold.

Some care has to be taken when setting up the masks: In order to avoid large errors at the mask boundary, the gradient calculation with a [-1 0 1] filter is allowed only at those pixels which come from a smaller region, namely the morphological erosion of the mask with a 3x3 cross. Likewise the bilinear interpolation can only be done at pixels from a region being an erosion with a 2x2 square of the original mask.

After a frame is registered, the 'new' portion of it is added to the image mosaic using bilinear interpolation. This can be done rather fast since each frame adds only a small new region to the existing mosaic. Currently no special blending occurs but a blending strategy as reported in [5] can be easily incorporated.

3   Results

We tested our algorithm on short endoscopic video sequences. In this first step the goal was to measure its accuracy and to compare its performance with another well-known image mosaicing algorithm [3] applied to the same task. We created a short endoscopic video sequence (30 frames) where each frame is connected to the next by a known affine transform, for example translations up to 10 pixel, size changes up to 8% and combinations thereof. These transforms correspond to simple camera movements. The motion field differs from frame to frame. Figs. 2a and 2c show 4 frames out of these sequences.

We tested two algorithms: The first one is our method described in Sec. 2, based on Kourogi's algorithm [2] with acceptance threshold $T = 5$. The second one is based on the well known Szeliski image mosaicing algorithm [3]. Both algorithms work *fully automated* on video sequences, i.e. they had no other information than the sequence itself (no start parameters). The resulting image mosaic (panoramic view) gives the surgeon a much better overview than the single frames. It is free of mosaicing artefacts and close to the original base image in Kourogi's case (Fig. 2b and 2d). In the case of Szeliski's algorithm (not shown here) it has clear artefacts and errors in aspect ratio estimation.

In Fig. 3, we compare the frame-to-frame accuracy, measured as the mean motion error Δu (in pixel) between the true and the estimated motion field. Kourogi's method has much lower error and we do not have any outliers in the frame sequence. Szeliski's method has outliers (e.g. frames #1-4). This is

Fig. 2. Results: (a) 4 out of 30 frames from a facial video sequence, (b) image mosaic resulting with Kourogi's algorithm, (c) and (d) the same for the neuroendoscopic video sequence

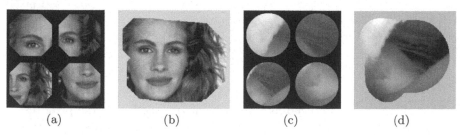

(a)   (b)   (c)   (d)

Fig. 3. Accuracy of Szeliski's and Kourogi's algorithm: (a) facial video, (b) neuroendoscopic video

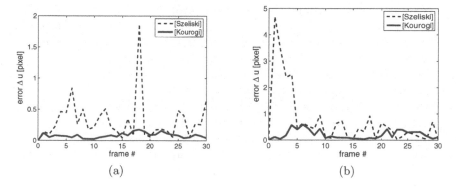

(a)   (b)

important because a single outlier will make all subsequent frames in the image mosaic wrong w.r.t. the frames before.

While having a 4 times better accuracy, the method of Kourogi is at the same time faster by a factor of 3 (Tab. 1). The computation time of 4.3 sec/frame is obviously not yet real time. But this is only due to the fact, that our current implementation is a first development step with slow Matlab code. We plan to rebuild the system in C or C++ and have no doubt that we can reach with today's standard PCs a performance of at least 10 fps as Kourogi [2] reported it 8 years ago.

4   Conclusion and Outlook

We have shown how to build image mosaics from endoscopic video sequences. Of course our work is only a very first step towards an integrated system for real-time endoscopic image mosaicing. Nevertheless this first step is promising, since the algorithm turns out to be robust, does not need any manual intervention or starting values, is faster and at the same time more accurate than comparable algorithms.

Table 1. Comparison of main features of both image mosaicing algorithms

	computation time	avg. frame-to-frame accuracy $< \Delta u >$	outlier frames $(< \Delta u > \; > 1$ pixel)
Szeliski	15.5 sec/frame	0.72 pixel	4
Kourogi	4.3 sec/frame	0.19 pixel	0
improvement	factor 3	factor 4	

We believe that the crucial feature of Kourogi's method is the pixel test in step (2.), which allows to base any estimate only on those pixels where the information seems reliable. This flexibility of the proposed algorithm has a further advantage when dealing with specular lights: If a system along the lines of [6] detects specular lights, these can be easily accounted for by marking them as 'non-acceptable' pixels during the registration process.

There are many directions we plan to investigate in the near future: The class of transforms should be extended from affine to projective to account for more general camera movements. The distorsion of an endoscope lens system has to be taken into account. We know from our previous work [7] how to calibrate an endoscope camera system and therefore believe that this step is quite straightforward. Changes in lighting should be accounted for: Global contrast and brightness will vary slowly from frame to frame, but specular lights can vary quite rapidly. We plan to port the system to a real-time environment and test it with real endoscope sequences, leading finally into the integration in our VN system [8]. Different strategies for combining videos to image mosaics will be explored and will be tested with respect to their ergonomic requirements by surgeons working in daily routine with endoscopic images.

References

1. Seshamani S, Lau WW, Hager GD. Real-time endoscopic mosaicking. Procs MICCAI 2006;4190:355–363.
2. Kourogi M, Kurata T, Hoshino J, et al. Real-time image mosaicing from a video sequence. In: International Conference on Image Processing. vol. 4; 1999. 133–137.
3. Szeliski R. Image mosaicing for tele-reality applications. Cambridge Research Lab; 1994.
4. Robinson JA. A Simplex-based projective transform estimator. In: Visual Information Engineering; 2003. 290–293.
5. Wald D, Reeff M, Székely G, et al. Fliessende Überblendung von Endoskopiebildern für die Erstellung eines Mosaiks. Procs BVM 2005; 287–291.
6. Vogt F, Klimowicz C, Paulus D, et al. Bildverarbeitung in der Endoskopie des Bauchraums. Procs BVM 2001; 320–324.
7. Konen W, Scholz M, Tombrock S. The VN-project: endoscopic image processing for neurosurgery. Computer Aided Surgery 1998;3(3):144–148.
8. Scholz M, Dick S, Fricke B, et al. Consideration of ergonomic aspects in the development of a new endoscopic navigation system. Br J Neurosurg 2005;19(5):402–408.

Haptische Interaktion zur Planung von Nasennebenhöhlen-Operationen

Arno Krüger[1], Kristina Stampe[1], Ilka Hertel[2], Gero Strauß[2], Bernhard Preim[1]

[1]Otto-von-Guericke-Universität Magdeburg, Institut für Simulation und Graphik
[2]Universitätskrankenhaus Leipzig, Abteilung HNO-Heilkunde
Email: krueger@isg.cs.uni-magdeburg.de

Zusammenfassung. Moderne Operationstechniken im Bereich der Nasennebenhöhlen bringen Vorteile für den Patienten, jedoch auch neue Herausforderungen für den Operateur mit sich. Durch die endoskopischen Verfahren ist die Navigation und Orientierung während des Eingriffs erschwert und setzt eine besonders gründliche Planung voraus. Bei Problemfällen ist die Nutzung von 2d-Schichtbildern, die traditionell Verwendung finden, schwieriger. Vor allem bei Rezidivoperationen fehlen oft zur Orientierung wichtige anatomische Landmarken. In diesem Paper wird ein System vorgestellt, das mit Hilfe virtueller Endoskopie eine patientenindividuelle Planung von endoskopischen Nasennebenhöhlen-Eingriffen unterstützt. Dabei wird besonderer Wert auf die Interaktion mit der 3d-Darstellung und eine intuitive Nutzerführung gelegt.

1 Einleitung

Für die Behandlung von chronischen Nasennebenhöhlen (NNH)- Entzündungen haben sich minimal-invasive Operationstechniken gegenüber der Radikalchirurgie durchgesetzt. Für die Durchführung endoskopischer Eingriffe ist Erfahrung, ein gutes räumliches Vorstellungsvermögen sowie manuelle Geschicklichkeit notwendig. Durch die eingeschränkte Sicht auf das Operationsfeld muss sich der Chirurg bei der Navigation durch die Hohlräume an antomischen Landmarken orientieren. Durch anatomische Variationen, pathologische Veränderungen oder vorangegangene Eingriffe kann die Orientierung während des Eingriffs erschwert sein. Eine exakte Planung der Eingriffe ist deshalb unverzichtbar. Dazu werden hoch aufgelöste 3d-Datensätze genutzt. Die Segmentierung ermöglicht die Darstellung der relevanten anatomischen Strukturen in Form von 3d-Modellen. Damit können komplexe Lagebeziehungen, anatomische Besonderheiten (stehende Schädelbasis) sowie Risikostrukturen (z.B. Nähe N. Opticus oder A. carotis interna) in einer vereinfachten und verständlichen Art und Weise hervorgehoben werden. Bei der Operationsplanung ermöglichen die Visualisierungen von Patientendaten die Minimierung von Risiken. Eine räumliche Repräsentation, ähnlich zu der während des späteren Eingriffs (Virtuelle Endoskopie), kann zusätzlich als Vorbereitung für die Operation dienen und damit die intraoperative Orientierung unterstützen. Eine wesentliche Schwierigkeit stellt jedoch die Interaktion mit derartigen 3d-Visualisierungen dar, weshalb ein 3d-Eingabegerät mit Kraftrückkopplung eingesetzt werden soll.

2 Stand der Forschung und Zielstellung

Die Anwendbarkeit der virtuellen Endoskopie für die Diagnose von NNH-Erkrankungen war bereits Gegenstand der Forschung ([1], [2], [3]). Die Darstellung der 3d-Informationen erfolgt dabei mittels eines Volumen- oder Surface-Renderings. Die Modelle werden genutzt, um Bilder und Videos verschiedener anatomischer Strukturen aus Sicht eines Endoskops für diagnostische Zwecke zu generieren. Die Vergleiche zwischen virtueller und optischer Endoskopie zeigen, dass die anatomischen Strukturen und Variationen der NNH ebenfalls gut am 3d-Modell erkennbar sind (vgl. [3]). Die Darstellung von pathologischen Veränderungen der Oberfläche hängt dabei jedoch von der Auflösung der Daten ab. Weiterhin erschweren fehlende Informationen die Identifizierung von krankem Gewebe [2]. Eine Untersuchung der Nasennebenhöhlen auf strukturelle Veränderungen ist auch bei Verschluss der Öffnungen möglich, solange der Hohlraum frei ist. Für das Training von NNH-Operationen sind verschiedene Prototypen entwickelt worden, die auf einer Kombination von visueller Repräsentation des Operationsgeschehens, gekoppelt mit haptischem Feedback basieren (z.B. [4], [5]). Neben einer möglichst realistischen Darstellung der Strukturen ist auch die Bedienung auf größtmögliche Realitätstreue hin optimiert. Pößneck u.a. [5] setzen ein für die Simulation von endoskopischen NNH-Eingriffen angepasstes Trainingssystem ein. Eine Segmentierungs- und Modellierungssoftware wird genutzt, um aus 3d-Daten ein verformbares polygonales Modell der NNH zu erstellen.

Bestehende Trainingssysteme lassen sich für eine patientenindividuelle Operationsplanung nur bedingt einsetzen. Neben dem hohen gerätetechnischen Aufwand ist vor allem die Vorverarbeitungszeit von Datensätzen ein Hinderungsgrund. Darüber hinaus ist eine exakte Simulation, z.B. von Gewebe für die Fragestellungen bei der Operationsplanung nicht nötig. Das STEPS-System [6] wurde zwar für die Planung von endoskopischen Tumoroperationen am Gehirn konzipiert, bietet jedoch planungstechnisch interessante Ansätze, die auch für NNH-Eingriffe anwendbar sind. Der Zugang zum Gehirn findet beim STEPS-System durch die gesunden NNH statt, wodurch keine Visualisierungs-Probleme mit Schwellungen oder krankhaft veränderten Strukturen auftreten können. Es werden direkt die CT-Daten des Patienten genutzt, und es besteht die Möglichkeit einer haptisch unterstützten Navigation mittels eines Force-Feedback-Joysticks.

Die hier vorgestellte Planung verfolgt die Zielstellung eine speziell für die NNH angepasste Operationsplanung zu schaffen, welche die Besonderheiten dieser sehr häufigen Eingriffe optimal unterstützt. Sowohl auf Seiten der Visualisierung als auch der Steuerung mit haptischer Unterstützung wird dem Chirurgen Vertrautes angeboten werden. Darüber hinaus wird für den praktischen Einsatz eine minimale Vorverarbeitungszeit der Patientendaten angestrebt.

3 Umsetzung

Für Untersuchungen der Hohlräume der Nase eignen sich egozentrische Interaktionsmetaphern, die eine Sicht aus der Ich-Perspektive ermöglichen. Exozentrische

Sichten können jedoch zusätzlich eine Übersicht vermitteln und die Orientierung erleichtern. Für die Realisierung der Kameraführung ist die Umsetzung einer geführten Navigation am geeignetsten, da sie dem Anwender eine individuelle Kameraführung ermöglicht, diese jedoch sinnvoll einschränkt. Eine automatische Berechnung eines idealen Kamerapfades für die Untersuchung der NNH ist aufgrund der Komplexität und Individualität der Anatomie nicht möglich. Hinzu kommt die besondere Schwierigkeit durch krankhafte Veränderungen. Eine Alternative ist die manuelle Bestimmung eines Kamerapfades zu den relevanten Strukturen, was jedoch den Aufwand im Vorfeld stark erhöht. Die Aufgabe des haptischen Feedbacks bei der geführten Navigation liegt in der Simulation des Kontaktes zwischen Kamera und Gewebe. Durch den Einsatz von 3d-Eingabegeräten kann die Positionierung von Messelementen bzw. virtuellen Instrumenten schneller durchgeführt werden. Haptisches Feedback kann die Präzision dieser Aktionen erhöhen, indem eine fühlbare Kollision mit der Oberfläche von Objekten über den Tastsinn des Benutzers simuliert wird.

Um eine größtmögliche Darstellungsgenauigkeit der filigranen Strukturen zu erreichen, eignet sich die Darstellung der Volumenmodelle über Direktes Volumenrendering (DVR). Die zeitintensive Generierung von Oberflächenmodellen entfällt bei diesem Ansatz. Für die Erzeugung von haptischem Feedback für die Planung von NNH-Eingriffen sind Volumenmodelle ebenfalls sehr gut geeignet. Kraftfelder werden z.B. vorberechnet und reduzieren damit den Rechenaufwand zur Laufzeit. Einige Algorithmen nutzen die Transferfunktion zum direkten Volumenrendering ebenfalls zur Bestimmung der haptischen Oberflächeneigenschaften [6]. Dieses Vorgehen erlaubt auch ein direktes visuelles und haptisches Rendern auf den originalen Volumendaten, stellt jedoch nur eine grobe Annäherung dar. Für die Interaktionsaufgabe der Kamerasteuerung eignen sich besonders Potentialfelder, die den Betrag der Abstoßungskräfte in Abhängigkeit von der Distanz zur Organoberfläche repräsentieren (vgl. [7]). Ein Eindringen in die Gewebeoberfläche wird damit verhindert und der Anwender erhält eine Sicht auf die Hohlräume. Während der Entwicklung wurde ein kommerziell verfügbares haptisches Eingabegerät PHANToM der Firma Sensable verwendet. Es besitzt in der Desktop-Version 6 Freiheitsgrade für die Eingabe und 3 für die Ausgabe.

4 Ergebnisse

Es wurde prototypisch ein System für die haptisch unterstützte virtuelle Endoskopie der NNH entwickelt. Als Plattform für die Umsetzung kam MeVisLab (www.mevislab.de) zum Einsatz. Dieses Rapid-Prototyping-System für medizinische Anwendungen beinhaltet viele der benötigten Bildverarbeitungs- und Visualisierungskomponenten in Modulform. Der Prototyp liegt in Netzwerken aus solchen Modulen vor. Dabei dient eines der Erzeugung der Datenstrukturen und ein weiteres für die virtuelle Endoskopie. Das neu entwickelte und für die Berechnung der Rückgabekräfte zuständige Modul setzt ein haptisches Rendering auf der Basis von Distanz- und Gradientenfeldern um. Das generierte

Abb. 1. Endoskopische Sicht (links), kombiniert mit den orthogonalen Navigationssichten sowie der Lage des Endoskops (rechts)

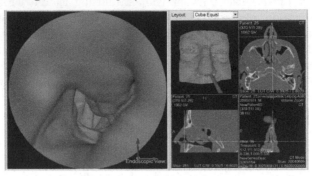

haptische Feedback dient als Benutzerführung und lässt sich bei Bedarf durch etwas stärkere Kraftaufwendung überwinden. Damit können auch Hohlräume, die keine direkte Verbindung zu den NNH besitzen, beispielsweise beim Verschluss oder Verlegung der Ostien durch Gewebe, untersucht werden. Die Visualisierung umfasst die Sicht des virtuellen Endoskops auf den Datensatz, orthogonale Schnittbilder für die Position des Endoskops und eine 3d-Übersicht, welche die Lage des Endoskops innerhalb des Datensatzes visualisiert (Abb. 1). Die Vorverarbeitung nimmt ca. 5 min in Anspruch, wobei die größte Zeitspanne für die Berechnung der Felder benötigt wird. Komplexe manuelle Anpassungen sind nicht erforderlich.

5   Evaluierung und Diskussion

Der Prototyp für die virtuelle Endoskopie wurde mit verschiedenen klinischen NNH-Datensätzen erfolgreich getestet. Es fand eine Evaluierung der Benutzerschnittstelle mit sechs Probanden im Alter zwischen 19 und 31 Jahren statt. Weiterhin haben HNO-Chirurgen und Experten im Bereich Computer Assisted Surgery das System beurteilt (Abb. 2). Die haptisch unterstützte Kamerasteuerung stellte sich bei den Tests gegenüber anderen (z.B. Maus oder SpaceMouse; 3d-Eingabe) als geeignetste Technik heraus. Die direkte Steuerung erleichterte die Orientierung und Positionierung des virtuellen Endoskops im NNH-Modell. Dieses äußerte sich in der Bewertung der Kriterien *räumliche Orientierung, Zufriedenheit* und *Erlernbarkeit*. Die Benutzerführung, die durch die Vermeidung von Kollisionen mit dem Gewebe unterstützt wird, ermöglicht eine effizientere Exploration der Daten als z.B. mit einer SpaceMouse. Die Navigation mit dem PHANToM ohne Rückgabekräfte wurde von den Probanden in einigen Punkten besser bewertet, als die Navigation mit der SpaceMouse, jedoch ist die freie Positionierung im Raum als anstrengend eingeschätzt worden. Bei der Interaktion mit dem System werden zukünftig auch kostengünstigere Eingabegeräte untersucht, die evtl. für die Operationsplanung hinreichende Möglichkeiten bieten.

Abb. 2. Evaluierung der Interaktionstechniken durch eine HNO-Ärztin

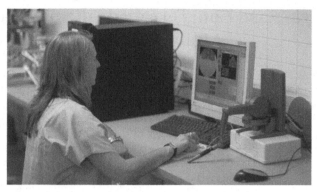

Weitere Entwicklungen erfolgen auch bei der Visualisierung, die aus ärztlicher Sicht noch zu wenig zwischen den Strukturen differenziert. Das betrifft vor allem die Unterscheidung zwischen knöchernem und weichem Gewebe und eine differenzierte Darstellung von z.B. Verschattungen der NNH. Dieses Ziel setzt zwangsläufig eine umfangreichere Vorverarbeitung der Daten (u.a. Segmentierung) voraus, ermöglicht dann jedoch eine noch detailliertere Planung.

Literaturverzeichnis

1. Rogalla P. Virtual Endoscopy of the Nose and Paranasal Sinuses. In: Rogalla P, van Scheltinga JT, Hamm B, editors. Virtual Endoscopy and Related 3D Techniques. Berlin [u.a]: Springer; 2001. 17–39.
2. Bisdas S, Verink M, Burmeister HP, Stieve M, Becker H. Three-Dimensional Visualization of the Nasal Cavity and Paranasal Sinuses: Clinical Results of a Standardized Approach Using Multislice Helical Computed Tomography. J Computer Assisted Tomography 2004;28(5):661 – 669.
3. Han P, Pirsig W, Ilgen F, Gorich J, Sokiranski R. Virtual Endoscopy of the Nasal Cavity in Comparison with Fiberoptic Endoscopy. European Archives of Oto-Rhino-Laryngology 2000;257(10):578–83.
4. Voss G, Ecke U, Bockholt U, Müller WK, Mann W. How to become the high score cyber surgeon: Endoscopic training using the nasal endoscopy simulator (NES). Procs CARS 2000; 290–293.
5. Pößneck A, Nowatius E, Trantakis C, Cakmak H, Maass H, Kühnapfel U, et al. A virtual training system in endoscopic sinus surgery 2002; 527–530.
6. Neubauer A, Wolfsberger S, et al MTForster. STEPS:An application for simulation of transsphenoidal endonasal pituitary surgery. Procs Conf Visualization 2004; 513–520.
7. Bartz D, Gürvit Ö. Haptic Navigation in Volumetric Datasets. Procs PHANToM User Research Symposium 2000.

Generation of Hulls Encompassing Neuronal Pathways Based on Tetrahedralization and 3D Alpha Shapes

Dorit Merhof[1,2], Martin Meister[1], Ezgi Bingöl[1],
Peter Hastreiter[1,2], Christopher Nimsky[2,3], Günther Greiner[1]

[1]Computer Graphics Group, University of Erlangen-Nuremberg, Germany
[2]Neurocenter, Dept. of Neurosurgery, University of Erlangen-Nuremberg, Germany
[3]Dept. of Neurosurgery, University of Erlangen-Nuremberg, Germany
Email: dorit.merhof@informatik.uni-erlangen.de

Abstract. Diffusion tensor imaging provides information about structure and location of white matter tracts within the human brain which is of particular interest for neurosurgery. The reconstruction of neuronal structures from diffusion tensor data is commonly solved by tracking algorithms based on streamline propagation. These approaches generate streamline bundles that approximate the course of neuronal fibers. For medical application, a 3D representation of streamline bundles provides valuable information for pre-operative planning. However, for intra-operative visualization, surfaces wrapping eloquent structures are required for integration into the OR microscope. In order to provide hulls tightly encompassing the neuronal structures obtained from fiber tracking, we propose an approach based on tetrahedralization. This technique reuses the sampling points derived from fiber tracking and therefore provides precise hulls which serve as basis for intra-operative visualization.

1   Introduction

In recent years, diffusion tensor imaging (DTI) data has gained increasing interest due to its capability to reflect location and structure of fibrous tissue such as white matter *in vivo*. For this reason, DTI data is of high value in neurosurgery enhancing the information obtained from standard magnetic resonance imaging (MRI) data. For pre-operative planning as well as intra-operative visualization, tract systems such as the pyramidal tract, the optical tract or the corpus callosum are reconstructed.

Commonly accepted techniques for fiber tract reconstruction from DTI data are fiber tracking algorithms. Respective tracking results indicate the location of white matter tracts within the human brain. In the context of neurosurgery, fiber bundles obtained from fiber tracking provide valuable information for diagnosis and therapy planning. However, for intra-operative visualization of fiber tract data, hulls tightly wrapping these structures are required. During surgery, the

Fig. 1. Microscope view: (a) tumor, (b) pyramidal tract in close neighborhood

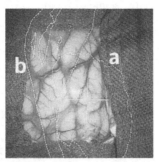

boundary curves of the hulls are displayed in the focus plane of the OR micro-scope and provide a direct relation between tumor tissue and neuronal structures (Fig. 1).

A first approach for wrapping fiber tracts [1] computes the centerline of the fiber bundle. In a second step, the center line is sampled equidistantly and planes perpendicular to the center line are considered. For each plane, the intersecting points of all fibers with the plane are computed. Finally, an ellipse encompassing all intersection points is defined for each plane and the ellipses of subsequent planes are connected using a triangular mesh. This approach provides hulls that fit the underlying fiber structure. However, the technique does not take into account branching fibers, requiring a splitting center line or a more sophisticated solution for defining ellipses and connecting them appropriately. In addition to that, the technique is restricted to elongated tract systems, where a centerline is well defined. For fiber tracts such as the corpus callosum encompassing fibers with significantly varying course and direction, the approach will fail.

For this reason, we present a novel hull algorithm overcoming these draw-backs. In order to provide precise hulls, the technique takes advantage of the sampling points of the tracked fibers to guarantee high precision. In a first step, a tetrahedral mesh is constructed from the sampling points based on 3D Delau-nay tetrahedralization. Since the tetrahedralization process results in the convex hull of the fiber tract, a variation of the 3D alpha shape algorithm has to be applied. As a result, the triangles on the surface of the remaining tetrahedral mesh describe a hull precisely encompassing the fiber tract.

2   Material

All datasets used in this work were measured using a Siemens MR Magnetom Sonata Maestro Class 1.5 Tesla scanner. The specifications of the gradient system were a field strength of up to 40 mT/m (effective 69 mT/m) and a slew rate of up to 200 T/m/s (effective 346 T/m/s) for clinical application.

DTI datasets were acquired using a field of view of 240 mm resulting in a voxel size of $1.875 \times 1.875 \times 1.9$ mm^3. For each of the six diffusion weighted datasets (gradient directions $(\pm 1,1,0)$, $(\pm 1,0,1)$ and $(0,1,\pm 1)$) and the reference dataset,

Fig. 2. 3D Delaunay tetrahedralization of a corpus callosum: (left) convex hull, (middle) subset with alpha = 10, (right) semi-transparent hull for alpha = 5 displayed with tracked fibers

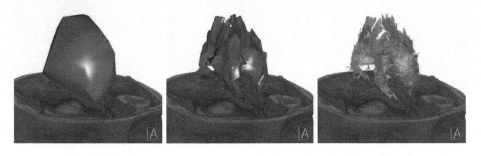

sixty slices with no intersection gap and an acquisition matrix of 128×128 pixels were measured.

3   Methods

In a first step, fiber tracts were computed using a streamline-based tracking approach incorporating trilinear tensor interpolation and fourth order Runge-Kutta integration [2]. Fractional anisotropy was used as termination threshold for fiber propagation. Single tract systems were obtained by incorporating ROIs (regions of interest) defined by a medical expert into the tracking process. As a result, fiber tracts corresponding to specific function such as the pyramidal tract (motor), the optical tract (vision) and the corpus callosum (connection between the two hemispheres) are obtained.

The point set comprising the sampling points of all fibers within the fiber tract is then used as input for the tetrahedralization algorithm. For the reconstruction of a tetrahedral mesh based on this point set, a 3D Delaunay [3] approach is applied. For points in general position, i.e. no geometric test is ambiguous, this tetrahedralization is uniquely defined and decomposes the convex hull of the point set into tetrahedra [3]. The tetrahedralization of a point set fulfills the 3D Delaunay criterion, if each sphere defined by the four points of a tetrahedron contains in its interior no other point of the point set. For implementation purposes, the 1000-5Delaunay3D class of the Visualization ToolKit (VTK) [4] was used (Fig. 2).

The output of the 3D Delaunay algorithm is a tetrahedral mesh filling the convex hull of the point set with volume elements. In order to obtain the subset of tetrahedra tightly enclosing the fiber tract, outer tetrahedra have to be removed in an iterative process. For this purpose, a variation of the 3D alpha shape algorithm is applied. The concept of alpha shapes [5] is a generalization of the convex hull, formalizing the intuitive notion of 'shape' for spatial point set data. Depending on the alpha value, which is a real number greater than zero, the alpha shape of an object encompasses only those tetrahedra with smaller or equal

Fig. 3. Hulls obtained from tetrahedralization and 3D alpha shapes (alpha = 5): (blue) pyramidal tract, (green) optic tract, (right) combination with the fibers

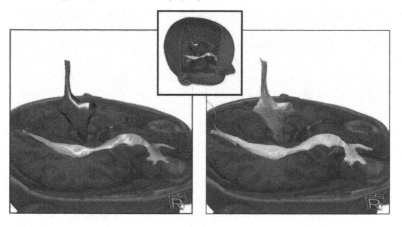

circumsphere than a sphere with diameter alpha. For sufficiently large alpha, the alpha shape is identical to the convex hull which is the original tetrahedral mesh. For decreasing values of alpha, approaching the step size used for fiber tracking, the alpha shape shrinks and gradually reveals the shape of the fiber tract.

When applying the alpha shape concept to the tetrahedral meshes obtained from 3D Delaunay tetrahedralization, holes may occur due to removal of inner tetrahedra. For this reason, a variation of the 3D alpha shape algorithm is used, where tetrahedra are only removed according to the alpha criterion, if they are on the surface of the current tetrahedral mesh. This is implemented by setting an alpha-flag for all tetrahedra which should be removed according to the alpha value, and a boundary-flag for all tetrahedra on the surface. In an iterative procedure, surface tetrahedra with valid alpha-flag are removed, and the boundary-flag of their neighbor elements is set. Sweeping through the tetrahedra data structure continues, as long as tetrahedra for removal are found.

After applying the 3D alpha shape algorithm, a tetrahedral mesh remains which exactly corresponds to the intuitive shape of the fiber tract. The triangular hull mesh is constructed from the outer faces of the surface tetrahedra.

4   Results

The novel technique for precise hull generation was applied to different tract systems, namely the pyramidal tract (motor), the optical tract (vision) and the corpus callosum (connection between the two hemispheres). For all tract systems, the algorithm succeeded to generate precise hulls following the shape of the fiber bundle (Figs. 2, 3).

In comparison to the initial approach for wrapping fibers [1], the presented technique provides higher precision which is an essential feature for the intended application. This is due to the fact, that points originating from fiber tracking are directly used for tetrahedralization and remain after application of 3D alpha shapes. Additionally, the algorithm is also able to wrap branching fiber tracts or tract systems with diverging fiber directions. With respect to computing times, the algorithm is more time consuming due to the reconstruction of the tetrahedral mesh. For a fiber tract comprising 7443 / 20139 / 70352 points (pyramidal tract / optical tract / corpus callosum), the 3D Delaunay tetrahedralization requires 2.3 / 8.5 / 80.2 seconds (on a PC equipped with a P4 3.0 GHz and 2 GB RAM).

5 Discussion

We presented a novel method for computing hulls encompassing neuronal pathways. As an advantage over existing techniques, the approach is capable to wrap tract systems of arbitrary shape such as branching or winding fiber tracts. In addition to that, the resulting hulls tightly fit the underlying fiber structure since the hull mesh is composed from sampling points derived by fiber tracking. Overall, the presented technique is able to wrap fiber tracts of any shape, and at the same time provides maximum wrapping precision. For medical application, this is of high value in order to obtain a precise visualization denoting the localization of white matter tracts.

Acknowledgments

This work was supported by the Deutsche Forschungsgemeinschaft in the context of SFB 603, Project C9 and the Graduate Research Center "3D Image Analysis and Synthesis". We thank Frank Enders for contributions to the visualization framework.

References

1. Enders F, Sauber N, Merhof D, Hastreiter P, Nimsky C, Stamminger M. Visualization of White Matter Tracts with Wrapped Streamlines. In: Proc. IEEE Visualization; 2005. 51–58.
2. Merhof D, Enders F, Vega F, Hastreiter P, Nimsky C, Stamminger M. Integrated Visualization of Diffusion Tensor Fiber Tracts and Anatomical Data. In: Proc. Simulation and Visualization; 2005. 153–164.
3. Delaunay B. Sur la sphère vide. Bulletin of Academy of Sciences of the USSR (VII) 1934; 793–800.
4. Schroeder W, Martin K, Lorensen B. The Visualisation ToolKit. Kitware; 2002. , URL: http://www.1000-5.org.
5. Edelsbrunner H, Mücke EP. Three-dimensional alpha shapes. ACM Transactions on Graphics 1994;13(1):43–72.

Surgical Cutting on a Multimodal Object Representation

Lenka Jeřábková and Torsten Kuhlen

Virtual Reality Group,
RWTH Aachen University, 52074 Aachen
Email: jerabkova@rz.rwth-aachen.de

Abstract. In this paper, we present the design of our surgery simulator under the aspects of multimodal object representation and parallelization on multicore architectures. Special focus is put on cutting. Surgical incisions can be accomplished interactively with force feedback.

1 Introduction

Surgical simulation is an important field of application in virtual reality (VR). A virtual surgery trainer can not only help to improve the skills of the surgeons, it also solves ethical issues related to training on animals or humans. Numerous surgical training systems have been developed in the last decade. The main requirement for a surgery simulator is the plausible deformation of the soft tissue in realtime and its interactive manipulation using a number of surgical instruments. An interactive cutting simulation is an essential feature of a surgery trainer. However, the interactive progressive cutting of a deformable object is still a challenging problem.

The majority of current surgical simulators use a polygonal approximation of the surface of the simulated object for visualization. The surface polygons are used to create a volumetric tetrahedral mesh needed by the finite elements method (FEM) in order to compute the tissue deformation. All vertices of the visualized geometry are placed at corresponding FEM mesh nodes. The interactive surgery simulation involves not only the simulation of the soft tissue deformation and its visualization, but also the processing of user interaction consisting of collision detection and response. In addition to that, force feedback is an indispensable part of user interaction. However, each of these tasks requires a different view of the data and different update rates in order to work efficiently.

An advantage of using dedicated representations of the simulated objects and the tools for each task enables the concurrent execution of the tasks. Parallelization used to be a domain of high performance computing on specialized computer architectures. However, the increase of performance of PCs due to the increase of the processor clock frequency reached its top. One of the most promising strategies for raising the performance of PCs is increasing the number of processor cores on a chip and on a board (multicore and multiprocessor architectures). However, the additional power can only be used if the application has been designed to run on a parallel architecture. Therefore, parallelization is becoming a crucial topic for all computationally intensive applications.

2 Related Work and Contribution

In this paper, we present the design of our surgery simulator under the aspects of multimodal object representation and parallelization. Special focus is put on cutting. The methods for surgical cutting published so far require the FEM elements to be aligned with the cut. This is achieved either by constraining the cut to the borders of existing elements [1] at the cost of creating unpleasing visual artifacts, or by splitting the elements along the cut [2], [3] or by snapping of the elements' borders to the cut [4] or by a combination of these methods [5].

All here mentioned approaches use the the polygonal boundary of the simulation mesh for visualization. As the tetrahedra are split along a cut, the visualization surface is updated to correspond to the new tetrahedra boundary. However, recent publications on interactive animation of deformable objects in computer graphics propose using a rougher resolution for the FEM simulation and a finer resolution for visualization [6], [7]. Moreover, the number and quality of the newly created FEM elements have a direct impact on the simulation performance and stability. Similarly, the newly created surface polygons influence the performance and quality of the visualization. Therefore, the main effort is to represent the cut using a small number of well shaped elements.

Our cutting approach is based on the discontinuous enrichment of the finite elements inspired by a method for crack modeling proposed by [8]. This method can effectively model discontinuity regions within an FEM mesh without remeshing. Our surgery simulator is based on four building blocks, each of them fulfilling a specific tasks (visualization, deformation, collision detection and force feedback) using dedicated representations of the simulated object and the surgical tools. The independence of the tasks allows their concurrent execution at task-specific update rates. In this paper, we describe the data coupling between collision detection, FEM simulation and the visual representation during an incision.

3 Methods

The structure of our surgery simulator is depicted in Figure 1. The visualization, deformation, collision detection and force feedback are four tasks run in parallel with different update rates.

- The visualization renders the polygonal approximation of the surface of the simulated object. Additionally, the surgical tools and an environment are rendered. A sufficient update rate for a smooth animation is about 20 Hz.
- The deformation process uses a mesh of tetrahedral elements approximating the volumetric object. Depending on the simulation time step, it has to be run up to several thousand times per second. The FEM deformation

Fig. 1. The structure of our surgery simulator. Each task uses a dedicated representation of the simulated object and surgical tool

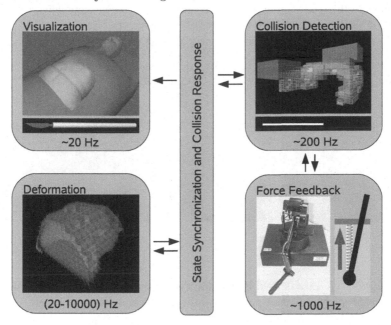

is the most computationally expensive task in this system. Therefore, it is parallelized internally.

– The collision detection uses primitives (e.g. bounding boxes) to approximate the tested surface and to quickly identify parts of the surface that the tool collides with. The tools are approximated using one or more line segments. The collision detection is processed about two hundred times per second.

– The force feedback process is usually run on a dedicated computer with a force feedback device attached to it. Here, a simplified local model of the simulated object is created. The force is proportional to the penetration depth and has to be updated about thousand times per second in order to provide smooth feedback without vibrations.

The multimodal object representation has to be kept consistent as the object undergoes deformation and topological changes. As the user perceives the system visually and haptically, it is crucial to provide the visual and haptical output at the specified rates. We synchronize the visualization, deformation and collision detection at the rate of the visualization, i.e. at about 20 Hz, so that the visualization renders the most current state of the objects. Any user interaction detected in the time between two synchronization steps is queued and processed simultaneously before the resulting changes are visualized. In the following, we will describe an interactive creation of an incision.

During a contact between the simulated object and a tool, the collision detection determines discrete points of contact and the tool penetration depth at

Fig. 2. Creating the visual representation of an incision. (a) the triangular mesh of the object surface (blue) with the desired cutting path (red line) and the vertices to be snapped to the (red points), (b) the situation with the cut completed, (c) the tool penetration depth is used to model the depth of the wound

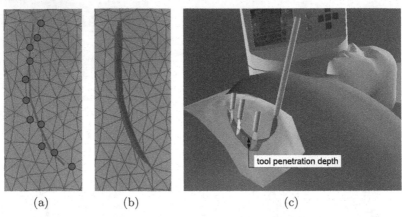

(a)   (b)   (c)

these points. This data is used by the haptics in order to give the user the feeling of a resistant surface. Moreover, the collision data is used to generate interaction forces leading to a local deformation of the simulated object. In the FEM, the deformation field is given by an interpolation of the nodal displacements within the elements using shape funcions. For a linear tetrahedron, this corresponds to the linear interpolation using barycentric coordinates. Each vertex of the detailed geometry surface is assigned to a tetrahedron and the barycentric coordinates of the vertex are computed in the non deformed state. The barycentric coordinates remain constant during the simulation and as the FEM mesh deforms, the positions of the geometry vertices are interpolated accordingly.

When a cut has to be created, the collision data is used to create a sequence of cutting planes aligned with the movement of the tool. The intersected FEM elements are enriched by a discontinuous function defining the location of the cut. The major advantage of the element enrichment is, that the structure of the simulation mesh does not change during the simulation. Each FEM element involved in a cut stores the definition of the respective cutting plane.

The incision has to be modeled in the geometry mesh as well. This can be achieved either by subdividing the triangles intersected by the cut or by snapping the existing vertices to the cut. The first method is more suitable for simulating fractures with small material slivers. For surgery simulation we prefer the latter method as it does not generate unnecessary faces along the cut. Both methods lead to triangles, that are either completely above or completely below the discontinuity. Figure 2a shows the geometry mesh before the cut with the desired cut and the vertices, that are going to be snapped to the cut marked in red. After the vertices have been snapped to the cut, their barycentric coordinates within the FEM mesh have to be updated. Further, these vertices are doubled and the copies are assigned to the respective side of the cut in order to create an opening. The copied vertices are still on the same positions as the originals, the created hole is opened by the physical simulation (Fig. 2b). In surgery simulation, volumetric objects are simulated. Therefore, the hole in the surface has to be closed properly by modeling a wound. Once the cut path on the surface and its depth below the surface are known, the wound can be modeled by moving a copy of the surface vertices involved in the cut according to the penetration depth (Fig. 2c). New faces are created between the vertices on the surface and below the surface.

4   Results and Discussion

The structure of a surgical simulator as described here takes advantage of the current development in the PC and workstations domain, utilizing multicore architectures. Dedicated representations of the simulated objects and the surgical tools are used in concurrently running tasks.

Surgical incisions can be accomplished interactively with force feedback. In the FEM mesh, the cut is modeled using discontinuous enrichment of the involved elements. As no new elements are created, the impact of an incision on performance and stability of the simulation is minimized.

The current prototype of our surgery simulator only allows for continuous cuts without branching, which has to be improved. Moreover, in order to increase realism of the surgery, different materials and internal organs have to be considered.

References

1. Cotin S, Delingette H, Ayache N. A hybrid elastic model for real-time cutting, deformations and force feedback for surgery training and simulation. The Visual Computer 2000;16(7):437–452.
2. Bielser D, Maiwald VA, Gross MH. Interactive cuts through 3-dimensional soft tissue. Procs Eurographics 1999;18(3):31–38.
3. Mor AB, Kanade T. Modifying soft tissue nodels: Progressive cutting with minimal new element creation. Procs MICCAI 2000; 598–607.
4. Nienhuys HW, van der Stappen AF. Supporting cuts and finite element deformation in interactive surgery simulation. Utrecht; 2001.
5. Steinemann D, Harders M, Gross M, Szekely G. Hybrid cutting of deformable solids. In: Procs IEEE VR; 2006. 35–42.
6. Müller M, Gross M. Interactive virtual materials. In: Procs Conference on Graphics Interface; 2004. 239–246.
7. Molino N, Bao ZH, Fedkiw R. A virtual node algorithm for changing mesh topology during simulation. ACM Transactions on Graphics 2004;23(3):385–392.
8. Belytschko T, Black T. Elastic crack growth in finite elements with minimal remeshing. Int J Numerical Methods in Engineering 1999;45(5):601–620.

Automatische Kamerapositionierung in komplexen medizinischen 3D-Visualisierungen

Mathias Neugebauer, Konrad Mühler, Christian Tietjen und Bernhard Preim

Institut für Simulation und Graphik, Otto-von-Guericke Universität Magdeburg
Email: muehler@isg.cs.uni-magdeburg.de

Zusammenfassung. In diesem Beitrag wird ein Verfahren vorgestellt, mit dessen Hilfe optimale Blickpunkte für die Betrachtung anatomischer Strukturen in komplexen 3D-Visualisierungen berechnet werden können. Der optimale Blickpunkt wird über verschiedene gewichtete Bewertungsparameter in Echtzeit ermittelt. Berücksichtigt werden u.a. Sichtbarkeit und Wichtigkeit der überdeckenden Strukturen. Das Verfahren wird in zwei Systemen für die medizinische Ausbildung und Therapieplanung angewendet.

1   Einleitung

Bei komplexen chirurgischen Eingriffen sind interaktive, dreidimensionale Darstellungen der patientenindividuellen Anatomie weitestgehend etabliert [1]. Nachteilig an dieser Darstellungsform ist jedoch, dass die einzelnen Strukturen sich gegenseitig verdecken können. Das Bestimmen eines günstigen oder gar optimalen Blickpunktes kann dadurch sehr zeitaufwendig sein.

Die Exploration von dreidimensionalen Darstellungen kann beschleunigt werden, indem für die einzelnen Strukturen Kamerapositionen automatisch berechnet werden und nicht vom Anwender selbst gesucht werden müssen. Die Kameraposition sollte dabei die anatomischen Strukturen von Interesse möglichst unverdeckt und aus einem für den Anwender gewohnten Blickwinkel zeigen.

Wir haben ein Verfahren entwickelt, welches automatisch Kamerapositionen in medizinischen Visualisierungen bestimmt. Dieses Verfahren besteht aus zwei Schritten: der Generierung von Sichtbarkeitsinformationen in einem Vorverarbeitungsschritt und der Berechnung der Kameraposition aus den jeweils aktuellen Gegebenheiten heraus in Echtzeit. Im Unterschied zur virtuellen Endoskopie, bei der die Kamera im Inneren von Strukturen navigiert wird, konzentriert sich diese Arbeit auf externe Ansichten auf anatomische Strukturen.

2   Stand der Forschung und Fortschritt durch den Beitrag

Der „Visibility Solver" [2] bestimmt die optimale Kameraposition ausgehend von einer aktuellen Kameraposition und einem Zielobjekt. Beim „Zoom Illustrator" [3] wird die Kameraposition aus einer relativ kleinen Menge von Sichtrichtungen ausgewählt, bei der die auf den Viewport projizierte Fläche der Fokusstruktur am größten ist. Ein exakter Ansatz ist das „Visibility Skeleton" [4], welches die Sichtbarkeitsverhältnisse innerhalb einer Szene anhand einfacher geometrischer Strukturen beschreibt. Ein Verfahren zur Bestimmung optimaler Sichten auf einzelne Objekte in Volumenvisualisierungen stellt [5] vor. Einen ausführlichen und aktuellen Überblick über weitere Verfahren zur Kamerasteuerung und Sichtbarkeitsbestimmung bietet [6]. Die Nachteile der einzelnen Verfahren sind jedoch ein oft hoher Berechnungsaufwand zum Ermitteln der Kameraposition [4], die Betrachtung nur einer Fokusstruktur [3], der lokale Charakter der Positionssuche [2] und die fehlende Berücksichtigung von Verdeckungen [5].

Das vorgestellte Verfahren ist effizient in seiner Berechnung, kann auf beliebige Strukturen einer Darstellung angewendet werden, findet eine global günstige Kameraposition und berücksichtigt neben anderem auch die Verdeckung von Objekten.

3   Methoden

Ziel des Verfahrens ist die Ermittlung von günstigen Kamerapositionen für Fokusstrukturen in medizinischen Visualisierungen. Fokusstrukturen können dabei einzelne krankhafte Veränderungen (z.B. Tumore oder vergrößerte Lymphknoten), Knochen oder Gefäßäste sein. Das Verfahren ist aber nicht auf bestimmte Strukturen beschränkt und lässt sich auf beliebige segmentierte Objekte einer Szene anwenden. Die meisten medizinischen Visualisierungen zur Operationsplanung sind kompakte Darstellungen der jeweiligen Körperregion, die von außen betrachtet werden (Abb. 1, links). Daher kann der Bereich der möglichen Kamerapositionen auf eine umgebende Kugeloberfläche eingeschränkt werden (Abb. 1, rechts). Die Blickrichtung der Kamera ist auf den Mittelpunkt der Kugel gerichtet. Die Kamerapositionen sind diskret auf der Kugeloberfläche verteilt. Dieser Ansatz liefert zwar keine vollständige Repräsentation aller möglichen Kamerapositionen, ist bei ausreichend kleiner Diskretisierung[1] mit Blick auf die Anwendungsziele aber ausreichend. Durch die beiden Einschränkungen lässt sich die Anzahl der zu berechnenden Kamerapositionen auf ein akzeptables Maß reduzieren.

3.1   Generierung der Sichtbarkeitsinformationen

Um Aussagen über die Sichtbarkeit einer Struktur und mögliche Verdeckungen treffen zu können, werden diese Informationen in einem Vorverarbeitungsschritt einmalig pro Szene generiert. Von jeder Kameraposition aus werden Informationen zur sichtbaren Fläche aller Strukturen, zu verdeckenden Strukturen sowie zur Größe der verdeckten Fläche ermittelt. Dieser Prozess erfolgt in zwei Schritten (Abb. 2):

---

[1] Positionen im Abstand von vier bis zehn Grad in horizontaler und vertikaler Richtung haben sich als praktikabel erwiesen.

Abb. 1. Sicht auf eine 3D-Visualisierung zur HNO-Operationsplanung (links), die Punkte stellen die möglichen Kamerapositionen auf der umgebenden Kugel dar (rechts)

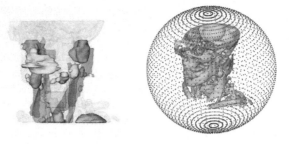

Abb. 2. z-Buffer einer einzelnen segmentierten Struktur: Knochen (links)), Auswahl der z-Buffer-Werte aller Buffer an einer einzelnen Pixelposition (rechts)

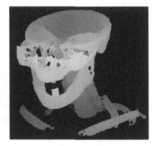 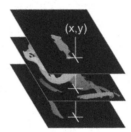

1. Erzeugen des z-Buffers und Zählen der Pixel für jede einzelne Struktur.
2. Sortieren der ermittelten z-Werte pro xy-Koordinate aller z-Buffer und Auswertung hinsichtlich jeweils verdeckender Strukturen.

3.2   Berechnung der optimalen Kameraposition

Die Berechnung der jeweils besten Kameraposition erfolgt in Echtzeit für die Szene unter Berücksichtigung der aktuellen Umgebungsparameter wie der momentanen Kameraposition. Dies geschieht beispielsweise, wenn der Nutzer eine Struktur in der Szene selektiert oder aus einer Liste auswählt. In die Berechnung der Kameraposition fließen verschiedene Bewertungsparameter ein. Jeder Bewertungsparameter stellt dabei eine zweidimensionale normierte Funktion auf der Kugeloberfläche der Form $b = f(x, y)$, $0 \le b \le 1$ dar. Die einzelnen Bewertungsparameter werden als gewichtete Summe in einer einzigen Bewertungsfunktion zusammengefasst,

$$K = \sum_{i=0}^{n} \alpha_i b_i(x, y) \quad , \quad 0 \le \alpha_i \le 1$$

wobei α_i der Bewertungsfaktor für jeden Bewertungsparameter b_i ist. Die Wahl des Bewertungsfaktors hängt von der jeweiligen medizinischen Fragestellung ab.

Das Maximum der Bewertungsfunktion K stellt die neue Kameraposition dar. Die Kamera wird automatisch zu dieser Position bewegt. Eventuell verdeckende Strukturen werden ausgeblendet, soweit sie nicht zur Kontextvisualisierung nötig sind. Dieses Konzept ist leicht um zusätzliche Bewertungsparameter erweiterbar. Momentan sind folgende Bewertungsparameter in unserem System implementiert:

– *Entropie*: Die Struktur soll aus einer Richtung betrachtet werden, von der möglichst viel zu sehen ist (z.B. längliche Strukturen von der Seite). Diese Entropie sowie verdeckende Strukturen und die Größe der verdeckten Fläche werden aus den vorberechneten Sichtbarkeitsdaten ermittelt und bilden eine „Visibility Map" (Abb. 3, links).
– *Wichtigkeit*: Abhängig von der Fragestellung hat jede Struktur eine Wichtigkeit für die Visualisierung (0 = geringe Wichtigkeit, 1 = hohe Wichtigkeit). Weil Strukturen geringerer Wichtigkeit nötigenfalls ausgeblendet werden können, geht die durch sie verdeckte Fläche gewichtet mit dem Reziproken ihrer Wichtigkeit in die Entropie ein.
– *Stabilität*: Eine Kameraposition ist stabil, wenn kleine Änderungen der Position zu nur kleinen Änderungen in der Sichtbarkeit des Fokusobjektes führen. Positionen im Zentrum von sichtbaren Bereichen werden daher höher gewichtet als Positionen an deren Rändern. Die Stabilität wird mit Hilfe einer Distanzfunktion auf der Entropie der Fokusstruktur berechnet (Abb. 3, Mitte und rechts).
– *Blickrichtung*: Es können beispielsweise äquatoriale oder anteriore Blickrichtungen als bevorzugt angegeben werden. Der Bewertungsparameter der gewohnten bzw. gewünschten Blickrichtung wird als Distanzfunktion beschrieben.
– *Kameranähe*: Um dem Nutzer große Veränderungen und Sprünge der Darstellung und dem damit einhergehenden Orientierungsverlust zu ersparen, sollten die Entfernungen zwischen den Kamerapositionen klein sein. Weiter entfernte Kamerapositionen und damit verbundene lange Kamerafahrten sind daher schlechter zu bewerten.

4   Ergebnisse

Es konnte ein Verfahren zur Bestimmung von optimalen Sichten auf anatomische Strukturen in medizinischen Darstellungen entwickelt werden. Dieses Verfahren arbeitet in Echtzeit und wurde in zwei Applikationen zur Operationsplanung und in ein System zur Animationserzeugung integriert [7, 8, 9]. Es konnten in Zusammenarbeit mit Ärzten im Bereich HNO-Chirurgie, Abdominal-Chirurgie und Orthopädie spezifische Wichtungsfaktoren für die einzelnen Bewertungsparameter gefunden werden. So werden die Blickrichtungen bei HNO-Visualisierungen stärker begrenzt und höher gewichtet als bei Abdominal-Ansichten. Die Nähe zur aktuellen Kameraposition ist bei Abdominal-Darstellungen von größerer Bedeutung und wird daher höher gewichtet, weil es hier schneller zu einem Orientierungsverlust kommen kann.

Abb. 3. Visibility Map: Die Kugel wird mittels Mercator-Entwurf auf eine ebene Fläche projiziert (links), Zwischenergebnis der Bewertungsfunktion an einer Kameraposition (Mitte), Ergebnis nach Anwendung einer Distanzfunktion auf das binarisierte Zwischenergebnis (rechts)

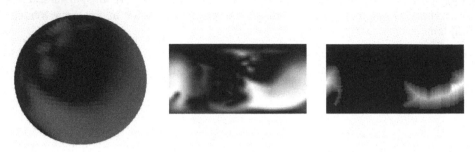

5   Diskussion

Das Konzept ist erweiterbar. So lassen sich neue Bewertungsparameter einfach hinzufügen. Das Verfahren wird derzeit um Funktionen zur Kamerapfadplanung erweitert, um mehrere Sichten auf verschiedene Strukturen durch einen Pfad effizient zu verbinden. Auch werden Möglichkeiten untersucht, optimale Sichten auf Gruppen von Objekten und auf minimale Abstände zwischen Objekten zu ermitteln. Eine Evaluierung mit einer größeren Gruppe von Probanden ist ebenfalls in Vorbereitung.

Literaturverzeichnis

1. Gering DT, Nabavi A, et al. An integrated visualization system for surgical planning and guidance using image fusion and interventional imaging. Procs MICCAI 1999; 809–819.
2. Halper N. Supportive Presentation for Computer Games. Ph.D. thesis; 2003.
3. Preim B, Raab A, Strothotte T. Coherent zooming of illustrations with 3D-graphics and text. In: Graphics Interface; 1997. 105–113.
4. Durand F, Drettakis G, Puech C. The visibility skeleton: A powerful and efficient multi-purpose global visibility tool. In: Procs SIGGRAPH; 1997. 89–100.
5. Takahashi S, Fujishiro I, Takeshima Y, Nishita T. A feature-driven approach to locating optimal viewpoints for volume visualization. Procs IEEE Visualization 2005; 495–502.
6. Christie M, Olivier P. Camera Control in Computer Graphics. In: Eurographics: State of the Art Reports; 2006. 89–113.
7. Bade R, Riedel I, Schmidt L, Oldhafer KJ, Preim B. Combining training and computerized planning of oncologic liver surgery. Procs BVM 2006; 409–413.
8. Krüger A, Tietjen C, Hintze J, Preim B, Hertel I, Strauß G. Analysis and exploration of 3D-visualizations for neck dissection planning. Procs CARS 2005; 497–503.
9. Mühler K, Bade R, Preim B. Adaptive script based animations for intervention planning. Procs MICCAI 2006; 478–485.

Quantifizierung und Visualisierung von Narbenbereichen des Myokards

Diana Wald[1,2], Stefan Wesarg[2], Stefanie Nowak[2]

[1] Uni Koblenz, Institut für Computervisualistik, Universitätsstr. 1, D-56070 Koblenz
[2] Fraunhofer Institut für Graphische Datenverarbeitung, Abteilung Cognitive Computing & Medical Imaging, Fraunhofer Str. 5, D-64283 Darmstadt
Email: diana.wald@uni-koblenz.de, Stefan.Wesarg@igd.fhg.de

Zusammenfassung. In diesem Beitrag wird ein automatisches Verfahren zur Quantifizierung von Narbenbereichen des Myokards aus MRT-Daten vorgestellt. Spezielles Augenmerk wird dabei auf die automatische Berechnung und die praxisnahe Präsentation der Analysedaten gelegt. Weiterhin werden dem Anwender verschiedene Möglichkeiten geboten, die Ergebnisse auf ihre Korrektheit zu überprüfen und wenn nötig zu korrigieren, um Fehldiagnosen zu vermeiden.

1 Einleitung

Der Herzinfarkt gehört zu den häufigsten Todesursachen in der westlichen Welt. Durch den Verschluss oder die Verengung eines Herzkranzgefäßes wird das Herzmuskelgewebe (Myokard) mit Sauerstoff unterversorgt und die Herzmuskelzellen sterben ab [1]. Dieser nekrotische Bereich wird als Infarktgewebe bezeichnet und kann nicht mehr aktiv zur Pumpleistung des Herzens beitragen. In diesem Beitrag wird ein automatisches Verfahren vorgestellt, das den Kardiologen bei der Diagnose durch eine detaillierte und eindeutige Analyse des Infarktgewebes unterstützen soll. Da das Bildmaterial in dreidimensionaler Technik aufgenommen wurde, ist es wünschenswert, eine räumliche Darstellung von Narbengröße, Transmuralitätsgrad und Lokalisation anzubieten.

In der klinischen Praxis wird das Infarktgewebe überwiegend manuell quantifiziert und analysiert. Heutzutage gehört neben den computergestützten bildgebenden Verfahren auch semi- oder vollautomatische Bildanalysesoftware zum klinischen Alltag eines Mediziners. Zur Verbesserung der Infarktdiagnostik wäre ein Verfahren von Vorteil, das die Infarktnarbe aus den Bilddaten extrahiert und anschließend quantifiziert. Als Datensätze stehen die Standardaufnahmen der Kardio-MRT für die Analyse zur Verfügung. Diese sind die dynamischen Cine-MRT-Daten und die statischen Late-Enhancement-Daten[1]. Für einen solchen Analyseprozess sind prinzipiell drei Schritte erforderlich: Im ersten Schritt werden die Bildinformationen der Narbe extrahiert; im zweiten Schritt werden

---

[1] Die Late-Enhancement-Daten sind Bilddaten, in denen das Narbengewebe aufgrund von Kontrastmittel hell hervorgehoben wird (vergl. [2]).

die quantitativen Parameter ermittelt; im dritten Schritt werden die Analyseergebnisse visuell präsentiert. Für die Extraktion von Informationen aus Bilddaten werden in [3], [4] und [5] spezielle Verfahren vorgestellt, die auf die Narbensegmentierung im Herzmuskel ausgerichtet sind. Diese Methoden unterscheiden sich in ihrer Anwendung. So werden in [3] und [4] Verfahren präsentiert, die auf einer manuellen Kontureinzeichnung des Anwenders basieren. In [5] werden verschiedene Schwellwertverfahren vorgestellt, die sich in ihrem Berechnungsablauf zwischen manuell, semi- und voll-automatisch unterscheiden. Die Quantifizierung des avitalen Gewebes erfolgt nach den für die Diagnose von Infarktnarben üblichen Parametern. Der Transmuralitätsgrad gibt dabei das lokale Verhältnis zwischen Herzwand- und Narbenbreite an. Das Percent Scar ist das Volumenverhältnis zwischen Narbengewebe und dem Volumen des gesamten Herzmuskels [5]. Diese Parameter werden aus den segmentierten Bilddaten berechnet. Die Darstellungen von Analyseergebnissen des Infarktgewebes sind in der Literatur sehr unterschiedlich gehalten. In [4] wurde das Bull's-Eye-Diagramm für die Darstellung der Transmuralität verwendet. Andere Verfahren setzen Liniendiagramme für die Ergebnisdarstellung ein (vgl. dazu [3]).

In diesem Beitrag werden Verfahren vorgestellt, die die Anforderungen einer automatischen Narbenquantifizierung erfüllen und das Ziel einer optimalen computergestützten Diagnose erreichen. Die Segmentierung des Narbengewebes erfolgt auf dem in [6] vorgestellten Verfahren der Segmentierung des linken Ventrikels und einem Multilevel-Otsu-Verfahren. Die Darstellungen der Analyseergebnisse sind praxisbezogen und gewährleisten eine geringe Einarbeitungszeit für den Kardiologen. Neben der Ergebnispräsentation sind Kontroll- und Korrekturmöglichkeiten der Resultate gegeben.

2   Methoden

Das Verfahren der Segmentierung besteht aus vier Schritten. Zuerst erfolgt eine Ausrichtung der LE-Daten zu den Cine-MRT-Daten durch eine rigide Registrierung [7]. Die Auswahl des zum Late-Enhancement akquirierenden Cine-Datensatzes basiert auf dem Wissen der Kardiologen, dass die Narbendaten auf 80% des Weges von und zur Enddiastole aufgenommen werden. Anschließend wird der linke Ventrikel durch das in [6] vorgestellte Verfahren segmentiert. Der nächste Schritt generiert eine Maske aus den berechneten Myokardrändern (Epi- und Endokardrand) und maskiert die registrierten LE-Daten. Das Ergebnis ist das segmentierte Myokard des linken Ventrikels in den Narbendaten. Der letzte Schritt hebt das avitale Gewebe durch ein Multilevel-Otsu-Schwellwert Verfahren hervor. Bei diesem Verfahren können mehrere Grenzwerte automatisch erzeugt werden. Die Einteilung in vier Klassen ergab bei allen Daten ein positives Ergebnis, wobei die hellste Klasse das Narbengewebe definiert. Die Berechnung der Parameter erfolgt auf dem binären segmentierten Narbenbild aus dem vorherigen Verarbeitungsschritt. Für die Verhältnisberechnung der Percent Scar müssen die beiden Volumina des linken Herzmuskels und die der Narbe bekannt sein. Die Größe des Herzmuskels wird anhand der binären Myokardmaske bestimmt, da genau diese den Herzmuskel umschließt. Die Berechnung des Narbenvolumens erfolgt auf dem binären Narbenbild der Segmentierung. In beiden Fällen werden die Objekt-Voxel in den Daten gezählt und mit der Voxeldimension multipliziert. Für die Bestimmung des Transmuralitätsgrades werden die Parameter der Wand- und Narbendicke vorausgesetzt. Die Wanddicke wurde bereits in der Funktionsanalyse aus [6] ermittelt. Die Berechnung der Narbendicke erfolgt auf dem Ergebnis der Narbensegmentierung und wird durch das Aussenden von Suchstrahlen detektiert. Die Suchstrahlen starten im Schwerpunkt des linken Ventrikels und verlaufen radial zum Bildrand. Die Berechnung der Narbendicke erfolgt durch den euklidischen Abstand zwischen dem ersten und letzten Schnittpunkt des Strahls mit der Narbe. Durchquert ein Strahl mehrere Narben, so werden alle Größen addiert. Dies ist vor allem für die Quantifizierung von "donut-signs" notwendig. Die Analyseergebnisse werden durch textuelle und visuelle Darstellungen dem Anwender präsentiert. Das Percent Scar wird textuell in einer Tabelle dargestellt. Dabei werden die Volumina der beiden Parameter Herzwand und Narbe sowie das Verhältnis zueinander ausgegeben (Abb. 1 (links unten)). Die Lokalität und das Ausmaß der Narbe wird in einem zweidimensionalen AHA[2]-konformen Bull's-Eye-Diagramm veranschaulicht. Anhand der berechneten Transmuralität, wird das Bull's-Eye-Diagramm je nach Narbenausdehnung eingefärbt. Die Farbkodierung lehnt sich dabei an die Visualisierungsanalyse von [8], wobei fünf Farbklassen erstellt werden. Für die Zuordnung der Farben ist eine Farbskala mit der dazu gehörigen Prozentangabe der Transmuralität eingefügt (Abb. 1 (links oben)). In dieser Visualisierung kann, durch die AHA-konforme Einteilung des Ventrikels, die Lokalität der Narbe und somit indirekt die erkrankte Koronararterie diagnostiziert werden. Darüber hinaus stehen dem Anwender für die Beurteilung der Narbe fünf verschiedene Visualisierungsarten zur Verfügung, die jeweils unterschiedliche Darstellungsaspekte verfolgen. Eine Visualisierungsart sind die Late-Enhancement-Daten, die für einen direkten Vergleich zwischen den berechneten Analysedaten des Bull's-Eye-Diagramms und den Originaldaten stehen. Hier besteht außerdem die Möglichkeit, Fehlinformationen[3], durch Setzen eines oder mehrerer Seed-Punkte ins Narbengewebe, aus den Analyseergebnissen zu entfernen. Die Korrektur basiert auf einem Region-Growing Algorithmus [7]. Die zweite Visualisierungsart ist ein $3D$ Modell des linken Ventrikels, welches das Größenverhältnis und die Beschaffenheit der Narbe im Verhältnis zum gesamten Herzmuskel präsentiert. Das Infarktgewebe wird anhand seines transmuralen Ausmaßes farblich hervorgehoben. Weiterhin wird ein Narbenmodell durch das Marching-Cubes Verfahren [9] erzeugt, welches die Beschaffenheit und äußere Form der Narbe illustriert. Die letzten beiden Visualisierungsarten verfolgen den Aspekt der Analysekontrolle, wobei zum einen die Abschätzung der Narbengröße und zum anderen die Ergebnisse der Registrierung und Maskengenerierung überprüft werden können. Dabei erfolgt

---

[2] American Heart Association

[3] Fehlinformationen bedeuten in diesem Zusammenhang, vitales Gewebe das als Narbe definiert wurde.

Abb. 1. Analysefenster. Die linke Seite beinhaltet die Quantifizierungsergebnisse. Das AHA konforme Bull's-Eye-Diagramm (Ausmaß, Transmuralität, Lokalität), sowie die textuelle Ausgabe der Percent Scar. Die rechte Seite beinhaltet die unterschiedlichen Visualisierungsarten (hier: Bildfusion zwischen Narbenmodell und LE-Daten)

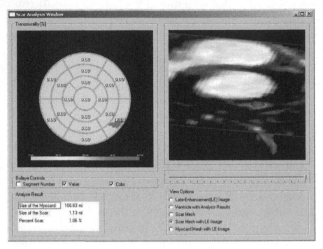

jeweils eine Bildfusion zwischen dem Narben- oder dem Myokardmodell mit den Late-Enhancement-Daten (Abb. 2).

3 Ergebnisse

Die Qualität des Verfahrens wurde an zwölf vorliegenden Datensätzen getestet und ausgewertet. In zehn von zwölf Fällen wird das Narbengewebe erfolgreich segmentiert und quantifiziert. Die Ursache für die Misserfolge lässt sich auf die Probleme der einfachen Registrierung zurück führen. Die Narbenquantifizierung ist zusammengefasst ein automatisierter Prozess, der die Narbe innerhalb von wenigen Sekunden (ø21.6s) in ihrer Beschaffenheit und dem lokalen Ausmaß quantifiziert. Die Visualisierungen der Analyseergebnisse basieren auf unterschiedlichen Aspekten der Informationspräsentation, wobei jede die Anforderung einer klaren visuellen Aussage erfüllt. Das in dieser Arbeit verwendete 2D-Bull's-Eye-Diagramm entspricht, im Gegensatz zu dem in [4] vorgestellten Diagramm, den AHA-Richtlinien. Diese Art der Darstellung ist bereits bei der Analyse der Myokardfunktion geläufig und hat somit den Effekt der problemlosen und schnellen Einschätzung der Narbe durch den Mediziner. Weiterhin werden die Kardiologen mit keiner für sie neuen Visualisierungsart konfrontiert, dass evtl. das Abschrecken gegenüber neuen Diagnose-unterstützenden Programmen verhindert. Durch den Vergleich zwischen dem Analyseergebnis und den Originaldaten können Fehlsegmentierungen schnell erkannt und durch Setzen eines Seed-Punktes korrigiert werden. Bei 8 von den 10 erfolgreichen Analyseergebnissen war eine Korrektur erforderlich, die im Durchschnitt 10s benötigt.

Abb. 2. Darstellung der fünf Visualisierungsarten: LE-Datensatz, Ausmaß der Narbe, Narbenmodell, Narbenmodell und LE-Daten, Myokardmodell und LE-Daten

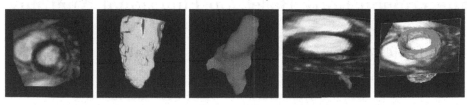

4 Diskussion

Bei der Beschaffenheit der Narbe wird zwischen einer geschlossenen und einer in ihrer Form geöffneten Struktur unterschieden. Bei den Offenen ("donutsign") kann das vitale Gewebe aufgrund des umliegenden nekrotischen Bereiches nicht zu der Pumpleistung des Herzens beitragen. Daher könnte von Interesse sein, diesen Bereich dem avitalen Gewebe hinzuzufügen, um das völlige Ausmaß der Kontraktionsdefizite einzuschätzen. Das Konzept der Narbenquantifizierung kann selbstverständlich auch auf die Analyse des rechten Ventrikel übertragen werden. Eine klinische Evaluation läuft bereits, um das Verfahren an weiteren Patientendaten zu testen.

Literaturverzeichnis

1. Grebe O. Kardiovaskuläre Magnetresonanztomographie. Stuttgart, New York: Schattauer; 2005. 375–388.
2. Judd RM, et al. Technology insight: assessment of myocardial viability by delayed-enhancement magnetic resonance imaging. Nature Clinical Practice Cardiovascular Medicine 2005;(2):150–158.
3. Säring D, et al. HeAT: A Software Assistant for the Analysis of LV Remodeling after Myocardial Infarction in 4D MR Follow-Up Studies. In: Informatik für Menschen - Band 1; 2006.
4. Breeuwer M. Quantification of atherosclerotic heart disease with cardiac MRI. Medica Mundi 2005;49(2):30–38.
5. Kolipaka A, et al. Segmentation of non-viable myocardium in delayed enhancement magnetic resonance images. In: The International Journal of Cardiovascular Imaging. vol. 21; 2005. 303–311.
6. Wesarg S, Nowak S. An automated 4D approach for left ventricular assessment in clinical cine MR images. In: in Informatics (LNI) LectureNotes, editor. Proc. of Softwareassistenten 2006 – Computerunterstützung für die medizinische Diagnostik und Therapieplanung; 2006.
7. Jaehne B. Digitale Bildverarbeitung. Berlin Heidelberg: Springer-Verlag; 2005.
8. Schuijf JD, other. Quantification of myocardial infarct size and transmurality by contrast-enhanced magnetic resonance imaging in men. The American Journal of Cardiology 2004;94:284–288.
9. Lorensen WE, Cline HE. Marching cubes: A high resolution 3D surface construction algorithm. Computer Graphics 1987;21:163–169.

Comprehensive Architecture for Simulation of the Human Body Based on Functional Anatomy

Sebastian Ullrich[1], Jakob T. Valvoda[1], Andreas Prescher[2], Torsten Kuhlen[1]

[1]Virtual Reality Group, RWTH Aachen University
[2]Institute for Neuroanatomy, University Hospital Aachen
Email: s.ullrich@rz.rwth-aachen.de

Abstract. In this paper we propose a structured approach for the simulation of the human body which is comprehensive and extendable. Our architecture resembles the human organism as defined by the systematic and functional anatomy to integrate a broad range of simulation algorithms. To share common data and to create interlinks between algorithms without modifying the algorithms themselves we introduce abstract control entities that mimic the basic setup of physiological systems. We utilize the model-view-controller pattern to establish a separation of algorithms and data. The structure was designed for the purpose of interactive simulation of the human body in virtual environments.

1 Introduction

The simulation of the human body is a challenging task that is still being broadly researched. Even though there are many simulators covering different medical areas, only few approaches are to a limited amount compatible between each other. Our goal is to create a framework to manage multiple algorithms for simulation of functional anatomy in order to create a virtual human patient that behaves realistically. The motivation is to provide an unified platform that allows to integrate already existing simulation algorithms and to prevent isolated solutions that are incompatible between each other. Ideally, the models and data sets of one approach should be interoperable and reusable for other approaches.

In order to achieve this goal, we adapt concepts from systematic and functional anatomy to software design. In systematic anatomy the human body is defined by a number of functional systems. The basic systems comprise the respiratory, cardiovascular, nervous, muscular, skeletal, and integumentary systems [1]. Further systems are digestive, excretory, endocrine, immune and reproductive. Each system fulfills a set of specific unique functions. These – often vital – tasks are accomplished by organs and other structural anatomical components. On a macroscopic or abstract level the interdependencies and actions are described by functional physiology.

Because this taxonomy differentiates between functional (physiological) and structural (anatomical) components, it is well suited to derive a structure for simulation of the human organism. For this reasons we have chosen systematic and functional anatomy as a blueprint for the creation of a comprehensive system that is capable of extension and integration, as well as, adaptable to subjects.

Fig. 1. Overview of the architecture for a virtual human organism, showing possible access mechanisms for simulation algorithms

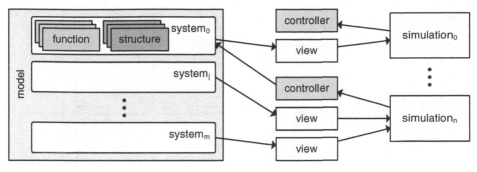

2   State of the Art and Motivation

Existing solutions are categorized by different fields of applications. Almost all surgical simulators focus on a set of procedures and implement simulations of restricted regions or specific layers of interest [2]. Current approaches for a unified simulation standard are still in early development. The international "'Digital Human"' consortium aims at combining micro- and macroscopic simulation [3]. Other examples are based on creating interactive anatomical atlases [4]. Cardenas et al. presented an extendible framework for medical image processing and visualization [5]. A comparable approach by Seifert et al. is used for surgical planning and also medical image processing [6]. The "'Digital Human"' project follows an intention similar to our approach, however, they have not proposed any system architecture yet. The other solutions presented above are restricted to one specimen (often the popular visible human data set) or to a limited amount of physiological systems. Until now, there is no systematic encapsulation of interindividually shared human anatomical and functional attributes.

Our structured approach allows to create comprehensive models of the human organism, based on functional systems, that strictly separates functionality from data. Thereby it enables individual, interoperable and reusable models that can be used by arbitrary simulation algorithms.

3   Methods

The architecture proposed in this paper consists of an abstract model for a human organism and defines access rules for simulation algorithms (Fig. 1). As mentioned before, we have adapted the distinction of functional systems and their inherent separation between physiology and anatomy, i.e., function and structure. Thus, the model consists of a set of functional systems. Furthermore, the data itself is stored in two types of interlinked containers: the functional and the structural component (Fig. 2). To provide access rules we use the model-

Fig. 2. Partial setup of four systems. Additional components per system and many attributes are not shown here but are derived from systematic anatomy accordingly

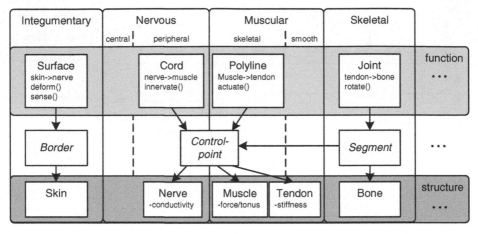

view-controller pattern to separate data from algorithms. Subsequent sections describe the system, as well as its components.

3.1 System Definition

The physiological systems are based on their real-world counterparts. The key idea is that there are negligible differences of the purely functional aspects of a physiological system between individuals. In addition interrelations and links between components differ only morphologically but not on an abstract level, e.g., *M. brachialis* is always innervated by *N. musculocutaneus*. This abstraction allows to exchange underlying data sets (i.e. patient-specific scans, cp. figure 3) with only minor changes of some individual functional parameters.

The basic responsibility of a system, in our definition, is to establish logical links between functional and structural components and manage data access. In order to solve prioritization of access from simulation algorithms, and concurrency issues we propose the following schema. Every algorithm is allowed to access the resources one time only during each iteration. The requests are processed by a priority queue, whereby the priorities are set by the developer. We use dirt-flag containers to manage data update notification for simulation algorithms. This means that when a simulation algorithm initially requests a component it is automatically registered in the system. Thus, it can be later notified of changes through a view. After each simulation cycle every system iterates over its anatomical components and looks for changes. These changes induced by specific simulation controllers are distributed to all linked components and trigger the views of other simulations in the next cycle.

Table 1. Example of a nerve stimulation procedure performed by two steps of user interaction and automatically following steps resolved by the respective systems (Fig. 2). The actions which are part of the functional components trigger attached simulation algorithms and thereby induce subsequent steps

Nr	Interaction	System	Action	Simulation algorithm
1	needle insertion into shoulder	integumentary	deformation	FEM
2	electric impulse from needle	nervous	stimulation	rule-based system
3	actuation of innervated muscles	muscular	contraction	biomechanics
4	pull of bone at insertion point	skeletal	rotation	kinematics

3.2 Functional & Structural Components

Following the idea motivated in previous sections to encapsulate anatomical knowledge, the *functional* components define logical connections between structural components. Usually, a function is associated with two structural components the actuator and the receptor and a specific action.

Opposed to the functional components the *structural* components contain no logical connections and are patient specific. As a result, to simulate a new subject only the structural components need to be exchanged. They store raw data of arbitrary format (i.e. spatial information, physical attributes, geometric or volumetric representations, etc.).

4 Results

The structure proposed in this paper has been used in several scenarios. We present two applications, one focusing on interactive musculoskeletal simulation, and the other on regional anaesthesia. Both systems have been designed for the use in virtual environments.

The musculature application provides a tool-set for interactive modeling, simulation and representation of musculature. We have refactored an existing application with a layered approach [7] that utilizes two functional systems: the muscular and the skeletal system. Several biomechanical, kinematic and representational algorithms access these systems accordingly.

In addition to new functional systems the regional anaesthesia simulator shares both systems of the aforementioned application. The simulator is composed of functional systems (Fig. 2). Thereby, existing structures and also relevant algorithms have been reused. The update sequence during a virtual peripheral blocking procedure (Tab. 1) illustrates the interrelation between the particular functional systems.

5 Discussion & Conclusion

We have presented a new data structure and architecture for simulation of virtual humans. Our approach is based on and motivated by systematic and functional anatomy. Even though there are various physiological systems with very

Fig. 3. Dissectional (*a*) and medical (*b*) imaging data are used within the components of systems (cp. figure 2) to form the base of a virtual simulated human body (*c*)

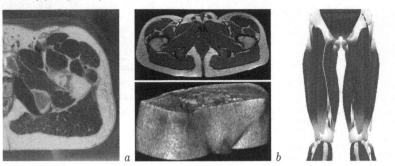

diverse functions we have established an abstract system base class with shared properties and common behavior for access management. Furthermore, we have provided a concept to allow for easy extension and creation of new systems by using functional and structural components.

Acknowledgments

This work was funded by the START-Programm (UK Aachen) and also supported by a grant from the German Research Foundation (DFG, KU 1132, LE 1108, RO 2000).

References

1. Leutert G, Schmidt W. Systematische und funktionelle Anatomie. 10th ed. Urban & Fischer; 2004.
2. Liu A, Tendick F, Cleary K, Kaufmann C. A survey of surgical simulation: Applications, technology, and education. Presence 2003;12(6):599–614.
3. of American Scientists Federation. Digital Human Project. http://www.fas.org/dh/index.html; 2006. Available from: http://www.fas.org/dh/index.html
4. Kriete A, Berger LC, Stallkamp J, Wapler M. Grundlagen eines interaktiv-funktionellen Atlanten der menschlichen Anatomie. In: Procs BVM. Heidelberg; 1999. 253–257.
5. Cardenas S CE, Braun V, Hassenpug P, Thorn M, Hastenteufel M, Kunert T, et al. Ein Framework für die Implementierung von Anwendungssystemen zur Verarbeitung und Visualisierung von medizinischen Bildern. Procs BVM 2001; 142–146.
6. Seifert S, Kussaether R, Henrich W, Voelzow N, Dillmann R. Integrating Simulation Framework MEDIFRAME. In: IEEE EMBC. Cancun, Mexico; 2003. 1327–1330.
7. Valvoda JT, Ullrich S, Kuhlen T, Bischof CH. Interactive biomechanical modeling and simulation of realistic human musculature in virtual environments. Procs BVM 2006; 404–408.

Segmentierungsfreie Visualisierung des Gehirns für direktes Volume Rendering

Johanna Beyer[1], Markus Hadwiger[1], Stefan Wolfsberger[2],
Christof Rezk-Salama[3] und Katja Bühler[1]

[1]VRVis Research Center
[2]Abteilung für Neurochirurgie, Medizinische Universität Wien
[3]Computergraphik und Multimediasysteme, Universität Siegen
Email: johanna.beyer@vrvis.at

Zusammenfassung. Direktes Volume Rendering (DVR) ist eine wichtige Technik zur 3D Visualisierung medizinscher Volumendaten, wie etwa von MRT oder CT Scans. Eines der größten Probleme des direkten Volume Rendering ist dabei die Verdeckung von möglicherweise interessanten Bereichen durch davor liegende Strukturen mit demselben Intensitätsbereich. Um etwa ein Gehirn zu visualisieren, das in einem MRT Datensatz abgebildet ist, musste man bisher auf eine Vorsegmentierung (das sogenannte Skull Stripping) zurückgreifen. In der vorliegenden Arbeit wird eine schnelle und direkte Methode zur Volumsvisualisierung des Gehirns vorgestellt, die keine vorherige Segmentierung des Gehirns benötigt. Dafür wird die Methodik des vor kurzem präsentierten "Opacity Peeling" erweitert und angepasst um optimal den (Robustheits-) Anforderungen neurochirurgischer Anwendungen zu genügen.

1 Einleitung

In der heutigen klinischen Praxis wird direktes Volume Rendering (DVR) zur 3D Darstellung von Bilddaten bereits routinemäßig eingesetzt [1]. Dabei bilden Transferfunktionen den Messwert der Originaldaten auf Farben und Opazitäten ab, um möglichst aussagekräftige Bilder zu generieren. Bei räumlich getrennten Bereichen eines Datensatzes mit gleichem Intensitätswert ist eine unterschiedliche Darstellung durch Transferfunktionen jedoch nicht möglich, und es kommt zur Verdeckung der hinterliegenden Strukturen. Ein Beispiel dafür sind MRT Datensätze des Kopfes, bei dem das Gehirn durch gleiche Messwerte stets von weiter aussen liegendem Gewebe verdeckt wird. Diese Arbeit beschreibt einen segmentierungsfreien Ansatz, der darauf basiert, dass das Problem der Verdeckung von der Betrachtungsposition abhängig ist. Zusätzliche Anwendungen sind die Darstellung von implantierten Elektroden vor Epilepsieoperationen und Tumore an der Hirnoberfläche (Abb. 1).

2 Stand der Forschung und Fortschritt durch den Beitrag

Seit der Publikation von direktem Volume Rendering (DVR) 1988 [1] wurden viele verschiedene Ansätze für DVR beschrieben. Seit dem Aufkommen program-

Abb. 1. Schnelle, segmentierungsfreie Visualisierung des Gehirns

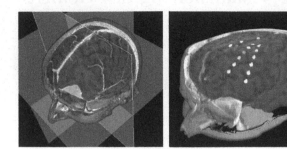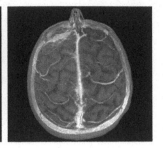

mierbarer Grafikkarten (GPUs) wurden schnellere, hardware-basierte Lösungen
entwickelt, wie etwa GPU-basiertes Raycasting [2].

Um das Gehirn aus MRT Daten in hoher Qualität zu rendern, musste bisher
auf Segmentierung zurückgegriffen werden. Die Komplexität des Skull Stripping
erkennt man jedoch bereits an der Anzahl der existierenden Methoden. In [3, 4]
werden verschiedene Ansätze beschrieben und ihre Performance evaluiert.

Opacity Peeling [5] wurde kürzlich präsentiert und ist eine DVR Methode
basierend auf Raycasting zur Visualisierung verdeckter Strukturen. Sobald die
akkumulierte Opazität eines Strahls einen Schwellwert T_1 übersteigt, werden
Farb- und Opazitätswert gespeichert und dann zurückgesetzt. Erst wenn der
Opazitätswert des aktuellen Samples unter einen Schwellwert T_2 sinkt, wird mit
der Akkumulierung fortgefahren. So können verschiedene Schichten des Datensatzes in einem Renderdurchlauf berechnet und anschließend dargestellt werden.
Confocal Volume Rendering [6] ist eine positionsabhängige Methode zur Visualisierung tiefer liegender Strukturen, bei der erst ab einer gewissen Tiefe und
nur für eine benutzerdefinierte Länge das Volumen dargestellt wird. Bruckner
et al. [7] haben illustratives kontexterhaltendes DVR vorgestellt, bei dem eine
Funktion aus Shading, Gradientenbetrag, Distanz zum Augpunkt und akkumulierte Opazität die Transparenz in gewissen Bereichen erhöht.

Bei all diesen Methoden zur selektiven Darstellung von verdeckten Strukturen ist jedoch das Ergebnis der Visualisierung kaum vorhersagbar oder kontrol-
lierbar. So kann sich die Größe des Gehirns durch kleine Schwellwertänderungen
gravierend ändern, was speziell im medizinischen Bereich gefährlich ist. Diese
Problematik wird durch die hier vorgestellte Methode behoben.

Unser Ansatz ist für die Neurochirurgie entwickelt und stellt schnell und ohne
komplizierte Benutzereingaben das Gehirn aus MR Daten dar. Die beschriebene
Methode basiert auf der Idee des Opacity Peeling, verwendet aber zusätzliche
Informationen aus einem registrierten CT Volumen. In vielen neurochirurgischen
Fällen stellt dies keinen erhöhten Akquisitionsaufwand dar, da ein CT schon für
die intraoperative Navigation vorhanden ist. Durch dieses Zusatzvolumen fallen
die Benutzereingaben des herkömmlichen Opacity Peelings weg, wodurch die
Qualität und Sicherheit der Visualisierung erhöht wird. Die Größe des Gehirns
kann also durch veränderte Schwellwerte nicht mehr variieren. Zusätzlich können

Abb. 2. Links: Original Rendering. Mitte: Problem des Clippings. Rechts: Korrekt geclipptes Volumen

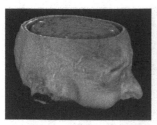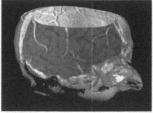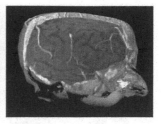

implantierte Elektroden zur Epilepsiediagnose aus registrierten CTs ebenfalls in Echtzeit visualisiert werden. Zur Operationsplanung kann ein operativen Zugang zum Gehirn simuliert werden, indem nur ein Teil des Gehirns freigelegt wird.

3 Methoden

3.1 Basis-Algorithmus

Unser Algorithmus basiert auf GPU-basiertem Raycasting [8], wobei MRT und CT Datensatz gleichzeitig geladen werden. Der Algorithmus akkumuliert Farb- und Opazitätswerte des MRTs. Zusätzlich wird bei jedem Abtastwert der Strahls auch der Wert aus dem registrierten CT bestimmt. Übersteigt dieser den Schwell- wert für den Knochen, wird das Sample als Knochen gewertet. Nach Verlassen der ersten aufgefundenen Knochenschicht werden nun Farb- und Opazitätswerte des Strahls zurückgesetzt und neu akkumuliert, wodurch das Gehirn sichtbar wird. Dieser Basis-Algorithmus funktioniert gut für Fälle bei denen das Ge- hirn von Knochen umgeben ist. Der Ansatz ist frei von Benutzereingaben und löst somit das Problem des original Opacity Peelings, bei dem die Schwellwerte Auswirkungen auf die sichtbare Größe des Gehirns haben. Ist das Volumen aller- dings durch Clipping angeschnitten, treten Probleme auf. Da alle Bereiche vor dem Knochen quasi übersprungen werden, werden nur Strukturen hinter dem ersten Auftreten von Knochen dargestellt. Falls das Gehirn jedoch von keinem Knochen mehr umgeben ist (z.B. durch Clipping), wird es übersprungen und erst das Gewebe ausserhalb des Schädels wieder angezeigt (Abb. 2, Mitte). Die Lösung dieses Problems wird im nächsten Abschnitt behandelt.

3.2 Clipping

Damit bei geclippten Volumen, ohne Knochen vor dem Gehirn, nicht das ganze Gehirn übersprungen wird, erweitern wir den Algorithmus. Dazu wird der erste Treffpunkt des Strahls mit dem zu rendernden Volumen gespeichert. Wenn nun innerhalb eines bestimmten Abstandes zu diesem Punkt der Strahl nicht auf Knochen trifft, wird standard DVR durchgeführt. Dies führt zu einem korrekten Rendering bei geclippten Volumen (Abb. 2, rechts).

Abb. 3. Links: Tumor an der Hirnoberfläche. Mitte: Implantierte Elektroden. Rechts: Simulation eines Zugangs zum Gehirn

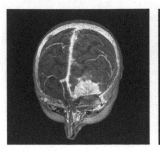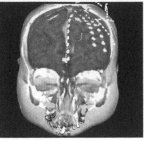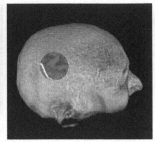

3.3 Visualisierung von Elektroden

Für die Visualisierung von invasiven Elektroden, zur Lokalisierung von epileptischen Anfällen, werden diese mittels Schwellwertsegmentierung markiert. Da die implantierten Elektroden oft etwas in die Hirnoberfläche einsinken, wird die ausreichende Sichtbarkeit der Elektroden gewährleistet, indem Farb- und Opazitätswerte des Strahls bei dem ersten Auftreffen auf eine Elektrode zurückgesetzt werden, sofern der Opazitätswert nicht schon maximal ist (Abb. 3, mitte).

3.4 Simulation von Zugängen zum Gehirn

Für die Planung neurochirurgischer Zugänge wird der beschriebene Algorithmus nur auf einem benutzerdefiniertem Bereich angewandt. Der Benutzer positioniert dabei eine kreisrunde Öffnung beliebigen Durchmessers, wodurch das Öffnen der Schädeldecke an der individuellen Anatomie simuliert wird (Abb. 3, rechts).

4   Ergebnisse

Der Algorithmus wurde auf einem Pentium IV 3,2 GHz PC und einer ATI X1800 Grafikkarte implementiert. Ein MR T1 Datensatz der Größe 512x512x154 kann dabei mit einer Geschwindigkeit von 14 fps dargestellt werden, was die Interaktivität unseres Ansatzes verdeutlicht.

Durch unsere Methode ist es möglich, die Ausbreitung oberflächlicher Tumore und umliegende Gefäße gut darzustellen (Abb. 3, links). Implantierte Elektroden zur Lokalisation von Epilepsiezentren sind in Abb. 3, Mitte zu sehen. Die Anwendung wurde in eine Umgebung für die 3D Planung neurochirurgischer Eingriffe integriert und getestet. Die einfache Art der Visualisierung, die eine langwierige Segmentierung des Gehirns überflüssig macht, wurde von Ärzten begeistert aufgenommen, ebenso wie die gute Sichtbarkeit der Gefäße. Die hier beschriebene Visualisierung von oberflächlichen Tumoren und Elektroden wird nahezu täglich eingesetzt, eine systematische Evaluierung muss jedoch erst durchgeführt werden.

5   Diskussion

Der vorgestellte Ansatz ist eine Methode zur schnellen, segmentierungsfreien Visualisierung des Gehirns aus MRTs. Eine Segmentierung des Gehirns wird dabei umgangen um mittels eines erweiterten Opacity Peelings verdeckte Strukturen zuverlässig anzuzeigen. Unsere Methode ist vor allem für zeitkritische Anwendungen gedacht, bei denen eine hochqualitative Segmentierung des Gehirns nicht möglich ist. Unser Ansatz ist nicht gänzlich frei von visuellen Artefakten (speziell im Bereich der Silhouette), eine Ausweitung des Verfahrens auf die Visualisierung anderer Strukturen, z.B. Gefäße innerhalb des Gehirns, ist jedoch denkbar.

Danksagung

Dieses Forschungsprojekt wurde durch das KPlus Projekt und AGFA Wien finanziert. Die Bilddaten stammen von der Abt. für Neurochirurgie der Med. Universität Wien.

Literaturverzeichnis

1. Levoy M. Display of surfaces from volume data. IEEE Comp Graph and Appl 1988;8:29–37.
2. Krüger J, Westermann R. Acceleration techniques for GPU-based volume rendering. In: Proc. of IEEE Visualization; 2003. 287–292.
3. Atkins MS, Siu K, Law B, Orchard JJ, Rosenbaum WL. Difficulties of T1 brain MRI segmentation techniques. Procs SPIE 2002;4684:1837–1844.
4. Song T, Angelini ED, Mensh BD, Laine A. Comparison study of clinical 3D MRI brain segmentation evaluation. In: Proc. of IEEE EMBS; 2004. 1671–1674.
5. Rezk-Salama C, Kolb A. Opacity peeling for direct volume rendering. In: Proc. of Eurographics; 2006. 597–606.
6. Mullick R, Bryan RN, Butman J. Confocal volume rendering: Fast segmentation-free visualization of internal structures. Procs SPIE 2000; 144–154.
7. Bruckner S, Grimm S, Kanitsar A, Gröller ME. Illustrative context-preserving volume rendering. In: Procs EuroVis; 2005. 69–76.
8. Scharsach H, Hadwiger M, Neubauer A, Wolfsberger S, Bühler K. Perspective ISO surface and direct volume rendering for virtual endoscopy applications. In: Procs EuroVis; 2006. 315–323.

Fast Interactive Region of Interest Selection for Volume Visualization

Dominik Sibbing and Leif Kobbelt

Lehrstuhl für Informatik 8, RWTH Aachen, 52056 Aachen
Email: {sibbing,kobbelt}@informatik.rwth-aachen.de

Abstract. We describe a new method to support the segmentation of a volumetric MRI- or CT-dataset such that only the components selected by the user are displayed by a volume renderer for visual inspection. The goal is to combine the advantages of direct volume rendering (high efficiency and semi-transparent display of internal structures) and indirect volume rendering (well defined surface geometry and topology). Our approach is based on a re-labeling of the input volume's set of isosurfaces which allows the user to peel off the outer layers and to distinguish unconnected voxel components which happen to have the same voxel values. For memory and time efficiency, isosurfaces are never generated explicitly. Instead a second voxel grid is computed which stores a discretization of the new isosurface labels. Hence the masking of unwanted regions as well as the direct volume rendering of the desired regions of interest (ROI) can be implemented on the GPU which enables interactive frame rates even while the user changes the selection of the ROI.

1   Introduction

Generating 2D images from volumetric datasets like MRI or CT scans is an important visualization task in medicine. These images help to understand anatomical structures, to make a diagnoses or to observe the healing process. They can be used for planning an operation or for surgical training. With modern graphics cards one can generate a 3D view of this data at interactive frame rates [1]. Unfortunately volumetric images often contain a lot of information, which one would not like to see all at once. Using only a transfer function which maps intensity values of the 3D image to colors and opacity values is not sufficient, because in most of the scans different tissues show similar intensity values. This often leads to the occlusion of the interesting components, for example the occlusion of the human brain by the skull. Therefore one has to separate somehow the interesting data for a certain application from the unimportant data [2]. We present a method which segments the volumetric image in an automated way using a set of isosurfaces. An isosurface is always closed and no isosurface can penetrate another isosurface. Applying a transfer function to the volumetric dataset does not change the set of isosurfaces (only their individual labels) and therefore one can consider this set of isosurfaces as an invariant geometric representation of the dataset.

The isosurfaces have a hierarchical structure which is induced by their inclusion relation. With this information the user can easily select regions like the human brain by simply peeling of the layers outside the ROI.

2 State of the Art and New Contribution

The common techniques for volume rendering are divided in direct and indirect methods. Direct methods render the voxels of the volumetric data and try to mask out those voxels that do not belong to the ROI. This method is preferable because it shows the original data and can therefore provide all the information of the original 3D image. One direct rendering technique is the registration of the input volume to a standard Talairach space and the usage of a template to mask the uninteresting voxels, see e.g. [3]. Unfortunately this is limited to healthy human brains and to a fixed set of templates. Another direct rendering technique uses a transfer function which maps intensity values to colors and opacities [1]. As said before this can lead to occlusions so the ROI is not visible anymore.

A marching cubes algorithm [4] which can be used for indirect volume rendering computes a polygonal representation of an isosurface, that can be rendered. Unfortunately the extraction of an isosurface surrounding the ROI often is a trial and error method. A more advanced technique is it to use active contours [5] which evolve until they approximate the boundary of the ROI. However, to control the stopping criterion is a hard task, see also [6], so active contours will not always produce a good approximation. Similar to that is the usage of deformable models for generating a certain ROI. But they are also limited to a fixed set of templates and cannot be used for arbitrary volumetric datasets.

Our method is a direct volume rendering method in the sense that we render the original volumetric data (OVD) in interactive framerates. But for the segmentation and visual improvement of the volumetric dataset we use techniques from indirect volume rendering, based on the extraction of isosurfaces. By combining both techniques we obtain the best of both worlds, i.e. the structure and geometry control from indirect methods and the flexibility and performance of direct methods.

3 Methods

The idea of our method is to first extract a large set of isosurfaces with the well known marching cubes algorithm [4], which provide the geometric information contained in the OVD independent from a transfer function. After separating these isosurfaces in connected components we relabel these components based on their inclusion relation, and store them in a tree data structure. In this tree component A is parent of B iff A encloses B. This will later allow the user to easily mask out the irrelevant components, by selecting nodes from the tree (Fig. 1) similar to the navigation in a hierarchical file system. In our experiments we extracted 64 isosurfaces for various gray levels between the minimum and

Fig. 1. Calculation of new labels, by traversing an thereby uniquely relabeling the nodes of a tree in a depth first order

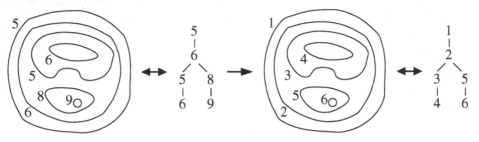

maximum voxel value. As we will show, these isosurfaces can be stored in a very memory efficient way.

The new labels are assigned by a depth first traversal in the tree and are used to generate an additional volumetric dataset where voxels are labeled by the smallest isosurface in which they are contained. Both the OVD and the new labeled volumetric data (LVD) are stored in the memory of the graphics card. For displaying the tree we designed an interface similar to a file browsing system, which is capable to visualize large structures in an easy way. One Click on one of the nodes toggles the visibility of the whole subtree. During interactive display, we only send the information which labels are visible to the graphics card, and decide for each fragment if it is visible or not by looking up its label in the LVD. After that we can render the fragment according to the value stored in the OVD using a simple transfer function. This allows for interactive frame rates.

The setup for the algorithm is as follows. We call an edge of the voxel grid x-edge if the adjacent grid point differ by one in the x-coordinate.

For building the tree and calculating the LVD we need two important procedures. The *'IsIn'*-Test which decides whether a surface is inside another surface and a scanline algorithms which line by line assigns the new labels for the voxels.

3.1   *IsIn*-Test and Scanline Algorithm

To test whether a surface A lies inside a surface B we first locate the point $p \in A$ with the highest x-coordinate. Note that p always lies on an x-edge. From p we shoot a ray in x-direction and count the number N of intersections with surface B. We observe

$$A \ inside \ B \Leftrightarrow N \, mod \, 2 = 1 \tag{1}$$

Due to the linear interpolation between the voxel samples, one (and only one) intersection with B happens for each x-edge which connects two voxel with values $V^- \leq B < V^+$.

For setting the values in the LVD we use a scanline algorithm, which traverses rays along the positive x-direction. Everytime we enter a surface s, we activate s. If we leave s we deactivate it. Then a voxel will get the label of the last surface we marked so far.

Fig. 2. Results: Direct volume rendering with high performance but occlusions may occur (a);i Indirect volume rendering based on Isosurfaces but finding the right labels is a trial and error method with low interactivity (b); Combining the best of both methods lead to a flexible and efficient direct volume renderer which is capable to distinguish every connected voxel component (c); Integrating lighting and shadows further improve the 3D impression of the image (d)

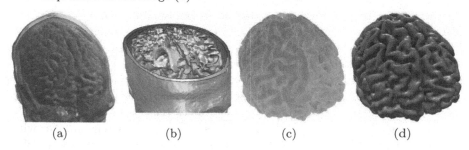

(a)   (b)   (c)   (d)

To put it more precisely, we process one of the $n_y \cdot n_z$ scanlines by first initializing a stack with label 0 on top. For every voxel $p = (x, y, z)$ we encounter, we first set the label to the value stored on top of the stack. We update the stack by looking at all the intersections on the next x-edge right of p. Intersecting a surface which has the same label as stored on top of the stack will remove the element on top of the stack. In the other case we push the label of the intersected surface on the stack. Note that each x-edge can intersect only once with a specific surface, because the marching cube algorithm linearly and hence monotonically interpolates between adjacent grid points to generate a vertex of the surface.

3.2 Efficient Storage of the Isosurfaces

As said before isosurfaces provide a lot of information, like vertex positions in 3D and the connectivity of the mesh. For our purpose we don't need all of the information. All we have to ensure is that the '*IsIn*'-Test and the scanline algorithm work. We observe that in both procedures we shoot a ray along x-edges of the grid. Because the marching cube algorithm only generates vertices on the edges of the grid we only can enter or leave a surface by passing a vertex on a x-edge. So we only store those vertices in form of an offset in x-direction w.r.t the left grid point, which extremely reduce the memory consumption. Both procedures can be executed very efficient if we store for every grid point a list of vertices which lie on the right x-edge and a list of their corresponding surfaces.

4   Results

We generated all results with an AMD64 with 2.2GHz, 2GB RAM and a NVidia GeForce 7800 GTX graphics card. The images 2a-d were generated from a MRI scan with a resolution of 256x256x170. The extraction of 64 isosurfaces and the calculation of the tree and the new labels took less than 15 Min. Fig. 2c and d show our method in comparison to a direct (Fig. 2a) and an indirect (Fig. 2b) method.

5   Discussion

The advantage of this method is that it works on differend kind of volume images. Nevertheless these images should not contain too much noise, because then it is difficult to extract smooth isosurfaces. In our case we use a bilateral filter [7] to denoise the intensity distribution of the OVD. The selection of the interesting regions is very intuitive, because the result of each selection can be seen immediately. If the user wants to see a deeper layer, he simply traverses the tree downwards. But for a large set of isosurfaces the tree can get rather large. Therefore we allow the user to decimate this tree, by discarding surfaces which have approximately the same volume as the parent surface, i.e. we can combine the nodes {1,2}, {3,4} and {5,6} in the example of Fig. 1.

6   Acknowledgement

This work is supported by the DFG (IRTG 1328).

References

1. Engel K, Hadwiger M, Kniss JM, et al. Real-time volume graphics. In: ACM SIGGRAPH 2004 Course Notes; 2004. 29.
2. Wang L, Zhao Y, Mueller K, et al. The magic volume lens: An interactive focus+context technique for volume rendering. In: IEEE Visualization; 2005. 47.
3. Collins DL, Neelin P, Peters TM, et al. Automatic 3D intersubject registration of MR volumetric data in standardized talairach space. J Comput Assist Tomogr 1994;18(2):192–205.
4. Lorenson W, Cline H. Marching cubes: A high resolution 3D surface construction algorithm. Computer Graphics 1987;21(4):163–169.
5. Davatzikos C, Prince J. An active contour model for mapping the cortex. IEEE Trans Med Imaging 1995;14:65–80.
6. Bischoff S, Kobbelt L. Sub-voxel topology control for level set surfaces. In: Procs Eurographics; 2003. 273–280.
7. Tomasi C, Manduchi R. Bilateral filtering for gray and color images. In: Procs ICCV; 1998. 839–846.

Hybrid Navigation Interface
A Comparative Study

Philipp Stefan[1], Joerg Traub[1], Sandro M. Heining[2], Christian Riquarts[2],
Tobias Sielhorst[1], Ekkehard Euler[2], Nassir Navab[1]

[1]Chair for Computer Aided Medical Procedures (CAMP), I-16, Technische
Universität München, Boltzmannstraße 3, 85748 Garching b. München, Germany
[2]Trauma Surgery Department, Klinikum Innenstadt, Ludwig Maximilian Universität
München, Nußbaumstraße 20, 80336 München, Germany
Email: stefanp@cs.tum.edu

Abstract. Since the introduction of computer aided surgery, many visualisation techniques for intraoperative navigation have been proposed. Systems employing multi planar reconstruction for the visualisation of volumetric imaging data are commercially available and frequently used. In these systems, three-dimensional biomedical data is generally displayed on a two-dimensional computer monitor as orthogonal planar sections defined by the orientation of a surgical instrument. In-situ visualisation, that was introduced as an alternative approach for intraoperative navigation, superimposes three-dimensional imaging data directly on the surgical object, typically using a stereoscopic display device, e.g. a head mounted display. In this paper, we compare monitor based navigation with video see-through augmented reality visualisation regarding performance and usability. Furthermore, we compare each with a hybrid of both systems that was recently introduced. We created an experimental setup to simulate an exemplary application for trauma and orthopedic surgery and conducted the experiment with three trauma surgeons with different levels of experience using all three approaches.

1 Introduction

The aims of computer aided surgery are the improvement of patient care by utilising computational tools during treatment. This includes the guidance of the surgeon during the intervention using intraoperative navigation systems, that visualise volumetric biomedical imaging data with respect to the orientation of surgical instruments.

Multi planar reconstruction (MPR) is a commonly used visualisation technique for such volumetric datasets. A tracked instrument defines planar sections through the reconstructed volume, that are visualised on a computer monitor display. Commercially available navigation systems, that employ MPR exist for more than a decade. The drawbacks of state-of-the-art navigation systems, based on preoperative or intraoperative imaging data, are, that a) the visualisation is focused on a small region of interest and does not give an overview of the surgical workspace, b) the guidance information based on three-dimensional data is presented on two-dimensional display devices, and c) the navigational information is not visualised directly at the operation site, forcing the surgeon to obtain the navigational information from a location unrelated to his surgical workspace.

Augmented reality (AR) using stereoscopic display devices, e.g. head-mounted displays (HMDs), has been discussed in the community as an alternative three-dimensional visualisation technique for navigated surgery in the last decade by different groups [1, 2, 3]. In this approach the navigational information, derived from the same volumetric dataset, that is used in MPR based navigation, is superimposed onto the surgeon's view of the real world.

Navigation systems based on MPR or AR, respectively, have been presented as concurrent approaches and were never compared in evaluations using *the same* experimental setup. We implemented a MPR based navigation interface displayed on a computer monitor and an AR navigation interface displayed on a HMD. Furthermore, we propose to fuse both interfaces into a single three-dimensional user interface and developed a *hybrid navigation interface* as a combination of both technologies. In order to evaluate the possible advantages of a hybrid navigation interface compared to its two complementary components, we conducted an experiment on the performance of computer guided instrument placement with three surgeons of different levels of experience.

2   Materials and Methods

We use an optical tracking system with four cameras fixed to the ceiling for precise real-time localisation of the instrument and the surgical object. The tracking system is capable of tracking the targets in our setup with an accuracy of $< 0.35[mm]$ RMS. The MPR-navigation system uses an off-the-shelf PC for visualisation (Fig. 2(b)). The AR system uses a stereoscopic video see-through HMD similar to a system described by Sauer et al. [3]. The display is equipped with two colour cameras to obtain images of the observed scene and a tracking camera, rigidly attached to the colour cameras, for head pose estimation using a marker frame as a reference (Fig. 2(a)(G)). The reason for the preference of a video-see-through display to an optical-see-through device is, first of all, that these systems achieve a perfect synchronisation of video and head pose data since all cameras are genlocked, eliminating any lag between the images of the cameras. Secondly, we have more options for merging virtual and real objects, while optical systems offer only a brightening augmentation.

The transformation from the coordinate system of the external tracking device to the two-dimensional coordinates in the overlay image is given by

$$H_{\text{Target}}^{\text{Overlay}} = H_{\text{Cam}}^{\text{Overlay}} H_{\text{Frame}}^{\text{Cam}} \left(H_{\text{Frame}}^{\text{Ext}}\right)^{-1} H_{\text{Target}}^{\text{Ext}} \tag{1}$$

The transformations $H_{\text{Frame}}^{\text{Ext}}$, $H_{\text{Target}}^{\text{Ext}}$ are provided by the external tracking system. $H_{\text{Frame}}^{\text{Cam}}$, $H_{\text{Cam}}^{\text{Overlay}}$ are derived using Tsai calibration. The instrument was calibrated and the patient registered as described in [4].

Fig. 1. Illustration of the experimental setup. X-ray dense, IR reflecting markers (E) attached to the phantom (D) and the drill (C) are tracked with an external optical tracking system (A). The visualisation (B) is displayed on an monitor, shown in figure (b) and respectively on the HMD (F) in figure (c). In the AR-system (a) a reference frame (G) is used to establish the transition between the external tracking system (A) and the single camera tracking system of the HMD (F)

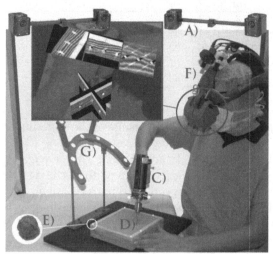
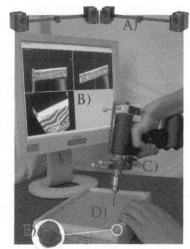

(a) Setup of the in-situ visualisation   (b) Setup of the MPR-navigation

To achieve a fully automatic patient registration we used a reference target consisting of fiducials, that are automatically detectable in the imaging data and using the external tracking system, in the physical space.

The navigation interfaces were implemented using a software framework [5] that ensures sychronisation of video and tracking data, eliminating any perceivable drift of the augmentation. The three different navigation methods designed for this study are shown in figure 2. We have decided to employ a in-situ visualisation method where two orthogonal slices are rendered along the longitudinal axis of an instrument, as this is, according to previous studies [6], a convenient guidance aid, especially regarding lateral positioning.

3   Experiment and Result

A phantom that consists of a wooden block with metal spheres of $4[mm]$ diameter implanted at depth of approximately $40[mm]$ was constructed. The surface was covered with a silicone rubber compound with properties similar to human skin. We estimated a maximum target registration error (TRE) of the implanted metal spheres of $0.24\ [mm]$ and a mean error of $0.17\ [mm] \pm 0.03\ [mm]$.

Three surgeons conducted the experiment ten times for each of the three navigation methods. The distance between the surface of the implanted metal sphere and the distal end of the drill was recorded along with the time required to

Table 1. Results of an experiment conducted by surgeons, regarding speed and accuracy. The navigation methods evaluated are monitor based navigation (MPR), in-situ visualisation (AR) and a hybrid combination of both (HYBRID). * denotes an experiment performed with the same surgeons under comparable conditions [6]

Navigation	Surgeon A error [mm]	time [s]	Surgeon B error [mm]	time [s]	Surgeon C error [mm]	time [s]
MPR	0.75 ± 0.68	71 ± 35	1.12 ± 0.52	66 ± 36	0.58 ± 0.44	51 ± 11
AR	0.84 ± 0.48	47 ± 17	0.69 ± 0.44	48 ± 21	0.66 ± 0.49	29 ± 8
HYBRID	0.58 ± 0.44	48 ± 14	0.97 ± 0.46	63 ± 20	0.68 ± 0.44	30 ± 9
AR*	2.3 ± 0.9	98 ± 24	1.7 ± 0.6	57 ± 52	3.1 ± 2.9	47 ± 28
HYBRID*	1.6 ± 0.6	95 ± 28	1.9 ± 0.5	84 ± 17	1.9 ± 0.2	26 ± 12

position the drill and reach the given target region. The results of the experiment are summarised in table 1.

Subject A is an inexperienced surgeon, who is not familiar with navigated surgery, subject B is a chief surgeon for trauma surgery, who performs navigated surgeries on a regular basis and subject C is a surgeon, who performs navigated surgeries and is involved in the development of systems for navigated surgery, that utilise AR technologies.

All experiments were performed within the accuracy of $1[mm]$ using a rigid, non deformable phantom. This result is acceptable according to the accuracy requirements for applications in orthopedic and trauma surgery. In order to be able to apply our methods to computer aided surgery however, additional challenges have to be accomplished to achieve the same accuracy for tracking and registration as we do in our lab environment.

4   Conclusion

The experiment indicates that a monitor based navigation interface has several disadvantages compared to in-situ visualisation. It is not intuitively usable, especially for surgeons, who never performed a computer assisted surgery, since it

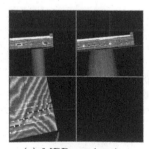 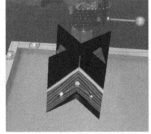 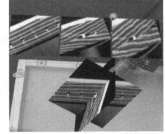

(c) MPR navigation   (d) In-situ visualisation   (e) Hybrid visualisation

Fig. 2. Different navigation modes displayed on a monitor (c) and in a HMD (d), (e)

requires enormous comprehensive skills to mentally transfer the obtained information to the surgical environment. The experiment supports our thesis, that AR visualisation does not improve accuracy of surgical interventions, but, due to a more intuitive interaction, their speed. Throughout the experiment all three surgeons preferred the hybrid interface, that was described by them as intuitive and as accurate and safe as the monitor based system. The results affect our future research in the field of surgical navigation with AR technologies. We believe that a successful integration of surgical navigation in the operation theatre strongly depends on the intuitiveness of the user interface. Augmented reality can be a step towards fulfilling this premise. The presented hybrid navigation interface can benefit from the intuitiveness of in-situ visualisation and the well proven accuracy of conventional navigation.

Acknowledgment

Special thanks to Frank Sauer, Ali Khamene and Sebastian Vogt from Siemens Corporate Research for providing us with the RAMP system. Additionally, we would like to thank Josef Schweiger for his help on the design of the phantom. Last but not least, we would like to thank Stefan Wiesner and K. Schweiger for moral support and company. This work was granted by the BFS within the NARVIS project (www.narvis.org).

References

1. King AP, Edwards PJ, Maurer CR Jr, de Cunha DA, Hawkes DJ, Hill DLG, et al. A system for microscope-assisted guided interventions. IEEE Trans Med Imag 2000;19(11):1082–1093.
2. Birkfellner W, Figl M, Huber K, Watzinger F, Wanschitz F, Hummel J, et al. A head-mounted operating binocular for augmented reality visualization in medicine: Design and initial evaluation. IEEE Trans Med Imag 2002;21(8):991–997.
3. Sauer F, Khamene A, Bascle B, Rubino GJ. A head-mounted display system for augmented reality image guidance: Towards clinical evaluation for iMRI-guided neurosurgery. In: Proc. of MICCAI. Springer-Verlag; 2001. 707–716.
4. Traub J, Stefan P, Heining SM, Sielhorst T, Riquarts C, Euler E, et al. Towards a hybrid navigation interface: Comparison of a slice-based navigation system with in-situ visualization. In: Proc. of MIAR. Springer-Verlag; 2006.
5. Sielhorst T, Feuerstein M, Traub J, Kutter O, Navab N. CAMPAR: A software framework guaranteeing quality for medical augmented reality. In: Proc. of CARS; 2006.
6. Traub J, Stefan P, Heining SM, Sielhorst T, Riquarts C, Euler E, et al. Hybrid navigation interface for orthopedic and trauma surgery. In: Proc. of MICCAI. Springer-Verlag; 2006. 373–380.

3D-Brain Model Software
A New Interactive Real-Time Graphics Visualization for Rat Brain

W. Ovtscharoff jr.[1], A. Riedel[1], C. Kubisch[1], S. Stoyanov[3], C. Helmeke[1],
A. Herzog[2], B. Michaelis[2] and K. Braun[1]

[1]Deptartment of Zoology/Developmental Neurobiology
[2]Institute for Electronics, Signal Processing and Communications
[1,2]Otto-von-Guericke-University Magdeburg, 39016 Magdeburg
[3]Department of Internal Medicine 1, University Hospital Heidelberg,Germany
Email: ovtscharoff@ifn-magdeburg.de

Abstract. The project's main goal is the development of an interactive
3D atlas, that allows detailed exploration of the rat brain as well as
illustration of interactions and information flows between various brain
structures. Compared to other software on the market, this tool will focus
more on the specific needs of scientists and students. Simplicity of use is
one of its keys features. Students and scientists should be able to easily
manipulate and view data that the system provides. Especially scientists
should be able to import or add results and compare or illustrate them
within a unified framework. The software will run on normal consumer
hardware and not require expensive workstations, so that students can
use it for learning purposes at home, as well as scientists being able to
add data from their regular work PCs. Despite not having high hardware
requirements, it will make use of various visualization effects.

1 Introduction

Brain atlas research was originally based on accurate localization of specific
structures and regions and supply the research with static profile. 3D atlas have
a potential to provide virtual model, better visualization and interpretations.
Such information is highly valuable for neuroanatomists and surgical procedures
[1]. 3D reconstruction of structures and cells has remained largely manual despite
the rapid development of computer technology. Current techniques for mapping
are too slow to support a adequate quantitative analysis of brain morphology at
cellular and tissue level.

To date very limited amount of detailed 3D data from brain to single cell
populations is available in electronic form to supply sufficient scientific information. With some exceptions like works of "Rutgers University"[2], which developing a major brain regions (reference brain) and containing outlines. Works
on a 3D atlas of spinal cord of rat done by Prof. Paxinos and Dr. Koutcherov
[3] proved how important ca be a detailed information. At ultrastructural level

"Synapse Web"(www.synapses.bu.edu), developing a powerful tools for reconstructions and visualization of fine structures of CNS which we take in account for our own model. We are developing a tool to help improve data collection, preparing and visualization of quantitative results. Structural presentation as 3D cordinate space is in use in many brain imaging researches. We creating a tool which can be adapted to cover large field of anatomy and teaching activities.

2   State of the Art and New Contribution

Compared to similar 3D viewing programs from the past, today's consumer graphics hardware is powerful widely available and not limited to workstations. Various visualization effects will make viewing our 3d atlas more exciting and present the models more vividly. When targeting students with our software (Fig. 1, 2), it should not have the "sterile"look of aged software, which simply didn't have the power to do further effects, but present the data in a form that is appealing to the current and coming generation of neuroscientists. The effects will not be used for the effects sake but to illustrate information flows, selections and objects . To make use of hardware accelerated viewing, OpenGL is used for rendering. It also allows portability of the application to various platforms, although for the beginning only Microsoft Windows-based systems are intended.

Most of today's top medical visualization software is very advanced and allows high-level application, however its functionality is not always easily accessible, and the software might be too expensive to be used for students as learning software at home. Once 3D atlas is created entirely it can be used for many purposes and can be associated with database. It make sense to develop the work further for localizations of expression of certain receptors of cellular proteins [4, 1].

3   Methods

For the development of the 3D rat brain we use "luxinia", a scriptable 3D engine, written by two students of the Otto-von-Guericke University of Magdeburg. The application code is written in LUA script, developed by Pontifical Catholic University of Rio de Janeiro, Brazil. Scripting languages, allow faster and easier development of software, due to them being high-level, compared to the low-level languages such as C or C++. However as low-level languages allow greater performance, the engine itself was written in C. The users of the rat brain viewer will also benefit from the use of a high-level language, as they can extend the software on their own, and do not need to write low-level code. Compared to similar 3D engines, luxinia's hardware requirements are still fairly low, but allow various effects even on older graphics hardware. There is also support for sound and physics and it is free for non-commercial use.

At first we were constructing the surface models of the brain structures. To achieve this, we uses a series of photographs taken from Nissl stained brain sections of Sprague Dawley rats, which have been traced and vectorized to spline

Fig. 1. 3D model surface presentation and 2D-3D atlas sectioning (left); Snapshots from user modus (right)

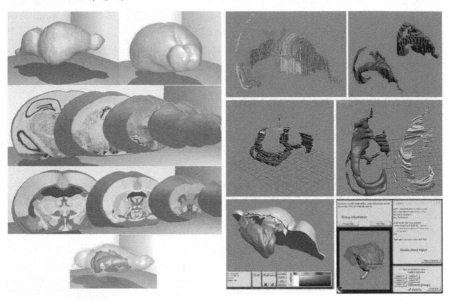

data. Every structure is made of a series of spline layers, where each layer has thickness of 0,75 mm. Surface creation from the spline layers is done in Autodesk 3dsmax. A tool written in maxscript and C++ generates a polygon mesh from the input data. Maxscript is the proprietary scripting language of 3dsmax and allows object creation, as well as workflow enhancement and many other tasks, as it often allows direct access to 3dsmax's objects. The aim is the ease of use, especially when it comes to creation of graphical user interfaces, which makes creation of artist friendly tools easier. On startup the user can define the location of the input files and set distance between layers, as well as starting layer location. After the import each layer is turned into a 2D polygon and rasterized using a C++ plugin. As result of the rasterization, a voxel representation of the model is being created. These voxels are then turned into a polygon hull mesh, with customizeable resolution. Various modifiers of 3dsmax can be applied to the hull mesh. Such as the generation of a relaxed surface, which is smooth and does not have the typical voxelized hard-edged look. While a certain precision loss compared to the original volume data comes with the use of triangle meshes and using voxels as base, the advantage is performance for the interactive 3d viewer. Triangle meshes are easily accelerated on most of today's graphics hardware, which is necessary for the software having low hardware requirements. However precision can also be raised with finer ray-shooting. 3dsmax also comes with various LOD methods to further lower the triangle count of the mesh, for improved interactive framerates. A high-resolution mesh could still be used as reference for advanced real-time rendering methods, such as local-space normal mapping. Another benefit from creating the data within 3dsmax also means it can be exported to various other file formats, or can be used for illustrative renderings and animations. Another method, creating the surface model from connecting the splines, did not yield good meshes, and was not so well suited for automatic use, as the voxel method is. As mentioned before the final meshes can be used for offline rendering of images and animations, however for this project the data will be exported to the 3D engine's format as indexed triangle meshes.

Real-time glow effects are used to enhance selection and illustration processes. Per-pixel Gooch-shading allows better perception of curvature. To illustrate volume data within the brain's substructures, a form of billboard rendering was chosen, which also allows shading on the normally flat billboards. Another method, which might be implemented additionally, is the use of 3D textures and view-aligned planes.

4   Results

Our 3D tool should not feel like a CAD application, but more like a virtual space. The classic three-views and wire frame depiction of the models, is less suited for transporting the spatial information of the "bigger picture" easily and fast, hence focus will be on perspective viewing. Light and environment effects, such as fog, should help giving the viewer enough depth cues to get familiar with the dimensions of the structure. Mouse interaction and a graphical user interface with proper icons should be sufficient. Students could be asked to click certain regions themselves, as a test. Furthermore the viewer must give easy access to detailed information about each structure, not just their names and functions, but also interaction between them. Structures should be categorize able and hide able. It would be needed to color-code them based on their influence towards certain effects. Particle systems, or other effects such as animated surface textures, glows and alike will be used to represent this data. Each 3D model can carry different calibrations depending on the age of animals. We are planing to incorporate a tool to view and use also a 2D atlas (Fig. 1) for fast orientation and moving. Once cell populations and connectivity been reconstructed they can be placed into virtual environment to visualize the dense neuronal forests and morphology [5]. A real-time rotating and zooming view will represent a cell population distribution using a voxel rendering technique. Our tool representing brain regions which are unique fill color coded and can divergent depending on cell (sub region) specification (Fig. 2).

5   Discussion

The tool which we are developing is a step along the way to improve data access and 3D visualization instead of static view. While students would rather consume this data, scientists would feed the data into the system. Scientists especially need to be able to create data sets of influence and flow values within the model's substructures. It must be easy for them to enter text or automatically

352   W. Ovtscharoff jr. et al.

Fig. 2. Snapshots from 3D detail analysis (neuronal population presented in blue)

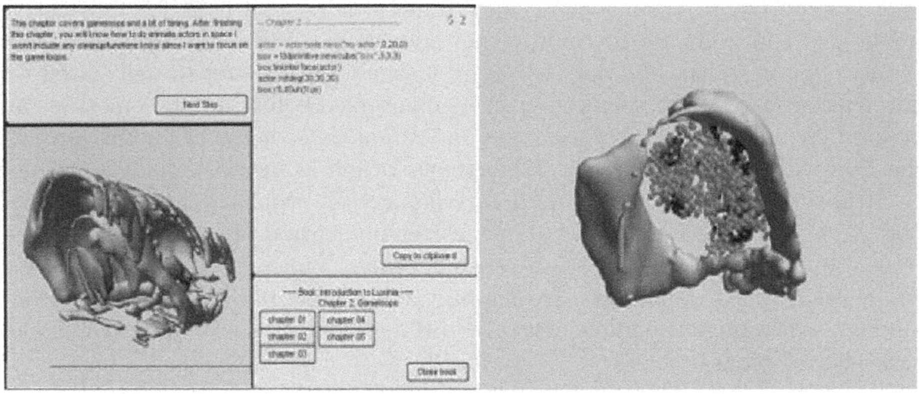

add values based on external data, e.g. Excel data files and alike. That way they could use the benefits of a unified viewer of their results, and also compare results against each other. For teaching purposes used in a similar way by the group of Sundstein [6], the system allow packing information in chapters. Each chapter can give information about a substructure or its interaction with others. Animated sequences could further illustrate effects. The advantage of being able to interact with the scene must be made use of, compared to the classic use of static images / pre-rendered animations. We presenting a tool simplified the way of data presentation and deriving a quantitative information. We creating a tool which presenting a anatomical and functional data, to manipulate and detect patterns in resulting image database. Thus will reflect in better understanding brain functions and support the scientists.

Acknowledgement

This work was supported by LSA Grant FKZ 3431B/0302M.

References

1. Toga AW, Tompson PM. Measuring, maping, and modeling brain structures and function. Procs SPIE 1997;3033.
2. Group Zaborsky. Ratbrain project. wwwratbrainorg.
3. Paxinos G, Koutcherov Y. Three-dimensional (3D) atlas of the rat spinal cord. Spinal injuries research centre at the "Prince of Wales Medical Research Institute".
4. Timsari B, Tocco G, Bouteiller JM, M Baudry, R Leahy. Accurate registration of autoradiographic images of rat brain using a 3-D atlas. In: CISST; 1999.
5. Burton BP, Chow TS, Duchowski AT, et al. Exploring the brain forest. Neurocomputing 1999;26-27:971–980.
6. Sundsten JW, Kastella JG, Conley DM. Videodisc animation of 3D computer reconstructions of human brain. J Biomed Comm 1991;18:45–49.

Finite Element Simulation of Moving Targets in Radio Therapy

Pan Li, Gregor Remmert, Jürgen Biederer, Rolf Bendl

Medical Physics, German Cancer Research Center, 69120 Heidelberg
Email: pan.li@dkfz.de

Abstract. Among other options, radiotherapy plays an increasing role for the treatment of lung cancer. This has raised the need for strategies to compensate for respiratory motion of the target. Sophisticated techniques such as tracking of the tumour position have become feasible. However, calculations for adequate dose delivery to moving targets with maximum preservation of healthy tissue require understanding the principle of soft tissue deformation In this paper, we introduce a new approach using non-linear finite element method to simulate lung tissue displacement during respiration. The geometric non-linearity and the material non-linearity were applied. The respiration movement was regarded as steady gradual process with equal velocity, and was simulated statically. Boundary condition was set on lung's surface, and the deformation of whole volume could be calculated. Simulation of diaphragm breathing was compared with 4DCT of ventilated porcine lung inside a chest phantom. The average difference of internal point movement was 3 mm vertically. Our vision is to integrate the concept of FEM simulation of respiratory motion into motion adapted radiotherapy planning.

1 Introduction

Among other options, radiotherapy plays an increasing role for its treatment. The key strategy of radiotherapy is to maximize local dose at the target, while at the same time minimizing damage to adjacent normal tissue. The easiest approach to account for target movement with respiration is to define larger planning target which covers the malignant lesion at any point of its course during the respiratory cycle. Meanwhile, techniques for gated irradiation at certain positions or for tracking the tumour during the respiratory cycle should principally allow for smaller planning target volumes. To understand the principle reason of soft tissue deformation due to external force has become a key for defining planning target volumes for motion-adapted radiation. Over the last three decades the biomechanism of soft tissue has been thoroughly investigated. Based on theoretical knowledge and recent technique of CT, MRI, biomedical simulation has been widely used in surgical planning system, functional assessment of organ (e.g. heart) or molecular biological simulation. However, less work has been done to simulate lung movement. The objective of this work is to introduce a new approach of finite element simulation to describe lung tissue deformation and to integrate it in radiotherapy planning.

2   State of the Art and New Contribution

Segars [1] describe structures inside the torso with a set of spline-based geometrical primitives. But he did not give any physical law for that model. Wu [2] implemented an adaptive FEM model for soft tissue. But no further work in lung simulation was given. In our FEM simulation we will study the internal deformation of lung.

3   Methods

Normal lung can be considered as homogeneous, isotropic, non-linear compressible object. Its non-linearity can be divided as geometric non-linearity (non-linear strain) and non-linear material property. Since no *in vivo* material law for lung was published so far, we employed simpler hyperelastic law. Another material which is more reasonable for soft tissue, was introduced by Veronda and Westermann [3]. This was also integrated in our work.

3.1   3D Volume Mesh

A FEM pre-processor was developed to generate 3D tetrahedron volume mesh and assign material properties. The 3D mesh was achieved firstly by initiating volume of interest (VOI) with volume grower segmentation algorithm, retrieving surface mesh with marching cube, and decomposing volume in tetrahedron elements with Netgen [4]. Assigning material properties was done in a graphic interactive process. According to its neighbourhood, each element on the boundary was labelled with one material index which represents its neighbour organ, e.g. elements which share boundary with diaphragm, were set with diaphragm index. All internal elements have the same index. Usually, meshing program, especially Delauny algorithm, couldn't assure mesh quality. Since FEM simulation works with volume mesh data, it has high demand for the mesh quality. We implemented a so-called steepest descendent approach to improve mesh quality. With V, L referring to volume and length of edges and C is the normalizing factor, the measure referring to tetrahedron quality was defined as

$$Q = C \frac{V}{L^3} \tag{1}$$

3.2   Finite Element Method

Here, we briefly introduce the problem which need to be solved. $\varOmega 0$ is the undeformed state of the elastic object. The principle of virtual work in the total lagrangian formulation is given by

$$\int_{\varOmega 0} {}_0^{t+\Delta t}S\delta_0^{t+\Delta t}\varepsilon d^0V = {}^{t+\Delta t}R \tag{2}$$

where $_0^{t+\Delta t}S$ is second Piolar Kirchhoff stress tensor, $_0^{t+\Delta t}\varepsilon$ is lagrangian strain tensor, operator δ indicates small virtual displacement. $^{t+\Delta t}R$ denotes to external virtual work. The small 0 means each item is related to referential configuration. Based of its non-linear property, equation (2) must be solved in an incremental way. t refers to any arbitrary time point, Δt implies time increment. The incremental decomposition of the non linear strain representing geometry non-linearity turned out to be an incremental part and a part related to the last time step. The incremental part can be further decomposed as linear and non-linear components. After linearizing the higher-order term in the non-linear component, we obtain the final equation of motion with $_0C$ denoting the material elastic tensor

$$\int_{\Omega 0} {}_0C e \delta_0 e d^0V + \int_{\Omega 0} {}_0^t S \delta_0 \eta d^0V + \int_{\Omega 0} {}_0^t S \delta_0 e d^0V = {}^{t+\Delta t}R \qquad (3)$$

Biomedical material always shows non linear, non elastic properties. Wu included both Mooney-Rivlin and Neo-Hookean material law which depict linear relation of strain energy and Cauchy deformation tensor. Veronda and Westermann introduced another material law which can express the feature of soft tissue through a exponential term. We included both Neo-Hookean and Veronda Westmann material law.

4   Results

We tested our finite element simulator with ventilated ex-vivo system. The phantom experiment used a diaphragmatic pump for the exactly reproducible ventilation of animal lung explants inside a dedicated porcine chest phantom [5]. Before CT scanning 8 markers were injected into the left and right lung, respectively 4 markers in each side. 4DCT lung image data was segmented to generate mesh in the following steps. Then the segmented region was labelled with a gray value, and the rest of the image cube was set with zero. In the next step the labelled image cube was transferred to a surface retrieving module. A water tight iso-surface triangle mesh was retrieved by using marching cube algorithm. Finally, the volume surrounded by the triangle surface mesh was decomposed into tetrahedron 3D mesh with software Netgen. To verify the conformity of our 3D lung model to the real lung, we compared it with the original 3D surface image reconstructed by a in house developed software.

Figure 1a shows segmentation of the right lung in one slice. Figure 1a indicates, there is no great mismatch between the real lung surface image and the 3D model. Figure 2a illustrates a kind of tetrahedron element with bad quality which is called sliver. Figure 2b gives the result of improved quality after 10 iterations. After obtaining 3D volume mesh, material properties were set to surface elements regarding their direct neighbours. Figure 3a depicts the boundary conditions.

First, we tried pseudo-simulation of diaphragm inspiration. Normally, it's difficult to measure the external surface force during the lung ex- or inspiration. Therefore, we defined surface nodes displacement for diaphragm instead

Fig. 1. Lung contour (a) and model (b): original (red), model (green)

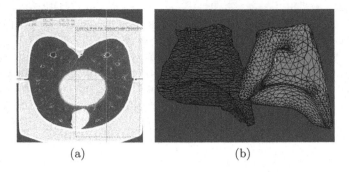

(a)   (b)

Fig. 2. Tetrahedon optimization: top tetrahedron with bad volume edge length behaviour (a) and optimized tetrahedon (b)

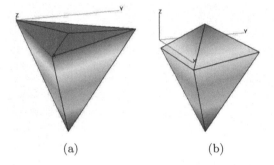

(a)   (b)

of setting external force. The whole body deformation was driven by its continuous surface nodes displacement. To simulate diaphragm inspiration, we drove down all surface nodes on diaphragm vertically with different increments. The sliding of other surface nodes along the pleural membrane was simulated by the displacement allowed only parallel to their surface planes.

Figure 3b illustrates the whole process of FEM simulation. Figure 3c demonstrates the deformed state. In Table 1 the result (in mm) was compared with 4DCT data.

The simulation was done in 250 steps. The computation of each incremental step took around 6 seconds for 5190 elements, which corresponds to 3 Newton iterations.

5 Discussion

The pseudo diaphragm inspiration was simulated by vertically moving surface nodes on diaphragm. However, in real anatomy the situation is far more complex. The pleural sliding between lung bottom and diaphragm must be considered. And no node moves only in one direction. There are two approaches to improve our simulation. First, inspiration can be considered as driven by external force.

Fig. 3. Boundary conditions (a), incremental solution (b) and deformed state (c) with diaphragm (green), lung (red), upper part (white) and small elements (yellow)

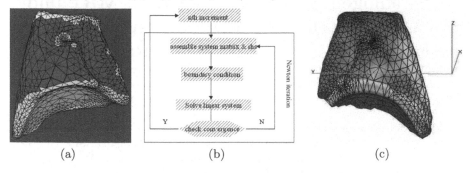

(a)   (b)   (c)

Table 1. Results: number of implants (N), displacement (x, y, z)

N	displacement in CT [mm]			Result of FEM simulation [mm]		
	x	y	z	x	y	z
1	1.170	0.000	-22.4	0.653	0.043	-19.6
2	-1.170	2.350	-18.4	0.677	-0.110	-20.0
3	0.000	-0.560	-13.6	-1.020	-1.040	-10.3
4	-2.340	1.760	-20.6	0.176	1.337	-17.0

In this case we have to calculate surface traction and its contribution to each surface node. Second, we can include diaphragm in our model and deal with frictionless contact problem between lung and diaphragm. Soft tissue always shows viscoelastic property. Lung should not be modelled only with hyperelastic material law. New material law must be studied. These will be done in our future work. Noted in the introduction, our goal is to apply the new FEM simulation to predict invisible tumor movement. Since techniques for the tracking of respiratory motion with external markers are available, it remains a challenge to use this signal for the calculation of invisible internal tumor movement with FEM simulation. Our vision is to generate a virtual 3D model for motion adapted radiotherapy planning based on the presented technology.

References

1. Segars WP, et al. Modeling respiratory mechanics in the MCAT and spline-based MCAT phantoms. IEEE Trans Nucl Sci 2001;48(1):89–97.
2. Wu X, et al. Adaptive nonlinear finite elements for deformable body simulation using dynamic progressive meshes. Procs Eurographics 2001;20(3):349–358.
3. Veronda DR, Westmann RA. Mechanical characterization of skin-finite deformations. J Biomech 1970;3:111–124.
4. Schöberl J. Netgen; 2007. http://www.hpfem.jku.at/netgen/.
5. Biederer J, et al. Reproducible simulation of respiratory motion in porcine lung explants. Fortschr Röntgenstr 2006;178:1067–72.

Ermittlung der Korrelation zwischen den postradiogenen Veränderungen im MRT und den Dosiswerten des Bestrahlungsplans bei der extrakraniellen stereotaktischen Radiotherapie

Thomas Lambertz[1], Regina Pohle[1], Iris Ernst[2] und Peter-Silvan Lücking[3]

[1]Fachbereich Elektrotechnik und Informatik, Hochschule Niederrhein, 47805 Krefeld
[2]Klinik für Strahlentherapie – Radioonkologie, Universität Münster, 48149 Münster
[3]Klinik für Strahlentherapie und Radiologische Onkologie,
Klinikum Krefeld, 47805 Krefeld
Email: regina.pohle@hsnr.de

Zusammenfassung. In den letzten Jahren hat sich die extrakraniel-le stereotaktische Radiotherapie (ESTR) als ein spezielles Verfahren in der Strahlentherapie etabliert. Durch die Besonderheit, dass hier in wenigen Fraktionen hohe Strahlendosen verabreicht werden, sind bei allen Patienten, die mit dieser Methode behandelt wurden, zeitlich befristete Bestrahlreaktionen im gesunden Gewebe zu beobachten. Diese treten besonders deutlich in den nach der Bestrahlung angefertigten MRT-Kontrollaufnahmen hervor. Zur Aufklärung der Ursachen dieser Veränderungen wird die Korrelation dieser Reaktionen zu den verabreichten Strahlendosen ermittelt. Um dies zu erreichen, muss eine 3D-Registrierung der Kontrollbilddaten und der Dosisverteilungen vorgenommen werden. Die Ermittlung der Korrelation erfolgt anschließend semiautomatisch durch eine Überlagerung ausgewählter Isodosenverläufe über die Kontrollaufnahmen. Der Einsatz des Programms zur Korrelationsbestimmung in der Praxis hat gezeigt, dass eine sehr viel schnellere und einfachere Aufdeckung der bestehenden Abhängigkeiten möglich wurde.

1 Einleitung

Die extrakranielle stereotaktische Radiotherapie (ESTR) ist eine Hochdosis-strahlentherapie [1]. Indikationen für die ESTR sind vor allem medizinisch inoperable Lungentumore früher Stadien, primäre Leber- und Gallengangstumore sowie Lungen- und Lebermetastasen. Die zu verabreichende Strahlendosis wird bei diesem Verfahren einmalig oder in wenigen Fraktionen in den Tumor oder in die Metastase appliziert. Da hier mit höheren Dosen als bei der herkömmlichen Strahlentherapie gearbeitet wird, ist ein höherer medizinischer und technischer Aufwand notwendig, um das Normalgewebe maximal zu schonen. Nach der Durchführung der ESTR am Klinikum Krefeld bei über 30 Patienten wurden Bestrahlreaktionen im gesunden Gewebe beobachtet. Deren Ursachen sollen in dem beschriebenen Projekt genauer untersucht werden.

Abb. 1. Ablauf der Korrelationsanalyse zur Evaluation der ESTR

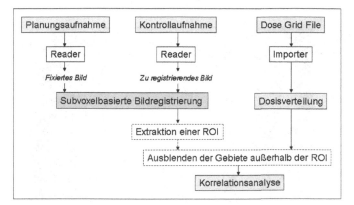

2 Stand der Forschung und Fortschritt durch den Beitrag

Die ESTR wird erst seit wenigen Jahren in der Praxis eingesetzt. Mit ihr kann bei bestimmten Tumoren bei moderaten Nebenwirkungen eine lokale Tumorkontrollrate zwischen 78-100 % erreicht werden [2]. Damit lässt sich je nach Art des Primärkarzinoms das Gesamtüberleben der behandelten Patienten statistisch signifikant verlängern. Zur weiteren Durchsetzung der Behandlungsart auch für andere Fragestellungen ist es wichtig, die Nebenwirkungen besser abschätzen zu können. Im Rahmen einer Evaluation der ESTR unter Nutzung von Verfahren der Bildverarbeitung sollen genauere Kenntnisse über die Ursachen der Bestrahlreaktionen und damit möglicher Nebenwirkungen erlangt werden. Zu Beginn des Projekts soll die Korrelation zwischen den Reaktionen und der eingebrachten Strahlendosis ermittelt werden.

3 Vorgehensweise und Materialien

Der Ablauf der vorgenommenen Korrelationsanalyse ist in Abb. 1 dargestellt. Die Auswertung stützt sich dabei auf drei unterschiedliche Datenmaterialien.

So werden zur Korrelationsbestimmung zum einen CT-Daten verwendet, die vor der Strahlenapplikation angefertigt wurden. Diese axialen Schnittbilder, auch als Planungsaufnahme bezeichnet, bilden die Grundlage für die Berechnung der Dosisverteilung im Körper (Abb. 2). Wegen der im Vergleich zur herkömmlichen Bestrahlung höheren Einzeldosen muss bei der ESTR die Strahlendosis mit einer sehr hohen Ortsgenauigkeit in den Körper appliziert werden. Die im Krefelder Klinikum praktizierte Lagerung des Patienten mit dem Bodyframe®, einer individuell an den Patienten angepassten Vakuummatratze kombiniert mit einer Abdominalkompression und einem speziellen Atemtraining zur Reduktion der Atemverschiebung garantieren das Erreichen einer Lagergenauigkeit von ⩽ 3 mm in allen Raumkoordinaten. Somit kann man davon ausgehen, dass die bei der Bestrahlung eingebrachte Dosisverteilung auch mit den Orten der geplanten Strahlendosisverteilung übereinstimmt.

Abb. 2. Planung der Dosisverteilung für die ESTR auf der Grundlage der axialen CT-Daten

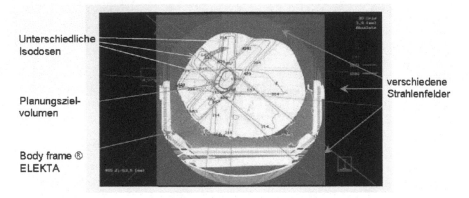

Abb. 3. MRT-Aufnahmen mit Bestrahlungsreaktionen im gesunden Gewebe [3]

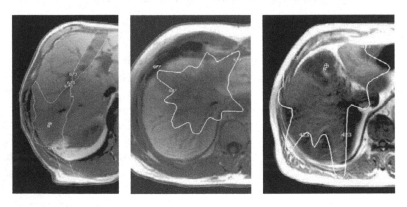

Neben den CT-Daten werden zur Korrelationsbestimmung noch die geplanten 3D-Dosisverteilungen verwendet (Abb. 2). Diese Daten werden vom Planungsprogramm für jeden Patienten in einem ASCII-Format abgelegt und lassen sich später von der im Korrelationsbestimmungsprogramm enthaltenen Routine jeweils schichtweise wieder einlesen.

Schließlich erfolgt zur Einschätzung der Wirksamkeit der ESTR die Anfertigung von CT- und MRT-Aufnahmen mit und ohne Kontrastmittelgabe zu bestimmten definierten Zeitpunkten nach der Bestrahlung. Diese Kontrollaufnahmen, die innerhalb von drei Monaten nach der Bestrahlung angefertigt wurden, enthielten die bei allen untersuchten Patienten beobachteten fokalen transienten Reaktionen (Abb. 3). Während die CT-Daten mit demselben Gerät erzeugt wurden, wodurch die Ortsauflösung bei den Planungsaufnahmen und den Kontrollaufnahmen identisch ist, ist dies bei den MRT-Aufnahmen nicht der Fall. Hinsichtlich der Positionierung treten in beiden Fällen Abweichungen zwischen den Aufnahmen vor und nach der Bestrahlung auf.

4   Methoden

Das Korrelationsbestimmungsprogramm wurde in C++ unter Benutzung der Programmbibliotheken VTK und ITK implementiert. Während die Planungs- und Kontrollaufnahmen im DICOM-Format vorliegen, und somit das Einlesen mit den Standardbibliotheksprogrammen erfolgen konnte, musste für das Einlesen des Dose Grid Files ein Importer implementiert werden. Für spätere Verarbeitungsschritte wurde ein Abspeichern der aus den Dosisdaten erzeugten Bilddaten im DICOM-Format vorgesehen.

Der wichtigste Schritt zur Gewährleistung der Vergleichbarkeit der Datensätze ist die Registrierung der Planungsaufnahmen mit den MRT- bzw. CT-Daten, die nach der Bestrahlung erhoben wurden. Im ersten Ansatz wurde hierzu eine vollautomatische Lösung für das multimodale Registrierungsproblem gesucht. Aufgrund einer geänderten Lagerung des Patienten zu den beiden Aufnahmezeitpunkten und teilweise auch aufgrund anatomischer Veränderungen im Laufe der Behandlung erwies sich eine Nonrigid Transformation als notwendig. Probleme für die Registrierung ergaben sich, da die Schichtdicken in den Planungsdatensätzen innerhalb eines Datensatzes variieren. Die Bibliotheksroutinen in ITK setzen jedoch feste Gitterabstände in den Bilddaten voraus. Um die Bibliotheksroutinen verwenden zu können, musste somit eine Interpolation zur Erzeugung von Zwischenschichten in den CT-Daten durchgeführt werden. Die gesamten aufgetretenen Probleme minderten das Ergebnis der Registrierung derart, dass trotz eines großen Rechenzeitaufwands nur noch eine sehr grobe Ausrichtung der Kontroll- an den Planungsdaten zu verzeichnen war.

Eine Verbesserung der Qualität der Planungsaufnahmen durch Verwendung gleicher Schichtdicken über den gesamten Datensatz als Lösung des Problems wurde aus klinischer Sicht verworfen, da sich damit zwar das Ergebnis der Registrierung verbessern ließe, jedoch der manuelle Aufwand im klinischen Alltag auf ein nicht vertretbares Maß ansteigen würde.

Aus diesem Grund wurde im zweiten Ansatz eine teilautomatische Lösung implementiert. Hierbei findet der Importer auf Basis der Dosiswerte automatisch das Isozentrum in den Dosisdaten. Das Isozentrum in den Kontrollaufnahmen muss vom Benutzer manuell angegeben werden. Zur Erleichterung dieser Eingabe werden neben den Kontrolldaten auch noch die Planungsdaten, in denen das Isozentrum markiert ist, angezeigt. Außerdem werden dem Benutzer von Seiten der Software Werkzeuge zur Abstandsbestimmung zur Verfügung gestellt. Nach der Festlegung des Isozentrums werden die beiden Aufnahmen gegeneinander drehbar im Isozentrum fixiert und mit variabler Transparenz überlagert dargestellt, um bei der manuellen Registrierung eine möglichst hohe Übereinstimmung zu erzielen.

Nach der Bildregistrierung kann im Ablauf der Korrelationsanalyse wahlweise eine ROI (Region of Interest) durch Setzen von Stützpunkten markiert werden, um später nur die interessierenden Bildbereiche in die Korrelationsberechnung einzubeziehen. Im jetzigen Stadium dient dieser Schritt ausschließlich der Erhöhung der Übersichtlichkeit der Darstellung.

Die eigentliche Korrelationsanalyse erfolgt bisher noch visuell. Man hat hier die Möglichkeit, einzelne Isodosiskurven als Overlay über die Kontrollaufnahmen einzublenden. Die Eingabe der Dosiswerte erfolgt dabei über einen Slider, so dass die Werte so lange variiert werden können, bis der Isodosisverlauf mit der Grenze der Gebiete der Bestrahlreaktion übereinstimmt.

5   Ergebnisse

Mit dem erstellten Programm war es möglich, für die einzelnen Daten der 30 untersuchten Patienten im Gegensatz zur bisherigen Vorgehensweise am Klinikum sehr einfach eine Korrelationsuntersuchung durchzuführen. In einem großen Teil der Daten war eindeutig visuell eine Übereinstimmung der Bestrahlreaktionen zu den Isodosisverläufen erkennbar. Die optimale Einstellung konnte jedoch zumeist nur für einige Schichten eingestellt werden, da Variationen in der Stärke der Sichtbarkeit der Bestrahlreaktion über die Schichten des Datensatzes auftraten. Somit zeigte sich, dass die visuelle Abschätzung nur ein erster Schritt bei der Korrelationsuntersuchung sein kann.

6   Diskussion

Da die bisherigen Ergebnisse aufgrund der visuellen Abschätzung der Korrelation eine sehr starke subjektive Komponente besitzen, ist im Weiteren zur Verbesserung der Auswertung und zur Objektivierung der Aussagen eine statistische Analyse geplant. Um diese Berechnungen jedoch durchführen zu können, müssen die Areale der Bestrahlreaktion in den Bilddaten zuvor segmentiert werden. Da diese Bereiche sich zumeist nur sehr wenig von den benachbarten Regionen abzeichnen, ist hierfür der Einsatz eines semiautomatischen Segmentierungsverfahrens, wie z.B. des Life-Wire-Verfahrens auf ausgewählten Schichten mit anschließender Interpolation vorgesehen.

Literaturverzeichnis

1. Münter MW, Debus J. Aktuelle technische Entwicklungen in der Strahlentherapie. Onkologe 2003;9(10):1130–1143.
2. Ernst I, Lücking PS, Eickmeyer F. Extrakranielle stereotaktische Radiotherapie (ESRT): Eine Übersicht unter besonderer Berücksichtigung von ESRT und LITT in der Behandlung von Lebermetastasen. Zentralblatt für Gynäkologie 2006;128:71–75.
3. Ernst I, Eickmeyer F, Lücking PS. Extracranielle stereotaktische Strahlentherapie der Leber: postradiogene Veränderungen im Leber-MRT. In: Procs 12. Jahreskongress Dt Ges f Radioonkologie; 2006. 1.

Evaluation of Electromagnetic Error Correction Methods

Correcting Distortion Fields for Appliance in the Radiation Therapy Room

Joerg Traub[1], Sukhbansbir Kaur[1], Peter Kneschaurek[2], Nassir Navab[1]

[1]Chair for Computer Aided Medical Procedures (CAMP), TU Munich, Germany
[2]Radiation Therapy Department, Klinikum rechts der Isar, TU Munich, Germany
Email: traub@cs.tum.edu

Abstract. Electromagnetic tracking is currently the only available technology to track flexible instruments inside the human body without the use of real time imaging technology such as ultrasound or mobile c-arms. The limitation of electromagnetic tracking is its accuracy and sensibility to the environment, especially in the presences of ferromagnetic material and electronic devices. Navigation systems based on these technologies were recently introduced especially flexible endoscopy. One design goal for setting up such navigation systems is the removal of all material from the close environment that can perturb the magnetic field. In our scenario, within the radiation therapy room, we can not eliminate the gantry. Thus, existing methods for electromagnetic tracking error estimation and correction algorithms were reviewed, implemented, and adopted to the special requirement for navigation during prostate cancer treatment.

1 Introduction

Electromagnetic tracking systems are the only method to estimate the pose of flexible instruments inside the patient's body without the use of imaging data. Navigation systems based on this tracking technologies were introduced for endoscopic procedures [1] and bronchoscopic interventions [2, 3]. One core requirement for image-guided medical procedures is high precision in the measured pose of objects, instruments and imaging devices. The pose estimation of objects with electromagnetic tracking system is highly dependent on the environment. Their sensitivity to the ferromagnetic metals and electronic materials that are in a close neighborhood of the field generator and/or sensors result in distortion of the reported pose. This is often referred to as tracking error. The tracking error could be reduced either by taking preventive measures or by corrective measures. Using preventive measures all materials that can perturb the electromagnetic field are eliminated from the close environment and replaced by equipment that does not affect the magnetic field. However, in several cases this is not practical e.g. in the radiation therapy room where it is not possible to remove the gantry. In case those objects can not be eliminated from the environment the only solution is to evaluate the corrective measures in order to correct the tracking errors reported by the electromagnetic tracking system. This has to be done within two steps. Firstly, estimating the distortion field by sampling measurements with a more precise pose estimation system or with well known ground truth data grid. Secondly, applying the estimated error function in real time to the erroneous measurements. Several methods were introduced in the past for corrective measures for electromagnetic tracking systems [4, 5, 6]. Kindratenko [7] provides an overview and extensive summery of existing methods.

2   Methods

The corrective measures are based upon the estimation of electromagnetic field distortions followed by the compensation of tracking errors [7]. The distortion field is estimated by a set of correspondences of exact (true sensor pose) and distorted (measured or reported sensor pose) values. These correspondences are stored in a lookup table. In this work a sampling lattice (indirect method) is used for the collection of the lookup table similar to the methods introduced by Bryson [8] and Zachmann [5]. In a second step the measured tracking pose is corrected in real time by the means of interpolation using this previously created displacement field (lookup table). Two different interpolation schemes have been implemented and evaluated. The first method is a local approach based on trilinear interpolation [8]. The second method is based on a global interpolation schemes [9]. The effects of certain parameters on the correction accuracy by the global interpolation scheme have been assessed and are discussed in the results.

The electromagnetic tracking system was physically mounted within the radiation therapy room in a close distance to the gantry. It was placed such, that the tracking volume covered the entire abdominal area of the patient.

3   Results

The lookup table collection procedure using sampling lattice is accurate and simple both in terms of apparatus and computation, but time consuming for building larger 3D lookup tables (7-12 minutes for 121 points within 10cm^2). Out of the two position error correction methods for magnetic tracking system, the correction method based on the global scattered data interpolation has proved to be better in terms of accuracy (97%)(see figure 1), smoothness of interpolant function and flexibility of arrangement of lookup table data. The method was tested in the radiation therapy environment with the gantry as a not removable source of distortion. The mean error after the application of local and global method is improved by 89.9% and 97.2% respectively (see figure 2). The correction performed with the global method is independent of the separation distance of the sensor from the transmitter and the local distortion of the magnetic field. For the local method, it varies from 4mm-21mm at different positions and for global

Fig. 1. Error metrics before and after correction. On x-axis, the method applied is specified. None corresponds to the uncorrected values. On y-axis, error metrics mean error, maximum error, minimum error and standard deviation are plotted in millimeters. Standard deviation is plotted as a bar that shows the limits for deviation from a measured value

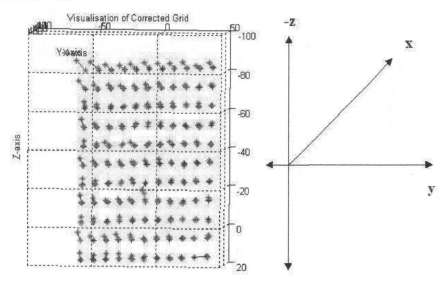

method it is within 4mm at all positions. However, the correction provided by the global correction method depends on certain parameters. The optimal parameter selection and preconditioning of the distortion function (in some cases) is required and has a crucial influence on the error correction.

4   Conclusion and Discussion

Global correction method was proved to be better in terms of accuracy, flexibility in the collection of data for distortion estimation, and ease of operation. The current work has shown that electromagnetic tracking errors could be corrected adequately. With the implemented methods we show an improvement of 97% in the radiation therapy environment with magnetic field generator mounted close to the gantry. Medical applications especially where flexible instruments are tracked with electromagnetic tracking systems can benefit from this error correction. Special evaluation need to be performed before applying the correction methods in each distingt environments to provide the best and most accurate available tracking results for each scenario and adjust the parameters of the correction. Further studies within the correction of electromagnetic field distortion will be conducted in the direction of a more feasible ground truth collection using a second, more accurate, tracking system (e.g. optical tracking). We discussed only the possibility of corrective measures by means of a not

Fig. 2. Vector field view of the correction. Ground truth values (blue asterisk), corrected values with trilinear interpolation method (red asterisks) and corrected values with HMQ method (magenta asterisks) are plotted in the yz plane of the tracking system coordinate system as shown in the plot of axes

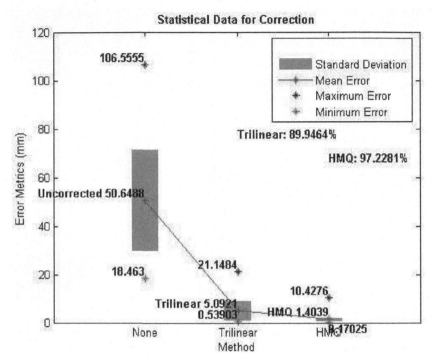

alternating distortion field dynamically. An extension will be to integrate additionally a system to detect changes in the environment in real time to ensure the safety and robustness of navigation system based on electromagnetic tracking. A complete integration of all there error detection and correction approaches will be the fundamental technology to enable accurate, safe, and reliable navigation, especially during procedures with flexible instruments.

References

1. Guiraudon G, Moore J, Jones D, et al. Augmented reality for closed intracardiac interventions. In: International Workshop for Augmented Environments for Medical Imaging and Computer-aided Surgery (AMI-ARCS); 2006.
2. Hautmann H, Schneider A, Pinkau T, Peltz F, Feussner H. Electromagnetic catheter navigation during bronchoscopy: Validation of a novel method by conventional fluoroscopy. Chest 2005;128:382–387.
3. Solomon SB, Jr PWhite, Wiener CM, et al. Three-dimensional CT-guided bronchoscopy with a real-time electromagnetic position sensor: A comparison of two image registration methods. Chest 2000;118:1783–1787.

4. Livingston MA, State A. Magnetic tracker calibration for improved augmented reality registration. Presence: Teleoperators and Virtual Environments 1997;6(5):532–546.
5. Zachmann G. Distortion correction of magnetic fields for position tracking. In: Procs Computer Graphics International; 1997.
6. Ikits M, Brederson JD, Hansen C, Hollerbach J. An improved calibration framework for electromagnetic tracking devices. IEEE Virtual Reality 2001.
7. Kindratenko VV. A survey of electromagnetic position tracker calibration techniques. Virtual Reality: Research, Development, and Applications 2000;5(3):169–182.
8. Bryson ST. Measurement and calibration of static distortion of position data from 3D trackers. Procs SPIE 1992;1669:244–255.
9. Hardy RL. Multiquadric equations of topography and other irregular surfaces. J Geophys Res 1971;76:1905–1915.

Pose Estimation of Eyes for Particle Beam Treatment of Tumors

B.P. Selby[1], G. Sakas[1], S. Walter[1], W.-D. Groch[2], U. Stilla[3]

[1]Cognitive Computing and Medical Imaging, Fraunhofer IGD, Darmstadt, Germany
[2]Fachbereich Informatik, University of Applied Sciences, Darmstadt, Germany
[3]Photogrammetry and Remote Sensing, Technische Universität Muenchen, Germany
Email: pselby@medcom-online.de

Abstract. To assure a correct position and orientation of the patient's eye in radiation treatment, a new approach in image-guided radiotherapy is used to determine the misalignment of the eye and the respective correction for the patient support devices. New methods allow correcting the misalignment of the patient's eye full-automatically. Therefore, metallic clips attached to the patient's eyeball are detected in a CT and in two digital X-ray images. Corresponding pairs of clip positions found in the X-ray images are then transferred into the 3D space of the CT volume via inverse projection and compared to the clips found in the CT slices. If several combinations of correspondences are possible, we use a temporary pre-registration to assure that the correct back-projections will be obtained. A rigid, point-set based 6 degrees of freedom registration of the back-projected clip positions with the CT clips allows determining the misalignment of the eye tumor which consists of three shifts and three rotations. These transformations are transformed into parameters for a treatment chair and an eye fixation designated to control placement and orientation of the eye during treatment.

1 Introduction

Modern particle beam based treatment techniques allow an accurate application of the treatment dose onto carcinogen tissue. A tumor can be treated by a proton beam line by line with a geometric accuracy much better than 1.0 mm. This is advantageous for radio-oncological treatment of organs where sensible tissue near the treatment target has to be saved from being irradiated, as for example the optic nerve in the treatment of eye tumors.

This accuracy is limited by treatment position set-up errors originating from aberrations of the location of the planned radiation target relative to the particle beam. Strategies like tracking of external markers or fixation of the patient's body do not suffice the requirement of high set-up precision and are not applicable in the case of eye tumor treatment. Besides that, the eye orientation may change according to patient movements, during a time consuming manual set-up procedure.

To overcome these problems, a new approach exploits the high-resolution slices of a planning CT for eye treatment and two X-ray images acquired from within the treatment device. About 5 clips of tantalum or titanium, attached to the treated eye are detected in the CT and the X-ray images acquired shortly before the treatment takes place or during the treatment session, to verify the correctness of the eye alignment.

Based on an automatic registration of the clip positions, an alignment correction for the eye is calculated in 6 degrees of freedom, 3 shifts and 3 rotations, with a very high precision and reliability.

2   State of the Art New Contribution

The correctness of the position of a patient's eye undergoing particle beam treatment relies on the fixation equipment and the X-ray images that are compared to a CT image series in order to detect remaining misalignments. While the fixation equipment assures an initial set-up preciseness of about 0.5mm [1], a fine-tuning is done by manual step-by-step correction, reducing the remaining misalignment between CT and X-ray images [2]. This procedure can be time consuming and therefore limits the throughput of patients in a commercial health center and it leads to a high number of X-ray acquisitions and the respective application of X-ray doses on the patient. Set-up errors from the manual correction cannot be eliminated, as the correctness of the alignment depends on the operator's judgment.

Automatic position correction procedures [3, 4] based on mutual information registration are not applicable in the scope of eye treatment, as they strongly rely on bony structures instead on the relatively homogenous tissue of the eyeball.

The automatic detection and registration of eye clips proposed herewith allows a very fast and accurate position and orientation correction for the eye in 6 degrees of freedom.

3   Methods

The automatic procedure consists of the following working steps: Segmentation of clips in a CT volume; Segmentation of clips in two X-ray images; Back projection of the clip positions from the X-rays; Registration of the resulting point-sets; Translation of the registration result into appropriate set-up correction parameters.

3.1   Clip Segmentation in CT Series

To enable a very fast detection, clips are segmented in the CT data using different levels of the volume resolution. The CT is resampled to a 4D pyramid containing several instances of the volume, each with a different resolution. The search for a clip starts at a low-resolution level. As soon as a potential clip voxel is found, the search continues at a higher resolution. To determine if a voxel belongs to a clip, two Hounsfield thresholds are used. A voxel between those thresholds is

Fig. 1. Results of segmentations with different thresholds (left); Patient chair (right)

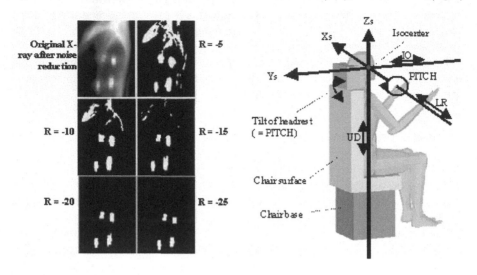

considered to belong to a clip. As soon as one clip is found the thresholds are adapted, assuming, that upcoming clips are of the same material and will be represented by similar Hounsfield values. If no clip is found, the thresholds are modified and the search continues.

3.2   Clip Segmentation in X-ray Images

For detecting the clips in the X-ray images, two different approaches are combined. Using a Harris Corner Detector [5] potential clip corners are identified. Then several segmentations are performed. In each segmentation a different gray value threshold is used to identify potential clip pixels. In addition the distance of a potential clip pixel to its next non-clip border is evaluated. Again different thresholds R are used for the accepted distance of a potential clip pixel to its border pixel (Fig. 1, left).

The information about area and periphery of all segmentations for one clip is combined and the results most likely representing a clip are maintained.

3.3   Back Projection

To compare the clips detected in the X-ray images with the clips from the CT, an inverse projection is performed for corresponding pairs of both X-rays.

Because it is not always clear, which clips correspond to each other, it is possible that one clip becomes a member in several back projection results. This is the case, if several clips are projected onto a horizontal line in the plane of one flat panel. Performing a separate registration for each possible result set of the inverse projection solves this problem. Only the registration that tends to result in an acceptable patient set-up is used for the final set-up correction.

3.4   Registration

Two sets of points in the 3D space of the CT are used to calculate 3 shifts and 3 rotations, which map one point-set onto the other as good as possible. The remaining mapping error serves as an indicator for the quality of the patient set-up calculation. We use a Downhill Simplex optimization [6] to minimize an error for the misalignment between back projected point-set A and the original CT clip positions B. The error metric bases on the undirected Hausdorff Distance [7]

$$H(A, B) = H(B, A) = \max(h(A, B), h(B, A)) \tag{1}$$

with $h(A, B) = \max_{a \in A} \min_{b \in B}(\|a - b\|)$ and $h(B, A) = \max_{b \in B} \min_{a \in A}(\|b - a\|)$

To avoid local minima we use the square sum of the undirected Hausdorff Distance of rank 0 to k, where k denotes the minimum of the number of clips detected in the X-ray images and the CT slices.

3.5   Calculation of the Correction

The patient support consists of the patient chair, an adjustable headrest and a fixation light. The patient is advised to focus the fixation light, so it can be used to modify the orientation of the eyeball.

The results from the registration are now used to compute a correction for the set-up parameters of these devices (Fig. 1, right). The possible degrees of freedom are:

- Chair rotation around vertical axis and translation along X-, Y- and Z-axis
- Tilt of the headrest
- Fixation light height and tilt angle to the left or the right

As chair parameter adjustment can be redundant to the eye alignment, it is possible to set preferences for the set-up parameters. A simulated annealing algorithm [6] is used to adjust the chair parameters step by step to model the eye transformation.

A remaining eye torsion, which is a rotation of the eye around the vector in viewing direction, cannot be corrected by patient support adjustment. Together with the remaining error of the registration point-set mapping, a large eye torsion value is used to indicate a bad patient alignment.

4   Results

Tests have been performed, using CT datasets (0.2mm slice distance) and X-rays of a pig's eye attached with 4 and 5 tantalum clips (Fig. 2). In all cases it was possible to detect all clips and to perform a correct mapping of the back projected clip positions (Tab. 1).

Table 1. Correction results for different set-up errors

Number of clips	Total (intended) set-up error (Rotation /Shift)	Remaining error after Correction (Rotation/Shift)	Indicated quality (0 to 100%)	Calculation-time in seconds
4	2° / 2mm	0.05° / 0.20mm	87%	1
4	5° / 10mm	0.09° / 0.25mm	90%	1
4	10° / 20mm	0.20° / 0.20mm	88%	2
5	2° / 2mm	0.05° / 0.21mm	95%	2
5	5° / 10mm	0.05° / 0.13mm	91%	3
5	10° / 20mm	0.18° / 0.18mm	87%	3

5 Discussion

It becomes apparent, that the automatic correction is superior to conventional manual correction techniques and allows accomplishing a correction with only one single set of X-ray images, which reduces the X-ray radiation applied to the patient. The proposed methods are suitable for accurate and reliable position

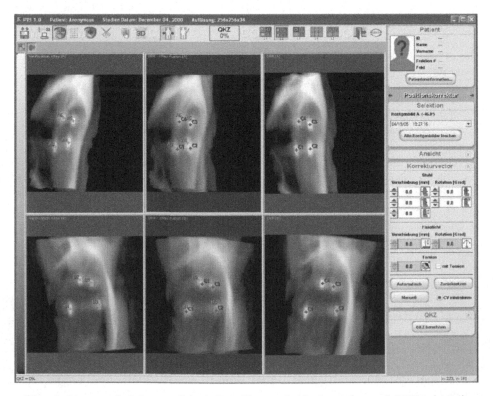

Fig. 2. Images of pig's eye with 4 clips: X-rays (left), fused (center) DRRs (right)

correction within seconds. The results show, that an increasing number of clips leads to a slightly more accurate correction, but increases the calculation time. Evaluations in real treatment situations still have to be done. Remaining errors result from the slice distance of 0.2mm. For higher accuracy, usage of CTs with a higher resolution is suggested.

The methods have been tested with 2.5mm tantalum clips, which could be detected relatively easy. Further efforts have to be done to assure a correct detection for the wide variety of applicable metal clips. Under adverse circumstances, as when clips are occluded by other clips or by bony structures of the skull, not all clips can be detected, which results, depending on the total number of clips used, in results less accurate.

References

1. Verhey LJ, Goitein M, McNulty P, Munzenrider JE, Suit HD. Precise positioning of patients for radiation therapy. Int J Radiation Oncology Biol Phys 1982;8(2):289–294.
2. Heufelder J, Cordini D, Fuchs H, et al. Fuenf Jahre Protonentherapie von Augentumoren am Hahn-Meitner-Institut Berlin. Z Med Phys 2004;14(1):64–71.
3. Thilmann C, Nill S, Tücking T, et al. Correction of patient positioning errors based on in-line cone beam CTs: Clinical implementation and first experiences. Int J Radiation Oncology Biol Phys 2005;63(1):550–551.
4. Pluim J, Maintz J, Viergever M. Mutual information based registration of medical images: A survey. IEEE Trans Med Imaging 2003;22(8):986–1004.
5. Harris C, Stephens M. A combined corner and edge detector. In: Procs Alvey Vision Conference; 1988. 147–152.
6. Press WH, Teukolsky SA, Vetterling WT, Flannery BP. Numerical Recipes in C. vol. 2. Cambridge University Press; 1992.
7. Huttenlocher DP, Klanderman GA, Rucklidge WJ. Comparing images using the Hausdorff distance. IEEE Trans PAMI 1993;15(9):850–863.

Bewegungsenergien zur Quantifizierung der Körpereigenbewegungen sedierter Patienten während der Intensivtherapie

Sven Friedl[1,2], Helmut Schwilden[1], Günther Braun[1] and Thomas Wittenberg[2]

[1] Klinik für Anästhesiologie, Friedrich-Alexander-Universität Erlangen-Nürnberg
[2] Fraunhofer Institut für Integrierte Schaltungen IIS, Erlangen
Email: sven.friedl@kfa.imed.uni-erlangen.de

Zusammenfassung. Der Einfluss der Eigenbewegungen eines Patienten auf den Verlauf der Intensivtherapie ist weitgehend unbekannt. Neben weiteren Faktoren wird dennoch auch die Unruhe eines Patienten genutzt um dessen Sedierungszustand zu schätzen. Um objektive Kriterien zur Bewertung der Unruhe und Bewegung des Patienten zu erhalten sowie den Einfluss auf den Therapieverlauf quantifizieren zu können, muss das Bewegungsaufkommen analysiert und ausgewertet werden. Im klinischen Alltag stellt sich dies als nicht-triviales Problem heraus. In dieser Arbeit wird ein Verfahren zur bildbasierten Bewegungsanalyse für den Einsatz in der Intensivtherapie adaptiert. Zudem werden Probleme identifiziert, die sich im klinischen Alltag ergeben. Es werden Möglichkeiten aufgezeigt, wie die interessierenden Bewegungsmuster herausgestellt und in einen medizinischen Zusammenhang gebracht werden können.

1 Einleitung

Patienten auf der Intensivstation befinden sich zumeist in einem gesundheitlich sehr ernsten Zustand. Zudem begleiten starke Schmerzen, Ängste und eine enorme Unruhe begleiten zudem ihren Aufenthalt. Die Sedierung und Analgosedierung der Patienten ist daher ein wesentlicher Bestandteil der Intensivtherapie. Im Gegensatz zu einer durchgehend starken Sedierung kann eine genaue Einstellung und gezielte Variation der Sedierungstiefe den Therapieverlauf erheblich verbessern [1, 2]. Die dadurch ermöglichte Eigenbewegung des Patienten ist dabei ein interessanter Faktor der Intensivtherapie. Der Einfluss der Bewegung auf den Therapieverlauf ist jedoch weitgehend unbekannt. Dennoch wird, neben anderen Faktoren wie Herzfrequenzvariabilität, EEG und weiteren Biosignalen, auch die Unruhe sowie die resultierende Eigenbewegung des Patienten in der klinischen Praxis für eine Schätzung der Sedierungstiefe genutzt [3].

Um jedoch objektive Kriterien zur Bewertung der Unruhe und Bewegung eines Patienten und demnach auch für die Skalierung der Sedierungstiefe zu erhalten sowie den Einfluss von Bewegung auf den Therapieverlauf quantifizieren zu können, muss das Bewegungsaufkommen möglichst automatisiert aufgezeichnet und ausgewertet werden.

Abb. 1. Bewegungsenergien $e_\tau(t)$ im Zeitraum 6 bis 18 Uhr für den gesamten Bildausschnitt und verschiedene spezifizierte Regionen

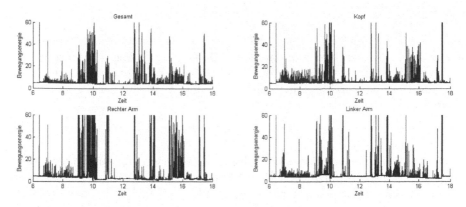

2 Stand der Forschung und Fortschritt durch den Beitrag

Um Bewegungen von Menschen messen und analysieren zu können, existieren verschiedene Möglichkeiten. Da jedoch in der klinischen Routine eine Beeinträchtigung des Patienten weitgehend vermieden werden soll, wurden anstelle von elektromechanischen Verfahren optische Sensoren eingesetzt um die Bewegungen berührungslos zu messen. Mittels einer Kamera kann die Bewegung der Patienten erfasst und aufgezeichnet werden.

In [4] wurden Verfahren der Bewegungsanalyse für den Einsatz bei sedierten Patienten vorgestellt und evaluiert, die auch ohne den Einsatz künstlicher Marker am Patienten auskommen und somit eine Beeinflussung vollständig vermeiden. Erfahrungen im klinischen Alltag fehlten jedoch bisher weitgehend.

In dieser Arbeit wird ein adaptiertes Verfahren zur Bewegungsanalyse für den Einsatz in der Intensivtherapie eingeführt, welches die Eigenbewegungen eines Patienten messen und quantifizieren kann. Anhand der im klinischen Alltag erfassten Daten werden damit zusammenhängende Probleme identifiziert und Möglichkeiten aufgezeigt wie die interessierenden Bewegungsmuster herausgestellt und in einen medizinischen Zusammenhang gebracht werden können.

3 Methoden

Bewegung in Bildsequenzen stellt sich als Intensitätswertänderung in aufeinander folgenden Bildern dar. Um das Bewegungsaufkommen an einem Bildpunkt zu erfassen, kommt in dieser Arbeit ein modifiziertes Differenzbildverfahren [5] zum Einsatz.

Für eine definierte Zeitspanne τ werden für aufeinander folgende Bilder $I[t]$ der Dimension $x \times y$ einer Sequenz Differenzbilder

$$\Delta I[t] = |I[t] - I[t-1]| \tag{1}$$

berechnet und mit

$$E_\tau[t] = \sum_{i=t-\tau}^{t} \Delta I[t-i] \qquad (2)$$

ein Bewegungsenergiebild $E_\tau[t]$ erzeugt, welches das Bewegungsaufkommen pro Bildpunkt über die Zeitspanne darstellt. Mit Hilfe eines Schwellwertes werden geringe Differenzen unterdrückt, die durch Bildrauschen entstehen. Durch Integration des Energiebildes wird nun die gesamte Bewegungsenergie zum Zeitpunkt t

$$e_\tau[t] = \sum_{x,y} E_\tau[t] \qquad (3)$$

ermittelt. Diese gibt Aufschluss über das gesamte Bewegungsaufkommen innerhalb der gewählten Zeitspanne τ. Durch eine isolierte Betrachtung verschiedener Bildregionen wie beispielsweise Kopf, linker oder rechter Arm können die Bewegungsmuster, wie in Abb. 1 weiter differenziert werden. Anhand dieser Kurven können Veränderungen der Aktivität im Tagesverlauf visualisiert und ausgewertet werden.

4   Ergebnisse

Im Rahmen des Projektes werden Patienten über einen Zeitraum von zwei bis fünf Tagen jeweils von 6 bis 18 Uhr beobachtet und mit einer Bildfrequenz von 3,75 Bildern pro Sekunde kontinuierlich aufgenommen. Zur Berechnung der Bewegungsenergien wurde eine Zeitspanne von 4 Bildern entsprechend etwa 1 Sekunde gewählt. Somit lässt sich das Bewegungsaufkommen sehr genau analysieren. Zur Datenreduktion können aufeinander folgende Energiewerte zusammengefasst werden. Für diese Arbeit wurden die Daten von fünf verschiedenen Patienten ausgewertet.

In der Praxis ergeben sich für die Bewegungsanalyse diverse Schwierigkeiten. Insbesondere in der Intensivtherapie ist der Patient immer wieder therapeutischen und pflegerischen Maßnahmen ausgesetzt. Dabei kommt es häufig zur Verdeckung des Patienten durch Personal oder technischen Hilfsmitteln wie zum Beispiel einem Tubus zur künstlichen Beatmung. Wird der Patient bei den Pflegemaßnahmen vom Personal bewegt kommt es zu sogenannten Passivbewegungen, die die Auswertung der Eigenbewegungen verfälschen. Das pflegende und behandelnde Personal verursacht zudem massive Fremdbewegungen in den Bildsequenzen.

Für die Auswertung der Eigenbewegungen ist es erforderlich die interessierenden Bewegungen innerhalb einer Sequenz zu annotieren. Eine manuelle Annotation zur Zeit der Aufnahme ist aus Gründen des klinischen Workflows nicht möglich und eine nachgelagerte manuelle Auswertung sehr aufwändig. Eigenbewegungen unterscheiden sich jedoch von Fremd- und Passivbewegungen insbesondere anhand ihrer Intensität, wie in Abb. 3(a) zu erkennnen ist. Die Analyse des Histogramms der Bewegungsenergien in Abb. 3(b) oben zeigt, dass

Abb. 2. Bewegungsenergien mit Passiv- und Fremdbewegungen (a) und Histogramm der originalen Bewegungsenergien und die isolierten Eigenbwegungen (b)

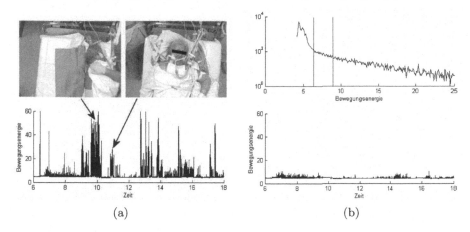

(a)   (b)

die interessierenden Bewegungsintensitäten innerhalb eines eingegrenzten Intervalls liegen. Somit können die Eigenbewegungen semiautomatisch annotiert und wie in Abb. 3(b) unten isoliert dargestellt werden. Unterstützend kann durch die isolierte Betrachtung des Bereiches außerhalb des Bettes anhand von dort auftretender Bewegung auf Pflegemaßnahmen geschlossen werden.

Eine alternative Darstellung der auftretenden Bewegungen ergibt sich aus dem kumulativen Integral der Bewegungsenergien wie in Abb. 3. Mit Hilfe dessen lassen sich die Veränderungen der täglichen Aktivität eines Patienten über einen Zeitraum mehrerer Tage vergleichen. Somit kann die Korrelation der Eigenbewegungen mit dem therapeutischen Verlauf der Intensivtherapie analysiert werden. Es ist erkennbar wie die gesamte Eigenbewegung von Tag 1 zu Tag 2 abnimmt jedoch am Nachmittag von Tag 2 verstärkt zunimmt. Dies steigert sich zu einer maximalen Unruhe an Tag 3 und endet mit einer wieder geringeren Aktivität an Tag 4. Die dokumentierte Veränderung der geschätzten Sedierungstiefe stimmt an den Tagen mit den Variationen des Bewegungsaufkommens überein. Eine Korrelation zur Medikation ist aber aufgrund der langen Nachwirkungen eher schwierig zu gewinnen.

5   Diskussion

Mit Hilfe eines adaptierten Verfahrens zur Bestimmung von Bewegungsenergien konnte die Eigenbewegung von Patienten während der Intensivtherapie bestimmt und analysiert werden. Ein Vergleich der Aktivität des Patienten an verschiedenen Tagen lässt sich in Einklang mit der pflegerischen Dokumentation bringen und stellt somit eine Möglichkeit dar, einen Zusammenhang mit der Sedierung des Patienten und dem Einfluss auf den Therapieverlauf herzustellen.

378 S. Friedl et al.

Abb. 3. Vergleich der kumulativen Bewegungsenergien eines Patienten an vier aufeinander folgende Tagen

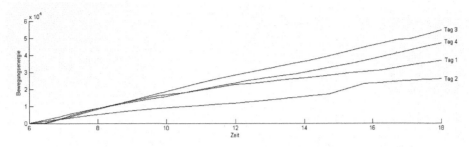

In dieser Arbeit wurden insbesondere Schwierigkeiten identifiziert, wie sie sich im klinischen Alltag ergeben. Insbesondere die intensiven therapeutischen und pflegerischen Maßnahmen stellen in der Intensivmedizin ein Problem für die Bewegungsanalyse dar. Die gewonnenen Daten lassen sich aber nutzen um Bewegung im Zusammenhang mit der Intensivtherapie weiter klinisch zu erforschen.

Neben der hier vorgestellten Möglichkeit Bewegungsenergien aus Differenzbildern zu gewinnen und somit Aussagen über das Bewegungsaufkommen zu treffen, würden sich auch Trackingverfahren zur Verfolgung von Kopfbewegungen [6] anbieten. In weiteren Untersuchungen sollen auch diese intensiver ausgewertet werden.

Literaturverzeichnis

1. Brook AD, Ahrens TS, et al. Effect of a nursing-implemented sedation protocol on the duration of mechanical ventilation. Crit Care Med 1999;27(12):2609–2615.
2. Kress JP, Pohlmann AS, et al. Daily interruption of sedative infusions in critically ill patients undergoing mechanical ventilation. N Engl J Med 2000;342(20):1471–1477.
3. Chernik DA, Gillings D, et al. Validity and reliability of the observer's assessment of alertness/sedation scale: Study with intravenous midazolam. J Clin Psychopharmacol 1990;10(4):244–251.
4. Wittenberg T, Fröba B, et al. Evaluierung von Ansätzen der Bewegungsdetektion und -verfolgung sedierter Patienten. In: Proc. BVM; 2004. 244–248.
5. Bobick AF, Davis JW. The recognition of human movement using temporal templates. IEEE PAMI 2001;23(3):257–267.
6. Fröba B, Küblbeck C. Face detection and tracking using edge orientation information. Procs SPIE 2001; 583–594.

Atembewegungssimulator für die in-vitro Evaluation von Weichgewebe-Navigationssystemen in der Leber

Lena Maier-Hein[1], Frank Pianka[2], Sascha A. Müller[2], Alexander Seitel[1], Urte Rietdorf[1], Ivo Wolf[1], Bruno M. Schmied[2], Hans-Peter Meinzer[1]

[1]DKFZ, Abteilung für Medizinische und Biologische Informatik
[2]Uni Heidelberg, Abteilung für Allgemein-, Visceral- und Unfallchirurgie
Email: l.maier-hein@dkfz.de

Zusammenfassung. In diesem Beitrag stellen wir einen neuartigen Atembewegungssimulator vor, welcher Experimente in bewegten Schweine- und Menschenlebern ermöglicht. Der Simulator ist mit relativ geringem Aufwand nachbaubar und eignet sich insbesondere zur in-vitro Evaluation von Weichgewebe-Navigationssystemen. Er besteht im Wesentlichen aus einem vereinfachten Modell des Korpus, welches die Befestigung einer Menschen- oder Schweineleber an ein künstliches Zwerchfell (Plexiglasscheibe) vorsieht. Das Anschließen einer Beatmungsmaschine an das Modell bewirkt eine periodische Bewegung der Leber. Durch Platzierung optisch trackbarer Nadeln in drei verschiedenen Schweinelebern zeigen wir, dass die durch den Simulator erzeugte Bewegung dieser Lebern im Korpusmodell mit der Bewegung einer Menschenleber im Körper qualitativ übereinstimmt: (1) Die Leber wird entlang aller drei Achsen bewegt, jedoch hauptsächlich axial und (2) die Leber wird nicht nur rigide verschoben, sondern echt deformiert.

1 Einleitung

Minimal-invasive Eingriffe im Abdominalraum sind inzwischen fester Bestandteil der klinischen Routine. Da das Erreichen der Zielstruktur durch erschwerte Orientierung in der Regel einen hohen Zeitaufwand erfordert, arbeiten zurzeit zahlreiche Forschergruppen an Systemen, welche minimal-invasive Eingriffe in Weichgewebe computergestützt erleichtern und beschleunigen sollen (z.B. [1, 2]). Um diese Systeme in realistischer Umgebung zu evaluieren, wird ein Modell der Zielregion benötigt, welches die Bewegung durch die Atmung berücksichtigt. Damit teure und ethisch umstrittene Tierversuche in diesem Zusammenhang vermieden werden können, stellen wir einen Atembewegungssimulator vor, der in-vitro Experimente in bewegten Menschen- und Schweinelebern ermöglicht.

2 Stand der Forschung und Fortschritt durch den Beitrag

Die Literatur zur Evaluation von Navigationssystemen für Weichgewebe ist spärlich. Die bislang zu diesem Zweck entwickelten Phantome eignen sich vornehmlich zur Simulation von Eingriffen an starren Strukturen, da sie die Bewegung der

Zielstruktur durch die Atmung unberücksichtigt lassen. Lediglich Banovac *et al.* entwickelten einen Atembewegungssimulator, der eine Evaluation am *bewegten* Modell erlaubt [1]. Die Zielstruktur wird hier durch eine Silikonleber modelliert.

Mit diesem Beitrag stellen wir den unserer Kenntnis nach ersten Atembewegungssimulator vor, der *in-vitro* Experimente in einer realitätstreu bewegten Leber erlaubt.

3   Material und Methoden

3.1   Aufbau und Funktionsweise des Atembewegungssimulators

Der Atembewegungssimulator ist am Aufbau des menschlichen Körpers orientiert. Er wurde so konstruiert, dass er sich mit relativ geringem Aufwand nachbauen lässt und besteht aus den folgenden Hauptkomponenten (Abb. 1):

- Einer Plexiglasplatte, welche das Zwerchfell modelliert
- Zwei künstlichen Lungen als Lungenflügel
- einer Haut aus Neopren
- einem Schaumstoffblock als Füllmaterial für den Abdominalraum
- einer Kunststoffkiste als Korpusmodell, welche die einzelnen Komponenten enthält

Die Benutzung des Atembewegungssimulators erfordert die Befestigung einer (Schweine- oder Menschen-) Leber an der Plexiglasplatte. Dazu werden Reste des am Organ verbliebenen Zwerchfells mit Hilfe von Löchern im Zwerchfellmodell an dieses angenäht. Zudem kann mittels Klettverschluss optional eine Haut über der Leber befestigt werden wie Abbildung 3a illustriert.

Zur Simulation der Atembewegung wird eine Beatmungsmaschine an die künstlichen Lungen geschlossen. Werden diese mit Luft gefüllt, so wird die Plexiglasplatte und somit die Leber um einige Zentimeter in kranio-kaudale Richtung

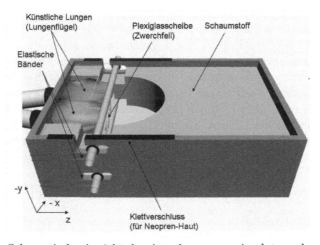

Abb. 1. Schematische Ansicht des Atembewegungssimulators ohne Haut

Abb. 2. Atembewegungssimulator ohne Haut in End-Exspiration (a) und End-Inspiration (b) mit optisch trackbaren Nadeln

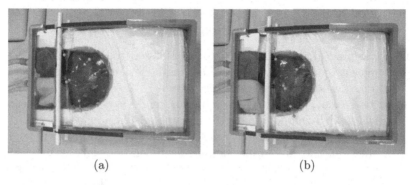

(a)   (b)

Abb. 3. Befestigung der Neopren-Haut am Simulator (a) und Referenztool (grau) zur Bestimmung der Bewegung einer Leber entlang der Achsen des Simulator-Koordinatensystems (b)

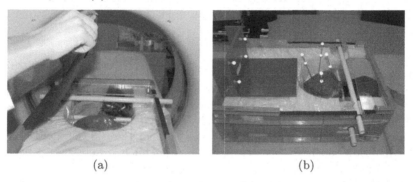

(a)   (b)

verschoben (Abb. 2b). Sobald die Luft wieder aus den künstlichen Lungen entweicht, wird die Platte durch elastische Bänder zurück in die ursprüngliche Lage gezogen (Abb. 2a).

3.2 Bewegungsanalyse des Simulators

Zur Messung der durch den Simulator erzeugten Bewegung einer Leber werden vier optisch trackbare Nadeln in die Leber eingebracht wie beispielhaft in Abbildung 2 veranschaulicht. Anschließend werden drei Messungen durchgeführt:

1. *Kontinuierliche Messung:* der Simulator wird beginnend in End-Exspiration für 30 s aktiviert und die Bewegung der Nadeln kontinuierlich gemessen.
2. *Exspiration ▷ Exspiration:* ein Timer mit der Periode der Beatmungsmaschine wird benutzt, um die Nadelpositionen in zehn aufeinanderfolgenden End-Exspirationsphasen zu messen. Hierdurch kann beurteilt werden, wie zuverlässig der Simulator die Leber wieder in die Ausgangsposition zurückbringt.

3. *Exspiration ▷ Inspiration:* die Positionen der Nadeln wird mittels eines Timers zunächst in End-Exspiration und anschließend in zehn aufeinanderfolgenden End-Inspirationsphasen gemessen. Durch dieses Experiment kann die maximale durch den Simulator erzeugte Bewegung analysiert werden.

Durch Verwendung eines optisch trackbaren Referenztools (Abb. 3b) kann für jedes Experiment die Bewegung der Nadeln entlang der drei Achsen des Koordinatensystems des Simulators bestimmt werden.

Um zu beurteilen, ob die Leber nicht nur rigide verschoben, sondern echt deformiert wird, wird eine landmarkenbasierte Registrierung durchgeführt: Für jeden Zeitpunkt der Aufnahme (d.h. jedes aufgenommene Sample) werden Landmarken entlang der Nadeln verteilt – jeweils beginnend bei der Spitze bis zu 3cm darüber, was etwa dem Eintrittspunkt in die Leber entspricht. Anschließend wird für jedes Sample aus den zugehörigen Landmarken und den zu den Inititalpositionen der Nadeln (d.h. zum ersten Sample) korrespondierenden Landmarken eine rigide Transformation berechnet. Aus der ermittelten Transformation kann der Fiducial Registration Error (FRE) bestimmt werden, welcher in diesem Fall ein Maß für den Grad der Deformation darstellt (FRE = 0 bedeutet rein rigide Transformation).

4   Ergebnisse

Die in Abschnitt 3.2 vorgestellten Experimente wurden für drei Schweinelebern mit jeweils drei verschiedenen Nadelkonfigurationen durchgeführt. Dazu wurden die Nadeln nach einem bestimmten Muster in dem Bereich der Leber verteilt, welcher der Höhe nach am ehesten mit der menschlichen Leber vergleichbar ist (Abb. 2). Die Ergebnisse der Bewegungsanalyse zeigt Tabelle 1.

Die Lebern bewegten sich entlang aller Achsen des Simulatorkoordinatensystems, vornehmlich jedoch in z-Richtung, also axial. Die maximale Auslenkung, d.h. der Betrag der Positionsänderung zwischen Inspiration und Exspiration, beträgt im Mittel 14.96 ± 4.65 mm. Der FRE zwischen Exspiration und Inspiration von 2.72 ± 1.40 mm lässt zudem darauf schließen, dass die Leber echt deformiert und nicht lediglich rigide verschoben wird. Dennoch nimmt die Leber die Ausgangsposition zuverlässig wieder ein, wie an den betragsmäßig kleinen Werten in Spalte 2 erkennbar ist. Den Arbeiten von [3] und [4] zufolge entspricht das genannte Verhalten qualitativ dem Verhalten der menschlichen Leber in-vivo.

5   Diskussion

Wir konnten zeigen, dass die durch den Simulator erzeugte Bewegung von Schweinelebern der Bewegung der Leber im menschlichen Körper ähnelt. Unser Modell ist folglich für die in-vitro Evaluation von Navigationssystemen geeignet.

Eine ortsabhängige Analyse der durch den Simulator erzeugten Bewegung könnte man durch zwei Kontrastmittel-Aufnamen einer perfundierten Leber in

Tabelle 1. Ergebnisse der Bewegungsanalyse für die Experimente aus Abschnitt 3.2 in drei Schweinelebern. Bewegung entlang der drei Achsen des Simulators ($B_{x/y/z}$), Mittelwert (MW), Standardabweichung (SA), Root-Mean-Square (RMS) Abstand und maximaler (MAX) Abstand von der Ursprungsposition (Betrag der Bewegung) sowie Fiducial Registration Error (FRE) für die rigide Registrierung

	Kontinuierlich	Exsp ▷ Exsp	Exsp ▷ Insp
Bewegung entlang Achsen			
B_x ($MW \pm SA$)	-0.53 ± 1.40	-0.03 ± 0.27	-1.06 ± 2.10
B_y ($MW \pm SA$)	-0.41 ± 1.98	-0.07 ± 0.32	-1.90 ± 3.09
B_z ($MW \pm SA$)	5.38 ± 7.59	0.34 ± 1.00	**14.24 ± 4.87**
Betrag der Bewegung			
MW	7.48	0.86	**14.96**
SA	6.07	0.75	**4.65**
RMS	9.64	1.14	15.66
MAX	26.02	4.46	**23.91**
Fiducial Registration Error			
MW	1.46	0.25	**2.72**
SA	1.27	0.27	1.40
RMS	1.93	0.37	3.06
MAX	6.56	1.86	6.39

End-Exspiration und End-Inspiration erreichen. Durch Markieren korrespondierender Punkte wäre die Berechnung eines Deformationsfeldes über die gesamte Leber möglich.

Danksagung

Diese Arbeit wurde im Rahmen des von der Deutschen Forschungsgemeinschaft unterstützten Graduiertenkollegs 1126: "Intelligente Chirurgie" durchgeführt.

Literaturverzeichnis

1. Banovac F, et al. Precision targeting of liver lesions using a novel electromagnetic navigation device in physiologic phantom and swine. Medical Physics 2005;32:2698–2705.
2. Maier-Hein L, et al. In-vitro evaluation of a novel needle-based soft tissue navigation system with a respiratory liver motion simulator. Procs SPIE to appear.
3. Clifford MA, et al. Assessment of hepatic motion secondary to respiration for computer assisted interventions. Computer Aided Surgery 2002;7:291–299.
4. Rohlfing T, et al. Modeling liver motion and deformation during the respiratory cycle using intensity-based free-form registration of gated MR Iiages. Medical Physics 2004;31:427–432.

Texturbasierte Segmentierung von frühen Hautläsionen in Epilumineszenz-Aufnahmen

Timm B. Busshaus[1], Jürgen Kreusch[2], Siegfried J. Pöppl[1]

[1]Institut für Medizinische Informatik, Universität zu Lübeck
[2]Dermatologische Praxis, Lübeck
E-Mail: busshaus@imi.uni-luebeck.de

Zusammenfassung. Es wird ein Algorithmus zur Segmentierung sehr früher, teilweise unpigmentierter Hautläsionen in Epilumineszenz(ELM)-Aufnahmen beschrieben. Solche Läsionen werden mit farbbasierten Segmentierungsverfahren nicht vollständig erfasst. Gerade die Eigenschaften der unpigmentierten, nicht erfassten Bereiche sind aber für die klinische Diagnose relevant. Das vorgestellte Verfahren basiert auf der Berechnung von Textureigenschaften der lokalen Umgebungen einzelner Pixel unabhängig von Farbwertinformationen und wird ergänzend zu diesen zur Segmentierung eingesetzt. Dadurch werden Läsionsbereiche zum Segment hinzugefügt, welche in diesem frühen Stadium noch keine ausreichende Farbänderung aufweisen, aber bereits eine charakteristische Struktur durch die Veränderung auf Zellebene aufweisen. Diese erweiterte Segmentierung ist ein wesentlicher Schritt zur Vorbereitung der Klassifikation der frühen Hautläsionen.

1 Einleitung

Für die Klassifikation von Hautläsionen ist die vollständige Segmentierung des Läsionsbereiches von großer Bedeutung. Gerade bei sehr jungen Läsionen sind die Farbveränderungen noch sehr gering und unregelmäßig. Durch die Veränderung der Zellen innerhalb der Basalschicht ist aber eine Strukturänderung in

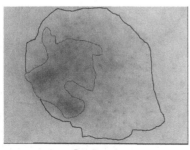 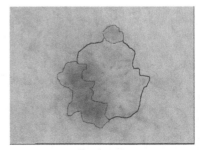

Läsion 1   Läsion 2

Abb. 1. Referenzsegmentierung: pigmentierte und unpigmentierte Bereiche wurden von einem Dermatologen getrennt segmentiert

Abb. 2. Farbbasierte Segmentierung: stabile Ergebnisse sind nur für die pigmentierten Bereiche erreichbar, ebenfalls zur Läsion gehörige rötlichen Areale werden nicht erkannt

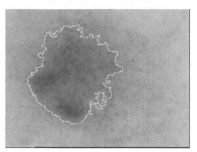
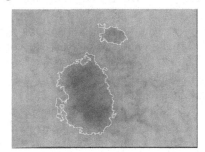

Läsion 1   Läsion 2

den ELM-Aufnahmen sichtbar. Die unpigmentierten Bereiche der Läsion spielen bei der visuellen Diagnose durch den Experten eine wichtige Rolle [1]. In den Beispielbildern sind Blutgefäße als kleine rote Punkte (pinpoint vessels) zu erkennen, welche ein sehr sicheres Zeichen für maligne Melanome sind (Abb.1). Im vorgestellten Verfahren wird deshalb zusätzlich zur Farbe die Texturinformation für die Segmentierung verwendet.

2   Stand der Forschung und Fortschritt durch den Beitrag

Zur vorliegenden Fragestellung wurden einige Verfahren zur Segmentierung von Hautläsionen implementiert und auf ihre Anwendbarkeit auf sehr frühe Läsionen getestet, z.B. die Segmentierung nach Leischner [2], Schmid [3] und Ganster [4]. Dabei stellte sich heraus, dass alle Verfahren der Läsion einen zu kleinen Bereich zuordnen und auch das Anpassen verschiedener Parameter nicht zu befriedigenden Ergebnissen führt (Abb. 2). All diese Algorithmen arbeiten nur mit Farbinformationen, was die Vermutung bestätigt, dass die Farbänderungen der frühen Läsionen für eine gute Segmentierung noch nicht ausreichend sind. Diese Fehlsegmentierung ist nicht tolerabel, da Strukturen zur Unterscheidung von Nävuszellnävi und Melanomen [1], wie pinpoint vessels oder Pseudopodien [5], gerade im Läsionsrandgebiet zu finden sind. Im neuen Verfahren werden zusätzlich Texturinformationen verwendet. Dadurch wird der Läsion ein Bereich zugeordnet, in welchem sich bereits Hautveränderung zeigen, ohne dass schon eine Farbänderung auftritt.

3   Methoden

Für die Lösung des Problems werden Texturinformationen für die Segmentierung eingesetzt, welche normalerweise zur Klassifikation der Segmente berechnet werden [6, 7]. Im V-Kanal des Bildes im HSV-Farbraum wird die Textur in der Umgebung jedes Pixels analysiert und die Texturparameter dem jeweiligen Pixel zugeordnet. Es entstehen multispektrale Texturkarten des Helligkeitskanals. In der

Testphase wurden Haraliksche Texturparameter und Laws Texturenergien berechnet [8, 9, 10]. Dabei ergaben sich für die ELM-Aufnahmen der Haut sehr interessante Ergebnisse, vor allem die Laws-Energie E3-E3 zeigte Ergebnisse, welche nach Schwellwertbinarisierung bereits nahezu vollständige Segmentierungen der Hautläsionen darstellten. Im vorliegenden Algorithmus wird Farbsättigung und Laws-Textur E3-E3 auf V verwendet. Zuerst werden pixelweise die Laws-Texturwerte berechnet und in einem Grauwertbild als Intensitäten gespeichert. Die Klassifikation der Pixel erfolgt mit dem Fuzzy C-Means Algorithmus [3]. Die Klassenanzahl wird manuell festgelegt, meist liefert der Algorithmus für 2 Klassen gute Ergebnisse, in Einzelfällen sind 3 Klassen notwendig. Eine automatische Bestimmung der Klassenzahl ist denkbar durch morphologische Analyse der Cluster im Bildraum. Alle Zusammenhangskomponenten (ZHK) mit weniger als 10% der Fläche der größten ZHK werden gelöscht. Durch morphologische Operatoren wird das Ergebnis bereinigt und geglättet. Der Algorithmus wurde in JAVA implementiert und auf digitale Bilder aus dem MicroDerm-System [11] und der Danaos-Studie [12] sowie eingescannte analoge Aufnahmen angewendet.

4 Ergebnisse

Läsionsgebiete werden bei teilweise unpigmentierten Läsionen meist vollständig erfasst, ohne dass zu viel angrenzende gesunde Haut mit segmentiert wird. Die unterschiedliche Farbe der Bilder hatte keinen Einfluss auf das Segmentierungsergebnis. Die Ergebnisse der Segmentierung wurden an Beispieldaten validiert. Der Datensatz enthielt 144 Läsionen, davon 74 maligne Melanome, davon 7 mit teilweise unpigmentiertem Läsionsgebiet. Geprüft wurde die Zuordnung aller Pixel zum Läsionsgebiet (positiv) oder zur umgebenden Haut (negativ) (Abb. 4). Für jedes Bild wurden die Sensitivität und Spezifität berechnet (Tab. 1). Für die vorliegende Fragestellung wird eine hohe Sensitivität angestrebt, bei Inkaufnahme einer geringeren Spezifität. Die besten Ergebnisse lieferte die Kombination von Farbsättigung und Laws-Textur E3-E3 (Abb. 3). Die Ergebnisse für die

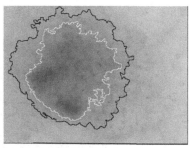 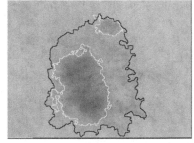

Läsion 1   Läsion 2

Abb. 3. Ergebnisse der Verfahren: pigmentierte Regionen farbbasiert segmentiert (weiß), unpigmentierte Bereiche texturbasiert segmentiert (schwarz); vergleiche Referenzsegmentierung (Abb. 1)

Abb. 4. Segmentierungsfehler (grün = richtig positiv, gelb = falsch positiv, rot = falsch negativ, schwarz = richtig negativ): Die Größe der falsch negativen Bereiche (rot) soll minimiert werden, falsch positive Bereiche (gelb) sind weniger kritisch

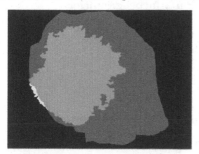

Läsion 1 farbsegmentiert

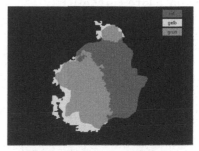

Läsion 2 farbsegmentiert

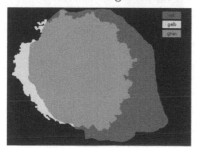

Läsion 1 texturbasiert

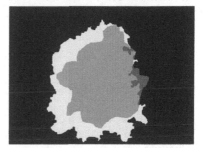

Läsion 2 textursegmentiert

Läsionen 1 und 2 sind in Tabelle 1 dargestellt. Bei beiden Bildern lieferte die texturbasierte Segmentierung eine höhere Sensitivität als die rein farbbasierte. Die Unterteilung in Läsionszentrum und -randgebiet wurde hier nicht beachtet. Eine Validierung der Ergebnisse der Klassifikation der Bilddaten nach klinischer Diagnose bzw. histologischem Befund wurde noch nicht durchgeführt. Die Merkmalsextraktion und Klassifikation dieser sehr frühen Läsionen ist zur Zeit Gegenstand unserer Forschung. Verfahren, welche auf der ABCD(E)-Regel [13] oder den ELM-7-Merkmalen [1] basieren, liefern voraussichtlich keine befriedigende Arbeitshypothese, da laut Aussage der Dermatologen die diesen Verfahren zugrundeliegenden Merkmale so früh noch nicht ausgebildet sind.

5   Diskussion

Das Verfahren ist geeignet, die beschriebenen, teilweise unpigmentierten Hautläsionen zu segmentieren. Da das Gesamtsystem zur Analyse von Hautläsionen später in Echzeit Ergebnisse liefern soll, spielt die Laufzeit der Algorithmen eine Rolle. Der vorgestellte Segmentierungsalgorithmus ist mit weniger als einer Sekunde Laufzeit unter JAVA auf einem Pentium 4 mit 2 GHz sehr schnell. Für eine optimale Unterteilung der Läsionen in Zentrum und Läsionsrandgebiet ist eine Kombination von textur- und farbbasierter Segmentierung denkbar (Abb. 3). Dies ist zur Zeit Gegenstand unserer Forschung.

Tabelle 1. Automatische Segmentierungen im Vergleich zur manuellen Referenz; prozentualer Anteil der Regionen

Läsion 1 farbsegmentiert:

auto\ref	Läsion	Umgebung	
segmentiert	23	2	25
nicht segm.	30	45	75
Summe	53	47	[%]

Sensitivität: 43%
Spezifität: 96%

Läsion 2 farbsegmentiert:

auto\ref	Läsion	Umgebung	
segmentiert	12	3	15
nicht segm.	11	74	85
Summe	23	77	[%]

Sensitivität: 52%
Spezifität: 96%

Läsion 1 textursegmentiert:

auto\ref	Läsion	Umgebung	
segmentiert	37	4	41
nicht segm.	17	42	59
Summe	54	46	[%]

Sensitivität: 68% (Δsens = +25%)
Spezifität: 91%

Läsion 2 textursegmentiert:

auto\ref	Läsion	Umgebung	
segmentiert	21	12	33
nicht segm.	2	65	67
Summe	23	77	[%]

Sensitivität: 91% (Δsens = +39%)
Spezifität: 84%

Literaturverzeichnis

1. Blum Andreas, Kreusch Juergen, Bauer Juergen, Garbe Claus. Dermatoskopie von Hauttumoren. Darmstadt: Steinkopf; 2003.
2. Leischner Carsten. Bildanalytische Methoden zur Charakterisierung pigmentierter Hautläsionen. Universität zu Lübeck; 2002.
3. Schmid P. Segmentation of Digitized Dermatoscopic Images by Two-Dimensional Color Clustering. IEEE Trans Med Imaging 1999;18(2).
4. Ganster H, Gelautz M, Prinz A. Initial Results of Automated Melanoma Recognition. TU Graz, Inst. f. Computer Graphics; 1995.
5. Kreusch Juergen, Koch Frauke. Auflichtmikroskopische Charakterisierung von Gefäßmustern in Hauttumoren. Der Hautarzt 1996;47(4):264–272.
6. Brock C, Flach B, Kask E, Osterland R. Objektsegmentierung durch Textur- und Randextraktion. TU Dresden Institut für KI; 1996.
7. Dhawan AtamP, Sicsu Anne. Segmentation of Images of Skin Lesions using Color and Textur Information of Surface Pigmentation. Comp Med Imag Graph 1992;16(3):163–177.
8. Haralick RM, Shanmugam K, Dinstein I. Textural Features for Image Classification. IEEE Trans Syst Man Cybern 1973;3(6):610–621.
9. Laws KI. Rapid Texture Identification. Procs SPIE 1980; 376–380.
10. Handels Heinz. Medizinische Bildverarbeitung. Teubner, Stuttgart; 2000.
11. Visiomed AG Bochum. microDERM; 2000. Http://www.visiomed.ag.
12. Hoffmann K, Gambichler T, Rick A, et al. Diagnostic and neural analysis of skin cancer (DANAOS). Br J Dermatol 2003;149(4):801–809.
13. Kreusch Juergen, Rassner Gernot. Auflichtmikroskopie pigmentierter Hauttumoren: Ein Bildatlas. Stuttgart: Thieme; 1991.

Automatische Segmentierung des Corpus Callosum aus sagittalen Schichten von kernspintomographischen Datensätzen

Ralf Schönmeyer[1,2], Anna Rotarska-Jagiela[1,2], David Prvulovic[1,2], Maria Athelogou[3], Corinna Haenschel[1,2] und David E.J. Linden[2,4]

[1]Brain Imaging Center, Universität Frankfurt am Main,
Schleusenweg 2-16, 60528 Frankfurt am Main
[2]Labor für Neurophysiologie und Neuroimaging, Universitätsklinikum Frankfurt,
Zentrum der Psychiatrie, Heinrich-Hoffmann-Str. 10, 60528 Frankfurt am Main
[3]Definiens AG, Trappentreustraße 1, 80339 München
[4]School of Psychology, University of Wales, LL57 2AS Bangor, U.K.
Email: schoenmeyer@bic.uni-frankfurt.de

Zusammenfassung. In dieser Arbeit stellen wir einen voll-automatisierten Algorithmus vor, der in der Lage ist, die Struktur des Corpus Callosum aus sagittalen Schichten von T1-gewichteten kernspintomographischen Datensätzen des menschlichen Gehirns zu segmentieren. Die Segmentierungsergebnisse werden dabei für die Untersuchung morphometrischer Merkmale in einer Studie zur Schizophrenie in definierte Abschnitte unterteilt, um sie im weiteren Verlauf statistisch auswerten zu können. Der Algorithmus wurde unter Zuhilfenahme der Cognition Network Technologie implementiert, die eine regelbasierte und kontextsensitive Handhabung der Bilddaten erlaubt, und dabei nur wenige Voraussetzungen über die Beschaffenheit und Qualität der zu verarbeitenden Datensätze macht. Das Verfahren scheitert im Rahmen einer Testreihe bei einem von 50 Datensätzen und erzielt ansonsten einen Dice-Koeffizienten von 0,97 im Vergleich zu manuell segmentierten Ergebnissen.

1 Einleitung

Durch die immer größere Verfügbarkeit von Kernspintomographen in der klinischen Forschung und die damit einhergehende steigende Anzahl der zu verarbeitenden Datensätze wird es zunehmend wichtiger, Arbeitsschritte zu automatisieren und unabhängig von manueller Interaktion zu machen. Dabei bilden Segmentierungs- und Partitionierungsaufgaben oftmals den „Flaschenhals" der Verarbeitungskette, da automatische Lösungen oft nur unzureichende Ergebnisse liefern und manuelle Verfahren sehr zeit- und personalaufwändig sind. Um die im Rahmen einer Studie zur Schizophrenie [1] benötigten umfangreichen Segmentierungsarbeiten des Corpus Callosum (CC) aus kernspintomographischen Datensätzen zu unterstützen, wurde mit Hilfe der „Cognition Network Technology" (CNT) der Firma Definiens AG, München, ein Algorithmus und Workflow entworfen, der die geforderten Aufgaben weitgehend automatisiert.

2 Stand der Forschung

Die manuelle Segmentierung definiert in der psychiatrischen Forschung mit bild-gebenden Verfahren immer noch den Goldstandard [2, 3, 4]. Bei der manuellen Segmentierung des CC dauert die Markierung in der erforderlichen Güte mindestens eine Minute pro Bild, so dass in den meisten Studien nur die zentrale sagittale Schicht eines MR-Datensatzes des menschlichen Kopfs herangezogen wird. Es existieren automatisierte Ansätze (z.B. [5]) und Softwarepakete (z.B. [6]), die in der Lage sind das CC zu segmentieren und zu vermessen, allerdings liefern diese andere als die erforderlichen Maße und setzen in der Regel manuell durchgeführte Normalisierung und individuell angepasste Filterung der Datensätze voraus, um zufriedenstellende Ergebnisse zu erlangen.

3 Wesentlicher Fortschritt durch den Beitrag

Die vorliegende Arbeit zeigt erstmals im Bereich der psychiatrischen Forschung anhand einer konkreten Studie, wie mit der CNT innerhalb einer Entwicklungszeit von rund 2 Arbeitswochen, von der ersten Idee bis zur kompletten Umsetzung, Segmentierungsaufgaben nahezu komplett automatisiert werden können, die manuell zu bearbeiten ansonsten einen zu großen Aufwand bedeutet hätten. Der Algorithmus wurde so konzipiert, daß keinerlei Vorverarbeitung wie Filterung, Homogenisierung oder Normalisierung der zu verarbeitenden MR-Datensätze vorausgesetzt wird. Die aus den Eingangsbilddaten generierten Ergebnisse werden so aufbereitet, daß sie sich nahtlos in den Workflow der weiteren Auswertung der zugrundeliegenden Studie eingliedern. Dies umfasst auch eine ergonomisch Möglichkeit der visuellen Inspektion und ggf. Korrektur.

4 Methoden

Die CNT ist ein objekt- und regelbasierter Ansatz, mit dessen Hilfe es möglich ist, Algorithmen für die automatisierte Bildanalyse auf der Basis von Expertenwissen zu entwerfen. Im vorliegenden Fall wird damit aus zentralen sagittalen Schnitten von T1-gewichteten kernspintomographischen Aufnahmen des Kopfs die Struktur des CC (Abb. 1a) extrahiert. Die Daten stammen dabei hauptsächlich aus MPRAGE (magnetization-prepared rapid acquisition gradient echo-Sequenz)-Messungen eines 3-Tesla Kernspintomographen (Siemens Magnetom Trio, TR = 2000 [ms], TE = 2.6 [ms], base resolution: 256x256 bei 160 slices, Voxelgröße: 1x1x1 [mm]^3, Dauer: 7 Minuten). Der Einsatz der CNT stützt sich dabei auf den in [7] vorgestellten Workflow zur Verarbeitung von 2D-Schichten aus 3D-Volumendatensätzen. Die maßgeblichen Arbeitsschritte seien hier kurz skizziert: Zunächst wird das Eingangsbild mit einem in der CNT implementierten Partitionierungsverfahren [8] in Objekte unterteilt, die homogene Grauwerte und auch Größenkriterien erfüllen. Danach entscheidet eine Klassifikation, ob in der Menge dieser Objekte bereits potentielle Objekte vorhanden sind, die das spätere CC bilden könnten. Diese charakterisieren sich durch relativen

Abb. 1. Ausschnitt einer sagittalen Beispiel-Schicht, die das Corpus Callosum enthält ohne (a) und mit (b) Segmentierungsergebnis für den Hauptkörper des CC (grau), dessen Umriß (schwarz), sowie dem hier mit dem CC verbundenen Fornix (weiß)

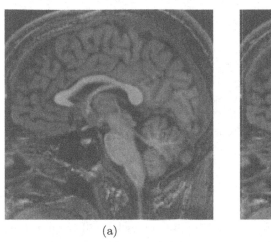 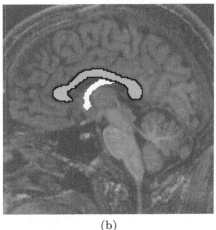

(a)   (b)

Grauwert-Kontrast zur Umgebung und zum gesamten Bild, sowie Dichte- und Formkriterien (die Bounding Box der gesuchten Struktur ist rund doppelt so lang wie breit und horizontal ausgerichtet), der Größe (gefordert sind zwischen 300 und 1500 Pixel) und Lage (Distanz zum Bildzentrum nicht größer als 40 Pixel). Falls keine solchen Objekte gefunden werden, wiederholt sich die Prozedur der Partitionierung mit strengeren Größenkriterien und weniger strengem Homogenitätskriterium. In der Regel konvergiert dieses Verfahren innerhalb von drei bis fünf Iterationen, bis sich potentielle CC-Objekte finden. Eine technische Schwierigkeit besteht nun darin, den in manchen Fällen augenscheinlich mit dem CC verbundenen Fornix (Abb. 1b) wieder abzutrennen. Dazu wird das gesamte bislang ermittelte CC-Objekt untergliedert und der „Zweig" abgetrennt, der die relativ zur Länge geringste Fläche repräsentiert, da das Fornix schmaler als der Hauptkörper des CC ist. Übrig bleibt das ggf. korrigierte CC-Objekt, das anschließend in neun Abschnitte unterteilt (Definition nach [9], siehe Abb. 2) und vermessen wird. Die daraus ermittelten Volumenberechnungen werden dann in Tabellenform der weiteren statistischen Auswertung der Studie zugeführt.

5   Ergebnisse

Es konnte ein Algorithmus gefunden werden, der auf der zentralen sagittalen Schicht, sowie wie gefordert auf den beidseitig drei benachbarten sagittalen Schichten die Aufgabe in weniger als fünf Minuten pro Datensatz löst. Nach Sichtkontrolle werden für ca. 95% aller Eingangsbilder (auf der Basis von über 750 Bildern aus bislang rund 100 Datensätzen) Ergebnisse geliefert, die ohne

Abb. 2. Unterteilung des CC nach [9] in neun Abschnitte: In (a) sind die Proportionen im Verhältnis zur Gesamtlänge L des CC angegeben. (b) veranschaulicht ein nach diesem Schema automatisch unterteiltes Segmentierungsergebnis anhand eines Beispieldatensatzes

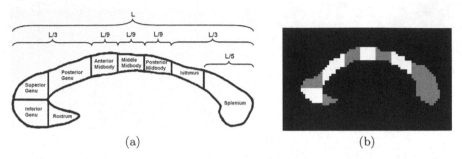

(a)   (b)

manuelle Korrekturen weiterverwendet werden können. Die Segmentierungsergebnisse eines Studienabschnitts mit 50 Datensätzen wurden näher quantitativ untersucht: In einem Fall scheiterte das Verfahren komplett, da das CC eine ausgeprägte morphologische Anomalie (Istmus) aufwies. Für die restlichen 49 Datensätzen konnte im Vergleich zu den von einem Experten manuell korrigierten Daten ein mittlerer Dice-Koeffizient von 0,97 mit einer Standardabweichung von 0,051 erzielt werden. Von den insgesamt 350 untersuchten Schichten wiesen dabei 13 „geringere" und 11 „gravierendere" Fehlsegmentierungen auf, die über 11 bzw. 6 Datensätze verteilt waren. Die geringeren Fehler zeichneten sich dabei dadurch aus, daß sie sich während der visuellen Inspektion in unter 10 Sekunden manuell korrigieren ließen. Die gravierenderen Fehler konnten in ca. 30 Sekunden pro Bild behoben werden. Neben den 7 Schichten der kompletten Fehlsegmentierung scheiterte der Algorithmus noch auf weiteren 4 einzelnen Schichtbildern, deren Korrektur in rund einer Minute pro Bild erledigt werden konnte.

6   Diskussion

Das vorgestellte Verfahren arbeitet genügend robust auf T1-gewichteten Datensätzen unterschiedlicher Sequenzen, wie insbesondere MPRAGE und der immer weiter verbreiteten MDEFT [10]. Der Algorithmus passt sich dabei automatisch den in der klinischer Diagnostik und Forschung vorkommenden unterschiedlichen Qualitäten der Bilddaten hinsichtlich Helligkeit, Kontrast und Signal-zu-Rausch-Verhältnis an. Um die Ergebnisse der Vermessung des CC für die statistische Auswertung der Studie besser vergleichen zu können, wird vorausgesetzt, daß die Datensätze in die AC (commissura anterior)-PC (commissura posterior)-Achse rotiert sind. Dies stellt den einzigen manuellen Vorverarbeitungsschritt dar, der für weniger genaue Untersuchungen nicht nötig ist. Der Workflow für das Postprocessing wurde so gestaltet, daß eventuelle Segmentierungsfehler gleich während der visuellen Inspektion korrigiert werden können, um die weitere Verarbeitungskette nicht länger zu unterbrechen. Die gewonnenen Erkenntnisse lassen sich auch für die Analyse von weiteren Strukturen ggf. auch aus anderen Modalitäten (z.B. CT) übertragen. Die Ergebnisse dieser Arbeit stellen der zugrundeliegenden Schizophrenie-Studie für vorhandene und alle künftig erhobenen Datensätze nahezu vollständig-automatisiert Parameter zur Verfügung, um diese in einem Umfang auswerten zu können, wie dies mit manueller Segmentierung nicht ohne deutlichen Mehraufwand möglich wäre. Damit können statistische Aussagen der Studie detaillierter und mit mehr Signifikanz angegebene werden und fügen ihr damit einen erheblichen Mehrwert zu.

7 Danksagung

Die Autoren danken der Alzheimer Forschung Initiative e.V. für die finanzielle Unterstützung. Das Brain Imaging Center Frankfurt am Main wird gefördert durch das Bundesministerium für Bildung und Forschung (DLR 01GO0203).

Literaturverzeichnis

1. Rotarska-Jagiela A, Schoenmeyer R, Oertel V, Haenschel C, Maurer K, Linden DEJ. Strukturelle Integrität des Corpus Callosum bei schizophrenen Patienten – untersucht mit Diffusion Tensor Imaging. In: DGPPN (submitted and accepted). Berlin; 2006.
2. Narr KL, Thompson PM, Sharma T, Moussai J, Cannestra AF, Toga AW. Mapping morphology of the corpus callosum in schizophrenia. Cereb Cortex 2000;10(1):40–9.
3. Luders E, Narr KL, Zaidel E, Thompson PM, Jancke L, Toga AW. Parasagittal asymmetries of the corpus callosum. Cereb Cortex 2006;16(3):346–54.
4. Ota M, Obata T, Akine Y, Ito H, Ikehira H, Asada T, et al. Age-related degeneration of corpus callosum measured with diffusion tensor imaging. Neuroimage 2006;31(4):1445–52.
5. Lee C, Huh S, Ketter TA, Unser M. Automated Segmentation of the Corpus Callosum in Midsagittal Brain Magnetic Resonance Images. Optical Engineering 2000;39(4):924–935.
6. Magnotta VA, Harris G, Andreasen NC, O'Leary DS, Yuh WT, Heckel D. Structural MR image processing using the BRAINS2 toolbox. Comput Med Imaging Graph 2002;26(4):251–64.
7. Schönmeyer R, Prvulovic D, Rotarska-Jagiela A, Dallmann K, Haenschel C, Athelogou M, et al. Automatisierte Segmentierung der Seitenventrikel des menschlichen Gehirns aus kernspintomographischen Datensätzen. In: BVM; 2005. 83–87.
8. Schäpe A, Urbani M, Leiderer R, Athelogou M. Fraktal hierarchische, prozeß- und objektbasierte Bildanalyse. In: Procs BVM; 2003. 206–210.
9. Highley JR, Esiri MM, McDonald B, Cortina-Borja M, Herron BM, Crow TJ. The size and fibre composition of the corpus callosum with respect to gender and schizophrenia: a post-mortem study. Brain 1999;122 (Pt 1):99–110.
10. Deichmann R, Schwarzbauer C, Turner R. Optimisation of the 3D MDEFT sequence for anatomical brain imaging: technical implications at 1.5 and 3 T. Neuroimage 2004;21(2):757–67.

Parametrisierung geschlossener Oberflächen für die Erzeugung von 3D-Formmodellen

Mareike Schönig, Tobias Heimann und Hans-Peter Meinzer

Abteilung für Medizinische und Biologische Informatik,
Deutsches Krebsforschungszentrum, 69120 Heidelberg
Email: m.schoenig@dkfz.de

Zusammenfassung. Statistische Formmodelle sind eine populäre Methode um den Segmentierungsprozess in der medizinischen Bildverarbeitung zu automatisieren. Dafür ist es notwendig, zuerst korrespondierende Landmarken auf den Oberflächen von Trainingsformen zu finden. Ein erfolgversprechender automatischer Ansatz hierzu [1] basiert auf Parametrisierungen: Dabei werden die dreidimensionalen Punkte auf den Trainingsformen zweidimensionalen Punkten auf der Einheitskugel zugeordnet. In dieser Arbeit erweitern wir ein Parametrisierungsverfahren für Voxeldaten [2] auf triangulierte Gitternetze. Durch Nutzung von Diffusionsgleichungen entsteht ein einfaches, schnelles und robustes Parametrisierungsverfahren. Damit können wir statistische Modelle auch von Formen wie dem Unterkieferknochen erzeugen, für die der bisher verwendete Parametrisierungsalgorithmus keine Lösung fand.

1 Einleitung

Die Segmentierung von 3D-Daten ist in der medizinischen Bildverarbeitung ein essentieller Schritt für die Diagnose- und Therapieunterstützung bei der Behandlung von Tumorpatienten. Ein rein manueller Segmentierungsprozess nimmt viel Zeit in Anspruch, während automatische Verfahren oftmals ungenügende Ergebnisse liefern. Als vielversprechende automatische Methode sollen in der Abteilung MBI des DKFZ statistische Formmodelle [3] für die Organsegmentierung eingesetzt werden.

Um statistische Formmodelle zu erzeugen, werden eine Anzahl von Trainingsdatensätzen benötigt, aus denen jeweils das gleiche Organ vorsegmentiert wurde. Mit Hilfe des Marching-Cubes-Algorithmus entsteht pro Trainingsdatensatz ein trianguliertes Gitternetzmodell (Mesh), welches die Oberfläche des segmentierten Organs darstellt. Auf den unterschiedlichen Formen der Trainingsdatensätze müssen nun eine Anzahl korrespondierende Punkte (Landmarken) gefunden werden, aus denen das statistische Formmodell erzeugt wird. Ein erfolgreiches Verfahren zur automatischen Erzeugung von Landmarken [1] basiert auf Parametrisierungen: Hierbei wird jedem beliebigen Punkt auf dem Mesh ein anderer Punkt auf der Einheitskugel zugeordnet. Über die inverse Funktion kann eine Menge von Punkten von der Kugeloberfläche auf die parametrisierten Meshes abgebildet werden. In [1] werden die initialen Parametrisierungen mit Hilfe von Warping modifiziert, um die minimale Beschreibungslänge (MDL) zu minimieren und die optimal korrespondierenden Landmarken zu erstellen. Voraussetzung ist, dass zuerst eine initiale Parametrisierung für jeden Trainingsmesh erstellt wird.

2 Stand der Forschung und Fortschritt durch den Beitrag

Es existiert eine Vielzahl verschiedener Ansätze für die Parametrisierung von geschlossenen dreidimensionalen Objektoberflächen [4]. Bei der Erstellung von Parametrisierungen sind zwei Eigenschaften von Bedeutung: Winkel- und Flächentreue. Bei triangulierten Meshes bilden drei Punkte auf der Oberfläche des Organs ein Dreieck, welches pro Ecke einen bestimmten Winkel aufweist und eine spezifische Fläche hat. Geht durch die Parametrisierung einer dieser Werte verloren, ist die Parametrisierung winkel- oder flächenverzerrend. Im Allgemeinen kann maximal eine der beiden Eigenschaften erhalten werden.

Gu et al. [5] beschreiben ein einfaches Verfahren für winkeltreue Parametrisierungen, welches in der Praxis aber für stark konkave Formen (wie Unterkieferknochen) nicht funktioniert. Die Methode nach [2] ist ebenso einfach und sogar robuster als [5], doch bisher nur für Voxeldaten beschrieben. In diesem Beitrag wird das Verfahren auf triangulierte Gitternetzmodelle erweitert. Es ist auf Genus-0 Topologien (kugelförmige Oberflächen) beschränkt.

3 Methoden

Der Parametrisierungsvorgang nach [2] gliedert sich in drei Schritte: Initialisierung, Breitengrad- und Längengradbestimmung. Zuerst werden bei der Initialisierung zwei Punkte des Meshes als Nord- bzw. Südpol bestimmt (p_n und p_s). In dieser Arbeit verwenden wir dafür die beiden Punkte mit dem größten Abstand bezüglich der x-Achse.

Das Problem der Breitengradbestimmung kann durch die Laplace'sche Gleichung

$$\nabla^2 \cdot \theta = 0 \tag{1}$$

formal beschrieben werden. Im diskreten Fall wird es durch Differenzen approximiert und durch folgendes Gleichungssystem dargestellt:

$$A \cdot \boldsymbol{\theta} = \boldsymbol{b} \tag{2}$$

Jeder Punkt $p(i)$ hat über die von ihm ausgehenden Kanten eine Menge $N(i)$ direkter Nachbarpunkte. Während bei dem Originalverfahren (auf isotropen Voxeldaten) alle Kanten gleich lang sind, weisen wir den Kanten im Mesh individuelle Gewichte entsprechend dem Kehrwert ihrer Länge zu. Für die Matrix A gilt: An die Diagonale a_{ii} wird die Summe der Kantengewichte zu den direkten Nachbarn gesetzt:

$$a_{ii} = \sum_{j \in N(i)} \frac{1}{|p(i) - p(j)|} \tag{3}$$

Das negative Gewicht der Kante zwischen dem Punkt $p(i)$ und dem Nachbar $p(j)$ wird in a_{ij} geschrieben:

$$a_{ij} = -\frac{1}{|p(i) - p(j)|} \qquad (4)$$

Der Vektor b erhält in allen Zeilen i, die direkte Nachbarn des Südpols sind, das Produkt aus π und dem Gewicht der Kante zwischen ihnen.

$$b_i = \frac{\pi}{|p(i) - p_s|} \qquad (5)$$

Der Rest wird auf 0 gesetzt. Der Lösungsvektor θ des Gleichungssystems 2 spezifiziert dann für jeden Punkt im Mesh den zugehörigen Breitengrad.

Für das Problem der Längengradbestimmung kann ebenfalls Gleichung 1 genutzt werden. Es gilt:

$$C \cdot \phi = d \qquad (6)$$

Für Matrix C gilt: Die Werte von A werden übernommen und etwas modifiziert. Für Punkte $p(i)$, die direkte Nachbarn des Nord- bzw. Südpols sind, wird das Gewicht zwischen dem Punkt und dem jeweiligen Pol von der Diagonalen abgezogen, also

$$c_{ii} = a_{ii} - \frac{1}{|p(i) - p_s|} \qquad (7)$$

für den Südpol und entsprechend für den Nordpol p_n. Wegen der Regularität muss die additive Konstante $2\phi_1 = 0$ zu einer beliebigen Zeile summiert werden. Im Gegensatz zum Breitengrad ist der Längengrad ϕ ein zyklischer Parameter. Der Längengrad nimmt im Verlauf auf einer Breitengradlinie stetig bis 2π zu und fällt am Nullmeridian auf 0 zurück. Dieser Meridian umfasst alle Punkte, an denen der Längengrad den Wert 0 besitzt und windet sich vom Nord- zum Südpol. Die Berechnung des Vektors d hängt vom Verlauf des Nullmeridians ab.

Der Nullmeridian wird mit Hilfe von drei Kontrollpunkten (*here*, *prevPos* und *nextPos*) bestimmt. Von *here* ausgehend wird *nextPos* als direkter Nachbar mit dem größten Breitengrad gewählt; *prevPos* ist der direkte vorangehende Punkt auf dem Meridian. Das erste *here* ist breitengradhöchster, direkter Nachbar des Nordpols. Dies wird solange wiederholt, bis die Wahl von *nextPos* auf den Südpol trifft. Die Ansammlung von *here* spezifiziert die Punkte des Nullmeridians auf dem triangulierten Gitternetzmodell.

Punkte $p(i)$, die auf dem Nullmeridian liegen, reduzieren die Werte aus b_i für den Vektor d_i um 2π multipliziert mit dem Gewicht der Kante. Es gilt:

$$d_i = b_i - \sum_{j \in N_{ost}(i)} \frac{2\pi}{|p(i) - p(j)|} \qquad (8)$$

Die direkten östlichen Nachbarn $N_{ost}(i)$ der Punkte des Nullmeridians $p(i)$ dagegen addieren 2π multipliziert mit dem Gewicht der Kante zwischen den Nachbarpunkten $p(j)$:

$$d_j = b_j + \frac{2\pi}{|p(i) - p(j)|} \qquad (9)$$

Abb. 1. Skizze zur Bestimmung der Punkte östlich des Nullmeridians

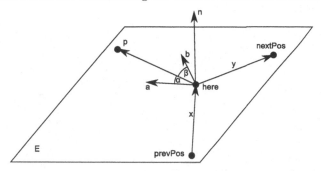

Um zu erkennen, ob ein Nachbarpunkt östlich oder westlich des Nullmeridians liegt, haben wir folgendes Verfahren entwickelt: Jeder Punkt auf dem Nullmeridian besitzt einen Normalenvektor n zu einer durch seine Nachbarn festgelegten Ebene E (siehe Abb. 1). Mit den Vektoren x und y aus den nach E projizierten Punkten *prevPos* und *nextPos* wird $a = n \times x$ und $b = n \times y$ berechnet. In dieser Situation kann a links von b liegen oder umgekehrt. Ist das Ergebnis von $(a \times b) \cdot n < 0$, so liegt a links von b. Tritt ein Skalarwert > 0 auf, liegt a rechts von b. Der zu überprüfende Nachbarpunkt wird nach E projiziert und dort als p bezeichnet. Zu a bildet er den Winkel α und zu b den Winkel β. p liegt östlich des Meridians, wenn a links von b liegt und gilt:

$$\alpha < \frac{\Pi}{2} \vee \beta < \frac{\Pi}{2} \tag{10}$$

Liegt a rechts von b, dann liegt p östlich des Nullmeridians falls:

$$\alpha < \frac{\Pi}{2} \wedge \beta < \frac{\Pi}{2} \tag{11}$$

4   Ergebnisse

Das beschriebene Parametrisierungsverfahren wurde auf Oberflächenmodellen von mehreren anatomischen Formen getestet, u.a. Leber, Lungenflügel und Unterkieferknochen. Für die Leber und den Unterkieferknochen sind die berechneten Längen- und Breitengrade in 2 visualisiert. Der zeitliche Aufwand einer Parametrisierung hängt proportional von der Anzahl der gegebenen Punkte im Mesh ab und dauert nur wenige Sekunden.

5   Diskussion

Die vorgestellte Methode ist ein einfaches, schnelles und robustes Verfahren für die Parametrisierung von triangulierten Gitternetzen. Auch die Oberflächen, bei

Abb. 2. Verlauf der Breiten- und Längengrade auf einer Leber und einem Unterkiefer-knochen. Die Breitengrade sind zusätzlich farblich von rot zu gelb kodiert

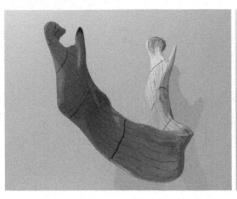
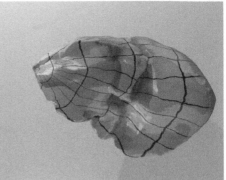

denen das iterative Verfahren nach [5] bisher nicht konvergierte, können so para-metrisiert werden und für die Erstellung von statistischen Formmodellen genutzt werden.

Um mit dem beschriebenen Verfahren noch weniger verzerrte Ergebnisse zu erzielen, werden wir in Zukunft die Auswahl der beiden Pole zu Beginn des Verfahrens optimieren: Die beiden Punkte, die unter allen Punkten im Mesh den maximalen geodätischen Abstand zueinander haben, führen zur minimal-sten Verzerrung. Diese beiden Punkte können z.B. mit einer Graphensuche auf dem Gitternetz des Meshes gefunden werden. Eine exakte Aufrechterhaltung der Winkel- und Flächentreue ist für die in [1] verwendete Methode nicht notwendig, da im nachfolgenden Schritt der Korrespondenzoptimierung alle Parametrisie-rungen sowieso modifiziert werden.

Literaturverzeichnis

1. Heimann T, Wolf I, Williams T, Meinzer HP. 3D active shape models using gradient descent optimization of description length. In: Procs IPMI; 2005. 566–577.
2. Brechbühler C, Gerig G, Kübler O. Parametrization of closed surfaces for 3-D shape description. Comp Vis Image Underst 1995;61:154–170.
3. Cootes TF, Taylor CJ, Cooper DH, Graham J. Active shape models: Their training and application. Comp Vis Image Underst 1995;61(1):38–59.
4. Floater MS, Hormann K. Surface parameterization: A tutorial and survey. In: Dodgson NA, Floater MS, Sabin MA, editors. Advances in Multiresolution for Geo-metric Modelling. Mathematics and Visualization. Springer; 2005. 157–186.
5. Gu X, Wang Y, Chan TF, Thompson PM, Yau ST. Genus zero surface conformal mapping and its application to brain surface mapping. In: Procs IPMI; 2003. 172–184.

Topology Correction for Brain Atlas Segmentation Using a Multiscale Algorithm

Lin Chen and Gudrun Wagenknecht

Central Institute for Electronics, Research Center Jülich, Jülich, Germany
Email: l.chen@fz-juelich.de

Abstract. In medicine and neuroscience, the reconstruction of anatomical structures from brain MRI images is an important goal, especially for regions in the human cerebral cortex. Topological correctness is important because it is an essential prerequisite for brain atlas deformation and surface flattening. We propose a new approach to repair a binary volumetric brain segmentation so that it becomes topologically equivalent to a sphere. A morphological multiscale approach which acts on foreground and background simultaneously divides the segmentation into several connected components, and subsequent region growing guarantees convergence to the correct spherical topology and changes as few voxels as possible. In addition to existing graph-based procedures, this provides an alternate approach which has several advantages, including high speed, ease of operation without graph analysis, and measuring the size of a handle, cutting a handle or filling the corresponding tunnel based on their sizes.

1 Introduction

Several methods for correcting the topology of brain segmentation have recently been developed. Shattuck and Leahy [1] and Xiao Han et al. [2] introduced graph-based methods for topology correction. Shattuck and Leahy examined the connectivity of 2D segmentations between adjoining slices to detect topological defects and minimally correct them by changing as few voxels as possible. Building on their work, Han et al. developed an algorithm to remove all handles from a binary object under any connectivity. Successive morphological openings correct the segmentation at the smallest scale. This method is effective for small handles, but large handles such as ventricles may need to be edited manually. Chen and Wagenknecht [3] localized handles by simulating wavefront propagation on the volume and the handles were deleted by a local region growing method. One drawback of this method is that the correction is 3D, but the handle localization is oriented along the Cartesian axes. Wood et al. [4] proposed a different approach. Handles in the tessellation are localized by simulating wavefront propagation on the tessellation and they are detected where the wavefronts meet twice. The size of a handle is the shortest non-separating cut along such a cycle, which helps retain as much fine geometrical detail of the model as possible. The region growing models are adopted by Kriegeskorte et al. [5] as topology correction methods. They start from an initial point with the deepest distance to the surface, and then grow the point by adding points that will not change the topology. One drawback of this approach is that the result strongly depends on the order in which the points are grown from the growing points set. Our method provides a fully automatic topology correction mechanism.

2   Methods

Some basics of digital topology will be given here (see [6] for details). The initial segmentation is a 3D binary digital image composed of a foreground object X and an inverse background object $\bar{X}$. From the conventional definition of adjacency, three types of connectivity are considered: 6-, 18- and 26-connectivity. For example, two voxels are 6-adjacent if they share a face, 18-adjacent if they share at least an edge, and 26-adjacent if they share at least a corner. In order to avoid topological paradoxes, different connectivities n and $\bar{n}$ must be used for the foreground and background objects. This leaves four pairs of compatible connectivities: (6, 18), (6, 26), (18, 6) and (26, 6). Considering a digital object, the calculation of two numbers (criteria) is sufficient to check if the modification of one single point will affect the topology. These topological numbers introduced by Bertrand [6] are an elegant way to classify the topology type of a given voxel. The following definitions are from [6].

Definition 1 (n-path) *An n-path of length $l > 0$ from p to q in X is a sequence of distinct points $p = p_0, p_1, ..., p_l = q$, where p_i is n-adjacent to p_{i+1}, for $i = 0, 1, ..., l - 1$. An n-path $p_0, p_1, ..., p_l$ is an n-closed path if and only if p_0 is n-adjacent to p_l.*

Definition 2 (Geodesic Neighborhood) *Denote the n-neighborhood of a point x with x removed by $N_n^*(x)$. The geodesic neighborhood of x with respect to the object X of order k is the set $N_n^k(x, X)$ defined recursively by: $N_n^1(x, X) = N_n^*(x) \cap X$, $N_n^k(x, X) = \{N_n^*(y) \cap N_{26}^*(x) \cap X, y \in N_n^{k-1}(x, X)\}$.*

Definition 3 (Topological Numbers) *An object is said to be n-connected, if and only if for any two points of the object, there exists an n-path between these two points within the object. Denote the set of all n-connected components of X by $C_n(X)$. The topological numbers of a point x relative to X are: $T_6(x, X) = \#C_6(N_6^2(x, X))$, $T_{6+}(x, X) = \#C_6 (N_6^3(x, X))$, $T_{18}(x, X) = \#C_{18}(N_{18}^2(x, X))$, $T_{26}(x, X) = \#C_{26}(N_{26}^1(x, X))$, where $\#$ denotes the number of n-connected components of a set C_n.*

Definition 4 (Simple Point) *For a point x, it is a simple point if and only if $T_n(x, X) = T_{\bar{n}}(x, \bar{X}) = 1$. Adding or removing a simple point will not change the topology of the object.*

Note, that in the definition of topological numbers there are two notations for 6-connectivity, where the notation "6^+" implies 6-connectivity whose dual connectivity is 18, while the notation "6" implies 6-connectivity whose dual connectivity is 26. This distinction is necessary in order to correctly compute topological numbers under 6-connectivity with different dual connectivities.

An object X has a handle if and only if there exists a closed n-path in X that can not be compressed to a point through a connected deformation. For example, as shown in Fig. 1a, the closed path $abcdefa$ can be compressed to a point. For an object X, the existence of handles depends on the chosen pairs of connectivities. As shown in Fig. 1a, when $n = 6$ and $\bar{n} = 26$, there exists a handle since the closed 26-path $\bar{a}\bar{b}\bar{c}\bar{d}\bar{e}\bar{f}\bar{g}\bar{a}$ can not be compressed to a point; when $n = 6^+$ and $\bar{n} = 18$, points a and b are not 18-connected, there exists no handle. In Fig. 1b, it has been illustrated that, when $n = 18$ or $n = 26$, the n-closed path $abcdefga$ can not be compressed to a point, there exists a handle; when $n = 6$ or $n = 6^+$, there exists no handle.

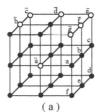 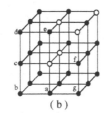

(a)   (b)

Fig. 1. Illustration that the existence of a handle depends on the chosen pairs of connectivities

The foreground object X and its inverse background object $\bar{X}$ have exactly the same number of handles in case a pair of compatible connectivities is used. Therefore, the tunnel associated with a handle of X is a handle in $\bar{X}$, where there exists a closed $\bar{n}$-path in $\bar{X}$ that cannot be deformed to a point through connected deformation. The number of handles of an object is called the genus of the object.

There are two types of filters which can be used to correct the topology of an input segmentation: foreground filters and background filters. Handles removed by a background filter correspond to tunnels filled in the foreground object. In the algorithm described here, both filters are applied at continuously increasing scales until all topology errors are fixed. Figure 2 shows the idea behind the development of each step. Morphological opening is used as a multiscale analyzer to detect handles at different scales. Figure 2b shows how the opening operation divides the foreground object into two classes.

Points in the largest connected component of the opened object are called body points, and points in the residue of the original object and body set are called residue points (Fig. 2c). Thus, the body set consists of one and the residue set of many connected components. This method was designed to transfer as many points as possible from the residue back to the body component. Unfortunately, with complex shapes as in brain segmentations, opening can create "false" tunnels in the body component. Thus, the body set must be grown without introducing handles, but with filling the "false" tunnels. This can be done by

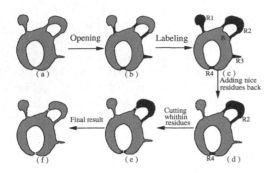

Fig. 2. Illustration of the basic idea behind the approach [7]

only adding nice points [2] from the residue set. The nice points can be detected like the simple points defined in [6].

Definition 5 (Nice Point) *Suppose that we add a point from the background object $\bar{X}$ to the foreground object X. It is a nice point if and only if $T_n(x, X) = 1$. It is equivalent to say that the n-components of X are preserved.*

The concept of nice points is necessary because morphological opening can introduce tunnels in the body, and these should be filled. Since a simple point must satisfy two topological criteria – $T_n(x, X) = T_{\bar{n}}(x, \bar{X}) = 1$ – and a nice point only needs to satisfy one, $T_n(x, X) = 1$, adding a simple point to the body preserves the topology of the body, but adding a nice point allows a tunnel in the body to be filled. The morphological opening was done by using a distance transform. The distance of a point within the object to its surface is the length of the shortest line to the surface. The chamfer distance transform is a quick way to calculate this distance. The morphological opening sequentially applies morphological eroding and morphological dilating: The erosion with a threshold r removes all points of the object with a distance less than or equal to r. This distance is the scale r. The dilation adds all points of the background with a distance less than or equal to r to the surface after the erosion. If there are regions within a handle which cannot fit a ball of radius r, then the handle can be broken into body and residue parts. For each residue component R, we performed the following iterative procedure:

Algorithm 1. Residue Component Expansion (RCE):

1. Recursively add each point of R to the body set B if it is a nice point. If each point of R is added back, then stop; otherwise, go to step 2 (Fig 2d).
2. From R, find the set S of residue points that are adjacent to the body B.
3. Find and label all connected components in the set S.
4. Take the largest connected component L.
5. For each point of L, add it back to B if it is a nice point (Fig. 2d-f).
6. If no points can be added back, stop; otherwise, go to step 2.

Note that in steps 2-5, the largest set of border points (if there are nice points) is added to the body. The criterion of nice points ensures that the final

Fig. 3. WM/GM surface before and after topology corrections

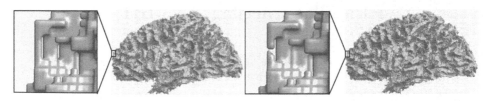

residue points are not added back to the body and are positioned at the thinnest parts of the handles.

3   Results and Discussion

We applied the method to the labeled version of the ICBM single subject MRI anatomical template (www.loni.ucla.edu/ICBM/ICBM_BrainTemplate.html). The image size is $304 \times 362 \times 309$ voxels. Cortical gyri, subcortical structures and the cerebellum are assigned a unique label.

Processing time for each volume was between 0-7 minutes except the white matter segmentation on an Intel Pentium IV 3.0-GHz CPU. Processing time for the white matter segmentation volume was about 14 minutes. The tessellation of each topologically corrected segmentation has the topology of a sphere, i.e, it has an Euler characteristic of two [2], corresponding to a genus of zero. Fig. 3 shows two sample rendered surfaces before and after topology correction. This algorithm changed between 0.0% and 1.8% of the voxels for each of the segmented volumes of the labeled ICBM atlas, with an average of 0.05%.

References

1. Shattuck D, Leahy M. Automated graph-based analysis and correction of cortical volume topology. IEEE Trans Med Imaging 2001;20(11):1167–1177.
2. Han X, Xu C, Neto U, Prince JL. Topology correction in brain cortex segmentation using a multiscale, graph-based algorithm. IEEE Trans Med Imaging 2002;21(2):109–121.
3. Chen L, Wagenknecht G. Automated topology correction for human brain segmentation. Procs MICCAI 2006;2:316–323.
4. Wood Z, Hoppe H, Desbrun M, Schroeder P. Removing excess topology from isosurfaces. ACM Transactions on Graphics 2004;23:190–208.
5. Kriegeskorte N, Goebel R. An efficient algorithm for topologically correct segmentation of the cortical sheet in anatomical MR volumes. NeuroImage 2001;14:329–346.
6. Bertrand G. Simple points, topological numbers and geodesic neighborhoods in cubic grids. Pattern Recognition Letters 1994;15:1028–1032.
7. Chen L, Wagenknecht G. Topology correction in brain segmentation using a multiscale algorithm. Advances in Medical Engineering, in Proceedings in Physics 2006.

Semi-automatic Segmentation of the Patellar Cartilage in MRI

Lorenz König[1], Martin Groher[1], Andreas Keil[1], Christian Glaser[2],
Maximilian Reiser[2], Nassir Navab[1]

[1]Chair for Computer Aided Medical Procedures, Technische Universität München
[2]Department of Clinical Radiology, Ludwig-Maximilians-Universität München
Email: koenigl@in.tum.de

Abstract. A software system for semi-automatic segmentation of the patellar cartilage is introduced. Providing tools for sub-pixel accurate edge tracing, automatic contour completion, and adequate visualization we achieve a remarkable speed-up of the physician's segmentation process. The exactness for cartilage segmentation can be reached if expertise and automation are merged in a meaningful way.

1 Introduction

Damage to the articular cartilage is an early and decisive step in the development of osteoarthritis (OA) a major socio-economic burden nowadays. This disease is among the ten leading causes of continued disability world-wide and annual costs associated with OA are estimated to amount up to the equivalent of 1 % of total productivity in the USA. This is the motivation to develop and to continuously refine therapies dedicated to cartilage repair contributing to at least postpone and to slow down the development and progression of OA. This, in turn, creates a strong need for non-invasive, accurate, and valid tools to establish appropriate indications for new treatment options, to monitor the disease process and to control therapeutic efficacy. MRI, especially with recent advances in scanner, coil and sequence design, is ideally suited for non-invasivly evaluating the cartilage. In this respect and especially in view of statistical discriminatory power, quantitative data are desirable in contrast to more or less subjective semiquantitative evaluation by scoring methods. Such data would be cartilage volume, thickness and the size of the cartilage bone interface, all of these parameters being directly related with the disease process.

2 State of the Art

Several methods and tools for segmentation of the patellar cartilage in MR images have been presented so far [1, 2, 3]. Some of them fully rely on manual segmentation, which makes them cumbersome for daily routine. Some tools perform the segmentation more or less automatically and require the user only to define a region of interest, for instance. In general, non-manual segmentation methods rely on gradient information from the image.

Depending on the MRI sequence used in the aquisition, however, slices with no contrast between the patellar cartilage and the adjacent femoral cartilage have to be segmented. In these cases, the radiologists have to rely on their experience for segmenting the cartilage and therefore must be in full control of the segmentation process. Tools not allowing for that will hardly be accepted among physicians.

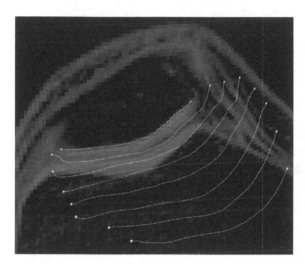

Fig. 1. MRI of the knee with poor contrast between the patellar (above) and femoral (below) cartilages: the perspective visualization of the segmented cartilage bone interface is visualized throughout the slices.

3   Method

We present a robust system to support radiologists in semi-automatically segmenting patellar cartilage in MRI images in daily routine, which does not restrict manual control of the segmentation process but at the same time facilitates this task.

We work on three-dimensional one-channel data sets as supplied by the MRI scanners. The data is organized as an array of slices $s^z(x, y)$. The ratio of slice distance to in-slice pixel distance is about 5 to 10, and the slices are in most cases oriented perpendicular to the bone cartilage interface and cartilage surface. We therefore decided to do the segmentation in 2D slice by slice. Accordingly, the preprocessing (3.1) is done in 2D.

The segmented regions in each of the slices are described by their sub-pixel accurate boundaries. The boundaries are in turn represented by a sequence of fragments, any of which can be manually drawn (3.2) or semi-automatically computed (3.3) as well as corrected (3.4) at any time.

To support review of the results of segmentation, we provide a view of the current slice superimposed with the segmentation of adjacent slices (using an orthographic projection) as well as a perspective visualization of the segmentation as in fig. 1. In Section 3.5, we introduce a unified projection matrix, which allows for smooth transitions between orthographic and perspective projection without the user getting lost.

3.1 Sub-pixel Edge Detection

Sub-pixel edge detection is an important preprocessing step of the proposed system. Edge detection is done in 2D separately for each slice $s^z(x, y)$ using a 2D facet model [4]. The idea is to find the maxima in the gradient image

$$g(x, y) = |\mathfrak{g}(x, y)| = \left| \begin{pmatrix} s_x^z(x, y) \\ s_y^z(x, y) \end{pmatrix} \right| = \left| \begin{pmatrix} \frac{\partial}{\partial x} s^z(x, y) \\ \frac{\partial}{\partial y} s^z(x, y) \end{pmatrix} \right|$$

which is obtained using the Sobel operator. In the following, we describe the algorithm for one pixel at (i, j).

Based on the 3×3 environment of (i, j), the gradient image g is locally approximated by a second degree polynomial in two variables $p(x, y)$. The maximum of p along the straight line defined by the gradient vector $\mathfrak{g}$ indicates a point E on the edge in the original image s. If E lies within the boundaries of the pixel at (i, j), we accept E as an edge point for further processing. We also label it with the value of $g(i, j)$ to indicate the sharpness of the edge at this point.

This is done for all the pixels in every slice. The result is a set of edge points and their respective sharpness for each slice.

3.2 Manual Tracing of Contours

As a first interaction step, we provide tools to manually trace edges for segmentation. This can be accomplished by drawing with the mouse (also with sub-pixel accuracy), as well as by relying on the previously computed edge points. In the latter case, for every point the mouse cursor passes, the edge points in a window around the cursor are weighted depending on the distance to the cursor and the sharpness of the edge they represent. Thus, the contour made up by these points is close to the trace of the mouse cursor, and is located on a sharp edge of the current slice with sub-pixel accuracy.

3.3 Semi-automatic Tracing and Propagation of Contours

We also provide the user with a tool to semi-automatically find the contours of the patella. User interaction is minimized to the input of a starting point A and an end point B of the contour fragment to be traced. Between A and B, a guiding contour c is constructed either from previously segmented contours in adjacent slices, if there exist any. Otherwise, we simply use a straight line. The contour fragment f to be found is initialized with A. Let E denote the last point of f.

The guiding contour is then discretized into a sequence of control points C_i at steps of one third of a pixel. For each C_i, the following steps are performed: (1) A set of edge points having a distance of less than 5 pixels to the end E of f is computed. (2) These edge points are weighted with respect to (a) their respective gradient magnitude, (b) their distance from E, (c) their position relative to E compared to the direction of c in the environment of C_i, (d) their position relative to E compared to the direction of f at E, and (e) whether they are farther from C_i than E. The weight for (e) increases as C_i gets closer to B. (3) The edge point with the highest weight is appended to f, if it is different from its current end point E.

Thus, a contour fragment f is constructed, that consists of rather uniformly spaced edge points with high magnitude, is shaped smoothly and similar to the guiding contour c.

3.4   Correction and User Interaction

Correction of segmentation results (be they generated automatically or manually) is simply done by re-drawing the part of the contour that is to be corrected. Similar to the manual segmentation, re-drawing can be done either fully manually or based on the previously calculated edge points. For the first and last point of a newly drawn contour fragment, the respective closest point on an existing contour is determined. If they belong to the same contour, the section in-between is replaced with the new contour. Similarly, open contours can be extended and shortened.

3.5   Unified Projection Matrix

Standard OpenGL projection matrices are limited either to orthographic projection or perspective projection. We therefore propose a unified projection matrix depending on a parameter p to control perspective foreshortening and on parameters d_x, d_y to control perspective displacement (Fig. 2). If $p = 0$, the unified projection matrix is of the same shape as an orthographic projection matrix. If $p > 0$, perspective foreshortening is enabled and the projection becomes perspective.

$$
\begin{bmatrix} * & 0 & 0 & * \\ 0 & * & 0 & * \\ 0 & 0 & * & * \\ 0 & 0 & 0 & 1 \end{bmatrix}
\qquad
\begin{bmatrix} * & 0 & * & 0 \\ 0 & * & * & 0 \\ 0 & 0 & * & * \\ 0 & 0 & 1 & 0 \end{bmatrix}
\qquad
\begin{bmatrix} * & 0 & d_x & 0 \\ 0 & * & d_y & 0 \\ 0 & 0 & * & * \\ 0 & 0 & -p & 1 \end{bmatrix}
$$
$$
\text{(a)} \qquad\qquad \text{(b)} \qquad\qquad \text{(c)}
$$

Fig. 2. Standard OpenGL orthographic projection matrix (a) and perspective projection matrix (b) compared to unified projection matrix (c)

4 Results

Tools and algorithms were implemented in C++ using a Qt-based User Interface and OpenGL as graphics engine. We segmented a set of MR images of healthy patellae, which were acquired using a FLASH sequence.

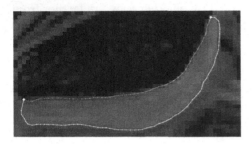

Fig. 3. Segmentation of the patellar cartilage in one slice with sub-pixel accuracy. The contour fragments show the cartilage bone inteface (gray, top) and cartilage surface (white, bottom) respectively. The nodes in the contour indicate the edge points that were determined in the preprocessing step.

Semi-automatic tracing and propagation of contours turned out to be highly effective on the cartilage bone interface (fig. 3). This technique was also successfully conducted on the cartilage surface in some cases, whereas in cases like the one in fig. 1 manual segmentation was required.

5 Discussion

We introduced a semi-automatic segmentation system for patellar cartilage extraction. Its slice-by-slice approach corresponds to the way radiologists are used to look at anatomy and thus enables radiologists to directly transfer their day-to-day experience in the segmentation process without any relevant training period. The focus of the system lies on user-friendliness instead of purely automatic procedures. We believe this to be more vital for a speed-up in segmentation, which is expected by clinicians to save 50 % of the time used on the segmentation task nowadays, using fully manual tools.

References

1. Stammberger T. Entwicklung von Bildverarbeitungsmethoden zur quantitativen Analyse des Gelenkknorpels in der Magnetresonanztomographie. Ph.D. thesis. Institut für Radiologische Diagnostik der Ludwig-Maximilians-Universität München; 1999.
2. Pirnog CD. Articular Cartilage Segmentation and Tracking in Sequential MR Images of the Knee. Ph.D. thesis. ETH Zürich; 2005.
3. Cohen ZA, McCarthy DM, Kwak SD, Legrand P, Fogarasi F, Ciaccio EJ, et al. Knee cartilage topography, thickness, and contact areas from MRI: In-vitro calibration and in-vivo measurements. Osteoarthritis Cartilage 1999;7(1):95–109.
4. Haralick RM, Shapiro LG. Computer and Robot Vision. vol. 1. Reading, Massachusetts, USA: Addison-Wesley; 1992.

Angiographic Assessment of Myocardial Perfusion Using Correlation Analysis

Yu Deuerling-Zheng[1], Jan Boese[1], Stephan Achenbach[2] and Josef Ludwig[2]

[1]Siemens Medical Solutions, Forchheim, Germany
[2]Cardiology, Friedrich-Alexander-University, Erlangen, Germany
Email: yu.deuerling-zheng@siemens.com

Abstract. Although angiography was originally designed as a morphological imaging modality, it is increasingly demanded to retrieve functional information from conventional angiograms. As X-ray angiography provides only 2D projection images, its most significant advantage over volumetric imaging modalities is its high temporal resolution. Thus the angiographic functional imaging relies mainly on the analysis of the temporal variation of single pixels or local regions. In order to assess the myocardial perfusion, the myocardium has to be recognized at first. This can be solved similarly with analysis of the time-intensity curves. Compared to most approaches in which the characteristic of the time-intensity curves are classified, our proposed method based on correlation analysis has the advantage of using all the sampled data points so that it is more robust against noise or outliers. As the correlation coefficient considers only the colinearity of two curves, we add the information about the amplitude and the numerical range of the curves, which further improves the recognition of the myocardium.

1 Introduction

Percutaneous coronary intervention (PCI) – also known as coronary angioplasty – is an established treatment strategy for acute myocardial infarction (AMI). The goal is to open the occluded infarct artery to facilitate prompt reperfusion of ischemic myocardium. Since the introduction of PCI, much effort has been done to retrieve functional information out of angiograms for the assessment of reperfusion.

Due to the high concentration of the contrast agent in the arteries, initial efforts were focused on measuring the blood flow in the coronary arteries. However, it has been shown that the opening of the stenosis in the epicardial artery does not necessarily lead to improvement of the microvascular circulation. To assess the perfusion directly at the capillary level, two dedicated measures are proposed: TIMI Myocardial Perfusion Grade (TMPG) [1] and Myocardial Blush Grade (MBG) [2]. TMPG emphasizes the dynamic of the contrast enhancement while MBG characterizes the contrast enhancement rather by its density or brightness.

Clinical trials have shown that both TMPG and MBG are independent pre-dictors for the long-term outcome of patients with AMI [1, 2]. They correlate well with other non-angiographic measures and the mortality. However, these two measures are assessed nowadays only visually in a few core labs worldwide. An automated and objective tool for angiographic assessment of myocardial perfusion has recently become the research of interest for both physicians and computer scientists.

2   State of the Art

Recognition of the myocardium is the essential prerequisite for the (re-)perfusion assessment. While the coronary arteries filled with dye show normally high con-trast and sharp edges, the myocardium is usually rather low-contrasted with the ground-glass appearance ("blush") without clear boundaries. Therefore, recog-nition of the myocardium remains a challenging task for angiographic perfusion assessment.

Principally, the efforts for the recognition of myocardium can be divided into two categories:

1. *Morphological approach*: outline the region of interest (ROI) for the blush out of a single frame based on morphological analysis and track the ROI in the consecutive frames [3]. The drawback of this approach is that the blush must show sufficient contrast to ensure its differentiation from other structures.
2. *Temporal approach*: retrieve the time-intensity curve for each pixel or local region and differentiate the myocardium according to the characteristics of the time-intensity curves, such as the maximum amplitude and the time to maximum amplitude [4, 5]. This approach is preferable because it directly analyzes the temporal information, which emphasizes the basic advantage of angiography. However, it is also inherently sensitive to object misalignment between the frames, which is unavoidable in coronary angiograms due to respiratory and cardiac motion. Motion compensation is thus one of the main research interests in this field nowadays [4, 5].

3   Methods – Correlation Analysis

Structures in angiographic series can be differentiated from each other by clas-sifying the features of their time-intensity curves (Fig. 1). The most commonly used features are the maximum amplitude and the time to maximum amplitude. This requires that the features are extracted in a robust manner, for instance with previous elimination of outliers, which is however in practice computation-ally highly intensive. In this work, an approach based on correlation analysis of the time-intensity curves is presented. This approach has been applied to separate pulmonary arteries and veins in 3D MR angiography [6]. After manu-ally selecting a region of interest (ROI) to define the reference, the correlation

Fig. 1. Time-intensity curves of contrast-enhanced coronary artery, myocardium and non contrast-enhanced background structures

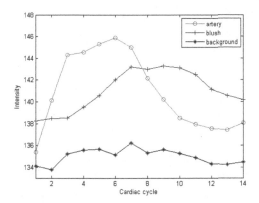

coefficient between time-intensity curve of the reference and those of all the local regions is computed. This is then used as a similarity measure between the reference and local regions. This approach has the advantage by using all the sampled data points in the time-intensity curve, which makes it less sensitive against outliers.

Let X and Y be the vectors containing the values of two time-intensity curves, $\bar{x}$ and $\bar{y}$ the mean of X and Y, respectively. The correlation coefficient between X and Y can be computed as in (Eq. 1). $c(X, Y)$ assumes values between -1 and $+1$ with the magnitude indicating the strength of the dependence. The correlation is positive if both X and Y increase or decrease together, and negative if Y decreases when X increases. If X and Y are said to be independent or uncorrelated, $c(X, Y)$ disappears

$$c(X, Y) = \frac{\sum_{i=1}^{n} (x_i - \bar{x})(y_i - \bar{y})}{\sqrt{\sum_{i=1}^{n} (x_i - \bar{x})^2 \sum_{i=1}^{n} (y_i - \bar{y})^2}} \qquad (1)$$

The correlation coefficient is *normalized*, i.e., it measures the similarity between X and Y only by considering their colinearity, with the magnitude of X and Y being ignored. Moreover, X and Y are shifted to the zero mean so that the actual numerical range is not considered either. However, the time-intensity curves of different tissues differ not only in the phase but also in the amplitude and the value range of the intensity. For the purpose of an accurate discrimination, it is important to take into account as many as possible discriminating features, for instance as following

$$F_a = \frac{\min(A_x, A_y)}{\max(A_x, A_y)} \qquad F_g = \frac{\min(\bar{x}, \bar{y})}{\max(\bar{x}, \bar{y})} \qquad c'(X, Y) = F_a^p \cdot F_g^q \cdot c(X, Y) \qquad (2)$$

where A_x and A_y are the amplitude (difference between the maximal and minimal intensity) of X and Y, respectively. Both F_a and F_g assume values in $(0,1]$ with p and q as weighting exponents.

4   Results

The angiographic data sets used in this work are acquired with a C-Arm system (AXIOM Artis, Siemens Medical Solutions). Analyzing time-intensity curves of single pixels or local regions assumes that the frames of an angiographic series are spatially aligned. To avoid respiratory motion, angiograms are acquired with patient breath holding. To avoid cardiac motion, a retrospective ECG-gating is performed to select only the frames corresponding to a certain cardiac phase. The resulting time-intensity curves contain normally 10-20 data points.

The correlation coefficient illustrated in Section 3 serves as a similarity measure between two time-intensity curves. To outline the myocardium, a reference curve needs to be determined. This can be done either empirically out of a sufficient large number of data sets, or with user interaction by mouse clicking in the region of the myocardium. The latter is applied in this work since it can adjust variations between different acquisitions with only minimal user interaction. The correlation coefficient between the time-intensity curve of the reference and those of all the local regions is computed (which returns the so-called correlation coefficient map). The regions where the correlation coefficient is larger than a certain threshold are classified as myocardium.

Our experiments on 5 angiographic sequences of the right coronary artery show that the myocardium can be recognized with the proposed approach. Fig. 2 shows the result of an example. The contrast enhancement in the original angiogram is hardly visible while the correlation map shows a rather clear, connected bright area indicating high correlation with the reference curve. The myocardium could be recognized after thresholding of the correlation coefficient. It can also be seen that there are sporadically distributed regions in the background which are falsely recognized as myocardium.

5   Discussion

As mentioned in Section 3, correlation analysis has the advantage of using all the data points in the time-intensity curve, which is more robust against noise and outliers. Outliers in the time-intensity curve occur quite often because motion during coronary angiography can usually not be avoided or corrected completely by breath-holding and ECG-gating. Therefore, to reduce noise or outliers, the time-intensity curve is retrieved not for single pixels but for a local region of pixels, with the mean of the local region as one data point in the curve. Dedicated approach for motion compensation is currently under working process. Similarly, for the sake of a reliable reference curve, it is to be recommended that the reference defined by a sufficient large region of interest.

Fig. 2. (a) A frame of the original angiogram acquired after contrast injection in the right coronary artery (RCA). The related myocardium is slightly darker than the surrounding structures, which is however hardly visible. (b) The correlation coefficient map showing local correlations with a reference region selected within the myocardium, bright for high correlation and dark for low correlation. (c) The recognized myocardium: regions with a correlation coefficient larger than a threshold of 0.5 are marked with red blocks

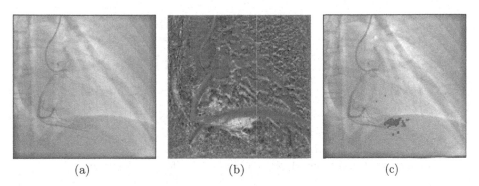

(a)   (b)   (c)

We have shown that correlation analysis is a feasible approach to recognize contrast-enhanced myocardium in angiograms. This is the first step for the further perfusion assessment of the myocardium. Correlation analysis can be applied to assess the myocardial perfusion as well. As MBG emphasizes the perfusion mainly by the strength of the blush which corresponds to the amplitude of the time-intensity curve, correlation analysis is more advantageous for the assessment with TMPG. Nevertheless, it should be pointed out that correlation analysis can not be used to recognize static objects whose time-intensity curve is flat. In case of TMPG=0 where no contrast agent enters the myocardium, special consideration must be taken into account.

References

1. Gibson C, et al. Coronary and myocardial angiography: Angiographic assessment of both epicardial and myocardial perfusion. Circulation 2004;109(25):3096–3125.
2. van't Hof A, et al. Angiographic assessment of myocardial reperfusion in patients treated with primary angioplasty for acute myocardial infarction: Myocardial blush grade. Circulation 1998;97(23):2302–2306.
3. Condurache A, et al. User-defined ROI tracking of the myocardial blush grade. Procs IEEE Southwest Symposium on Image Analysis and Interpretation 2006; 66–70.
4. Esbacher M, Dickhaus H, Kücherer H. Computergestützte Auswertung koronarangiographischer Bildfolgen hinsichtlich des Myocardialen Blushgrades. Procs BVM 2006; 241–245.
5. Malsch U, Dickhaus H, Kücherer H. Quantitative Analyse von Koronarangiographischen Bildfolgen zur Bestimmung der Myokardperfusion. Procs BVM 2003; 81–85.
6. Bock M, et al. Separation of arteries and veins in 3D MR angiography using correlation analysis. Magn Reson Med 2000; 481–487.

Towards Automated OCT-based Identification of White Brain Matter

Lukas Ramrath[1], Ulrich G. Hofmann[2], Gereon Huettmann[3],
Andreas Moser[4] and Achim Schweikard[5]

[1,5]Institut für Robotik und Kognitive Systeme,
[2]Institut für Signalverarbeitung und Prozessrechentechnik,
[3]Institut für Biomedizinische Optik,
[4]Klinik für Neurologie, UK-SH, Campus Lübeck, 23538 Lübeck
Email: ramrath@rob.uni-luebeck.de

Abstract. A novel model-based identification of white brain matter in OCT A-scans is proposed. Based on nonlinear energy operators used in the classification of neural activity, candidates for white matter structures are extracted from a baseline-corrected signal. Validation of candidates is done by evaluating the correspondence to a simplified intensity model which is parametrized beforehand. Results for identification of white matter in rat brain *in vitro* show the capability of the proposed algorithm.

1 Introduction

Optical coherence tomography (OCT) is a powerful, real-time technique for investigating depth structure of biological tissue. Since entering the field of medical imaging it has been well established for imaging purposes in certain medical disciplines e.g. ophthalmology and dermatology [1]. Major advantages are the high resolution, the video-rate scanning capability, and the non-invasive nature of OCT-imaging. Recent research results show that OCT is also applicable to image brain morphology ex vivo and in vitro [2]. This motivates the usage of OCT for identification of brain structure which is of interest in other neurosurgery applications. As white matter provides a high-contrast structure in brain tissue, it is one of the best candidates for OCT-based identification. This contribution concentrates on an automated identification of white matter based on OCT-signals. Based on a simplified signal model of OCT and spike detection algorithms from neural acitivity analysis, a two-stage identification process is proposed. Capability of the algorithm is shown by identifying white matter in a coronal section of a rat brain.

2 State of the Art and New Contribution

Although OCT has been widely used to image tissue structures, little work has been done on brain imaging. Possible identification of white matter in OCT images has been shown for rat brains *in vitro* [3]. The authors analyzed the light intensity and attenuation coefficient of the backscattered signal based on Beer's law

$$I(z) = I_0 e^{-2\mu_t z} \tag{1}$$

where I_0 is the initial intensity, μ_t denotes the attenuation coefficient and z corresponds to the penetration depth. Results showed that I_0 and μ_t for a wavelength of 1300nm differ for various tissue structures (e.g cortex, external capsule) allowing a clear distinction of white and grey matter. In [4], the authors used a catheter-based OCT probe to examine the possibility of optical guidance in placing a deep brain stimulation electrode. OCT images were acquired by advancing the probe on characteristic tracks in human brains *in vitro*. Their results show that myelinated fibres are strong backscatterers of light and that penetration of light is shallow. Evaluation of OCT scans in both cases has been done manually and only for exclusive areas of white or grey brain matter. In areas where structures with different optical properties are scanned, Beer's law in equation (1) does not hold for the entire scan range. If multiple fibres of white matter are embedded into gray matter the signal features multiple peaks which are superimposed to the exponential decay. This establishes a backscattered signal featuring spiking intensity characteristics. Unfortunately, OCT images are subject to speckle noise which considerably distorts the acquired signal. Speckle noise is usually modeled as multiplicative Rayleigh distributed noise causing a signal-to-noise ratio (SNR) with a value of up to 1. This motivates the use of spike sorting and classification algorithms developed for analysis of neural activity where the signal-to-noise ratio is very low. Based on the model given in equation (1), a method of automated identification of white matter brain structures is proposed. It significantly improves the processing of OCT images of brain structures. This can be used to support an online validation of a desired path, to detect important areas or to improve consecutive steps like segmentation and registration to e.g. histology informations. Automated identification therefore leads to a better integration of OCT into neuronavigation settings.

3   Methods

Brain from a freshly decapitated rat was dissected in an ice-cold Krebs-bicarbonate buffer. A coronal section crossing the cortex, the external capsule and the striatum was scanned by a Swept Source OCT Microscope System (Thorlabs, Inc., Newton, USA) with a center wavelength of 1325nm and an axial scan rate of 16kHz. The field of view was was 2.14mm in depth (y), 3mm in transverse direction (x) and 5mm in dorsal direction (z). Figure 1 shows the coronal section and the intensities of a lateral OCT B-scan crossing the cortex, the external capsule and the striatum. Figure 2 shows an OCT scan at a lateral position of $x = 615\mu$m and the corresponding filtered and baseline-corrected signal. It can be seen that white matter corresponds to peaks in the local intensity neighborhood. As trauma reduction in neurosurgery applications is crucial, OCT probes are required to be as small as possible leading to a relatively small field of view.

Fig. 1. Coronal section and B-Scan of rat brain. Arrows mark corresponding structures

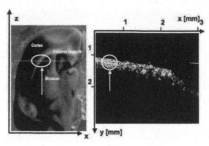

Fig. 2. (top) Log intensity versus penetration depth of a single A-scan and the corresponding baseline (bottom) baseline corrected and filtered signal

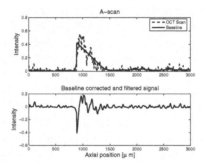

Peak identification in A-scans therefore presents a promising approach to find candidates for automated identification of white matter structures. Detection and sorting of spikes in noisy signals under very low signal-to-noise ratios has been extensively researched in the analysis of neural activity. In [5], the authors use a nonlinear energy operator (NEO) in order to extract action potentials from a recorded signal. The NEO-operator is given as

$$\psi_{\mathrm{NEO}}(x(n)) = x^2(n) - x(n+1)x(n-1) \tag{2}$$

where $x(n)$ denotes the measured signal at time or location n. Another extraction operator is introduced in [6]. The shift and multiply operator (SAM) is given by

$$\psi_{\mathrm{SAM}}(x(n)) = x(n-3)x(n-2)x(n-1)x(n) \tag{3}$$

Both operators have been used for the analysis of spiky waveforms in neural recordings which motivates the use of NEO and SAM to identify candidates of white matter structures in OCT signals. The subsequent classification of a spike is done by thresholding.

The proposed algorithm consists of 3 steps where the first step preprocesses the data by baseline correction. The baseline was determined by fitting a linear regression curve into the linear descent of the intensity curve. The baseline before and after the descent was calculated by taking the mean within a window of

Fig. 3. Detection of white matter: (top) proposed peaks; (bottom) validated peaks

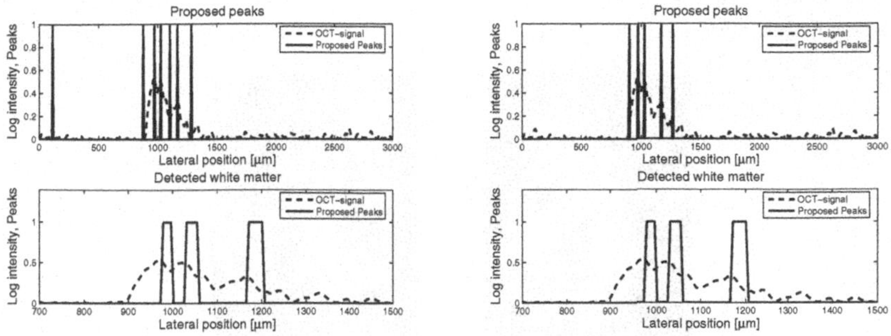

(a) NEO   (b) SAM

117.2μm. In a second step, the proposed operators are used to identify spikes in the baseline-corrected signal. This leads to a set of potential candidates for white matter structures. The third step is used to validate a potential spike and to determine the size of the structure by analyzing the slope in a local neighborhood of the spike candidate. Applying the log-operator on equation (1) yields a linear dependency of the log-intensity and the attenuation coefficient μ. For white matter, μ_t takes a characteristic value. The value $\mu_{t,ref}$ for white brain matter which can be identified by evaluating a set of test images where the white brain matter is classified manually. The parameters I_0 and μ_t at the position $z = z_1$ are subsequently identified by a fitting a linear regression curve into the intensity curve within a local neighborhood of z_1 e.g. in the interval $[z_1 - c_1 \ldots z_1 + c_1]$ where c_1 denotes the size of the local neighborhood. Now, the regression result μ_t is compared to the manually classified $\mu_{t,ref}$. If μ_t lies in a user defined interval $[\mu - \sigma, \mu + \sigma]$, position z_1 is classified as white matter.

4 Results

The proposed algorithm was tested with the following parameter settings $\sigma_{NEO} = \sigma_{SAM} = 0.02$, $c_1 = 1$ and $\mu = 0.005$. Figure 3 shows the results of the detection by the NEO for one A-scan. It can be seen that both operators are able to identify peaks in noisy environment. The subsequent classification via slope identification excludes wrong propositions (e.g. the first proposition which corresponds to a negative spike in the baseline corrected signal). Figure 4 shows an automated identification for all A-scans of the acquired B-scan for the SAM operator. Identified white matter is shown as white dots in the total image. It can be seen that the detected white matter shows good correspondence to the manual classification.

Fig. 4. White matter detection for all A-scans: (left) original image with circles indicating white matter areas (right) automatically identified white matter with white dots indicate detection

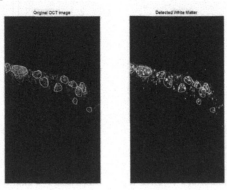

5   Discussion

The proposed algorithm is able to detect white brain matter reliably in speckle noise corrupted OCT A-scans. Tuning of the parameters, essentially the respective thresholds, based on heuristic experiences might lead to better performance. It is important to note that the algorithm is signal-based. Peaks resulting from the stochastic speckle distribution in the A-scan image might therefore be proposed falsely in the first place. The second step, however, provides a validation of a proposition by analysing the correspondance of the local neighborhood to a simplified OCT-intensity model. This results in a robust classification of white structures.

References

1. Bouma BE, Tearney GJ. Handbook Of Optical Coherence Tomography. Marcel Dekker, Inc.; 2002.
2. Boehringer HJ, Boller D, Leppert J, et al. Time-domain and spectral-domain optical coherence tomography in the analysis of brain tumor tissue. Lasers in Surgery and Medicine 2006;38:588–597.
3. Jeon SW, Shure MA, Baker KB, etal. Optical coherence tomography and optical coherence domain reflectometry for deep brain stimulation probe guidance. Procs SPIE 2005;5686:487–494.
4. Safri MS, Farhang S, Tang RS, et al. Optical coherence tomography in the diagnosis and treatment of neurological disorders. J Biomed Opt 2005;10(5):1–11.
5. Kim KW, Kim SJ. Neural spike sorting under nearly 0-dB signal-to-noise ratio using nonlinear energy operator and artificial neural-network classifier. IEEE Trans Biomed Eng 2000;47:1406–1411.
6. Menne KL. Computerassistenz zur Implantation von Tiefenhirnstimulatoren. Ph.D. thesis. University of Luebeck; 2005.

Vollautomatische Vorverarbeitung und rigide Registrierung zur Rekonstruktion von Bildern histologischer Stufenschnitte der Rattenleber

Anna Weinhold[1,2], Stefan Wirtz[1], Andrea Schenk[1], Tobias Böhler[1],
Xiaoyi Jiang[2], Uta Dahmen[3], Olaf Dirsch[4], Heinz-Otto Peitgen[1]

[1]MeVis Research, [2]Westfälische Wilhelms-Universität Münster,
[3]Universitätsklinikum Essen, [4]Klinikum der Universität Köln
Email: anna.weinhold@uni-muenster.de

Zusammenfassung. Im klinischen Einsatz ist die Leberlebendspende, bei der vom Spender ein Teil der Leber entfernt und dem Empfänger eingesetzt wird, bereits ein vielfach durchgeführter Eingriff. Die Leber ist eincs der wenigen Organe, das sich vollständig regenerieren kann. Der genaue Regenerationsprozess und die notwendigen Voraussetzungen dafür sind allerdings noch nicht geklärt. Im Laborversuch werden regenerierte Restlebern von Ratten histologisch untersucht, um so Einflussfaktoren der Regeneration genau studieren zu können. In dieser Arbeit wird erstmals cin Verfahren vorgestellt, dass die Verarbeitung der histologischen Schnitte von der vollautomatischen Vorverarbeitung bis hin zur rigiden Registrierung vereint. Dadurch wird der zeitaufwändige Prozess der Rekonstruktion nicht nur erheblich verkürzt, sondern auch robust und reproduzierbar gemacht.

1 Einleitung

Die Leber ist ein Organ, das in der Lage ist, sich vollständig zu regenerieren. Daher wird in der Leberchirurgie die Leberlebendspende durchgeführt, bei der der Empfänger statt einer vollständigen Leber nur einen Teil der Leber erhält, die sich dann zu einem vollwertigen Organ regenerieren kann. Ebenso regeneriert sich die Leber des Spenders. Um die Regenerationsleistung der Leber genau analysieren zu können, wurden bei dieser Studie im Laborversuch Rattenlebern untersucht. Den Ratten wird durch Resektion 90% des Lebervolumens entfernt. Nach einer Regenerationszeit von 24 bis 72 Stunden wird das regenerierende Organ vollständig entnommen und histologisch zu Stufenschnitten weiterverarbeitet [1]. Dazu wird die Restleber in Paraffin eingebettet und anschließend werden in axialer Ausrichtung in einem Abstand von $500 \mu m$ Schichten mit einer Dicke von $4 \mu m$ vom Paraffinblock abgeschnitten und mit Hämatoxilin-Eosin eingefärbt. Mit einem Videomikroskop werden die Gewebeschnitte mit einer Auflösung von $10 \mu m$ pro Pixel digitalisiert. Pro Datensatz entstehen 50-62 Farbbilder mit ca. (1000×800) bis (2200×1800) Pixeln. Eine direkte Superpositionierung der Schichten ist durch die manuelle Datenakquisition nicht möglich. Vor weitergehen-

Abb. 1. Eine Schicht aus der Serie der Bilder histologischer Schnitte zu verschiedenen Zeitpunkten der ersten Phase der Registrierung. (a) Original Farbbild mit Hintergrundrauschen durch Verunreinigungen und bei der Digitalisierung entstandenen schwarzen Rand. (b) Grauwertbild nach der Hauptachsentransformation der RGB-Kanäle. (c) Maskiertes Grauwertbild. Die Verunreinigungen wurden eliminiert und der Hintergrund auf einen homogenen Grauwert gesetzt

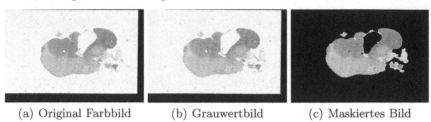

(a) Original Farbbild   (b) Grauwertbild   (c) Maskiertes Bild

den 3D-Analysen, z.B. einer Gefäßbaumextraktion, ist die Korrektur der Verformungen der Präparate essenziell. Durch den Herstellungsprozess entstehen Verunreinigungen durch Staub, Haare oder Fingerabdrücke, Verformungen und Unterschiede in der Repräsentierung durch unterschiedliche Färbung. Bei der Digitalisierung wird zusätzlich in jedem Bild ein unterschiedlich ausgeprägter schwarzer Randbereich (Abb. 1) erzeugt. Das vorgestellte Verfahren extrahiert den Hintergrund vollautomatisch, so dass eine dreidimensionale Rekonstruktion der Schnitte möglich wird.

2   Stand der Forschung und Fortschritt durch den Beitrag

Um eine dreidimensionale Rekonstruktion der Bilder zu ermöglichen, ist eine besonders zeitaufwändige Vorverarbeitung notwendig. Diese Vorverarbeitung wird in der Regel von Hand mit einem Grafikprogramm durchgeführt (siehe [2]), indem nach einer einfachen Konvertierung der Farb- in Grauwertbilder und der Beseitigung von Störungen im Hintergrund die Bilder gedreht und zentriert werden. Diese Arbeit ist daher nicht einfach reproduzierbar. Erst nach einer guten Vorverarbeitung und affiner Korrektur lassen sich High-Level Verfahren, wie in [3, 4, 5] vorgestellt, einsetzen. Der wesentliche Fortschritt durch diesen Beitrag besteht damit in der vollautomatischen Verarbeitung vom ersten Bild bis hin zur linearen Rekonstruktion. Anschließende Frei-Form-Registrierungen wie die elastische Registrierung lassen sich dadurch mit idealen und reproduzierbaren Voraussetzungen anwenden. Die Integration einer solchen Registrierung in den vollautomatischen Prozess ist in der Planung.

3   Methoden

Zur Konvertierung der Bilder in Grauwertdaten wird eine Hauptachsentransformation [6] auf den Farbkanälen durchgeführt, um die redundante Information in den RGB-Kanälen auf einen essentiellen Kanal zu reduzieren. Die Maskierung des Präparates wird in mehrere Schritte unterteilt. Zunächst wird der künstliche schwarze Rand im Hintergrund entfernt. Mit einem Laplacefilter wird das Objekt vom Hintergrund getrennt. Staub, Haare, Fingerabdrücke und andere Artefakte im Bereich des Hintergrunds bleiben neben dem Objekt zunächst erhalten. Eine geschickte Kombination verschiedener morphologischer Operatoren erlaubt die Verkleinerung, teilweise Eliminierung dieser Verunreinigungen. Anschließend werden zusammenhängende Komponenten detektiert und die Objekt-Komponenten anhand ihrer Größe ausgewählt. Die so entstandenen binären Masken werden morphologisch geglättet, um kleine Löcher und Randartefakte in den Masken zu beseitigen. Für die Registrierung der maskierten Grauwertbilder wird zunächst der Schwerpunkt des Präparats in jeder Schicht berechnet und eine Überlagerung dieser Schwerpunkte durch Translation erreicht. Im zweiten Schritt der Rekonstruktion wird für alle Schichten sukzessive eine rigide Transformation berechnet, wobei mit der Schicht mit dem größten Präparatsvolumen begonnen und zu den Enden der Leber hin fortgeschritten wird. Zur Registrierung wird eine Gauß-Newton Optimierung zur Minimierung des Least-Squares-Fehlers zwischen je zwei Schichten verwendet [7]. Zur weiteren Effizienzsteigerung, Beschleunigung und Umgehung lokaler Minima wird ein Multiresolutionsansatz, basierend auf einer Gaußpyramide, verwendet. Um die Schichten, die zueinander stark rotiert sind, korrekt registrieren zu können, werden insgesamt für eine Schicht vier Registrierungsdurchläufe gestartet, die sich ausschließlich in der Ausrichtung der zu registrierenden Schicht unterscheiden. Die Ausrichtung wird durch Rotation um den Schwerpunkt um 90°, 180° und 270° variiert. Das bzgl. des Fehlermaßes beste Ergebnis gilt dann als Korrektur (*best-of-four*-Registrierung). Um eine optische Kontrolle zu ermöglichen, werden die Ergebnisse dreidimensional durch ein Volumenrendering und zweidimensional in Orthogonalansichten dargestellt.

4   Ergebnisse

Die vorgestellte Methode wurde vollständig in MeVisLab [8] implementiert. Nach der Auswahl eines Datensatzes erfolgen alle Schritte der Rekonstruktion (Farbanalyse, Maskierung, Registrierung) vollautomatisch. Bei einem Datensatz wie in unseren Versuchsreihen mit 50-62 Bildern und einer Auflösung von bis zu (2200×1800) Pixeln pro Bild kann nach einer Rechenzeit von ca. einer Stunde auf einem PC die fertige Rekonstruktion analysiert werden. Die Analyse der Farbkanäle ergab im Mittel eine Gewichtung der Kanäle Rot, Grün und Blau von $(0.3223, 0.339, 0.3387)$. Die Maskierung des Präparates erfolgte zuverlässig. Verunreinigungen konnten eliminiert und abgetrennte Präparatstücke gefunden und mit einbezogen werden. In den drei durchgeführten Versuchsreihen, in denen Datensätze ohne weitere Vorverarbeitung dem Verfahren zugeführt wurden, konnten bei 93% der Schnitte die Artefakte vollständig eliminiert werden. Bei den übrig gebliebenen Schichten handelt es sich bei den Artefakten um Fingerabdrücke bzw. Farbflecken, die aufgrund ihrer Größe und farblichen Darstellung nicht vom Objekt automatisch unterschieden werden konnten. Eine visuelle Kontrolle durch einen Experten ergab, dass die Qualität der automatischen Objekt-

Abb. 2. 3D-Darstellung des gesamten Datensatzes: komplette Schichten nach Überlagerung der Schwerpunkte (a), maskierte Bilder (b), Rekonstruktion nach Registrierung mit glatter Oberfläche (c)

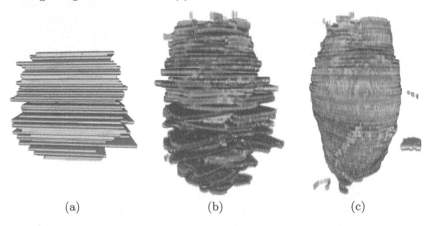

(a)   (b)   (c)

Abb. 3. Orthogonaler Schnitt durch das rekonstruierte Volumen: nach dem Schwerpunkt ausgerichtete Schichten (a), Schichten nach der Registrierung (b)

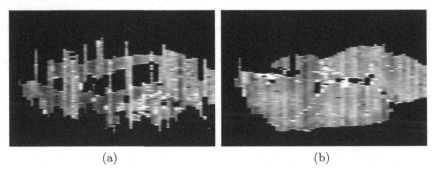

(a)   (b)

Hintergrund-Trennung eine Volumenanalyse ermöglicht. In Abb. 1c ist zu erkennen, dass die Maskierung sinnvolle Ergebnisse lieferte. Zur Bestimmung des Schwerpunktes wurde das Maskenbild verwendet und anschließend die Schwerpunkte der Bilder durch Translation in der Mitte neu ausgerichtet (bb. 2a). Nach Anwendung der Masken konnte in der dreidimensionalen Darstellung bereits die grobe Form der Restleber erkannt werden (Abb. 2b). Im nächsten Schritt wurden die verbliebenen Rotationen und Translationen durch die rigide *best-of-four*-Registrierung korrigiert, so dass die Schichten sich sehr gut überlagerten und insgesamt eine glatte Oberfläche erzeugt werden konnte (Abb. 2c). Wird zusätzlich zur Oberfläche auch das Innere des Volumens betrachtet, so lassen sich feine Strukturen und Gefäße gut erkennen (Abb. 3).

5 Diskussion

Es wurde ein vollautomatischer Algorithmus zur Vorverarbeitung und rigiden Registrierung histologischer Schnitte entwickelt. Die vorgestellte Methode erlaubt eine schnelle und effiziente rigide Rekonstruktion eines 3D-Volumens aus den Bildern der histologischen Schnitte. Die Beurteilung der Ergebnisse erfolgte bislang optisch durch einen Experten. Weitere Analysen zur Genauigkeit stehen noch aus. Die Ergebnisse sind aufgrund der Automatisierung reproduzierbar und bieten damit eine zuverlässige Möglichkeit, histologische Präparate zu rekonstruieren. In weiterführenden Arbeiten werden die restlichen Verformungen in den Daten, die aufgrund des Herstellungsprozesses nur durch nichtlineare Methoden zu rekonstruieren sind, mit Hilfe eines elastischen Registrierungsverfahrens korrigiert. Zur Erhöhung der örtlichen Auflösung soll der Abstand zwischen zwei Schichten weiter verringert und damit die Gesamtzahl der Schichten erhöht werden. Dadurch lassen sich weitere Details wie kleinere Gefäße, etc. in der Rekonstruktion erkennen. Auf diesen verbesserten Daten lassen sich dann Gefäßsegmentierungen effizienter durchführen und damit eine genauere Analyse der Regenerationsleistung der Lebergefäße erzielen.

Literaturverzeichnis

1. Horn LC, Riethdorf L, Löning T. Leitfaden für die Präparation uteriner Operationspräparate. Der Pathologe 1999;20(1):9–14.
2. Em G, Vanderloos H. A semi-automatic computer-microscope for the analysis of neuronal morphology. IEEE Trans Biomed Eng 1965;12:22–31.
3. Braumann UD, Kuska JP, Eikel J, et al. Three-dimensional reconstruction and quantification of cervical carcinoma invasion fronts from histological serial sections. IEEE Trans Med Imaging 2005;24(10):1286–1307.
4. Ourselin S, Roche A, Subsol G, Pennec X, Ayache N. Reconstructing a 3D structure from serial histological sections. Image Vis Comp 2001;19(1):25–31.
5. Wirtz S, Fischer B, Modersitzki J, Schmitt O. Vollständige Rekonstruktion eines Rattenhirns aus hochaufgelösten Bildern von histologischen Serienschnitten. Procs BVM 2004; 204–208.
6. Alleysson D, Süsstrunk S. Spatio-chromatic PCA of a mosaiced color image. Procs European Conf on Color in Graphics, Imaging and Vision 2004.
7. Baker S, Matthews I. Lucas-Kanade 20 years on: A unifying framework. Int J Comp Vis 2004;56(3):221–255.
8. Rexilius J, Spindler W, Jomier J, et al. A Framework for algorithm evaluation and clinical application prototyping using ITK. The Insight Journal 2005.

Multiscale Fractal Analysis of Cortical Pyramidal Neurons

Andreas Schierwagen[1], Luciano da Fontoura Costa[2],
Alán Alpár[3], Ulrich Gärtner[3]

[1]Institute for Computer Science, University of Leipzig, D-04109 Leipzig, Germany
[2]Institute of Physics at São Carlos, University of São Paulo,
13560-970 São Carlos, SP, Brazil
[3]Department of Neuroanatomy, Paul Flechsig Institut for Brain Research,
University of Leipzig, D-04109 Leipzig, Germany
Email: schierwa@informatik.uni-leipzig.de

Abstract. The present study used 3D data on neuronal morphology images to quantitatively characterize the phenotype of transgenic neurons. We calculated the multiscale fractal dimension (MFD) of reconstructed neuronal cells. It was shown that in a specific mouse mutant changes in the complexity of neuronal morphology correlate with changes in the MFD of dendrites of pyramidal neurons. Neurons in the mutant strain have lower peak fractal dimension compared with the wildtype, and a greater variety of the cell morphological phenotype.

1 Introduction

During brain development, neurons form complex dendritic and axonal arbors that reach a characteristic pattern and size. The development of arbor shape is partly determined by genetic factors and partly by interactions with the surrounding tissue. Important means for understanding gene function are provided by transgenic mice mutations. In these mutants, gene overexpression may affect several organs and tissues, including the brain. In a specific mouse mutant introduced in [1] a permanently active Ras protein in post-mitotic neurons is expressed in the primary somatosensory cortex resulting in a dramatically enlarged dendritic tree. In both cortical layers II/III and V, the total surface area and the total volume of dendritic trees is greatly increased. This is mainly caused by increased dendritic diameter and tree degree [2]. Topological complexity of pyramidal neurons in layers II/III, however, appeared hardly affected: Sholl analyses of both basal and apical dendrites revealed no differences between transgenic and wildtype mice regarding any parameters considered, i.e. numbers of intersections, branching points (nodes) and tips (leaves) [2]. These results suggest a rather proportional increase of dendritic tree size, without distinct changes in the space-filling properties.

The present study was intended to substantiate these findings by analyzing fractal aspects of dendritic tree shape. There are several methods for describing trees by fractal measurements (e.g. [3, 4]). Multiscale fractal analysis [5] seems

Fig. 1. Retrogradely labelled pyramidal neurons in layers II/III of the primary somatosensory cortex (left), and a cell (transgenic neuron SE8, right) rendered with CVAPP

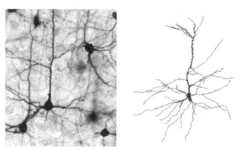

to be particularly suitable in the present case because the multiscale fractal dimension (MFD) is independent of size-related parameters like surface area and volume. The aim of this study is to show that observed changes in the complexity of neuronal morphology due to transgenic Ras activation in the primary somatosensory cortex of mice correlate with changes in the multiscale fractal dimensions of dendrites of pyramidal neurons.

2   Materials and Methods

Neurons of two samples (17 pyramidal neurons of wildtype and 26 of transgenic type) were reconstructed and digitized using Neurolucida^{TM}, as described in [2]. The morphology files obtained were processed with CVAPP, a freely available program [6] for cell viewing, editing and format converting (Fig. 1).

After thresholding 3D binary images were obtained with the neuron shape represented by the set of 1-voxels. The binary neuron images were used to calculate the MFD, a measure related to image complexity [7]. It has been computed through the Minkowski sausages approach which can be described as follows:

Let the neuron shape under study be represented by the set S of the Cartesian coordinates of each of its 1-voxels. Its exact dilation by a radius r is defined as the union of all spheres of radius r centered at each of the elements of S. A series of dilations on the image is made, with radii r_i equivalent to the intrinsic lattice distances, the so-called *exact distances*. At each dilation, the volume $V(r_i)$ of the image is computed.

The volume $V(r)$ of the shape S is therefore defined by

$$V(r) = \sum_{i=1}^{M} V(r_i)\, \delta(r - r_i) \tag{1}$$

where $\delta(.)$ is the Dirac delta function and M is the index of the largest exact distance being considered. As $V(r)$ is a discontinuous function on r, which is a consequence of the discrete nature of r_i, it is necessary to interpolate between the

Dirac deltas, which is here accomplished by convolving $V(r)$ with the Gaussian $g_\sigma(r) = 1/\sigma/\sqrt{2\pi} \exp\left(-0.5\left(r/\sigma\right)^2\right)$ yielding the following interpolated volume

$$v_\sigma(r) = \sum_{i=1}^{M} V(r_i) g_\sigma(r - r_i) \tag{2}$$

It is important to choose a suitable value of the standard deviation parameter, σ, that is large enough just to interpolate between the largest gaps between the exact radii, which occur for small values of r. The cumulative volume is defined as

$$C(s) = \int_{-\infty}^{s} v_\sigma(r)\, dr \tag{3}$$

The Euclidean distance is now represented in terms of its logarithm, leading to the spatial scale parameter $s = \log(r)$, so that the exact radii are expressed as $s_i = \log(r_i)$. The multiscale fractal dimension $f(s)$ of the set S of voxel elements then can be defined by

$$f(s) = 3 - \frac{d}{ds}\log\left(C(s)\right) = 3 - \frac{C'(s)}{C(s)} \tag{4}$$

While the traditional fractal dimension corresponds to a single scalar value, the MFD is a function of the spatial scale parameter s. Meaningful parameters of the MFD curve are: peak fractality, f_M, characteristic scale, s_M, and average fractality, $<f>$. For the computational implementation of this method, see [4].

3   Results

In Figure 2, an example calculation of multiscale fractal dimension for the transgenic cell SE8 displayed in Fig. 1 is shown. Following the scheme defined in Eqns. 1-4, the multiscale fractal dimension depending on s was obtained.

As shown in Fig. 2, the fractal dimension decreases at both micro and macro scales, and a peak fractal dimension value, f_M, is observed at an intermediate scale value, s_M. Another relevant parameter is the average fractal dimension, $<f>$.

The sample histograms of the three parameters utilized, f_M, s_M, and $<f>$, are presented in Fig. 3. For f_M, a two mode distribution for the transgenic cases results, while wildtype cells produced a single mode (Fig. 3a). The distribution of the spatial scales where the peak fractality s_M is observed suggests that the two types of cells are characterized by similar values of this parameter (Fig. 3b). Finally, the distributions of $<f>$ are bimodal in the case of transgenic cells, and unimodal for wildtype cells (Fig. 3c).

Fig. 4 shows the Gaussian densities after principal component analysis for the parameter combinations (f_M, s_M) and $(f_M, <f>)$, after normal statistical transformation (leading to null mean and unit variance in both cases). Obviously,

Fig. 2. The multiscale fractal dimension of a neuron (cell SE8)

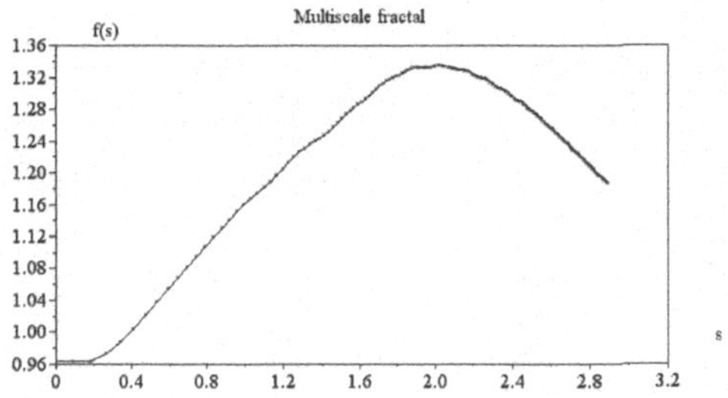

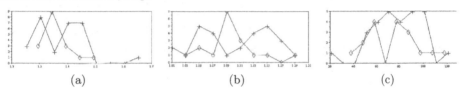

Fig. 3. Histograms: Peak fractal dimension f_M (a), maximum fractality scale s_M (b), average fractal dimension $<f>$ (c). Wildtype and transgenic cases are identified by diamonds and crosses, resp.

(a)   (b)   (c)

the parameter combination (f_M, s_M) enables a better separation of the two cell types. As indicated in Fig. 4 (left), transgenic cells tend to be less complex (lower fractality), expressing at the same time greater variance.

4   Discussion

The present study is one of the few which used 3D data on neuronal morphology to quantitatively characterize the morphological phenotype of neurons. We calculated the multiscale fractal dimension of neuronal cells reconstructed in 3D. The advantages of the multiscale fractal dimension (a function of the spatial scale) over the traditional fractal dimension (a single scalar value) reside in providing additional information about the analyzed shapes. Thus, we calculated complementing parameters such as the peak fractality, the spatial scale where it occurs, and the average fractality, for quantifying and characterizing the cell types.

Two sets of neurons, i.e. pyramidal cells from wildtype and transgenic mice, have been analyzed. The results obtained after principal component analysis mark transgenic neurons as slightly less complex, if measured by the peak fractal dimension, f_M, compared to their wildtype counterpart, while the other two parameters considered (maximum fractality scale, s_M, and average fractal dimension, $<f>$) did not reveal differences between the two types. Transgenic pyramidal neurons are characterized by increased dispersion when compared to the wildtype pyramidal neurons, suggesting that the enhanced Ras activity in transgenic mice may lead to greater variety of the cell morphological phenotype.

Fig. 4. Gaussian densities for (f_M, s_M) (left) and $(f_M, <f>)$ (right). Wildtype and transgenic cases are marked by diamonds and crosses, respectively

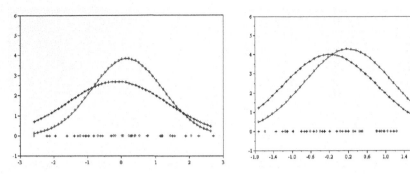

Neuronal shape analysis requires the specification of appropriate shape measures and corresponding computational methods. An important problem is the discriminative power of the particular shape measures. It is known that multiscale analyses tend to augment the resolution power of geometric descriptors [7]. In this context, our results suggest to consider the MFD as measure with discriminative strength. Only recently, we could confirm our findings with an alternative method, i.e. percolation analysis [8].

References

1. Heumann R, Goemans C, Bartsch D, et al. Constitutive activation of Ras in neurons promotes hypertrophy and protects from lesion-induced degeneration. J Cell Biol 2000;151:1537–1548.
2. Alpár A, Palm K, Schierwagen A, et al. Expression of constitutively active p21H-rasVal12 in postmitotic pyramidal neurons results in increased dendritic size and complexity. J Comp Neurol 2003;467:119–133.
3. Schierwagen A. Dendritic branching patterns. In: Degn H et al. Chaos in Biological Systems. Plenum, New York; 1987. 191–193.
4. Fernandez E, Jelinek HF. Use of fractal theory in neuroscience: Methods, advantages, and potential problems. Methods 2001;24:309–321.
5. Costa LF, Manoel ETM, Faucereau F, et al. A shape analysis framework for neuromorphometry. Comput Neural Syst 2002;13:283–310.
6. Cannon RC. Structure editing and conversion with cvapp; 2000. Available from: http://www.compneuro.org/CDROM/nmorph/usage.html
7. Costa LF, Jr RCesar. Shape Analysis and Classification: Theory and Practice. CRC Press, Boca Raton; 2001.
8. Costa LF, Barbosa MS, Schierwagen A, et al. Active percolation analysis of pyramidal neurons of somatosensory cortex: A comparison of wildtype and p21H-rasVal12 transgenic mice. Int J Mod Phys C 2005;16:655–667.

Das MediGRID Projekt
Gridcomputing in der medizinischen Bildverarbeitung

Michal Vossberg, Dagmar Krefting und Thomas Tolxdorff

Institut für Medizinische Informatik,
Charité – Universitätsmedizin Berlin, 12200 Berlin
Email: michal.vossberg@charite.de

Zusammenfassung. Aufgrund zunehmend höherer Anforderungen an Rechenleistung und Speicherplatz in der medizinischen Bildverarbeitung ist Gridcomputing auch für dieses Arbeitsgebiet eine vielversprechende Perspektive. Im Rahmen der D-Grid Initiative des BMBF wird durch das MediGRID-Projekt eine bundesweite Grid-Infrastruktur für die Lebenswissenschaften aufbaut, die insbesondere die hohen Anforderungen an Sicherheit und Zuverlässigkeit berücksichtigt. Das Modul Bildverarbeitung im MediGRID implementiert prototypische Anwendungen aus der medizinischen Bildverarbeitung und analysiert Möglichkeiten und Beschränkungen der Grid-Nutzung. Erste Algorithmen sind bereits im MediGRID implementiert und über ein Portal von jedem internetfähigen Webbrowser aus nutzbar.

1 Einleitung

Viele Anwendungen in der medizinischen Bildverarbeitung benötigen eine hohe Rechenleistung oder haben einen hohen Speicherplatzbedarf. Zusätzlich werden in der medizinischen Informatik Algorithmen entwickelt, die auch weiteren Nutzern zur Verfügung gestellt werden sollen. Diese Anforderungen kann ein Computergrid erfüllen, das den Zusammenschluss von räumlich verteilten Rechnern zu einem virtuellen Gesamtcomputer ermöglicht. Ein solches Grid soll bundesweit durch die D-Grid-Initiative aufgebaut werden, die derzeit mehr als 100 Einrichtungen gezielt in dem Bereich Grid-Forschung fördert.

MediGRID als Communityprojekt für die Medizin und biomedizinische Informatik hat das Ziel, in den kommenden Jahren schrittweise eine Grid-Infrastruktur für die biomedizinische Verbundforschung aufzubauen und nachhaltig zu betreiben. Aufgrund der besonderen Anforderungen an Sicherheit und Zuverlässigkeit sind Grid-Netzwerke im medizinischen Umfeld noch recht neu und werden vor allem in der Praxis noch nicht umfassend eingesetzt [1].

Das Modul Bildverarbeitung soll die wesentlichen Methoden medizinischer Bildverarbeitung sowie Datenstrukturen und -organisation auf das MediGRID bringen. Ziel ist es, wissenschaftliche Aufgabenstellungen in der medizinischen Bildverarbeitung effizienter zu lösen, neue Anwendungen zu erschließen und somit eScience im Bereich der Bildverarbeitung zu stärken. Das Methodenspektrum wird in drei praktisch relevanten Anwendungsszenarien exemplarisch in das MediGRID implementiert:

- Statistische Analyse funktioneller Hirnbilddaten,
- Virtuelle Gefäßchirurgie,
- 3D Ultraschallaufnahmen bei Prostatabiopsien.

Besondere Berücksichtigung finden dabei die sichere Bilddatenübertragung und -speicherung, effizienter (inhaltsbasierter) Zugriff auf Bilddaten und die Interoperabilität verschiedener Applikationen über den DICOM-Standard.

2 Stand der Forschung

Derzeit wird Gridcomputing vor allem von Forschungscommunities betrieben, die keine hohen Anforderungen an Benutzerfreundlichkeit und Datensicherheit stellen, beispielsweise die Hochenergiephysik. In der letzten Zeit sind jedoch verstärkt auch Benutzerschnittstellen und Konzepte zur sicheren Nutzung der Middleware entwickelt worden.

Auf der anderen Seite werden medizinische Bildverarbeitungsprobleme zurzeit hauptsächlich durch für eine Modalität oder Organ hochspezialisierte und optimierte Algorithmen gelöst. Diese sind von einer Gruppe oder Organisation lokal implementiert. Oft sind aber viele Teilschritte universeller einsetzbar und könnten auch von anderen Forschergruppen vorteilhaft eingebracht oder genutzt werden. Zusätzlich gibt es viele Dienste die völlig unabhängig vom Bildmaterial sind oder parallel zum Hauptworkflow laufen.

Einzelne Bildverarbeitungsschritte aus der medizinischen Forschung sind bereits in verschiedenen Grid-Projekten implementiert worden [2, 3]. Jedoch sind die Lösungsansätze aufgrund mangelnder nachhaltiger Infrastruktur, nichtstandardisierter Middleware und der oben genannten besonderen Anforderungen nicht weiterverfolgt worden und haben keine weitere Verbreitung in der Bildverarbeitungscommunity gefunden.

Alle drei ausgewählten Szenarien der medizinischen Bildverarbeitung beinhalten komplexe, rechenintensiven Algorithmen und umfassen große Datenmengen. Das hier ausgewählte Projekt zur Bildverarbeitung von 3D-Ultraschallbildern von Prostatabiopsien umfasst in seinem vollen Umfang neben Segmentierungs-, Registrierungs-, Klassifikations- und Visualisierungsalgorithmen auch die Anbindung an ein PACS, den Zugriff auf eine Datenbank innerhalb des Grids sowie den Anschluss an ein Image Retrieval System [4].

Ziel des Projektes ist die Bestimmung der räumlichen Lage der Gewebeproben im Prostatavolumen zur besseren Diagnose und Therapieplanung von Prostatakarzinomen, eine der häufigsten Krebserkrankungen von Männern. Besonders rechenintensiv ist die 2D-3D-Registrierung der Ultraschallaufnahmen. Desweiteren wird die Segmentierung der Biopsienadel auf zahlreiche Bildsequenzen angewendet, die ohne Parallelisierungsaufwand auf mehrere Computer aufgeteilt werden können. Die Vorteile einer Benutzung von MediGRID liegen deshalb auf der Hand:

1. Schnellere Ausführung der rechenaufwändigen Algorithmen durch Aufteilung des Problems und Verteilung auf Hochleistungsrechner im Grid,

2. Nutzung zusätzlicher Methoden, wie Klassifizierung oder Segmentierung, ohne Eigenentwicklung oder umständliche Hard- und Softwareinstallationen,

3. Nutzung verteilten Speicherplatzes zur Speicherung der voluminösen 3D Bilddatensätze und -filme.

3 Methoden

Die Algorithmen des Ultraschallprojektes, die bisher ins Grid implementiert sind, sind Teilschritte der Segmentierung und der Registrierung. Die Segmentierungsalgorithmen sind in Matlab 7.1. geschrieben, die Registrierung verwendet ITK 2.9. Für die Verwendung im Grid sind die Matlab-Skripte compiliert und können so lizenzfrei als ausführbare Programme auf die Gridrechner verteilt werden. Die Algorithmen werden so angepasst, dass sich die Aufgaben durch Angabe entsprechender Parameter in kleinere Teilprobleme zerlegen lassen. Diese Teilaufgaben sind unabhängig voneinander und können beliebig auf die zur Verfügung stehenden Gridrechner verteilt werden.

Die Gridversionen der Algorithmen werden in einem lokalen Testbed, bestehend aus vier Arbeitsplatzrechnern, entwickelt und anschließend auf das MediGRID gebracht. Beteiligte Gridrechner sind in der derzeitigen Anfangsphase bei MediGRID zwei Hochleistungsrechencluster am Konrad-Zuse-Zentrum, Berlin und an der Gesellschaft für wissenschaftlichen Datenverarbeitung mbH in Göttingen. Prinzipiell wird freie Software eingesetzt, die unter GNU- oder ähnlichen Lizenzmodellen laufen. Als Middleware wird das weitverbreitete Toolkit Globus [5] in der Version 4.0 eingesetzt. Vorteile des Globus Toolkits ist einerseits seine starke Verbreitung und andererseits die konsequente Umsetzung moderner, diensteorientierter Technologien, wie beispielsweise WebServices. Der Datentransfer wird über das gridftp-Protokoll gewährleistet. Diese FTP-Variante ist optimiert für Zugriffe in Gridnetzwerken und besonders sicher und effizient für höchsten Datendurchsatz. Beim Datenmanagement kommt der SRB zum Einsatz [6], der es erlaubt, transparent Dateien auf entsprechenden Datenservern zu speichern und wieder zu laden. Der Datenbankzugriff erfolgt über OGSA-DAI, das einen effizienten und sicheren Zugriff auf SQL-Datenbanken im Grid ermöglicht. Die Authentifizierung und Authorisierung der Benutzer und beteiligten Rechner wird über Globus-GSI mithilfe von DFN-Zertifikaten realisiert. Dieser Sicherheitsstandard findet unter anderem auch im Signaturgesetz Verwendung und bietet nach derzeitigen Erkenntnissen ausreichend Sicherheit zur Authentifikation der beteiligten Benutzer und zur Autorisierung ihrer gewünschten Handlung. Der Zugang zum Grid und die Steuerung der Anwendungen erfolgt über ein Webportal, das als webbasierte Anwendung von jedem internetfähigem Webbrowser aus verfügbar ist. Das in MediGRID verwendete Webportal basiert auf einem Gridsphere-Server [7]. Neben dem Zugang zum Grid und seinen Basisdiensten bietet das Webportal auch den Zugang zu den einzelnen Anwendungen. Die Entwicklung der anwendungsspezifischen Oberflächenkomponenten und ihre Integration ins Gesamtportal erfolgt in Java nach dem JSR168-Portlet Standard. Die Algorithmen, die ebenso wie die entsprechenden Bibliotheken auf den Gridrechnern installiert sein müssen, werden über einen Webservice angesprochen.

Abb. 1. Snapshot des MediGRID-Webportals

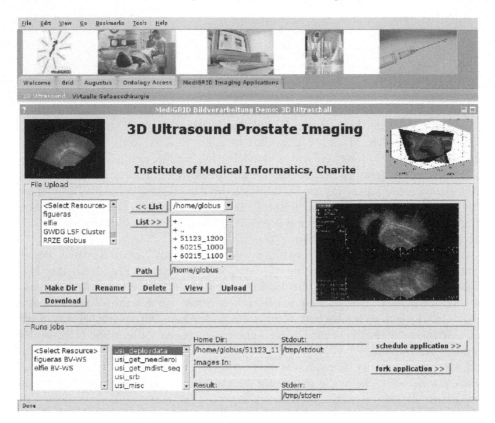

4   Ergebnisse

Seit einigen Monaten werden sukzessive Teilschritte der Ultraschall-Anwendung
für die Arbeit mit MediGRID umgesetzt und von uns für die Experimente benutzt. Die Umsetzung beinhaltet sowohl die Anpassung der Algorithmen, die
Entwicklung der Webservices als auch die Portalentwicklung (Abb. 1). Konkret
lassen sich derzeit über das Webportal Bilddaten im Grid ablegen, Jobs sowohl
im Batchbetrieb als auch direkt auf manuell ausgewählten Rechnern starten, ihre
Ausführung überwachen und nach Beendigung auf die Ergebnisse zugreifen. Weiterhin ist es möglich, die Ergebnisse in der Dokumentationsdatenbank im Grid
eintragen zu lassen oder abzufragen. Zusätzlich besteht nun die Möglichkeit,
auf die Anwendung von jedem internetfähigem Webbrowser aus zuzugreifen. So
können die Experimente nun einfach und ohne größere Installationen von zu-
hause, unterwegs oder anderen Büros aus gestartet und kontrolliert werden.

5 Diskussion

Zusammenfassend können wir im Fall des Ultraschallprojektes schon nach kurzer Zeit sehr positive Erfahrungen mit der Benutzung von MediGRID ziehen. Mit geringem Entwicklungsaufwand können die angebotenen Hochleistungs-Ressourcen im Grid genutzt und die Anwendung einer breiteren Benutzerschicht, wie beispielweise den an dem Projekt beteiligten Ärzten, zugänglich gemacht werden. Da allerdings das Sicherheitskonzept bisher noch nicht vollständig im MediGRID umgesetzt ist, können zur Zeit nur anonymisierte Daten verarbeitet werden. Neben zahlreichen Erweiterungen, die in MediGRID geplant sind, etwa eine Workflowengine zur automatischen Aufteilung und komfortablen Überwachung von Jobs im Grid, stehen speziell im Modul Bildverarbeitung die folgenden Entwicklungen an: Nach den ersten Erfahrungen wird die Anwendung 3D-Ultraschall nun weiter ausgebaut, und um diagnoseunterstützende Dienste erweitert. Der Schwerpunkt hierbei wird weniger im Zeitvorteil liegen als in der Tatsache dass es überhaupt möglich sein wird diese Anwendungen ohne lokale Implementationen zu nutzen. Außerdem wird im Bereich Datenmanagement an der Umsetzung des DICOM Protokolls, dem weltweiten Standard zur Bildübertragung in der Medizin, im Grid zur Anbindung von PACS Systemen gearbeitet. Neben dem vorgestellten Anwendungsszenario werden die schon beschriebenen zwei weiteren Projekte aus dem Modul Bildverarbeitung, Funktionelle Hirnbilddaten und Virtuelle Gefäßchirurgie, implementiert, um einen möglichst umfassenden Teil von typischen Methoden der Bildverarbeitung beispielhaft in MediGRID umzusetzen.

Danksagung

Diese Arbeit ist Teil des MediGRID Projektes und wird gefördert vom BMBF, Förderkennzeichen 01AK803F.

Literaturverzeichnis

1. MediGRID. GRID-Computing für die Medizin und Lebenswissenschaften; 2006. BMBF Förderkennzeichen 01AK803F, http://www.medigrid.de.
2. GEMSS. Grid-Enabled Medical Simulation Services; 2005. Http://www.ccrl-nece.de/gemss/index.html.
3. EGEE. Enabling Grids for E-science; 2006. Http://www.eu-egee.org.
4. IRMA. Image Retrieval in Medical Applications; 2005. Http://irma-project.org.
5. Foster I, et al. Globus toolkit version 4: Software for service-oriented systems. LNCS 2005;3779:2–13.
6. Rajasekar A, et al. Storage resource broker: Managing distributed data in a grid. Computer Society of India Journal 2003;33(4):42–54.
7. Novotny J, Russell M, Wehrens O. GridSphere: An Advanced Portal Framework. http://www.gridsphere.org; 2005.

Point-Based Statistical Shape Models with Probabilistic Correspondences and Affine EM-ICP

Heike Hufnagel[1,2], Xavier Pennec[1], Jan Ehrhardt[2],
Heinz Handels[2] and Nicholas Ayache[1]

[1] Institut National de Recherche en Informatique et en Automatique,
Asclepios Project, 06902 Sophia Antipolis, France
[2]Institut für Medizinische Informatik, Universität Hamburg, 20246 Hamburg
Email: Heike.Hufnagel@sophia.inria.fr

Abstract. A fundamental problem when computing statistical shape models (SSMs) is the determination of correspondences between the instances. Often, homologies between points that represent the surfaces are assumed which might lead to imprecise mean shape and variation results. We present a novel algorithm based on the affine Expectation Maximization - Iterative Closest Point (EM-ICP) registration method. Exact correspondences are replaced by iteratively evolving correspondence probabilities which provide the basis for the computation of mean shape and variability model. We validated our approach by computing SSMs using inexact correspondences for kidney and putamen data. In ongoing work, we want to use our methods for automatic classification applications.

1   Introduction

One of the central difficulties of analyzing different organ shapes in a statistical manner is the identification of correspondences between the shapes. As the manual identification of landmarks is not a feasible option in 3D, several techniques were developed to automatically find exact one-to-one correspondences. In order to automatically establish correspondences between surfaces represented by point clouds, some authors propose elaborate preprocessing methods [1, 2, 3]. Other approaches solve this with a search for the registration transformation using an atlas [4] or the ICP algorithm [5]. More recent methods directly combine the search of correspondences and SSM [6, 7, 8]. All of these enforce homologies between the shapes. However, exact correspondences can only be determined between continuous surfaces, not between point cloud representations of surfaces. Thus, when using imprecise homologies, the resulting variability model will not only represent the organ shape variations but also artificial variations caused by the wrongly assumed exact correspondences. The SoftAssign algorithm tries to solve this problem with an initial probabilistic formulation of the correspondences but it also ends up with one-to-one correspondences [9].

In order to solve for inexact correspondences, we pursue a probabilistic approach and base our work on an affine EM-ICP registration algorithm which proved to be robust, precise, and fast (see [10] for rigid EM-ICP).

2   Methods

The affine EM-ICP algorithm determines the affine registration transformation T to match a point set $M \in (\mathbb{R}^3)^{N_m}$ on $S \in (\mathbb{R}^3)^{N_s}$. Instead of assuming homologies, we focus on the probability of a transformed model point $T * m_j$ being a measure of an instance point s_i. If we knew that point s_i corresponds exactly to point m_j, the measurement process would be Gaussian (see eq. 1).

$$p(s_i|m_j,T) = \frac{1}{(2\pi)^{\frac{3}{2}}|\Sigma_j|^{\frac{1}{2}}} \exp(-\frac{1}{2}(s_i - T \star m_j)^T.\Sigma_j^{-1}(s_i - T \star m_j)) \quad (1)$$

where Σ_j represents the noise as the covariance of m_j.

However, point s_i can in fact be a measure of any of the model points, so the PDF of its spatial location is the mixture $p(s_i|M,T) = \frac{1}{N_m}\sum_{j=1}^{N_m} p(s_i|m_j,T)$. Unfortunately, even if we assume that all scene point measurements are independent, no closed form solution exists for the maximization of $p(S|M,T)$. A solution is to model the correspondences $H \in \mathbb{R}^{3N_s \times 3N_m}$ as *random hidden variables* and to maximize the likelihood efficiently using the EM algorithm. We denote $E(H_{ij})$ as the expectation of point s_i being an observation of point $T\star m_j$ (with the constraint $\sum_j^{N_m} E(H_{ij}) = 1$). In the E-step, we fix T and estimate the complete data likelihood log $p(S,H|M,T)$, thus calculating $E(H)$. In the M-step, we fix $E(H)$ and maximize the estimated likelihood with respect to T. This process is iterated until convergence. In order to easily reach the global minimum, we employ a variance multi-scaling. We begin with great variances σ^2 to ensure that shape positions, rotation and sizes are aligned and end with small variances to cover for shape details. We also implemented the EM-ICP for rigid transformations in order to be able to adapt to the data at hand.

The calculation of the mean shape point set M consists of two steps that are iterated until convergence: First, all N instances S_k of the data set are registered with the initial model $M^{(iter)} = M^{(0)}$ using the affine EM-ICP. As initial model we choose one of the instances of our data set which seems to have a 'typical' shape. Next, a new model $M^{(iter+1)}$ is calculated. Using the EM-ICP framework, we have to minimize the associated global criterion

$$C_{\text{global}}(T, E(H), M) = \sum_{k,i,j}^{N,N_{sk},N_m} E(H_{k_{ij}})(s_{ki} - T_k \star m_j)\Sigma_j^{-1}(s_{ki} - T_k \star m_j)(2)$$

where s_{ki} is a point of instance S_k, $E(H_{k_{ij}})$ the correspondence probability between model point m_j and instance point s_{ki}, and T_k the registration transformation from the model to S_k. The criterion is optimized alternately with respect to all T_k and $E(H_k)$ (EM-ICP) and M (which is determined by a simple derivation of equation (2)).

Fig. 1. The original objects S (dark grey) and their transformed versions S_T (light grey) before (a) $d(S, S_T) = 40, 3mm)$ and after (b) $d(S, S_T) = 0.5mm$) registration. For the EM-ICP, the kidney was decimated from 10466 to 510 points, we chose an initial sigma of 8mm, 30 EM-ICP iterations and a reducing factor of 0.9 (which leads to a final sigma of 0.38mm)

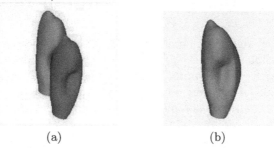

(a)   (b)

For the variability model we need to compute the principal modes of variation regarding all S_k and M. The usual method is to use the traditional PCA. However, we do not dispose of the exact correspondences between each model point and the instance points. Thus, we generate virtual correspondences $\breve{s}_{kj}$ for each m_j and each S_k by evaluating the mean position of the probabilistic correspondences. In that manner, the PCA results gain a certain independence of the positions of the initially chosen points of the instances.

$$\breve{s}_{kj} = \sum_i \frac{E(H_{k_{ij}})}{\sum_i E(H_{k_{ij}})} (T_k^{-1} \star s_{ik}) \tag{3}$$

These "virtual surface points" are then used as input for the PCA.

3   Results

In order to evaluate the performance of the affine EM-ICP registration, we applied it to synthetic registration problems. We tested for rigid, similitude, and affine T_{synth} with different numbers of points, variances, and iteration numbers. Our experiment object was a kidney S with $T_{\text{synth}} \star S = S_T$. To evaluate the results, we introduced a distance measure $d^2(S, S_T) = \frac{1}{N_S} \sum_{i=1}^{N_S} \|s_i - s_{T,i}\|^2$. The source S and the deformed version S_T were decimated using different parameters so that no exact correspondences existed between them and the number of points in the clouds were different (for the decimating algorithm see [11]). Thus, real conditions were simulated. We established that the affine EM-ICP finds very good results, needs no previous rigid registration for the affine case and converges quickly. For an evaluation example with distance values before and after registration see the affine case in figure 1.

We computed successfully SSMs for data sets of kidney CTs, brain structure MRs, and sulcal lines. In this article, we focus on the SSM results for the

Fig. 2. First image: Transversal slice of a CT volume of the brain where the putamen structures are marked in white. First and second row: The mean shape (middle images) of the left putamen and the principal deformations according to the first eigenvector (v_1) and second eigenvector (v_2). The images show a deformation of $-3\sqrt{\lambda_i}v_i$ (left) and $+3\sqrt{\lambda_i}v_i$ (right) respectively (with λ_i being the associated eigenvalues)

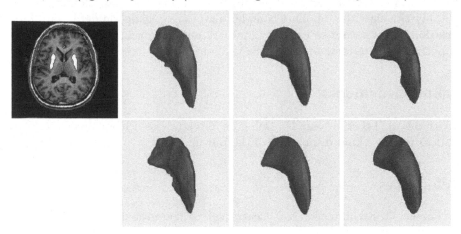

putamen, see figure 2. The data set consists of 24 right and left segmented instances (approximately $20mm \times 20mm \times 40mm$) which are represented by about 1000 points. The variance multi-scaling in the EM-ICP registration started with $\sigma_{initial} = 6mm$ and ended with $\sigma_{final} = 0.8mm$. Figure 2 shows the resulting mean shape and the deformations of the left putamen according to the variation modes. We then employ the SSM algorithm for an automatical classification of the putamen. The putamen data consist of 12 healthy and 12 pathological subjects. We want to determine if the disease causes significant shape deformations in the putamen. For the diseased and healthy data respectively, a mean shape and variability model are calculated. Then, the mean shapes and the variations of the shapes are compared. The results seem to show a shape difference between healthy and pathological putamen, but this needs to be confirmed by a statistical test.

4   Discussion

We proposed in this paper an EM-ICP framework to compute statistical shape models. We believe that our approach offers an advantageous method as it provides a resolution to the fundamental problem of homology identification between shapes. We proved that the algorithm is flexible and stable as it comes to good results for different types of organs. Currently, we are investigating the correspondence matrix as an indicator of the quality of the point distribution in the model with respect to the instances in the data set. This might help to choose an appropriate initial model. Secondly, we work on the replacement of the ad-hoc PCA as this approach is not coherent with the initial demand of inexact correspondences. At present, we are developing a proper probabilistic model including the mean shape *and* the variation modes in a global criterion. In future work on the applications, we will intensify our analysis of the putamen variability by extending the data set, conducting more experiments and implementing clustering techniques in order to finally realize an automatic classification. Besides, we plan to apply the algorithm on more complex shapes (e.g. ganglion data) with larger variations. As we want to carefully evaluate our approach, we need to compare its performance to state-of-the-art SSM algorithms.

Acknowledgments

We thank S. Lehéricy and C. Delmaire (Hôpital La Pitié-Salpêtrière, Paris, France) for their kind disposition of the putamen data.

References

1. Lorenz C, Krahnstoever N. Generation of point-based 3D statistical shape models for anatomical objects. Computer Vision and Image Understanding 2000;77(2):175–191.
2. Raynaud N. Segmentation d'Images Hépatiques par Analyses Statistiques. Master's thesis. DEA Mathématiques, Vision, Apprentissage – ENS Cachan; 2000.
3. Bookstein FL. Landmark methods for forms without landmarks: Morphometrics in group differences in outline shapes. Medical Image Analysis 1996;1:225–243.
4. Shelton CR. Morphable surface models. International Journal of Computer Vision 2000;38(1):75–91.
5. Besl PJ, McKay ND. A method for registration of 3D shapes. IEEE Trans Pat Anal and Mach Intel 1992; 239–256.
6. Davies RH, Twining CJ, Cootes TF. A minimum description length approach to statistical shape modeling. IEEE Transactions on Medical Imaging 2002;21(5).
7. Heimann T, Wolf I, Williams T, Meinzer HP. 3D active shape models using gradient descent optimization of description length. In: IPMI. vol. 3565; 2005. 566–577.
8. Zhao Z, Theo EK. A novel framework for automated 3D PDM construction using deformable models. Procs SPIE 2005;5747:303–314.
9. Rangarajan A, Chui H, Bookstein FL. The softassign procrustes matching algorithm. In: IPMI; 1997. 29–42.
10. Granger S, Pennec X. Multi-scale EM-ICP: A fast and robust approach for surface registration. LNCS 2002;2353:418–432.
11. Schroeder WJ, Zarge JA, Lorensen WE. Decimation of triangle meshes. Computer Graphics 1992;26(2):65–70.

Projection Technique for Vortex-Free Image Registration

Patrick Scheibe[1], Ulf-Dietrich Braumann[1,2], Jens-Peer Kuska[2]

[1]Translational Center for Regenerative Medicine (TRM)
[2]Interdisciplinary Center for Bioinformatics
University Leipzig, Germany
Email: mai99dnn@studserv.uni-leipzig.de

Abstract. One important application of image processing in medicine is to register tissue samples onto another. Registering these highly textured images with non-parametric methods sometimes leads to solutions which are known to be suboptimal. We show a projection technique for unwanted vortices in the displacement field. A new strategy is presented which does not change the registration method itself but continuously correct the solution during the registration process.

1 Introduction

Many variants of non-parametric image registration methods are known [1]. The basic goal is to find a transformation $u(x)$ so that the transformed template image $T(x - u(x))$ is *similar* to the reference image $R(x)$. This *similarity* which indirectly is expressed in the *difference* of the two images is not the only condition the searched transformation has to fulfill. Beside this, a *smoothing term* is part of the registration criterion which is physically motivated, whereas its task is to ensure the smoothness of the transformation. This method, which was introduced in [2], applied to high textured tissue samples still may lead to vortex-affected solutions.

One may ask how to know that these solutions are bad. The explanation is: In the way of getting the image data from the medical device, some kind of image deformations are very unlikely. Especially vortices which are often part of the solutions with high textured images are demonstrably false and should not be part of the displacement field $u(x)$. These are caused by the solution procedure when images with many similar structures are used. Tissue consisting of many cells is one example for highly textured data.

A first workaround for the vortex problem was presented by Kuska and Braumann [3]. Their method includes the suppression of vortices as weighted term in the variational problem.

In this paper we present a new method to get rid of these vortices. It is based on the idea of projecting them continuously out during the iterative steps of finding the solution $u(x)$.

2   Methods

Vortex-free image registration extends a curvature-based method that was introduced in [4] and later used in [1]. Braumann and Kuska discussed in [2] the
influences of the boundary conditions and gave a fast implementation for the
method. The registration follows a variational approach to find the transformation $u(x)$ that fulfills

$$\min_{u} \left(\mathcal{D}(u) + \alpha \mathcal{S}(u)\right) \tag{1}$$

with

$$\mathcal{D}(u) = \frac{1}{2} \int_{\Omega} \left(T(x - u(x))\right) - R(x))^2 dx$$
$$\mathcal{S}(u) = \frac{1}{2} \int_{\Omega} (\Delta u)^{\mathrm{T}} \cdot (\Delta u) dx \tag{2}$$

With the rules of the calculus of variations it follows a highly non-linear partial
differential equation which was solved by extending it toward a time dependent
function

$$\frac{\partial u}{\partial t}(x, t) = -\alpha \Delta^2 u(x, t) + f(x, u(x, t)) \tag{3}$$

with

$$f(x, u(x, t)) = (R(x) - T(x - u(x, t))) \cdot \nabla T(x - u(x, t)) \tag{4}$$

This function $u(x, t)$ converges with $\lim_{t \to \infty} u(x, t) = u(x)$. Equation 3 is solved
with an iterative algorithm. The only place where vortices can arise is the term
$f(x, u(x, t))$.

What our new method does is to project all vortices out of this term before the next time-step is calculated. This is possible using the theorem of
Helmholtz which states a vector field can be decomposed in its irrotational and
its solenoidal component. With this it is possible to calculate the solenoidal
part of $f(x, u(x, t))$ and subtract it. This vortex-free version is then used in the
calculation of the next time-step.

The extraction of the solenoidal part $\nabla \times p$ is again a variational problem
given by the functional

$$\mathcal{W}[p] = \frac{1}{2} \int_{\Omega} |\nabla \times p - f|^2 dx \tag{5}$$

The partial differential equation that is defined by this functional is a Poisson
equation for the third element of the vector potential $p = (0, 0, p)^{\mathrm{T}}$

$$\frac{\partial^2}{\partial x^2} p(x) + \frac{\partial^2}{\partial y^2} p(x) = \frac{\partial}{\partial y} f_1(x) - \frac{\partial}{\partial x} f_2(x) \tag{6}$$

Since we have digital images, we have to solve a discrete version of this equation.
To avoid the calculation of a linear system of equations in p we use the Fourier
transform with appropriate boundary conditions. Therefore only one equation
per point must be solved.

Fig. 1. The original image and the distorted image with the applied frog- eye transformation. The advantage of this transformation is the fact that the inverse is known and one can identify solution errors easily

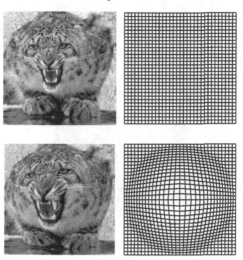

3   Results

As input for the first illustrative example an image is given that was distorted with a vortex-free transformation. Thus, the solution of the registration problem should not contain vortices either. Since the registration method may run into unwanted vortices when the image is highly textured, we have distorted a picture of a leopard whose coat is obviously textured enough (see fig. 1). In figure 2 the pictures in the upper row depicts the registration without vortex extraction. Notice that the high textured region of the leopards head causes the method to distort this area. That can be clearly seen looking at the line integral convolution [5] in the middle picture column. The difference between the transformation found by the method and the real inverse is given by the error plots in the right column of figure 2.

In contrast to that with our new strategy this critical region of the head of the leopard is handled very well. Only the error plot unveils where the method is not exactly. The human eye is not able to find differences between the original and the registered image.

In figure 3 we present the application of our new method on a realistic problem. The images show two HE-stained histological slices of the uterine cervix which are registered onto another. As one can clearly see, the right line integral convolution shows a much smoother displacement field. This was calculated using the new vortex-free registration.

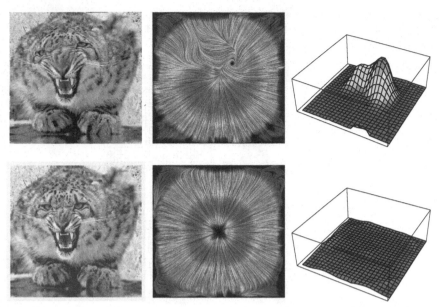

Fig. 2. Comparison of the method without (upper row) and with (lower row) vortex extraction: results after registration (left), line integral convolutions of the displacement fields (middle), error plots for the obtained displacement vector fields (right)

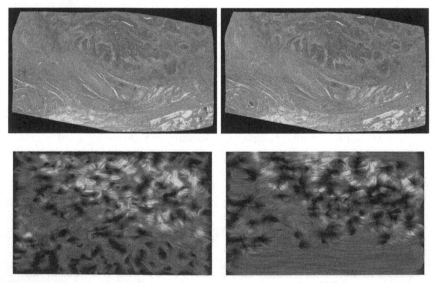

Fig. 3. Two HE-stained histological slices consecutively cut from a specimen of a squamous cell carcinoma of the uterine cervix, which are to be registered (top) and displacement field (bottom): without vortex extraction (left), using our new algorithm (right). As in fig. 2, blue denotes weak, green medium, and red strong displacements

4   Discussion

We have presented a projection technique for image registration that allows to force the displacement field to be vortex-free. This is appropriable in cases where it is known that the solution does not contain vortices. The method presented in [3] has several drawbacks compared to our new approach:

- The vortex suppression term in the functional can lead to situations where its influence is on a level disabling the terms for minimal distance and smoothness. Our strategy leaves the functional as is, so this situation is not possible.
- Even when the term for vortex suppression is rated high it is still possible that the calculation runs into a solution where vortices appear in the displacement field. Since we project them out of the partial solution and let the method find a good transformation in the space of vortex-free functions this can not happen.
- The projection that extracts all vortices does not need a weighting parameter like the vortex suppression term. Therefore our method has one less parameter to adjust.

Since the Helmholtz decomposition requires sufficiently smooth and fast decaying vector fields, the border of the images can be a bit problematic. For vortices near the border the decomposition does not work well but by adding extra space around the image it is likely that we can suppress this behavior.

Finally we can say that the presented algorithm surpasses our expectations and yields in all test cases better results than the underlying curvature-based registration.

References

1. Modersitzki J. Numerical Methods for Image Registration. Oxford University Press, USA; 2004.
2. Braumann UD, Kuska JP. Influence of the boundary conditions on the result of nonlinear image registration. In: Proceedings of the IEEE International Conference on Image Processing. IEEE Signal Processing Society; 2005. I-1129–I-1132.
3. Braumann UD, Kuska JP. A new equation for nonlinear image registration with control over the vortex structure in the displacement field. In: Proceedings of the IEEE International Conference on Image Processing. IEEE Signal Processing Society; 2006. 329–332.
4. Yali A. A nonlinear variational problem for image matching. SIAM Journal on Scientific Computing 1994;15(1):207–224.
5. Cabral B, Leedom LC. Imaging vector fields using line integral Convolution. In: Proceedings SIGGRAPH '93; 1993. 263–272.
6. Braumann UD, Kuska JP, Einenkel J, Horn LC, Löffler M, Höckel M. Three-dimensional reconstruction and quantification of cervical carcinoma invasion fronts from histological serial sections. IEEE Trans Med Imag 2005;24(10):1286–1307. http://dx.doi.org/10.1109/TMI.2005.855437.

Image Registration with Local Rigidity Constraints

Jan Modersitzki

Institute of Mathematics, University of Lübeck, Wallstraße 40, D-23560 Lübeck
Email: modersitzki@math.uni-luebeck.de

Abstract. Registration is a technique nowadays commonly used in medical imaging. A drawback of most of the current registration schemes is that all tissue is being considered as non-rigid. Therefore, rigid objects in an image, such as bony structures or surgical instruments, may be transformed non-rigidly. In this paper, we integrate the concept of local rigidity to the FLexible Image Registration Toolbox (FLIRT). The idea is to add a penalty for local non-rigidity to the cost function and thus to penalize non-rigid transformations of rigid objects. As our examples show, the new approach allows the maintenance of local rigidity in the desired fashion. For example, the new scheme is able to keep bony structures rigid during registration.

1   Introduction

The incorporation of pre-knowledge in registration is a key for getting meaningful results. For many registration tasks, the images inhibits an classification of soft and hard tissue. It thus seems to be natural to ask for transformations keeping hard tissue rigid. However, current registration schemes consider all parts of the tissue as non-rigid [1]. As a consequence rigid objects, such as bony structures or surgical instruments, can be transformed non-rigidly. Other consequences are that tumor growth between follow-up images may be concealed, or that structures containing contrast material in only one of the images may be compressed by the registration scheme.

Starting with the variational framework of the FLexible Image Registration Toolbox (FLIRT) [2, 3], we integrate the concept of local rigidity in terms of an additional penalty term. For a transformation, rigidity is measured by linearity, orthogonality, and orientation preservation.

We also compared our approach to the non-rigidity penalized but B-spline based scheme in [1]. As it turned out, the FLIRT approach gives visually more pleasing results: a perfect match (i.e. transformed template equals reference) is achieved with a much more regular transformation; see, e.g., Figure 1.

2   State of the Art and New Contribution

There are currently two main numerical approaches to image registration. The first one is based on an expansion of the wanted transformation in terms of

Fig. 1. Example from [1]: reference and template (first column), B-spline results taken from [1] without and with penalty (middle column), and FLIRT results without and with penalty (right column); all four transformations lead to a perfect match

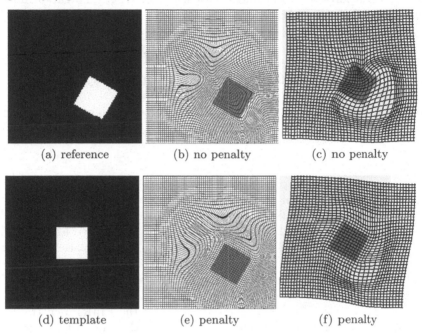

(a) reference   (b) no penalty   (c) no penalty

(d) template   (e) penalty   (f) penalty

B-splines [4] and the other one is based on the more general variational framework [3]. Both approaches principally allow for the integration of additional pre-knowledge in terms of a penalty, like, e.g. local rigidity. For the B-spline approach this has been implemented in [1], while the objective of this paper is the integration of a local rigidity penalty into FLIRT. In contrast to schemes with a spatially variant regularization parameter [5], where weights are given to local elasticity, the new approach explicitly penalizes non-rigidity.

The integration of application conform pre-knowledge like, e.g., local rigidity, is an important step towards improved registration. Users are much more confident to the results if important or obvious structures (like bones or surgical instruments) are transformed in a meaningful way.

3   Methods

We use the powerful variational framework for image registration, see [3, 6, 7] for details. The objective is to minimize a joint functional J with respect to the transformation y, where

$$J(y) = D(T(y), R) + \alpha S(y - y^{\text{kern}}) + \beta C(y) \tag{1}$$

Here R and T are the reference and template image, respectively, $T(y)$ is the transformed template image, D is a distance measure of choice, S is a regularizer (e.g. the elastic potential), y^{kern} models the kernel of the regularization, and α is a regularization parameter compromising between similarity and regularity. The new part is hidden in the penalty (or soft constraints) C, where in this paper we used local rigidity. Rigidity is measured via linearity ($\partial_{i,j} y_k = 0$), orthogonality ($\nabla y^\top \nabla y = I$), and orientation preservation (det $\nabla y = 1$), where ∇y denotes the Jacobian of the transformation. For a convenient implementation in a multi-level framework, the non-rigidity penalty is computed on a pixel/voxel basis and the final penalty is given as a weighted sum, where zero weights are assigned to regions which are not to be penalized; see Figure 3(j) for an example.

4 Results

We tested our implementation on a variety of examples. Due to page limitations, we can only present two intuitive and representative examples. Our first example is a repetition of the experiment performed in [1], see Figure 1. From these results, we see the effect of local rigidity constraints placed at non-zero locations in the moving template itself: as expected, both approaches keep the square rigid. However, a direct comparison of the two schemes is delicate. The B-spline implementation uses a backward interpolation scheme while the FLIRT implementation uses a forward scheme (in fact, for the FLIRT registration we interchanged reference and template in order to make the grids comparable). Moreover, the B-spline implementation obviously uses inappropriate vanishing Dirichlet boundary conditions (BC) (i.e. fixing the boundary of the domain), while the FLIRT approach is based on vanishing Neumann BC's. To be precise, the results of the FLIRT scheme is a global rigid transformation (which is the expected solution for this problem), but we didn't make use of the overall FLIRT capacities and do not use kernel information. Even under this artificial limitations, we find the FLIRT results superior to the B-spline results: the FLIRT transformations obtained with and without penalty are much smoother and local than the ones obtained by the B-spline approach.

A more realistic but still intuitive example is presented in Figure 2, see also [8, 3]. Note that the template image shows a global rotation of approximately 25 degrees which outrules the B-spline approach with Dirichlet BC. In this example we make the middle finger of the hand to be rigid (see Figure 3(j)). Figure 2 shows FLIRT results without ($\beta = 0$) as well as with penalty ($\beta = 0.01$). For both variants, we picked $\alpha = 500$. As it apparent, the penalized approach does keep the finger rigid while the unconstrained does not; see particularly the plots of det(∇y) (see Figure 3(m) and 3(n)).

5 Discussion

The incorporation of pre-knowledge in image registration is a key for reliable results. For many registration tasks, soft and hard tissue can often be identified

Fig. 2. Results for hand example: data and mask (first column), without penalty ($\alpha = 500$, $\beta = 0$; second column), with penalty ($\alpha = 500$, $\beta = 10^{-2}$; third column), map of $\det(\nabla y)$, where the "blockyness" is multi-level related (last row)

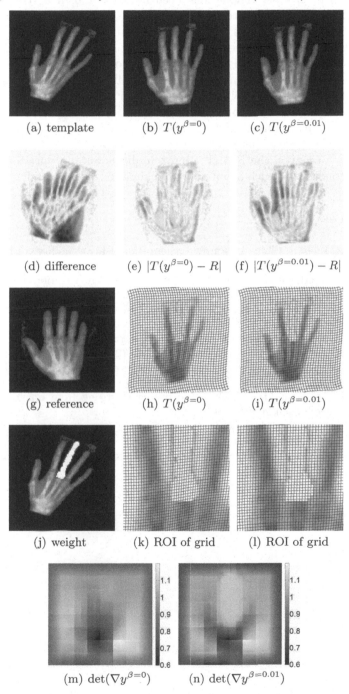

(a) template   (b) $T(y^{\beta=0})$ (c) $T(y^{\beta=0.01})$

(d) difference   (e) $|T(y^{\beta=0}) - R|$ (f) $|T(y^{\beta=0.01}) - R|$

(g) reference   (h) $T(y^{\beta=0})$ (i) $T(y^{\beta=0.01})$

(j) weight   (k) ROI of grid   (l) ROI of grid

(m) $\det(\nabla y^{\beta=0})$ (n) $\det(\nabla y^{\beta=0.01})$

and it seems to be natural to ask for transformations keeping the hard tissue rigid.

The concept of local rigidity has been implemented in a B-splines framework by [1]. The purpose of this paper is the integration into the more general variational FLIRT framework. Our results, of which only two representative are shown in this short paper, clearly indicates that the penalized approach keeps structures like bones locally rigid and thus leads to improved registration results. For the examples presented in [1] we obtain visually more pleasing results. Compared to the alternative B-spline approach, the FLIRT approach is much more flexible. For example, it also allows the incorporation of rigidity of nearby structures, where in the B-spline approach, one has to add "enough" control points in a possible "small" gap. This can lead to very dense and/or unstructured control point grids. Moreover, the FLIRT approach allows an appropriate handling of boundary conditions which again adds to a superior overall result.

References

1. Staring M, Klein S, Pluim J. Nonrigid registration using a rigidity constraint. Procs SPIE 2006;6144:1–10.
2. Fischer B, Modersitzki J. Flirt. A flexible image registration toolbox. LNCS 2003;2717:261–270.
3. Modersitzki J. Numerical Methods for Image Registration. Oxford University Press, 2004.
4. Rueckert D, Sonoda L, Hayes C, et al. Non-rigid registration using free-form deformations. IEEE Trans Med Imaging 1999;18:712–721.
5. Kabus S, Franz A, Fischer B. Variational image registration with local properties. LNCS 2006;92–100.
6. Fischer B, Modersitzki J. Large scale problems arising from image registration. GAMM Mitteilungen 2004;27:104–120.
7. E Haber, Modersitzki J. A multilevel method for image registration. SIAM J Sci Comput 2006;27:1594–1607.
8. Amit Y. A nonlinear variational problem for image matching. SIAM J Sci Comput 1994;15:207–224.

Ein numerisches Verfahren zur Kalibrierung von Gammakameras

Sven Barendt, Jan Modersitzki, Bernd Fischer

Institut für Mathematik
Universität zu Lübeck, 23560 Lübeck
barendt@math.uni-luebeck.de, http://www.math.uni-luebeck.de

Zusammenfassung. Die folgende Arbeit fasst die Entwicklung, sowie erste Ergebnisse eines Verfahrens zur Kalibrierung von Gammakameras, wie sie z.B. in Single Photon Emission Computed Tomography (SPECT) Geräten zum Einsatz kommen, zusammen. Um eine gleichbleibende Qualität von Gammakameraaufnahmen zu garantieren, ist es nötig die Gammakamera auf Homogenität und Linearität zu untersuchen. Werden Abweichungen festgestellt, müssen entsprechende Korrekturen berechnet werden. Dieses Korrekturproblem wird in der folgenden Arbeit auf ein nichtlineares Optimierungsproblem abgebildet und mit dem Gauss-Newton-Verfahren gelöst. Die Evaluation des neuen Verfahrens erfolgte in Zusammenarbeit mit einem Industriepartner.

1   Einleitung

Eine Gammakamera detektiert Photonen einer radioaktiven γ-Quelle und bestimmt die zweidimensionale Position des Zerfalls. Trotz gut eingestellter Hardware der Gammakamera und ihrer Komponenten treten sogenannte Inhomogenitäten und Nichtlinearitäten auf. Nichtlinearitäten sind dabei falsch berechnete Positionen von γ-Photon Interaktionen. Als Folge davon werden in bestimmten Bereichen der Aufnahme einer Gammakamera mehr γ-Photon Interaktionen gezählt (sogenannte Counts), als in anderen Bereichen. Diese dadurch entstehenden Unterschiede in der Dichte der Counts sollen Inhomogenitäten genannt werden. Nähere Beschreibungen zum Aufbau und der Funktionsweise einer Gammakamera sind [1] zu entnehmen.

Es soll ein Korrekturverfahren vorgestellt werden, welches anhand einer inhomogenen Aufnahme einer Gammakamera Änderungen an der Linearität einer Gammakamera vornimmt, so daß diese homogen ist.

2   Stand der Forschung und Fortschritt durch den Beitrag

Fast alle in der industriellen Praxis eingesetzten oder für den praktischen Einsatz vorgeschlagenen Korrekturverfahren benötigen direkt gemessene Linearitätsdaten einer Gammakamera (siehe [2, 3, 4]). Für solche Linearitätsmessungen sind Linearitätsaufnahmen mit Gitterstrukturen oder parallelen Linien nötig. Das mit

Abb. 1. Unterteilung der viereckigen Gitterflächen in Dreiecke der Art D1, D2, D3, D4

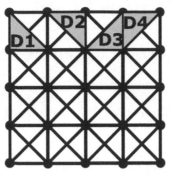

Gitter u

diesem Beitrag vorgestellte Korrekturverfahren bestimmt die Korrekturen der Linearität ausschließlich aus einer Homogenitätsaufnahme einer Gammakamera, die die Inhomogenitäten zeigt. Solch eine Aufnahme entsteht mit wesentlich weniger finanziellen sowie arbeitstechnischen Aufwand, da keine Anschaffungskosten für Phantome oder weitere Apparaturen anfallen, sowie diese auch nicht an den Einsatzort der Gammakamera transportiert werden müssen. Nicht zuletzt ist das neue Korrekturverfahren vollständig in eine Softwarelösung integrierbar.

3   Methoden

Das Problem eine geeignete Korrektur zu finden wurde auf ein nichtlineares Optimierungsproblem abgebildet und mittels des iterativen Gauss-Newton Verfahrens gelöst.

3.1   Das Modell

Das Modell des Korrekturverfahrens bildet ein Gitter, dessen Gitterknoten anfangs eine äquidistante Unterteilung eines gewählten Intervalles (beispielsweise $[0,1] \times [0,1]$) bilden und sich in ihrer Anzahl nach der Pixelzahl n der eingegebenen Homogenitätsaufnahme richten. Jede Pixelposition hat so eine Entsprechung in einem Gitterknoten gefunden. Die Gitterknoten werden dabei im Folgenden durch einen Vektor $u \in \mathbf{R}^{2n}$ bezeichnet, welcher alle horizontalen und alle vertikalen Positionen der Gitterknoten enthält. Jede der m viereckigen Gitterflächen wird nun in vier, sich zum Teil überlappende Dreiecke unterteilt, wie beispielhaft in Abbildung 1 dargestellt. Dies garantiert ein Erhöhen des Verhältnisses von Gleichungen zu Unbekannten und schließt in der Optimierung bestimmte, nicht praxisrelevante Gitterstrukturen in Verbindung mit einer geeigneten Zielfunktion aus. Jede Dreiecksfläche $D_i(u)$ ($i \in \{1, 2, ..., 4m\}$) bekommt nun eine Höhe Height$_i$ zugewiesen, welche direkt aus der Homogenitätsaufnahme gewonnen wird, indem diejenigen Grauwerte gemittelt werden, dessen Pixelpositionen eine Entsprechung in denen der Dreiecksfläche umgebenden Gitterknoten haben. Das Volumen V_i zu einer Dreiecksfläche kann nun als Produkt von Flächeninhalt einer Dreiecksfläche $D_i(u)$ und dessen Höhe berechnet werden. Unter der Bedingung, daß sich die Volumina V_i während der Korrektur nicht verändern dürfen (die Korrektur soll count-erhaltend sein), gilt es nun Gitterknoten u zu finden, so daß die Höhen $\text{Height}_i^* = \frac{V_i}{D_i(u)}$ für alle i möglichst ähnlich sind. Interpretieren kann man die so gefundenen Gitterknoten als Linearitätskorrektur, welche eine Homogenitätskorrektur zur Folge hat.

3.2 Die Zielfunktion

Die Umsetzung des im vorigen Abschnitt genannten Angleichens der Höhen Height_i^* bei geeigneter Wahl von u soll über die Optimierung folgender Zielfunktion erreicht werden

$$f(u) := \|D(u)\text{Height}_{\text{mean}} - V\|_2^2 \tag{1}$$

mit $D(u) = (D_1(u), D_2(u), ..., D_{4m}(u))^T$ und $V = (V_1, V_2, ..., V_{4m})^T$. Die skalare Größe $\text{Height}_{\text{mean}}$ ist das arithmetische Mittel aller Höhen Height_i. Bei minimalen Funktionswert von $f(u)$ sind so die Volumina $D_i(u)\text{Height}_{\text{mean}}$ über jeder Dreiecksfläche möglichst ähnlich denen aus der Homogenitätsaufnahme gewonnenen Volumina V_i. Gleichzeitig sind die Höhen, die sich aus der skalaren Division von V mit $D(u)$ ergeben möglichst ähnlich der Höhe $\text{Height}_{\text{mean}}$. Dies ist die mit dem Verfahren erreichte Homogenitätskorrektur unter Änderung der Linearität.

3.3 Optimierung

Das Problem, geeignete Gitterknoten zu finden, kann nun auf das nichtlineare Optimierungsproblem

$$f(u) = \|D(u)\text{Height}_{\text{mean}} - V\|_2^2 := \|F(u)\|_2^2 = \text{Min!} \tag{2}$$

abgebildet werden. Als Optimierungsverfahren kommt eine Implementierung des Gauss-Newton Verfahrens zum Einsatz, welches für eine Verbesserung der Konvergenzeigenschaften um die Armijo-Schrittweitenregel erweitert wird. Da die Lösungsmenge von (2) unendlich groß ist (wenn u^* eine Lösung von (P) ist, so ist $u^* + c$, $c \neq 0$ ebenso eine Lösung), wird zur Beschränkung der Lösungsmenge das Optimierungsverfahren um eine Tikhonov-Regularisierung erweitert. Ausführliches zum Gauss-Newton Verfahren, der Schrittweitensteuerung, sowie der Tikhonov-Regularisierung ist [5, 6, 7] zu entnehmen.

Es ergibt sich eine iterative Lösungsmethode, welche additive Updates $v^{(k)} \in \mathbf{R}^{2n}$, $k = \{0, 1, ...\}$ zu einem Startgitter u_0 über die Lösung von linearen Ausgleichsproblemen

$$\|F(u^{(k)}) + J_F(u^{(k)})v^{(k)}\|_2^2 + \tau\|v^{(k)}\|_2^2 = \text{Min!} \tag{3}$$

bestimmt ($J_F(u^{(k)})$ ist die Jakobimatrix von F an der Stelle $u^{(k)}$, für den Regularisierungsparameter τ gilt $\tau > 0$). In der ersten Iteration wird (3) mit $u^{(0)} = u_0$

Abb. 2. Regularisierungsparameter τ: 10; v.l.n.r: Iterationszahl: 0, 3; $f(u)$: 60.91, 4.95. Damit ergibt sich eine Verbesserung des Funktionswertes auf $\frac{1}{12}$ des Anfangswertes

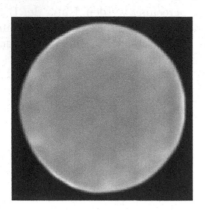 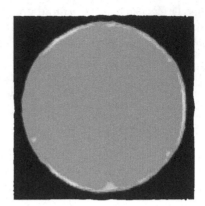

gelöst, in den folgenden Iterationen mit $u^{(k+1)} = u^{(k)} + v^{(k)}$. Die Lösung von (LAP) wird hier über die Normalengleichungen

$$(J_F(u^{(k)})^T J_F(u^{(k)}) + \tau I)v^{(k)} = -J_F(u^{(k)})^T F(u^{(k)}) \tag{4}$$

mit I als Identitätsmatrix, bestimmt. Somit hat das Korrekturverfahren einen Parameter τ, welchen es geeignet zu wählen gilt. Eine für die Evaluation des Korrekturverfahrens ausreichende Methode der Bestimmung von τ ist die Analyse des Einflusses von τ auf $\|F(u^{(0)}) + J_F(u^{(0)})v^{(0)}\|_2^2$ versus $\|v^{(0)}\|_2^2$ beim Lösen von (3) mittels der L-Kurve (siehe [8]).

4 Ergebnisse

In Tests des Korrekturverfahrens auf realen Homogenitätsaufnahmen einer Gammakamera ist eine gute Korrektur der Homogenität nachweisbar (Abb. 2). Desweiteren wurde eine erste Studie zur Berechnung der Homogenität und Linearität in den Aufnahmen einer korrigierten Gammakamera seitens des Industriepartners durchgeführt. So ist eine integrale Homogenität nach NEMA NU 1-2001 und IEC 789 / DIN EN60789 nach der Korrektur von 1,79 % (vor der Korrektur von 14,65 %) nachweisbar. Eine erste Auswertung der Linearitäten einer korrigierten gegenüber einer unkorrigierten Gammakamera ist in Tabelle 1 zusammengefaßt. So ist auch hier eine Verbesserung nachweisbar.

5 Diskussion

Die Ergebnisse, der im vorigen Abschnitt dargestellten ersten Auswertungen des neuen Korrekturverfahrens zeigen, nach Aussagen des Industriepartners, eine

Tabelle 1. Auswertung der Linearität vor der Korrektur (obige Tabellen) und nach der Korrektur (unten stehende Tabellen) in Millimeter. Da die Linearität mittels horizontalen und vertikalen Linearitätsphantomen bestimmt wurde, ergibt sich eine horizontale (linke Tabelle), sowie eine vertikale (rechte Tabelle) Abweichung. Die Kürzel UFOV und CFOV bezeichnen den **U**seful **F**ield **O**f **V**iew (gesamter Nutzbarer Sichtbereich der Gammakamera) und den **C**enter **F**ield **O**f **V**iew (mittig 75 % der Fläche des UFOV)

horizontal	UFOV	CFOV		vertikal	UFOV	CFOV
absolut	4,6	2,4		absolut	3,4	1,4
differentiell	1,4	0,9		differentiell	1,0	0,6

horizontal	UFOV	CFOV		vertikal	UFOV	CFOV
absolut	2,1	1,2		absolut	2,1	1,1
differentiell	0,3	0,2		differentiell	0,3	0,2

sehr gute Homogenitätskorrektur und eine gute, aber noch verbesserungswürdige Linearitätskorrektur. Dies bestätigt auch ein Vergleich mit denen in [9] genannten Auswertungen eines Korrekturverfahrens, welches ebenso alleinig auf einer Homogenitätsaufnahme die Korrekturen berechnet. Weitere Untersuchungen der Inhomogenitäten sind geplant und vielversprechend hinsichtlich einer verbesserten Linearitätskorrektur. An dieser Stelle ein Dank an das Unternehmen MiE in Seth für die Bereitstellung geeigneter Eingangsdaten, sowie für die Bewertung des Korrekturverfahrens.

Literaturverzeichnis

1. Krestel E. Bildgebende Systeme für die medizinische Diagnostik. Siemens; 1988.
2. Spector SS, Brookeman VA, Kylstra CD, Diaz NJ. Analysis and corrections of spatial distortions produced by the gamma camera. J Nucl Med 1972;13:307–312.
3. Muehllehner G, Colsher JG, Stoub EW. Scintillation camera uniformity correction through spatial distortion removal. J Nucl Med 1980;21:771–776.
4. Knoll GF, Schrader ME. Computer correction of camera nonidealities in gamma ray imaging. IEEE Trans Nucl Sci 1982;29:1272–1279.
5. Nocedal J, Wright S. Numerical Optimization. Springer; 1999.
6. Werner J. Numerische Mathematik, Band 2. Vieweg; 1992.
7. Björck AA. Numerical Methods for Least Squares Problems. SIAM; 1996.
8. Hansen PC. Analysis of discrete ill-posed problems by means of the L-curve. SIAM Review 1992;34:561–580.
9. Johnson TK, Nelson C, Kirch DL. A new method for the correction of gamma camera nonuniformity due to spatial distortion. Phys Med Biol 1996;41:2179–2188.

Effiziente Streustrahlberechnung für die volle 3-D Volumenrekonstruktion in der Positronen-Emissions-Tomographie mittels vollständig symmetriebasierter Indizierung von Projektionsvektoren und Volumenvoxeln

Christian Thies[1], Jürgen Scheins[1], Fritz Boschen[2] und Hans Herzog[1]

[1]Institut für Medizin, Forschungszentrum Jülich, 52425 Jülich
[2]Lehrstuhl für Allg. Elektrotechnik und Theor. Nachrichtentechnik
Bergische Universität Wuppertal, 42119 Wuppertal
Email: cthies@fz-juelich.de

Zusammenfassung. In dieser Arbeit wird ein Indizierungschema für die effiziente Bestimmung des Streuanteiles bei der Positronen-Emissions-Tomographie (PET) für die etablierte Single Scatter Simulation (SSS) vorgestellt. Dabei findet eine beliebige Verteilung der betrachteten Streupunkte, und somit eine entsprechend dichte Auswertung der Streuanteile an den gemessenen Koinzidenzen statt. Das Indizierungschema wird offline erstellt, und auf unkorrigiert rekonstruierte Daten angewandt. Es wird ein sechzehntel aller möglichen Projektionslinien explizit berechnet und auf alle anderen durch Symmetrieoperationen abgebildet. Auf aktuell handelsüblicher Hardware (Pentium 4, 3 GHz, 2GB RAM) werden für die eigentliche Streustrahlberechnung bei einem angenommenen Detektormodell mit 72 Kristallen, 8 Ringen und 3200 zufällig verteilten Streupunkten 60 Sekunden benötigt. Dabei wurden 304.178.944 Linienintegrale für 71.424 Projektionslinien in einem Volumen mit 250.000 Voxeln ausgewertet.

1 Einleitung

Die Korrektur des Streustrahlenanteils bei der PET bildet einen Schritt in der quantitativen Volumenrekonstruktion gemessener Zerfallsereignisse. Aufgrund von Compton Streuung kommt es auf dem Weg durch das Gewebe zur Ablenkung der entstandenen Gammaquanten, so dass eine gemessene Line-of-Response (LoR) nicht der wahren LoR entspricht. Dieser statistische Streuanteil wird mittels Single Scatter-Modellierung aus den gemessenen Daten bestimmt [1]. Dabei wird für jede LoR der Anteil aller einfachen Streuereignisse an zufällig im Volumen verteilten Streupunkten unter den entsprechenden Ablenkungswinkeln bestimmt. Die Anteile hängen von den integrierten Werten derjenigen Voxel ab, die von den Verbindungslinien eines Streupunkt zu den jeweiligen Endpunkten der LoR geschnitten werden. Im Gegensatz zur Computer-Tomographie fliegen Gammaquanten aus dem Patienten heraus in alle Raumrichtungen. Daher ist die Bestimmung all derjenigen LoR erforderlich, die sich aus den paarweisen Kristallkombinationen ergeben, die von einem Streupunkt aus als koinzident detektierbar sind. Detektierbar sind Ereignisse nur dann, wenn der Streuwinkel so klein ist, dass die Energie des gestreuten Gammaquants oberhalb der Energieschwelle des Detektors bleibt. Dies ist die eigentlich zeitaufwändige Operation der Streustrahlkorrektur, da sie für jede Berechnung eines Streustrahlvektors die geometrische Bestimmung der geschnittenen Volumenelemente und der entsprechenden Schnittlänge unter dem Akzeptanzwinkel erfordert. Da es sich bei Streuung signaltheoretisch um niederfrequentes Rauschen handelt, läßt sich die Zahl der betrachteten Kristalle und Streuereignisse jedoch erheblich reduzieren. Zur Ermittlung der "geeigneten" reduzierten Detektorgeometrie ist ein flexibles Verfahren für unterschiedliche Geometrien sinnvoll.

Zur Beschleunigung der dreidimensionalen SSS werden einmal berechnete Werte der Streustrahlintegrale gespeichert und bei der Auswertung der LoR wiederverwertet [1, 2]. Zur Volumenrekonstruktion stehen Indizierungsschemata zur Verfügung, in denen Voxel entlang der einzelnen LoR durch Umsetzten von Indizes für Rotations- und Transaxialsymmetrien abgebildet werden [3]. In dieser Arbeit wird die Kristall- und LoR-Verteilung im Detektorzylinder nun so indiziert, dass 4 Basissymmetrien nutzbar sind um die Streustrahlen effizient und frei, für die dreidimensionale Detektorgeometrie zu bestimmen. Es werden keine Anforderungen an die Verteilung der Streuzentren und die resultierenden Streustrahlen gestellt (Abb. 1).

2 Methoden

Die Implementierung trennt zwischen dem aufwändigen Berechnen des geometrieabhängigen Indizierungsschemas und dessen effizienter Anwendung auf unkorrigierte Volumendaten.

2.1 Detektorgeometrie

Die modellierte Detektorgeometrie ergibt sich aus dem Ringradius, der Anzahl der Kristalle pro Ring (#C), der Anzahl der Ringe (#R) sowie deren axialer Dicke. Zusätzlich wird ein Field-of-View (FoV) als Zylinder in Form von frei wählbarem Radius, und Länge innerhalb des Detektorzylinders bestimmt. Die Annahme, dass Kristalle und Ringe ohne Lücken vorliegen, bedeutet technisch keine Einschränkung, da eventuelle Lücken beim Aufbereiten der dreidimensionalen Daten für die Rückprojektion berücksichtigt werden. Die Kristalle werden gegen den Uhrzeigersinn durchnumeriert und für jeden Kristall die acht symmetrischen Zuordnungen zu entsprechenden gegenüberliegenden Kristallen, an der X-/Y-Achse sowie der Winkelhalbierenden vorberechnet (Abb. 1, (a)). Damit ist die Zahl der Kristalle auf ein Vielfaches von Acht festgelegt. Im Dreidimensionalen ergibt sich zu der planaren Nummerierung die Ringzugehörigkeit eines Kristalls in axialer Richtung (Z-Achse). Als Symmetrieebene dient hier die Ringebene zwischen den Ringen #R/2 und #R/2+1 (Abb. 1, (b)).

Abb. 1. Die 3 Ringsymmetrien X,Y,XY erfordern die Verwaltung eines Achtels aller Detektorkristalle #C pro Ring (a). Die Verwaltung der axialen Z-Symmetrie erfolgt für die Hälfte aller Ringe (b)

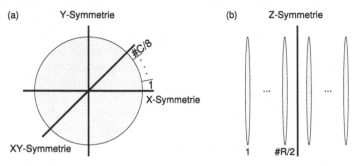

2.2 Projektionsgeometrie

Die Projektionsgeometrie ergibt sich aus denjenigen paarweisen Kristallkombinationen, deren Verbindung das FoV schneidet,wobei sich die Anzahl der LoR wie folgt berechnet:

$$\#LoR = \frac{\#C_F \cdot (\#C_F + 1)}{2} \cdot \#R^2 \tag{1}$$

Dabei ist $\#C_F$ die Anzahl der Kristalle pro Ring, die von dem maximal breiten Fächer aller LoR von einem gegenüberliegenden Kristall durch das FoV getroffen werden. Für das volle FoV in einem Scanner wie dem ECAT Exact HR+ von Siemens mit 576 Kristallen und 32 Ringen ergibt sich mit $\#C_F = 575$ und $\#R = 32$ somit eine theoretische Gesamtzahl von 169.574.400 LoR. Die Ringsymmetrien der einzelnen Kristalle dienen nun der Vorberechnung der entsprechenden Symmetrien der paarweisen Kristallkombinationen einer LoR. Aufgrund der Zylinderform übertragen sich die planaren Symmetrien und somit validen LoR in der XY-Ebene axial auf alle Ringe. Daher läßt sich die Z-Symmetrie entkoppelt von den XY-Symmetrien platzsparend modellieren. Für jede LoR bzw. Kristallkombination existiert damit ein eindeutiger Index bzw. eine Speicherstelle, auf die ohne zeitaufwendige geometrische Operationen zugegriffen wird.

2.3 Volumengeometrie

Die Volumengeometrie basiert auf dem frei wählbaren, äquidistanten Sampling eines dreidimensionalen Quaders in entsprechende Volumenelemente (Voxel). Die Werte der Voxel dienen sowohl der Beschreibung des unkorrigierten Emissions- als auch des Transmissionsbildes, die aus der Rückprojektion der entsprechend gemessenen Detektordaten bestimmt werden. Die Indizes der Voxel werden analog zu den Indizes der LoR in Form von 16 Symmetriefeldern mit dem gleichen Ursprung des Koordinatensystems wie Detektor und FoV angeordnet. Damit wird auch hier lediglich der sechszehnte Teil der Indizes zu den räumlichen Voxelgeometrien vorberechnet [3].

2.4 Streustrahlen-Template

Ein Template verwaltet die Indizes der Voxel aller Linien die den Streupunkt mit allen Kristallen verbinden, alle sich daraus ergebenden LoR sowie die Winkel zwischen den jeweiligen Endpunkten der LoR und dem Streupunkt. Das Datenfeld der Voxelindizes hat die Dimensionen: $\#R \cdot \#C \times 16 \times$ Voxel pro Linie. Es wird für einen Streupunkt, ein Volumen und einen maximalen Streuwinkel erzeugt (00). Die Linien werden für alle Kristalle und alle 16 Symmetriefelder bestimmt und so 16 Repräsentationen des Streupunktes generiert (01-04). Dabei werden nur die Kristalle jener LoR betrachtet, deren Winkel über den Streupunkt so groß ist, dass der davon abhängige streuungsbedingte Energieverlust die Energie eines Gammaquants nicht unter die untere Energieschwelle des Detektors drückt (05-11). Die Voxelindizes der beteiligten LoR und die jeweiligen Winkel werden unabhängig von konkreten Voxeldaten einmalig berechnet und gespeichert (12).

```
00  GenerateTemplate (Volume V, ScatterPoint S, MaxScatterAngle M)
01    for Crystal = 0 to #C * #R; Crystal++
02      for Sym = 0; Sym < 16; Sym++
03        (A,B) = getSymmetricLinePoints(S, CrystalCenterPoints[Crystal], Sym)
04        LineVoxelIndicies[Crystal][Sym] = getVoxelIndiciesForLine(A,B,V);
05    #CLoRs = 0
06    for LoR = 0 to #LoRs, LoR++
07      (A,B) = getLoRPoints(LoR);
08      if Angle(SA,SB) > M
09        ContributingLoRs[#CLoRs] = LoR
10        Angles[#CLoRs] = Angle(SA,SB)
11        #CLoRs++
12    Export LineVoxelIndicies, ContributingLoRs, Angles
```

2.5 Anwendung des Indizierungsschemas

Zur Anwendung wird ein gemessenes unkorrigiertes Volumen in der gleichen Dimension wie das vorberechnete Template benötigt (00). Ein Template für einen Streupunkt wird eingelesen (01) und dann zu allen Kristallen und Symmetrien, die entsprechenden Linienintegrale aus den Volumendaten berechnet (02-05). Das Feld der Integrale hat die Dimensionen $\#R \cdot \#C \times 16$ Es werden nur die Streubeiträge der LoR berechnet die tatsächlich im Template definiert wurden (06-11). Dabei wird der Streupunkt und mit ihm das Template automatisch in alle 16 Symmetriefelder gespiegelt. Auf diese Weise werden die Streuanteile aller LoR bestimmt, die von dem Streupunkt unter dem jeweiligen Winkel betroffen sind (10).

```
00  ApplyTemplate (Volume V)
01    Import LineVoxelIndicies, ContributingLoRs,Angles
02    for Crystal = 0 to #C * #R
03      for Sym = 0; Sym < 16; Sym++
04        for Voxel = 0; Voxel < #LineVoxelIndicies[Crystal][Sym]; Voxel++
05          Integrals[C][Sym] += V[LineVoxelIndicies[Crystal][Sym][Voxel]]
06      for LoR = 0 to #ContributingLoRs; LoR++
07        for Sym = 0; Sym < 16;Sym++
08          CurLoR = getSymmetricLoR(ContributingLoRs[LoR], Sym)
09          (A,B) = getLoRCrystals(CurLoR);
10          SSS = Scatter(Integrals[A][Sym], Integrals[B][Sym], Angles[LoR])
11          LoRScatter[CurLoR] = LoRScatter[CurLoR] + SSS;
```

Tabelle 1. Laufzeiten und Dateigrößen für zwei Projektionsgeometrien

#C	#R	Dateigröße	Zeit-Aufbau	# Linien	Zeit-Anwendung	# Integrale
120	16	737 MB	6 min	783.360	20 Min	2.804.006.464
72	8	119 MB	80 s	71.424	60 s	304.178.944

3 Ergebnisse

Für einen Radius von 825 mm und ein FoV von 583 mm wurde ein Volumen von $50 \cdot 50 \cdot 100$ Voxeln erzeugt. Darauf wurden Indizierungsschemata für eine Annahme, sowie sowie eine Referenzanwendung [2] berechnet (Tab. 1). Es wurden jeweils 200 Streupunkten im FoV angegeben und mittels der 16 Symmetrien auf 3200 Punkten angewandt, um die Dateigrößen und Laufzeiten zu untersuchen.

4 Diskussion

Die Größe der Datei mit den Streustrahlen-Templates hängt bei festgelegter Projektionsgeometrie von der Zahl der betrachteten Streupunkte ab und ist selbst mit 737 MB bei aktuell gängigen Plattengrößen von 300 GB vertretbar, zumal sie nur einmalig berechnet wird. Das vorgestellte Verfahren realisiert die notwendigen Operationen zur effizienten Datenauswahl für die dreidimensionale SSS ohne die in [2] angegebenen systematischen Einschränkungen in der Dimensionierung und Verteilung von Streupunkten und Detektorgeometrie. Die in [2] angegebenen Laufzeiten von 30-40 Sekunden auf einer Sun Ultra SPARC II mit 260 MHz liegen für 72 Kristalle und acht Ringe höher. Dafür wird das gesamte Volumen mit einer höheren Genauigkeit ausgewertet, da die Berechnung eine deutlich größere Anzahl im Raum verteilter LoR erfasst. Eine bessere Alternative sind lediglich noch zeitaufwändigere Monte Carlo Methoden.

Aufgrund der freien Skalierbarkeit ist eine flexible Anpassung an Detektorgeometrien möglich. Durch die Vorberechnung der Indizierung werden bei der Templateanwendung keine gleitkommabasierten Geometrieoperationen mehr benötigt. Die vorgestellte SSS lässt sich in ein iteratives Verfahren für die volle 3D Rekonstruktion integrieren [4].

Literaturverzeichnis

1. Watson CC. New, faster, image-based scatter correction for 3D PET. IEEE Trans Nucl Sci 2000;47:1587–1594.
2. Werling A, Bublitz O, Doll J, Adam LE, Brix G. Fast implementation of the single scatter simulation algorithm and its use in iterative image reconstruction of PET data. Phys Med Biol 2000;47:2947–2960.
3. Scheins J, Boschen F, Herzog H. Analytical calculation of volumes-of-intersection for iterative, fully 3D PET reconstruction. IEEE Trans Med Imaging 2006;25(10):1363–1369.
4. Hudson HM, Larkin RS. Accelerated image reconstruction using ordered subsets of projection data. IEEE Trans Med Imaging 1994;4(13):601–609.

Whole Body MRI Intensity Standardization

Florian Jäger[1], László Nyúl[1], Bernd Frericks[2],
Frank Wacker[2] and Joachim Hornegger[1]

[1]Institute of Pattern Recognition, University of Erlangen,
{jaeger,nyul,hornegger}@informatik.uni-erlangen.de
[2]Department for Radiology and Nuclear Medicine,
Charité, Campus Benjamin Franklin, Berlin,
{bernd.frericks,frank.wacker}@charite.de

Abstract. A major problem of segmentation of magnetic resonance images is that intensities are not standardized like in computed tomography. This article deals with the correction of inter volume intensity differences that lead to a missing anatomical meaning of the observed gray values. We present a method for MRI intensity standardization of whole body MRI scans. The approach is based on the alignment of a learned reference and the current histogram. Each of these histograms is at least 2-d and represents two or more MRI sequences (e.g., T1- and T2-weighted images). From the matching a non-linear correction function is gained which describes a mapping between the intensity spaces and consequently adapts the image statistics to a known standard. As the proposed intensity standardization is based on the statistics of the data sets only, it is independent from spatial coherences or prior segmentations of the reference and newly acquired images. Furthermore, it is not designed for a particular application, body region or acquisition protocol. The method was evaluated on whole body MRI scans containing data sets acquired by T1/FL2D and T2/TIRM sequences. In order to demonstrate the applicability, examples from noisy and pathological image series acquired on a whole body MRI scanner are given.

1 Introduction

For magnetic resonance imaging no protocol dependent intensity standard, like the Hounsfield units in computed tomography, is available due to magnetic field inhomogeneities in both B_0 and RF excitation fields. One type of variation is that intensities of the same tissue class differ throughout a single volume. In order to deal with that problem, a variety of algorithms for bias field correction were developed in the last decade. However, these methods do not solve the other type of problem: a certain measured intensity cannot be associated with a tissue class. The distinction of both kinds of variations is illustrated in Figure 1. For segmentation, a missing protocol dependent standard intensity scale has the disadvantage that for every new suspect an individual training of the used (statistical) model has to be performed. For this reason the clinical applicability of many algorithms is low due to runtime restrictions. Furthermore, visualization

Fig. 1. The distinction of both types of variations (inter and intra scan inhomogeneities). The first image shows the original FL2D scan of a patient. The second image shows the same slice after gain field correction. In the third image a threshold of 580 is applied to the gain field corrected slice. The last image shows a FL2D scan of another patient after gain field correction with the same threshold applied

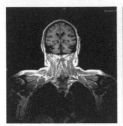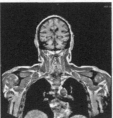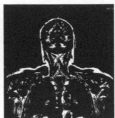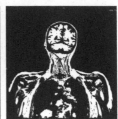

systems cannot use standard presets (e.g., transfer functions) to visualize certain organs or tissue classes. The settings have to be adjusted for every single scan. Hence, a second class of approaches dealing with inter-scan intensity standardization was developed by several authors. State-of-the-art algorithms, generally, standardize the observed intensities using a single image at a time and ignore spatially adjacent images. For many applications this is sufficient, because in many regions of the body a gray value in one image is associated with exactly one intensity in another sequence (e.g., the brain). In general, however, this is not the case. The algorithm presented in this article utilizes all acquired images for intensity standardization. With that, it is possible to separately correct tissue classes that have the same intensity in one image but can be distinguished using more data sets. Furthermore, the introduced approach does not rely on any assumptions about the shape of the joint histograms used. Thus the method is completely independent from the application, region of interest (brain, thorax, pelvis, etc.), scanning protocol (e.g., T1-, T2-weighted) as long as there are learned histograms available for the task.

In [1], a 1D histogram matching approach was presented. First, they detected some landmarks (percentiles, modes, ...) on the template and the reference histogram, matched them and finally interpolated linearly between the detected locations. Pierre Hellier presented in [2] a correction method for MRI brain images that estimates a mixture of Gaussians that approximates the histogram first. Then he computes a polynomial correction function that aligns the mean intensities of the tissues. A multiplicative correction field is estimated in [3], that adapts the intensity statistics of an acquired MR volume to a previously created model. This is achieved by minimizing the Kullback-Leibler divergence between the model and the template intensity distribution. In [4] a method including spatial information between the reference and the template image is presented. In order to match the images a non-linear registration algorithm was used. On the aligned images a scalar multiplicative correction weight is computed. How intensity standardization and bias correction influence each other is evaluated

Fig. 2. Schematic illustration of the intensity standardization. First, from the reference images a reference joint histogram is created. This is the training component of the approach. Then from the current MRI images a joint histogram is generated. In the next step these histograms are non-rigidly registered. Using the gained transformation function, the current images are standardized

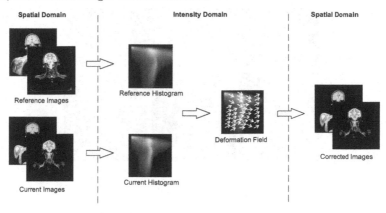

in [5]. The authors conclude that both steps are necessary but the correction of inhomogeneities has to be done beforehand.

2   Methods

The goal of the intensity standardization approach is to find a mapping between the intensities of a set of images $U = (U_1, U_2, \ldots, U_n)$, where n is the number of images and a reference set of images $R = (R_1, R_2, \ldots, R_n)$ so that an intensity vector $i \in \mathcal{I}^n$ describes the same tissue class in both sets with $\mathcal{I}^n$ being the intensity space of the image sets [6]. The main idea of this contribution is that this mapping can be approximated by the minimization of the distance between the joint relative histograms of the two sets of images. The required relative joint histograms have a dimensionality of n. The domain is $\mathbb{R}^n$. In general, however, it can be scaled to $[0, 1]^n$ due to the limited number of gray values observed. The relative joint histograms of the two tuples will usually never be equal (at least for real data sets) as the volume of the same tissue class in the image set U and R differs for inter- as well as for intra-patient measurements (e.g., partial volume averaging effects, positioning of the patient). Thus the search for a mapping between the intensity spaces is equivalent to finding the deformation between the relative joint histograms $\mathcal{H}(R)$ and $\mathcal{H}(U)$ so that they are closest with respect to a given distance measure. If the joint histograms are treated as images, this task can be viewed as non-rigid image registration [7].

The used whole body MRI data sets are very large, thus the influence of small local structures on the appearance of the histogram is very low. For this reason we split the volume in K sub volumes. These sub volumes are than corrected separately. However, in order to guarantee a common gray level standard, the

Fig. 3. First row: head region of the reference image (FL2D), the reference image (TIRM), the template image (FL2D) and the template image (TIRM). Second row: Thresholded images, FL2D protocol (Reference, Template, Result). The threshold for the binarization of all images is the same. The effect of the intensity standardization can be seen best in the brain area

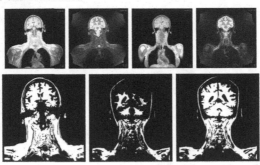

other $K-1$ histograms are used as additional regularizer. Consequently our new distance measure can be written as

$$\mathcal{D}^i[\mathcal{H}(R), \mathcal{H}(U); \boldsymbol{u}^i] = \sum_{k=1}^{K} a_{i,k}\mathcal{D}[\mathcal{H}(R^k), \mathcal{H}(U^k); \boldsymbol{u}^i], \quad \sum_{k=1}^{K} a_{i,k} = 1 \qquad (1)$$

where i is the current sub volume and $a_{i,k}$ is the influence of the force of sub volume k in the context of the standardization of block i. $\mathcal{D}$ is a distance measure like sum of squared differences or mutual information. R^k and U^k are the $k-th$ sub volumes and $\boldsymbol{u}^i$ is the current deformation field.

The result of the optimization is the transformation $T : \mathbb{R}^n \mapsto \mathbb{R}^n$. In the case of the registration of multi-dimensional relative joint histograms, it describes how to transform the gray values of one set of images U such that its intensity distribution best matches the reference distribution, with respect to the used distance measure and smoother. Here a curvature based smoother was used. Thus the intensity standardization can be done by $\boldsymbol{i}_{corr} = T(\boldsymbol{i}_{orig})$.

3   Results

All data sets were acquired on a Siemens Avanto 1.5 T whole body MRI scanner. The TIRM images had a resolution of $512 \times 512 \times 30$ (each block) with 0.98 mm^2 and 5.5 mm slice thickness and TE = 83 and TR = 1660 and the FL2D images had a resolution of $512 \times 410 \times 30$ (each block) with 0.98 mm^2 and 5.5 mm slice thickness and TE = 4.7 and TR = 291. The size of the composed whole body images was $542 \times 1746 \times 20$ for both protocols. Only the composed volumes were used for the experiments. All images were acquired in clinical routine. In total ten whole body MRI data sets were used for evaluation.

We divided the volumes in $K = 5$ blocks along the y-direction. Thus each block had a size of $542 \times 350 \times 20$. The size of a joint histogram was 128×128 pixel. The registration of one histogram took about one second. Using these settings, the overall computational time for the standardization was about seven seconds.

The difference μ_d of the mean intensities of the data sets was chosen as quality measure. For the TIRM images this resulted in a difference of $\mu_d = 6.4$ before and $\mu_d = 3.2$ after the standardization. As the TIRM images do not have many visible structures in the legs, the histograms are very blurred in these regions. Thus no reliable registration is possible. After removing these regions (block four and five) from the evaluation we got a difference of $\mu_d = 7.0$ before and $\mu_d = 2.3$ after standardization. Figure 3 illustrates the effect of the standardization.

4 Discussion

In this article we present a new method for MRI intensity standardization of whole body MRI scans. In contrast to most of the previously published methods, the proposed approach is independent from any prior knowledge about the structure of the data sets and it relies on the image statistics only. Hence, there is no prior registration or segmentation of the data sets necessary. Furthermore, the method is independent from the application, body region and imaging protocol, if learned joint histograms are available. The most important improvement is that the proposed method utilizes all acquired images jointly and does not perform the standardization of the images separately. However, if the image statistics are too different, the obtained results may not be satisfying. This is the case, for instance, for volumes disturbed by a strong bias field. This yields blurred histograms and thus no reliable registration is possible anymore.

References

1. Nyúl LG, Udupa JK, Zhang X. New variants of a method of MRI scale standardization. IEEE Trans Med Imaging 2000;19(2):143–150.
2. Hellier P. Consistent Intensity Correction of MR images. In: Procs ICIP. vol. 1; 2003. 1109–1112.
3. Weisenfeld NI, Warfield SK. Normalization of joint image intensity statistics in MRI using the Kullback-Leibler divergence. In: Procs IEEE ISBI. vol. 1; 2004. 101–104.
4. Schmidt M. A Method for Standardizing MR Intensities between Slices and Volumes. University of Alberta; 2005.
5. Madabhushi A, Udupa JK. Interplay between intensity standardization and inhomogeneity correction in MR image processing. IEEE Trans Med Imaging 2005;24(5):561–576.
6. Jäger F, Deuerling-Zheng Y, Frericks B, Wacker F, Hornegger J. A new method for MRI intensity standardization with application to lesion detection in the brain. Procs VMV 2006; 269–276.
7. Modersitzki J. Numerical Methods for Image Registration. Oxford University Press, Oxford New York; 2004.

Kategorisierung der Beiträge

Autorenverzeichnis

Stichwortverzeichnis